Polyphenols: Mechanisms of Action and Role in Cancer

Polyphenols: Mechanisms of Action and Role in Cancer

Edited by Bruce Booth

STATES
ACADEMIC PRESS
www.statesacademicpress.com

States Academic Press,
109 South 5th Street,
Brooklyn, NY 11249, USA

Visit us on the World Wide Web at:
www.statesacademicpress.com

ISBN: 978-1-63989-767-4

Cataloging-in-Publication Data

Polyphenols : mechanisms of action and role in cancer / edited by Bruce Booth.
p. cm.
Includes bibliographical references and index.
ISBN 978-1-63989-767-4
1. Cancer--Chemotherapy. 2. Polyphenols--Therapeutic use. 3. Polyphenols--Physiological effect.
4. Polyphenols--Health aspects. 5. Polyphenols--Therapeutic use--Effectiveness. I. Booth, Bruce.
RC271.C5 P65 2023
616.994 061--dc23

Table of Contents

Preface

This book has been an outcome of determined endeavour from a group of educationists in the field. The primary objective was to involve a broad spectrum of professionals from diverse cultural background involved in the field for developing new researches. The book not only targets students but also scholars pursuing higher research for further enhancement of the theoretical and practical applications of the subject.

Polyphenols are compounds that are derived from plant sources and are beneficial for the human body. These compounds have one aromatic ring along with attached hydroxyl (-OH) functional groups. They are divided into two types, namely, flavonoids and non-flavonoids. Lignans, phenolic acids and their derivatives, flavonoids, and stilbenes are among antioxidants that fall under the category of polyphenols. They inhibit carcinogenesis during the initiation of cell defense systems, including antioxidant and detoxifying enzyme systems, and inhibit anti-cellular and anti-inflammatory growth signaling pathways in cellular death. A diet rich in vegetables and fruits containing natural polyphenols can lower the risk of certain cancers. Dietary polyphenols have been demonstrated to influence the overall process of carcinogenesis through a variety of mechanisms. The effects of consuming dietary polyphenols might vary depending on tissue or cell type, and can also vary based on the quantity consumed. Polyphenols may also be recommended for cancer prevention and improving the existing cancer treatments. This book provides comprehensive insights into the role of polyphenols in treating cancer. It will provide comprehensive knowledge to the readers.

It was an honour to edit such a profound book and also a challenging task to compile and examine all the relevant data for accuracy and originality. I wish to acknowledge the efforts of the contributors for submitting such brilliant and diverse chapters in the field and for endlessly working for the completion of the book. Last, but not the least; I thank my family for being a constant source of support in all my research endeavours.

Editor

1

Polyphenols and DNA Damage: A Mixed Blessing

Amaya Azqueta [1,2,*] and Andrew Collins [3]

1 Department of Pharmacology and Toxicology, Faculty of Pharmacy, University of Navarra, C/Irunlarrea 1, 31009 Pamplona, Spain
2 IdiSNA, Navarra Institute for Health Research
3 Department of Nutrition, Institute of Basic Medical Sciences, University of Oslo, PB 1046 Blindern, 0316 Oslo, Norway; a.r.collins@medisin.uio.no
* Correspondence: amazqueta@unav.es

Abstract: Polyphenols are a very broad group of chemicals, widely distributed in plant foods, and endowed with antioxidant activity by virtue of their numerous phenol groups. They are widely studied as putative cancer-protective agents, potentially contributing to the cancer preventive properties of fruits and vegetables. We review recent publications relating to human trials, animal experiments and cell culture, grouping them according to whether polyphenols are investigated in whole foods and drinks, in plant extracts, or as individual compounds. A variety of assays are in use to study genetic damage endpoints. Human trials, of which there are rather few, tend to show decreases in endogenous DNA damage and protection against DNA damage induced ex vivo in blood cells. Most animal experiments have investigated the effects of polyphenols (often at high doses) in combination with known DNA-damaging agents, and generally they show protection. High concentrations can themselves induce DNA damage, as demonstrated in numerous cell culture experiments; low concentrations, on the other hand, tend to decrease DNA damage.

Keywords: polyphenols; flavonoids; human studies; in vitro; in vivo; DNA damage; DNA protection

---

1. Introduction

For many years now it has been recognised that fruits and vegetables play an important role in preventing or alleviating the effects of various chronic diseases, notably cardiovascular disease and various cancers. The mechanism(s) of this protection is still not clear. A common explanation is the so-called antioxidant hypothesis; oxidative stress is a factor in many diseases; fruits and vegetables contain various phytochemicals with antioxidant properties, and so these are likely to be the agents of protection. This is clearly a simplistic hypothesis; phytochemicals have been shown to have a wide array of influences on the physiological processes of human cells, and reducing them to sources of antioxidant activity is misguided and misleading. A meta-analysis of clinical trials indicates that antioxidant phytochemicals taken as supplements have no beneficial effect on mortality and may even increase it [1]. In natural plant foods, of course, phytochemicals of different kinds are present, acting in concert, often in all likelihood synergistically, and so studies of whole foods or extracts are particularly valuable. The reductionist approach (looking at individual components) is still popular, however, as evidenced by the large number of studies of individual phytochemicals, and by the growing catalogue of plant species that have been extracted and tested for potential health-promoting effects using a range of molecular markers. DNA damage is one of the most commonly employed such markers, in the reasonable belief that a decrease in DNA damage—as the initiating event of carcinogenesis—must signify a decrease in cancer risk.

Currently, the most popular assay for DNA damage at the cellular level is single cell gel electrophoresis, or the comet assay [2]. It is based on the ability of a strand break (SB) to relax supercoiling in a loop of DNA, thus allowing the DNA to extend to the anode during electrophoresis forming a comet-like image in which the relative intensity of the comet tail reflects the break frequency. Strand breakage is a feature of some but not all kinds of DNA-damaging agent. Reactive oxygen species, in particular, tend to cause damage to DNA bases. An example of base oxidation is 8-oxo–7,8-dihydroguanine (8-OH–Gua). This is converted to a SB by the action of formamidopyrimidine DNA glycosylase (Fpg)—a bacterial repair enzyme, and a simple modification of the comet assay, incorporating an enzymic digestion of the DNA after lysis of cells in agarose—allows the detection of oxidised purines. An analogous enzyme, endonuclease III (or Nth) converts oxidised pyrimidines to SBs. In the search for antioxidant protection of cells against such damage, it is surprising that so few published studies actually use the enzyme-modified comet assay.

The measurement of resistance to H_2O_2-induced damage is a good marker of cellular antioxidant status. Typically, cells are exposed in vitro to 50–100 μM H_2O_2 for a brief period, and the yield of SBs is measured with the basic comet assay; the lower the break frequency, the higher the antioxidant status.

The base 8-OH–Gua and the nucleosides 8-OH–Guo and 8-OH–dGuo can be detected in tissues, but are more commonly measured in urine, plasma or serum, using high performance liquid chromatography (often linked with mass spectrometry) and antibody-based techniques (ELISA or immunohistochemistry). In the tables and text that follow, we use the abbreviation 8-OH–G to cover all three compounds, as the oxidised base is the common factor. They are markers of oxidative stress [3,4]; free 8-OH–Gua can arise through cellular DNA base excision repair, though the origin of the oxidised nucleosides is not certain.

γ-H2AX is the phosphorylated form of histone H2AX, which appears at the site of DNA damage (particularly double SBs); it is detected by immunocytochemistry [5], or sometimes by immunofluorescence combined with flow cytometry [6], and is a sensitive damage indicator.

Unrepaired DNA damage can result in alterations at the level of chromosomes. Classically, chromosome aberrations (chrom abs) were studied as an index of genomic instability, but now the presence of micronuclei (MN: fragments of chromosomes or whole chromosomes that segregate as discrete bodies at mitosis) is a more common marker [7]. Both chrom abs and MN have been confirmed—in long-term human clinical studies—as prospective markers of cancer risk [8,9].

Here, we summarise the results of recent investigations of effects of polyphenols—a very broad class of phytochemicals—on DNA damage, at the level of humans, in animal experiments, and in in vitro studies using cultured (usually human) cells.

2. Methods

In this review, we have concentrated on papers published from 2010 to the present. We used PubMed with the followings terms in the title or abstract: polyphenols/polyphenol/flavonoids/flavonoid combined with DNA damage/DNA protection/DNA repair. We found a total of 386 papers. We have concentrated on papers where the effect of polyphenols, in the form of real food, plant extract or pure compound, is tested in cell culture, animals and humans. We have excluded papers where only gene expression was studied, papers specifically focused on other diseases than cancer, and papers, for example, with deficient experimental design. Papers in which the main interest is in the induction of apoptosis were also excluded.

The reports are summarised in tables according to whether they deal with whole foods (or drinks) (Table 1), with extracts of plants (Table 2), or with single phytochemicals (Table 3). Studies are further classified as 'in humans', 'in vivo' (animal studies), or 'in vitro' (experiments with cultured cells). Extracts and phytochemicals are, where possible, grouped according to functional, chemical or botanical relationships (such as 'tea and coffee related compounds', or 'flavonoids', or '*Lamiaceae*'). We have generally excluded in vitro experiments with plants or compounds appearing in just one or two publications, unless they fall into one of these groups.

Table 1. Effects of whole foods or drinks on various genetic damage endpoints, in humans, in animals ('in vivo'), and in cultured cells ('in vitro').

Reference	Material Tested	Analysis	Assays	System	Concentration/Dose	Result
				In Humans		
[10]	Orange juice	Polyphenols	8-OH-G in urine by ELISA	Overweight/obese humans	300 or 745 mg/day (12 weeks)	8-OH-G ↓
[11]	Aronia-citrus juice	Flavonones, flavones, antocyanins etc.	8-OH-G in plasma by UHPLC-MS/MS	Triathletes (supplemented and placebo groups)	200 mL/day (45 days)	Inconclusive—levels of DNA damage products too low
[12]	Dark chocolate	Polyphenols	Comet assay	Healthy subjects: PBMN cells	860 mg/day (2 weeks)	H_2O_2-induced SBs ↓ (short-term—2 h—only)
[13]	De-alcoholised wine	Anthocyanins, flavonols etc.	Comet assay with Fpg	Post-menopausal women; peripheral blood lymphocytes	500 mL/day (1 month)	No effect
[14]	Wild blueberry drink	Phenolic acids and anthocyanins	Comet assay + Fpg; H_2O_2resistance (comet assay); DNA repair (in vitro comet assay)	Subjects with cardiovascular risk factors: PBMN cells	375 mg anthocyanins/day (6 weeks)	No effect on DNA SBs. Fpg-sensitive sites ↓; H_2O_2 resistance ↑; no effect on repair
[15]	Green tea		Comet assay	Healthy subjects: PBMN cells 30, 60, 90 min after ingestion, exposed ex vivo to UV(A)/VIS radiation	Single 540 mL dose	Protection against UV(A)/VIS-induced DNA SBs seen in 'responders'
[16]	Honey	Phenolic compounds	Comet assay with EndoIII, Fpg	Pesticide-exposed humans	2-week honey supplementation (50 g/day)	DNA repair ↑, EndoIII and Fpg sites ↓
				In Vivo		
[17]	*Chrysobalanus icaco* fruit	Polyphenols, Mg, Se	Comet assay on blood and MN assay on bone marrow and PBMN	Rats + Dox	Up to 0.4 g/kg/day for 14 days	Blood cells; DNA SBs ↓. Bone marrow, blood cells; MN ↓
[18]	Green and black teas		8-OH-G on liver by HPLC	Swiss albino mice + Na arsenite	2.5% of 0.5 g dry leaves/5 mL of boiled water (equivalent to human consumption of 1 cup). 22 days.	Protection (8-OH-G ↓)
[19]	Piquia pulp	Phenolic compounds, carotenoids	Comet assay on liver, kidney, heart cells MN on bone marrow and PBMN cells	Rats + Dox	75, 150, 300 mg/kg/day for 14 days	Protection against DNA SBs and MN formation: lowest dose tends to be most effective
[20]	Açai pulp	Phenolic compounds, carotenoids	Comet assay on liver, kidney and PBMN cells: MN on bone marrow and PBMN cells	Mice + Dox	3.33,10, 16.7 g/kg/day for 1 or 14 days	Protection against DNA SBs and MN formation: 14 days pretreatment more effective
[21]	Cloudy apple juice	Polyphenols	Comet assay on liver cells	Rats	10 mL/kg/day for 28 days	DNA SBs ↑ and no effect on N-nitrosodiethylamine-induced damage

Table 1. *Cont.*

Reference	Material Tested	Analysis	Assays	System	Concentration/Dose	Result
[22]	Green tea	–	Comet assay on intestinal cells	Rats + As	10 mg/mL in water for 28 days	Claim protection
[23]	Spinach	Total polyphenols	Comet assay on leukocytes	Hyperlipidemic rats	5% (powder) in diet, for 6 weeks	H_2O_2-induced DNA SBs in leukocytes ↓
				In Vitro		
[24]	Green tea	–	Comet assay with Fpg	Human PBMN cells	7–71 μM catechins	DNA damage ↓ at lower concentrations but ↑ at highest concentration
[25]	Herbal preparation	Total phenolics	Comet assay	YAC-1 (mouse lymphoma) cells	1–13 mg/mL	DNA SBs ↑ at 8.7 mg/mL
				Rat fibroblasts	1–13 mg/mL	DNA SBs ↑ at 2.2 mg/mL
[26]	Various honeys	–	Comet assay	HepG2 (human liver carcinoma) cells treated with B(a)P, PhIP, nitrosamines	0.1–100 mg/mL	Slight decreases in DNA SBs in most cases, not dose-dependent

PBMN: peripheral blood mononuclear; SB: strand break; Fpg: formamidopyrimidine DNA glycosylase; UV: ultraviolet; VIS: visible; MN: micronucleus/micronuclei; Dox: doxorubicin; EndoIII: endonuclease III (Nth); 8-OH–G: 8-oxo–7,8-dihydroguanine; B(a)P: benzo(a)pyrene; PhIP: 2-amino-1-methyl-6-phenylimidazo[4,5-b]pyridine.

Table 2. Effects of plant extracts on various genetic damage endpoints, in humans, in animals ('in vivo'), and in cultured cells ('in vitro').

Reference	Material Tested	Analysis	Assays	System	Concentration/Dose	Result
				In Humans		
[27]	Green tea polyphenols		Urinary 8-OH-G by HPLC	Postmenopausal women with osteoporosis	500 mg/day (capsules, 6 months)	8-OH-G ↓ over 6 months
				In Vivo		
				Tea-Related		
[28]	Green tea polyphenols		8-OH-G in brain by Ab assay	Rats	400 mg/day (gastric intubation, 4 weeks)	8-OH-G ↓
[29]	Green tea polyphenols	Epicatechin derivatives	CPD on skin and lymph nodes by Ab assay	Mice (NER+ and-) + UV	0.2% in drinking water (7 days before UV irradiation)	Enhanced removal of CPDs in NER-proficient mice
[30]	Green tea extract		MN in polychromatic erythrocytes	Mice + Cr(VI)	30 mg/kg (one dose—gavage)	MN ↓
[31]	Green tea polyphenols		Comet assay with Fpg on blood; 8-OH-G in brain by HPLC	Rats + acrylonitrile	0.4% in diet (1 week before acrylonitrile and then throughout acrylonitrile treatment for 28 days)	↓ Fpg-sensitive sites and 8-OH-G ↓
[32]	*Calluna vulgaris* polyphenol extract		CPDs in skin by Ab assay	Mice + UV(B)	4 mg/cm^2 (30 min before exposure to UV, repeated on 10 days)	CPDs ↓
[33]	*Podophyllum hexandrum* extract	Total phenolics	Alkaline halo assay; DNA repair (SB rejoining—PCR assay)	Thymocytes from γ-irradiated mice	15 mg/kg (one dose, i.p.)	Protection against γ-ray-induced DNA SBs and accelerated rejoining
[34]	*Cotinus coggyria* extract		Comet assay on liver	Rats + pyrogallol	0.5–2 g/kg (single dose, i.p.)	SBs at highest dose of extract alone: protection against pyrogallol-induced SBs at 0.5 g/kg
				In Vitro		
				Tea-Related		
[35]	Green tea polyphenols		Comet assay	Melanoma cell lines	20–60 μg/mL (time)	40, 60 μg/mL; DNA SBs ↑
[36]	Green tea extract		Comet assay	Human laryngeal carcinoma cell line (HEp2) + drug-resistant cell line CK2	1× = 2 g/200 mL H_2O_2 Concentration tested = 0.1×	SBs ↑ at 72 h, not 48 h
				Lamiaceae		
[37]	Citrus and rosemary bioflavonoid extract	Total polyphenols	Comet assay	HaCaT (human keratinocytes) + UV(B)	100 μg/mL	Pre-treatment: UV(B)-induced DNA SBs ↓
			MN	Human lymphocytes + X-ray	1 mg/mL	X-ray induced MN ↓

Table 2. *Cont.*

Reference	Material Tested	Analysis	Assays	System	Concentration/Dose	Result
[38]	*Thymus vulgaris* extract		Comet assay and γ-H2AX by Ab	Human skin model exposed to UV(B)	1.8 μg/mL	Protection against DNA damage
[39]	*Thymus vulgaris* extract		Comet assay 24 h after UV	NCTC (human keratinocytes) + UV(A) or UV(B)	1.82 μg/mL	DNA SBs ↓
			MN			No effect seen
			γ-H2AX by Ab			No effect seen
[40]	Lemon balm extract	Polyphenols	Comet assay and γ-H2AX by Ab assay	Human keratinocytes + UV(B)	15–100 μg/mL	DNA SBs ↓ (100 μg/mL); γH2AX ↓ (15 μg/mL)
[41]	*Ocimum sanctum* extract ("Holy basil")	Total phenolics	Comet assay	SH-SY5Y (human neuroblastoma) cells	75 μg/mL	H_2O_2-induced DNA SBs ↓
[42]	Various *Lamiaceae* leaf extracts	Total polyphenols, flavonoids	Comet assay	HepG2 (human liver carcinoma) cells + $CdCl_2$	50–350 μg/mL for 4 h	Dose-dependent decrease in Cd-induced DNA SBs
				Fruits and Berries		
[43]	Strawberry extract	Anthocyanins	Comet assay	Human dermal fibroblasts exposed to UV(A)	0.05–0.5 mg/mL	Protection against DNA SBs at 0.25, 0.5 mg/mL
[44]	Strawberry extract	Total phenolics, flavonoids, anthocyanins, vitamin C, β-carotene	Comet assay	Human dermal fibroblasts exposed to H_2O_2	0.5 mg/mL	DNA SBs ↓
[45]	*Vaccinium* berries extract	Total polyphenols and anthocyanins	Comet assay	A549 (human lung adenocarcinoma) cells	21–167 μg/mL	Dose-dependent protection against DNA SBs induced by t-BOOH
[46]	Blackcurrant extract		Comet assay (H_2O_2 resistance)	TK6 (human lymphoblastoid) cells	0.5–3 mg/mL	H_2O_2-induced DNA SBs ↓
			MN ± H_2O_2		1 mg/mL	H_2O_2-induced MN ↓
[47]	Various apple polyphenol s extract	Monomeric polyphenols oligosaccharides and oligomeric procyanidins.	Comet assay with Fpg	Caco2 (colon carcinoma) cells	1–100 μg/mL	Menadione-induced DNA SBs and Fpg-sensitive sites ↓ Greatest protection at low concentrations; with some extracts, damage ↑ at high doses
[48]	Polyphenol extracts of Australian fruits	Phenolic acids and anthocyanins	MN	HT29 (human colon adenocarcinoma) cells	0.5–1 mg/mL	MN ↑ with one extract

Table 2. *Cont.*

Reference	Material Tested	Analysis	Assays	System	Concentration/Dose	Result
[49]	Red wine extract		Comet assay	HUVECs (human umbilical vein endothelial) cells + *t*-BOOH	25 μg/mL	DNA SBs ↓
				Honey-Related		
[16]	Honey extract	Phenolic compounds	Comet assay with EndoIII, Fpg	Bronchial epithelial and neuronal cells	5 μg/mL	Pesticide (glyphosate, chlorpyrifos)-induced damage (SBs, EndoIII and Fpg sites) ↓
			Cellular DNA repair			Protection against inhibition of repair of DNA SBs by pesticides
[50]	Propolis extr		Comet assay	Fibroblasts	0.1–0.3 mg/mL	γ-Ray-induced DNA SBs ↓
[51]	Propolis		Comet assay + Fpg, EndoIII	Human gastric cancer cell line AGS	0.3 μg/mL	High DNA damage, suppressed by antioxidants or catalase

Ab: antibody; CPD: cyclobutane pyrimidine dimer; NER: nucleotide excision repair; i.p.: intraperitoneal; *t*-BOOH: *tert*-butyl hydroperoxide; HUVEC: human umbilical vein endothelial cell.

Table 3. Effects of individual polyphenolic compounds on various genetic damage endpoints, in humans, in animals ('in vivo'), and in cultured cells ('in vitro').

Reference	Material Tested	Assays	System	Concentration/Dose	Result
In Humans					
[52]	Epigallocatechin gallate	8-OH–G in leukocyte DNA (HPLC/UV/MS)	Prostate cancer patients	800 mg/day (3 to 6 weeks before surgery)	Decrease in 8-OH–G not significant
[53]	Xanthohumol (drink)	Comet assay and urinary 8-OH–G (UPLC)	Cross over intervention trial, healthy subjects	12 mg/day for 14 days	FPG-sites ↓, H_2O_2-induced SBs ↓, 8-OH–G ↓
	Xanthohumol (pills)	Comet assay	Parallel intervention trial, healthy subjects		FPG-sites ↓, H_2O_2-induced SBs ↓
In Vivo					
[54]	Luteolin	Comet assay and MN on blood and bone marrow	Mice + ochratoxin A	2.5 mg/kg (one dose i.p.)	No effect
	Chlorogenic acid			10 mg/kg (one dose i.p.)	DNA SBs ↓; also MN ↓
	Caffeic acid			10 mg/kg (one dose i.p.)	DNA SBs ↓
[55]	Curcumin	Comet assay with FPG on bone marrow	Rats + etoposide	100 or 200 mg/kg/day (7 days, gavage)	Pretreatment → etoposide-induced DNA damage ↓
	Epicatechin			20 or 40 mg/kg/day (7 days, gavage)	Pretreatment → etoposide-induced oxidative DNA damage ↓ (less than with Curcumin) but not DNA SBs.
[56]	Ellagic acid	MN in polychromatic erythrocytes; alkaline unwinding	Swiss albino mice + cyclophosphamide	50/100 mg/kg/day (orally, 7 days)	Protection against MN formation and DNA SBs
[57]	Epigallocatechin gallate and theaflavin	Alkaline unwinding assay	Mouse skin + dimethylbenzanthracene	100 μg/mouse (topical application, 1 h)	Topical pretreatment → DNA SBs ↓
	Epigallocatechin gallate and theaflavin as NPs (PLGA)			5–20 μg/mouse (topical application, 1 h)	NP form has ~30-fold dose-advantage
[58]	Epigallocatechin gallate	γ-H2AX by Western blot and Ab and 8-OH–G by Ab assay	H1299 (human lung cancer cells) xenografts in mice	0.1%–0.5% in diet, 30 mg/kg/day injection	Dose-dependent ↑ in γ-H2AX and 8-OH–G
[59]	Silibinin	8-OH–G in various brain regions by ELISA	Diabetic mice	20 mg/kg/day i.p. (4 weeks)	8-OH–G ↓ in different regions of brain
[60]	Quercetin	MN in bone marrow and blood	Rats + PCBs	50 mg/kg/day for 25 days	PCB-induced MN ↓
[61]	Quercetin	Chrom abs and MN in bone marrow; Comet assay on blood	Mice + γ-irradiation	20 mg/kg/day for 5 days	Radiation-induced Chrom abs, SBs, MN ↓
	Rutin			10 mg/kg/day for 5 days	
[62]	Chrysin	Comet assay (hepatocytes and leukocytes)	Rats + methyl mercury	0.1, 1, 10 mg/kg/day for 45 days	MeHg-induced SBs ↓ at higher doses

Table 3. *Cont.*

Reference	Material Tested	Assays	System	Concentration/Dose	Result
[63]	Puerarin	8-OH–G in kidney by HPLC	Mice + CCl4	0.2 or 0.4 g/kg/day for 4 weeks	8-OH–G ↓
[64]	Quercetin	8-OH–G in kidney by HPLC	Rats + lead	10 mg/kg/day for 10 weeks	8-OH–G ↓
[65]	Myricitrin, Myricetin	MN (reticulocytes); Comet assay (liver, duodenum, stomach)	Mice	1, 1.5, 2 g/kg/day for 3 days	No increase in MN, SBs only in liver + myricetin
[66]	Quercetin	Comet assay on liver	Rats + DEN	10, 30, 100 mg/kg/day for 5 days	DEN-induced SBs ↓
[34]	Myricetin	Comet assay on liver	Rats + pyrogallol	255.5 µg/kg 2 h and 12 h before pyrogallol	SBs ↓ in liver
[67]	Quercitin	Comet assay on liver	Rats + acrylamide	10 mg/kg/day for 5 days	No effect of quercetin alone. Acrylamide-induced SBs ↓
		8-OH–G in liver by ELISA			No effect of quercetin alone. Acrylamide-induced 8-OH–G ↓
[68]	Naringin	Comet assay	Mice (hepatocytes and cardiocytes)	50, 250 or 500 mg/kg oral (one dose)	No effect
				50, 250 or 500 mg/kg oral (one dose) + Dau i.p.	DNA SBs induced by Dau ↓
[69]	Apigenin	Chrom abs and MN in bone marrow; comet assay on skin; DNA repair (removal of CPDs by Ab)	Mice + UV(B)	1.5–3 mg/cm^2 (24 h; during UV irradiation)	Chrom abs and MN ↓; tail length ↓. Removal of dimers apparently stimulated by apigenin
In Vitro					
Tea-Related					
[70]	Chlorogenic acid	Comet assay	HaCaT (human keratinocytes) cells + UV(B)	Not stated. Probably 5–80 µM	DNA SBs ↓
[71]	Chlorogenic acid	Comet assay	K562 (human leukaemia) cells	0.5–5 mM	DNA SBs ↑
		γ-H2AX by Ab	Chinese hamster AA8 cell line and K562	0.5 mM	γ-H2AX foci ↑
[73]	Ellagic acid	Comet assay	Prostate cancer cell lines LNCaP, DU145, BPH-1	4.5–300 µM	DNA SBs ↑ at 9 µM in BPH-1, 37 µM in DU 145, 150 µM in LnCap
[74]	Epicatechin gallate	Comet assay; MN	C6 astroglial cells	0.1–1 µM	H_2O_2-induced DNA SBs and MN formation ↓
[58]	Epigallocatechin gallate	γ-H2AX and 8-OH–G by Ab assay	H1299 (human lung adenocarcinoma) cells	50 µM	γ-H2AX and 8-OH–G ↑
[75]	Metabolites of quercetin, chlorogenic acid	Comet assay	LT97 (human colorectal adenoma) cells + cumene hydroperoxide	2.5 µM/5 µM	Decrease in DNA SBs

Table 3. *Cont.*

Reference	Material Tested	Assays	System	Concentration/Dose	Result
[76]	Epigallocatechin gallate	Comet assay	HeLa (human cervical cancer) cells, p53R (cells with p53 reporter)	10, 20 μg/mL	DNA SBs ↑
[77]	Ethyl gallate	Comet assay	Human carcinoma cell line KB	20–50 μg/mL	DNA SBs ↑
[78]	Tannic acid	Comet assay with Fpg	Human neutrophils	10–150 μM	DNA SBs ↑ (dose-dependent); weak effect (↑) in TPA-stimulated cells. Fpg sites also ↑, but ↓ in TPA-stimulated cells
	Resveratrol				DNA damage (SBs) ↑ (dose-dependent); but ↓ (dose-dependent) in TPA-stimulated cells. Same pattern with FPG sites
[72]	Chafuroside B (tea polyphenol)	CPDs by Ab	Human keratinocytes + UV(B)	1 μM	CPDs ↓ after 24 h
[36]	Epigallocatechin gallate; Epicatechin gallate	Comet assay	HEp2 (human laryngeal carcinoma cell line)	50 μM	With either ECG or EGCG, SBs ↓ at 48 h (from background); no effect at 72 h
			CK2 (drug resistant, from HEp2)		No effect at 48 or 72 h
Curcumin					
[79]	Curcumin; Ellagic acid	Comet assay	HeLa (human cervical cancer) cells	25 μM	DNA SBs ↑ (with both together; not significant alone)
[80];	Curcumin	Chrom abs and PCC	Human lymphocytes, with/without stimulation	0.14–7 μM	Radioprotective effects seen for both reagents in PCC assay (non-cycling cells) Radiosensitisation of cycling cells (chrom abs) by both reagents
	Resveratrol			2.2–220 μM	
[81]	Curcumin	8-OH–G by Ab assay	Smooth muscle cells	up to 10 μM	8-OH–G ↑
[82]	Quercetin; Curcumin	γ-H2AX by Ab assay	HT1080 human fibrosarcoma cell line	30 and 80 μM Quercetin; 10 and 15 μM Curcumin,	Significant increases in γ H2AX
		MN		30 μM Quercetin; 10 μM Curcumin	Significant increases in MN. (Quercetin less effective.)
[83]	Soy isoflavones	γ-H2AX by Ab assay	LNCaP (human prostate cancer) cells	10 μg/mL	No effect on H2AX
	Curcumin			25 μg/mL	γ-H2AX ↑
[84]	Polyphenols	Comet assay	Lymphocytes + B(a)P	5 μg/mL	DNA SBs ↓
	Curcumin			5 and 10 μg/mL	DNA SBs ↓
[85]	Curcumin	Comet assay	HCT-116 (human colon cancer) cells	50 μM	DNA SBs ↑
[86]	Curcumin	Comet assay	K562 (human leukaemia) cells	12.5–200 μM	DNA SBs ↑
Resveratrol					

Table 3. *Cont.*

Reference	Material Tested	Assays	System	Concentration/Dose	Result
[87]	Resveratrol	Chrom abs	Human lymphocytes + aflatoxin	10–100 μM	No effect of resveratrol alone. Dose-dependent decrease in aflatoxin-induced chrom abs
[88]	Resveratrol	MN; Comet assay	Human bronchial epithelial cell line HBE + Na arsenite	5 μM	↓ DNA SBs and MN induced by arsenite
[89]	Resveratrol	γ -H2AX by Ab assay	HCT-116 (human colon cancer) cells	25 μM	γ-H2AX foci ↑: DNA damage due to toposiomerase II poisoning
[90]	Resveratrol	γ -H2AX by Ab assay	Prostate epithelial cells	5 μM	Ionising radiation-induced damage enhanced
[91]	Resveratrol	Comet assay	Rat astrocytes + ethanol	1–10 μM	↓ DNA SBs induced by ethanol
Lamiaceae					
[39]	Thymol	Comet assay 24 h after UV	NCTC (human keratinocytes) + UV(A) or UV(B)	1 μg/mL	DNA SBs ↓
		MN			No effect seen
		γ-H2AX by Ab assay			No effect seen
Flavonoids					
[92]	Naringin	Chromosome aberrations	Human lymphocytes treated with Cd	1, 2 μg/mL	Cd-induced chrom abs ↓
		SCE			No significant effect on SCE
[93]	Rutin	Comet assay	Rat hepatic cell line HTC	10–810 μg/mL (24 h)	SBs at highest concentration
		MN			No significant increase in MN—but protection against MN induced by B(a)P
[94]	Quercetin; Rutin	ã-H2AX by Ab assay	V79 lung fibroblast hamster cells	100 μg/mL for 12 h	Massive foci, results of lethality
[95]	Kaempferol	Comet assay	HL-60 human leukemia cells	75 μM, 6–48 h	SBs induced
[96]	Quercetin	Comet assay	Lymphocytes from healthy subjects and colon cancer patients, + food mutagens PhIP and IQ	100, 250, 500 μM	SBs induced by PhIP or IQ ↓
	Rutin			50, 250, 500 μM	
[97]	Fisetin, Kaempferol; Galangin; Quercetin; Luteolin; Chrysin; 7-hydroxyflavone; 7,8-dihydroxyflavone; Baicalein; Rutin	Comet assay; MN	HepG2 (human liver carcinoma) cells + B(a)P	2.5–25 μM	SBs induced by B(a)P ↓ (all except rutin); MN induced by B(a)P ↓ (all except rutin); Fi>Qu>Ga>Ka>Lu (more effective group); Ch, 7Fl, 7,8Fl, Ba (less effective group)
[98]	Fisetin	Comet assay	Human hepatic Huh-7 cells	60 μM	SBs ↑
[99]	Kaempferol	Comet assay	Human osteosarcoma cells U2-OS	50, 100, 150 μM	SBs ↑ (not quantitated)
[65]	Myricitrin	MN	TK6 (human lymphoblastoid) cells	20–500 μg/mL for 24 h	MN ↑ (Dose-dependent)
	Myricetin			2.5–75 μg/mL for 24 h	MN ↑ (significant?)

Table 3. *Cont.*

Reference	Material Tested	Assays	System	Concentration/Dose	Result
[100]	Quercetin and rutin	Comet assay	Human hepatoma cell line HepG2	0.1, 1 and 5 μg/mL (2 h of treatment)	No induction of SBs (quercetin and rutin alone)
			HepG2 + Aflatoxin B, MMS, Dox	Pre-, co- and post-treatment	DNA damage induced by AFB1, MMS, Dox ↓ in all treatment conditions
[101]	Quercetin	Comet assay, 8-OH–G (HPLC)	Human hepatoma cell line HepG2 cells	0.1, 1 and 5 μg/mL (24 h of treatment)	No effect
			HepG2 cells + $HgCl_2$ and MeHg	Pre-, co- and post-treatment	DNA damage induced by $HgCl_2$ and MeHg ↓ in pre- and co-treatment
[102]	Quercitrin	Comet assay	Mouse epidermal cell line JB6 + UV(B)	10, 20 and 80 μM, 30 min	No effect
				10, 20 and 80 μM, 30 min + UV(B)	UV(B)-induced SBs ↓
[51]	Galangin, chrysin	Comet assay + FPG, EndoIII	AGS human gastric adenocarcinoma cells	20 μM (1 h)	Base oxidation ↑
[69]	Apigenin	Comet assay: Chrom abs; MN	HaCaT human keratinocytes + UV(B)	15–25 μg/mL	DNA damage ↓, Chrom abs ↓, MN ↓

PCB: polychlorinated biphenyls; chrom ab: chromosome aberration; DEN: diethylnitrosamine; Dau: Daunorubicin; TPA: tetradecanoyl phorbol acetate; ECG: epicatechin gallate; EGCG: epigallocatechin gallate; PCC: premature chromosome condensation; SCE: sister chromatid exchange; IQ: 2-amino-3-methylimidazo[4,5-f]quinolone; MMS: methylmethanesulphonate; AFB1: aflatoxin B1.

3. Results

3.1. *Whole Foods and Drinks*

Relatively few investigations of effects of whole foods on genetic damage endpoints have been published. A variety of fruit-derived drinks as well as tea (though this could be considered an extract), and dark chocolate, were tested in human supplementation trials. A decrease in urinary 8-OH–G was seen in overweight or obese adults supplemented with orange juice [10] but levels of plasma 8-OH–G in triathletes were too low to see any effect of Aronia-citrus juice [11]. De-alcoholised wine given daily for one month was without effect on DNA SBs or Fpg-sites in peripheral blood mononuclear (PBMN) cells of post-menopausal women [13]. However, a daily blueberry drink taken for 6 weeks protected PBMN cells from H_2O_2-induced damage, but had no effect on SBs or DNA repair capacity [14]. Malhomme de la Roche et al. [15] found that ingestion of green tea protected PBMN cells challenged ex vivo with UV(A)/VIS (ultraviolet(A)/visible) radiation, but only in some subjects, described as responders. Alleva et al. [16] gave a honey supplement to humans exposed to pesticides, and found, after two weeks' supplementation, lower levels of EndoIII- and Fpg-sensitive sites in lymphocytes as well as an enhanced capacity for DNA repair. Dark chocolate induced a transient protection against H_2O_2-induced DNA damage in PBMN cells ex vivo [12].

Most of the animal studies have looked at the possible protection afforded by polyphenol-rich foods or drinks against DNA damage induced by treating the animals (rats or mice) with known carcinogens such as doxorubicin (Dox), n-nitrosodiethylamine, or sodium arsenite. Protection was claimed with *Chrysobalanus icaco* fruit [17], Piquia pulp [19], Açai pulp [20], and tea [18,22]; but cloudy apple juice actually increased SBs and had no effect on nitrosamine-induced damage [21]. Treatment of hyperlipidemic rats with spinach increased the resistance of blood cells ex vivo to H_2O_2-induced damage [23].

Experiments with cultured cells and whole foods/drinks are understandably rarely performed. Incubation of PBMN cells with green tea decreased DNA damage at low concentrations but increased it at the highest concentration tested (representing 71 mM catechins) [24]. Various honeys afforded slight protection of HepG2 cells against SBs produced by treatment with certain organic carcinogens [26]. A Chinese herbal preparation caused SBs in mouse lymphoma cells and rat fibroblasts, but at extreme concentrations (1–13 mg/mL) [25].

3.2. *Extracts of Plants*

3.2.1. Tea-Related Extracts

One human trial and several animal experiments have been reported with tea-related extracts. Post-menopausal women with osteoporosis were supplemented with green tea polyphenols for 6 months; the level of urinary 8-OH–G decreased [27]. Xu et al. [28] found a decrease in 8-OH–G in rats given a very high dose of green tea polyphenols. Protective effects of green tea extracts against genetic damage were reported by Garcia-Rodriguez et al. [30] in mice treated with Cr(IV); and by Pu et al. [31] in rats treated with acrylonitrile. Katiyar et al. [29] found that green tea polyphenols promoted the repair of UV-induced DNA lesions in mice proficient in nucleotide excision repair (NER), but not in NER- mice. Two studies with cultured cells have found increases in DNA SBs induced by green tea extract; Prasad et al. [35] in melanoma cell lines (though at rather high concentrations), and Durgo et al. [36] in a human laryngeal carcinoma cell line.

3.2.2. Lamiaceae Family Plants

The *Lamiaceae* family includes many plants used as culinary herbs, and so they have been grouped together here. All publications in our search deal with effects in cell culture.

Calo et al. [39] tested an extract of *Thymus vulgaris* (and thymol in parallel) on keratinocytes irradiated with UV(A) or UV(B); they found a decrease in SBs, though no effect on MN or γ-H2AX foci. A similar protective effect was reported by Cornaghi et al. [38] in a human skin model exposed to UV(B). A citrus and rosemary extract (but at high concentrations) decreased the frequency of MN induced by X-rays in human lymphocytes, and decreased UV(B)-induced SBs in keratinocytes [37]. This last group also tested lemon balm extract on UV(B)-irradiated keratinocytes and found a decrease in SBs (at a high concentration) and in γ-H2AX foci at a more moderate concentration [40]. Thirugnanasampandan et al. [42] studied three *Lamiaceae* species; HepG2 cells were incubated for 4 h with an extract before treating with $CdCl_2$. Dose-dependent decreases in SBs were seen with all three (though even the lowest concentration tested was high). An extract of *Ocimum sanctum* (a form of basil) was tested by Venuprasad et al. [41] on human neuroblastoma cells; it protected against H_2O_2-induced SBs (at a high concentration).

3.2.3. Honey-Related Extracts

In parallel experiments to their human honey trial, Alleva et al. [16] showed that pre-treatment of cells with honey extract protected against pesticide-induced DNA damage and inhibition of DNA repair. Propolis extract (at high concentration) decreased the frequency of γ-ray-induced SBs in fibroblasts [50], and yet—at a much lower concentration—it caused oxidative damage (SBs measured with Fpg and EndoIII together in the comet assay) in a human cancer cell line, which was suppressed by antioxidants or catalase and so was imputed to the production of H_2O_2 [51].

3.2.4. Fruits and Berries

All papers on extracts of fruits and berries reviewed here describe cell culture experiments and with one exception they have made use of high to extremely high extract concentrations. The extract of one Australian fruit (among several studied) caused an increase in MN [48]. Other reports are of protection against oxidation damage caused by H_2O_2 [43,44,46]; or tert-butyl-hydroperoxide (t-BOOH) [45,49]. The exception to usage of high doses is a report by Bellion et al. [47] with apple polyphenol extracts; they found that 24 h pre-incubation of Caco2 cells decreased the DNA damage induced by menadione (low concentrations actually giving the greatest protection).

3.2.5. Miscellaneous Plant Extracts

Animal experiments with various plant extracts have shown protection against SB production in liver cells of pyrogallol-treated rats (at very high doses of extract) [34]; accelerated rejoining of γ-ray-induced DNA SBs [33]; and a decrease in pyrimidine dimers in the skin of UV(B)-irradiated mice [32].

4. Isolated Phytochemicals

4.1. Compounds Related to Tea and Coffee

Compounds tested—caffeic acid, chafuroside B, chlorogenic acid, ellagic acid, epicatechin, epicatechin gallate, epigallocatechin gallate, theaflavin.

One human trial with epigallocatechin gallate in prostate cancer patients showed no significant effect on 8-OH–G in leukocytes [52]. Animal studies with single polyphenols have generally involved treating mice or rats with a known DNA-damaging agent and looking for protection against DNA breaks, MN and chrom abs. Generally, protection is seen [54,57] though in some cases at rather high doses [56,63]. Pretreatment of rats with epicatechin reduced the level of DNA breaks induced in bone marrow cells by the topoisomerase poison etoposide [55]. High concentrations have also been used in in vitro experiments with cultured cells, and have given increases in SBs and γ-H2AX foci [71] and in γ-H2AX and 8-OH–G [58]. Kumar et al. [79] found that a combination of ellagic acid with curcumin (25 μM each) caused SBs while the separate compounds had no significant effect. A decrease in (background) SBs with epigallocatechin gallate or epicatechin gallate was reported by Durgo et al. [36] at 48 but not 72 h. At more reasonable concentrations, the results are mixed: decreases in UV(B)-induced SBs [70] and cyclobutane pyrimidine dimers [72]; decreases in H_2O_2-induced SBs and MN [74]; a decrease in SBs induced by cumene hydroperoxide [75]; but SBs and Fpg-sites increased in tetradecanoyl phorbol acetate (TPA)-stimulated neutrophils [78] and an increase in SBs with ellagic acid in prostate cancer cells was reported by Vanella et al. [73] at concentrations of 9 μM in one of the cell lines but higher concentrations in two other lines.

4.2. Curcumin

Curcumin was examined alongside epicatechin by Papiez [55]; at high concentration (up to 0.2 g/kg/day), it decreased DNA damage in the bone marrow of rats treated with etoposide. In cultured cells, curcumin at rather high concentrations caused SBs [85,86] and γ-H2AX foci [83]. The production of SBs in combination with ellagic acid was noted above [79]. Lewinska et al. [81] reported a pro-oxidant effect of curcumin at concentrations of 10 μM (and below), indicated by an increase in 8-oxo–G in smooth muscle cells. Sebastia et al. [80] compared effects of curcumin on human lymphocytes, both stimulated by TPA and unstimulated, and γ-irradiated. In non-cycling cells, the phytochemical was radioprotective (decreasing the level of premature chromosome condensation), whereas in cycling cells it acted as a radiosensitiser, increasing the frequency of chrom abs.

4.3. Resveratrol

At high concentration, in human lymphocytes, resveratrol decreased the frequency of chromosome aberrations caused by aflatoxin [87]. At a lower concentration, it protected human epithelial cells against SBs and MN induced by sodium arsenite [88], and rat astrocytes against SBs caused by ethanol [91]. However, a low dose enhanced the frequency of γ-H2AX foci after ionising irradiation of prostate epithelial cells [90]. A moderately high concentration applied to colon cancer cells caused γ-H2AX foci, apparently as a result of topoisomerase II poisoning [89]. SBs as well as Fpg-sites were increased in non-cycling cells but decreased in TPA-stimulated, cycling cells [78]. In contrast, Sebastia et al. [80] found that, as with curcumin, effects of resveratrol on irradiated lymphocytes differed depending on whether the cells were non-cycling (showing a decrease in premature chromosome condensation), or cycling (in which it had the opposite effect, acting as a radiosensitiser, increasing chromosome aberrations).

4.4. Flavonoids

Kozics et al. [97] performed a useful comparative study of 10 flavonoids, concluding that their effectiveness at protecting against B(a)P-induced SBs and MN depended on their chemical structure. Tested over a relatively low concentration range, fisetin, quercetin, galangin, kaempferol and luteolin (in order of decreasing effectiveness) were more effective than chrysin,7-hydroxyflavone, 7,8-dihydroxyflavone or baicalein, while rutin was without effect.

Among the flavonoids, quercetin appears most often in this survey. At low concentrations, SBs induced by aflatoxin B1 (AFB1), methyl methanesulphonate (MMS), Dox, $HgCl_2$ or methyl mercury in HepG2 cells were decreased [100,101]. At high concentrations, quercetin and also rutin (glycoside of quercetin with rutinose) caused massive γ-H2AX foci, probably reflecting lethality [94], and yet they decreased DNA damage (SBs) induced by food mutagens PhIP and IQ [96].

Quercitrin, the rhamnose glycoside of quercetin, protected mouse epidermal cells against UV(B)-induced SBs [102]. Rutin at low concentrations showed the same protective effect as quercetin on HepG2 cells treated with AFB1, MMS or Dox [100]; at much higher concentrations, it caused SBs, but still protected against MN induced by B(a)P [93].

The myricetin rhamnoside, myricitrin, at high concentrations, induced MN in TK6 cells; the aglycone myricetin, being more cytotoxic, was tested at lower concentrations, and gave equivocal results [65]. Kaempferol at high concentrations induced SBs [95,99], as did fisetin [98]. Galangin and chrysin caused base oxidation at the moderate concentration of 20 μM [51], while a low concentration of naringin was protective against cadmium-induced chromosome aberrations [92]. Apigenin at a high concentration decreased SBs, chrom abs and MN [69].

5. Discussion and Conclusions

Many of the papers that we have reviewed report experiments with high or very high concentrations of phytochemicals. When investigating the role of phytochemicals in normal human nutrition, the aim should always be to study concentrations close to those likely to be present in humans as a result of dietary intake. As a rule of thumb, we have assumed this concentration to be in the low micromolar range. Many papers quote concentrations in μg/mL. To convert these concentrations to micromolar, again as a rule of thumb, we have assumed a molecular weight of 500; then 1 μg/mL = 2 μM. We would regard a concentration of over 20 μM or 10 μg/mL as high, and over 50 μM or 25 μg/mL as very high. Clearly, in functional foods or phytochemical supplements, the concentration is likely to be higher than in natural foods, and experiments showing genotoxicity of phytochemicals at high doses should at least serve as a warning to designers of functional foods.

It is always instructive to carry out experiments over a range of concentrations. Often, in the case of micronutrients in general, the dose–response curve is U-shaped, i.e., a beneficial effect at low concentrations changes to a detrimental effect at higher concentrations, and this tendency is clear in many of the reports described here.

Of course, if genotoxicity is specifically directed to cancer cells while healthy cells are unaffected, it is regarded as beneficial, and it is evidently the aim of some of the papers that we have reviewed to identify plant extracts or particular polyphenols that have such targeted action and so might have potential value as therapeutic agents. The differential response of cycling vs non-cycling cells to certain polyphenols might be exploited therapeutically in targeting dividing cancer cells.

With such a wide-ranging set of phytochemicals, not to mention the variety of test systems, experimental designs and assays applied in their study, it is difficult to generalise. However, high concentrations are likely to show DNA-damaging effects, while also in many cases protecting cells against damaging effects of other agents, apparently acting as pro-oxidants when present alone, but as anti-oxidants in combination. This is not a novel observation: many years ago, Duthie et al. reported DNA-damaging effects of quercetin at 50 μM [103] alongside an ability to protect cells against H_2O_2-induced DNA damage at concentrations of 10–50 μM [104]. Low concentrations are generally protective, in some cases even decreasing the already low background level of cellular DNA damage.

To summarise, results reported in the recent literature, on the whole, lend support to the hypothesis that dietary polyphenols protect the body against the effects of reactive oxygen species on DNA integrity, but do so reliably only when present at low concentrations. We recommend that greater attention be paid to the concentrations used, particularly in in vitro experiments, if the results are to be extrapolated to issues of human health. An important consideration when extrapolating is that plant foods contain a variety of micronutrients which might be expected to act in concert, whereas most experiments are carried out with single compounds. In this respect, there are clear advantages in using plant extracts or whole foods, though this approach does present practical difficulties. We also recommend that, since oxidative damage to DNA, and its prevention, are of major concern, the modified comet assay incorporating Fpg or EndoIII should be employed, since it provides increased sensitivity and specificity.

Acknowledgments: A.A. thanks the Ministerio de Economía y Competitividad ('Ramón y Cajal' programme, RYC-2013-14370) of the Spanish Government for personal support. This work was also supported by the BIOGENSA project (AGL2015-70640-R) of the 'Ministerio de Economía y Competitividad' of the Spanish Government.

Abbreviations

SB	strand break
Fpg	formamidopyrimidine DNA glycosylase
EndoIII	endonuclease III (Nth)
8-OH–Gua (8-OH–G)	8-oxo–7,8-dihydroguanine
PBMN	peripheral blood mononuclear
NER	nucleotide excision repair
Ab	antibody
NP	nanoparticle
Dox	doxorubicin
B(a)P	benzo(a)phenol
CPD	cyclobutane pyrimidine dimer
t-BOOH	*tert*-butyl hydroperoxide
PCB	polychlorinated biphenyls
DEN	diethylnitrosamine
TPA	tetradecanoyl-phorbol acetate

References

1. Bjelakovic, G.; Nikolova, D.; Gluud, L.L.; Simonetti, R.G.; Gluud, C. Mortality in randomized trials of antioxidant supplements for primary and secondary prevention: Systematic review and meta-analysis. *J. Am. Med. Assoc.* **2007**, *297*, 842–857. [CrossRef] [PubMed]
2. Azqueta, A.; Collins, A.R. The essential comet assay: A comprehensive guide to measuring DNA damage and repair. *Arch. Toxicol.* **2013**, *87*, 949–968. [CrossRef] [PubMed]
3. Kasai, H. Analysis of a form of oxidative DNA damage, 8-hydroxy-2′-deoxyguanosine, as a marker of cellular oxidative stress during carcinogenesis. *Mutat. Res./Rev. Mutat. Res.* **1997**, *387*, 147–163. [CrossRef]
4. Kasai, H.; Kawai, K. 8-hydroxyguanine, an oxidative DNA and RNA modification. In *Modified Nucleic Acids in Biology and Medicine*; Jurga, S.E., Erdmann, V.A., Barciszewski, J., Eds.; Springer: Basel, Switzerland, 2016; pp. 147–185.
5. Sedelnikova, O.A.; Rogakou, E.P.; Panyutin, I.G.; Bonner, W.M. Quantitative detection of (125)idu-induced DNA double-strand breaks with gamma-h2ax antibody. *Radiat. Res.* **2002**, *158*, 486–492. [CrossRef]
6. Huang, X.; Darzynkiewicz, Z. Cytometric assessment of histone h2ax phosphorylation: A reporter of DNA damage. *Methods Mol. Biol.* **2006**, *314*, 73–80. [PubMed]
7. Fenech, M. Cytokinesis-block micronucleus cytome assay. *Nat. Protoc.* **2007**, *2*, 1084–1104. [CrossRef] [PubMed]
8. Bonassi, S.; Norppa, H.; Ceppi, M.; Stromberg, U.; Vermeulen, R.; Znaor, A.; Cebulska-Wasilewska, A.; Fabianova, E.; Fucic, A.; Gundy, S.; et al. Chromosomal aberration frequency in lymphocytes predicts the risk of cancer: Results from a pooled cohort study of 22,358 subjects in 11 countries. *Carcinogenesis* **2008**, *29*, 1178–1183. [CrossRef] [PubMed]
9. Bonassi, S.; El-Zein, R.; Bolognesi, C.; Fenech, M. Micronuclei frequency in peripheral blood lymphocytes and cancer risk: Evidence from human studies. *Mutagenesis* **2011**, *26*, 93–100. [CrossRef] [PubMed]
10. Rangel-Huerta, O.D.; Aguilera, C.M.; Martin, M.V.; Soto, M.J.; Rico, M.C.; Vallejo, F.; Tomas-Barberan, F.; Perez-de-la-Cruz, A.J.; Gil, A.; Mesa, M.D. Normal or high polyphenol concentration in orange juice affects antioxidant activity, blood pressure, and body weight in obese or overweight adults. *J. Nutr.* **2015**, *145*, 1808–1816. [CrossRef] [PubMed]
11. Garcia-Flores, L.A.; Medina, S.; Cejuela-Anta, R.; Martinez-Sanz, J.M.; Abellan, A.; Genieser, H.G.; Ferreres, F.; Gil-Izquierdo, A. DNA catabolites in triathletes: Effects of supplementation with an aronia-citrus juice (polyphenols-rich juice). *Food Funct.* **2016**, *7*, 2084–2093. [CrossRef] [PubMed]
12. Spadafranca, A.; Martinez Conesa, C.; Sirini, S.; Testolin, G. Effect of dark chocolate on plasma epicatechin levels, DNA resistance to oxidative stress and total antioxidant activity in healthy subjects. *Br. J. Nutr.* **2010**, *103*, 1008–1014. [CrossRef] [PubMed]
13. Giovannelli, L.; Pitozzi, V.; Luceri, C.; Giannini, L.; Toti, S.; Salvini, S.; Sera, F.; Souquet, J.M.; Cheynier, V.; Sofi, F.; et al. Effects of de-alcoholised wines with different polyphenol content on DNA oxidative damage,

gene expression of peripheral lymphocytes, and haemorheology: An intervention study in post-menopausal women. *Eur. J. Nutr.* **2011**, *50*, 19–29. [CrossRef] [PubMed]

14. Riso, P.; Klimis-Zacas, D.; Del Bo, C.; Martini, D.; Campolo, J.; Vendrame, S.; Moller, P.; Loft, S.; De Maria, R.; Porrini, M. Effect of a wild blueberry (vaccinium angustifolium) drink intervention on markers of oxidative stress, inflammation and endothelial function in humans with cardiovascular risk factors. *Eur. J. Nutr.* **2013**, *52*, 949–961. [CrossRef] [PubMed]
15. Malhomme de la Roche, H.; Seagrove, S.; Mehta, A.; Divekar, P.; Campbell, S.; Curnow, A. Using natural dietary sources of antioxidants to protect against ultraviolet and visible radiation-induced DNA damage: An investigation of human green tea ingestion. *J. Photochem. Photobiol. B Biol.* **2010**, *101*, 169–173. [CrossRef] [PubMed]
16. Alleva, R.; Manzella, N.; Gaetani, S.; Ciarapica, V.; Bracci, M.; Caboni, M.F.; Pasini, F.; Monaco, F.; Amati, M.; Borghi, B.; et al. Organic honey supplementation reverses pesticide-induced genotoxicity by modulating dna damage response. *Mol. Nutr. Food Res.* **2016**, *60*, 2243–2255. [CrossRef] [PubMed]
17. Venancio, V.P.; Marques, M.C.; Almeida, M.R.; Mariutti, L.R.; Souza, V.C.; Barbosa, F., Jr.; Pires Bianchi, M.L.; Marzocchi-Machado, C.M.; Mercadante, A.Z.; Antunes, L.M. Chrysobalanus icaco l. Fruits inhibit nadph oxidase complex and protect DNA against doxorubicin-induced damage in wistar male rats. *J. Toxicol. Environ. Health Part A* **2016**, *79*, 885–893. [CrossRef] [PubMed]
18. Sinha, D.; Roy, M. Antagonistic role of tea against sodium arsenite-induced oxidative DNA damage and inhibition of DNA repair in swiss albino mice. *J. Environ. Pathol. Toxicol. Oncol.* **2011**, *30*, 311–322. [CrossRef] [PubMed]
19. Almeida, M.R.; Darin, J.D.; Hernandes, L.C.; Aissa, A.F.; Chiste, R.C.; Mercadante, A.Z.; Antunes, L.M.; Bianchi, M.L. Antigenotoxic effects of piquia (caryocar villosum) in multiple rat organs. *Plant Foods Hum. Nutr.* **2012**, *67*, 171–177. [CrossRef] [PubMed]
20. Ribeiro, J.C.; Antunes, L.M.; Aissa, A.F.; Darin, J.D.; De Rosso, V.V.; Mercadante, A.Z.; Bianchi Mde, L. Evaluation of the genotoxic and antigenotoxic effects after acute and subacute treatments with acai pulp (euterpe oleracea mart.) on mice using the erythrocytes micronucleus test and the comet assay. *Mutat. Res.* **2010**, *695*, 22–28. [CrossRef] [PubMed]
21. Krajka-Kuzniak, V.; Szaefer, H.; Ignatowicz, E.; Adamska, T.; Markowski, J.; Baer-Dubowska, W. Influence of cloudy apple juice on n-nitrosodiethylamine- induced liver injury and phases i and ii biotransformation enzymes in rat liver. *Acta Pol. Pharm.* **2015**, *72*, 267–276. [PubMed]
22. Acharyya, N.; Sajed Ali, S.; Deb, B.; Chattopadhyay, S.; Maiti, S. Green tea (camellia sinensis) alleviates arsenic-induced damages to DNA and intestinal tissues in rat and in situ intestinal loop by reinforcing antioxidant system. *Environ. Toxicol.* **2015**, *30*, 1033–1044. [CrossRef] [PubMed]
23. Ko, S.H.; Park, J.H.; Kim, S.Y.; Lee, S.W.; Chun, S.S.; Park, E. Antioxidant effects of spinach (*Spinacia oleracea* L.) supplementation in hyperlipidemic rats. *Prev. Nutr. Food Sci.* **2014**, *19*, 19–26. [CrossRef] [PubMed]
24. Ho, C.K.; Siu-wai, C.; Siu, P.M.; Benzie, I.F. Genoprotection and genotoxicity of green tea (camellia sinensis): Are they two sides of the same redox coin? *Redox Rep. Commun. Free Radic. Res.* **2013**, *18*, 150–154. [CrossRef] [PubMed]
25. Kuhnel, H.; Adilijiang, A.; Dadak, A.; Wieser, M.; Upur, H.; Stolze, K.; Grillari, J.; Strasser, A. Investigations into cytotoxic effects of the herbal preparation abnormal savda munziq. *Chin. J. Integr. Med.* **2015**, *53*, 1–9. [CrossRef] [PubMed]
26. Haza, A.I.; Morales, P. Spanish honeys protect against food mutagen-induced DNA damage. *J. Sci. Food Agric.* **2013**, *93*, 2995–3000. [CrossRef] [PubMed]
27. Qian, G.; Xue, K.; Tang, L.; Wang, F.; Song, X.; Chyu, M.C.; Pence, B.C.; Shen, C.L.; Wang, J.S. Mitigation of oxidative damage by green tea polyphenols and tai chi exercise in postmenopausal women with osteopenia. *PLoS ONE* **2012**, *7*, e48090. [CrossRef] [PubMed]
28. Xu, Y.; Zhang, J.J.; Xiong, L.; Zhang, L.; Sun, D.; Liu, H. Green tea polyphenols inhibit cognitive impairment induced by chronic cerebral hypoperfusion via modulating oxidative stress. *J. Nutr. Biochem.* **2010**, *21*, 741–748. [PubMed]
29. Katiyar, S.K.; Vaid, M.; van Steeg, H.; Meeran, S.M. Green tea polyphenols prevent uv-induced immunosuppression by rapid repair of DNA damage and enhancement of nucleotide excision repair genes. *Cancer Prev. Res.* **2010**, *3*, 179–189. [CrossRef] [PubMed]

30. Garcia-Rodriguez Mdel, C.; Carvente-Juarez, M.M.; Altamirano-Lozano, M.A. Antigenotoxic and apoptotic activity of green tea polyphenol extracts on hexavalent chromium-induced DNA damage in peripheral blood of cd-1 mice: Analysis with differential acridine orange/ethidium bromide staining. *Oxidative Med. Cell. Longev.* **2013**, *2013*, 486419. [CrossRef] [PubMed]
31. Pu, X.; Wang, Z.; Zhou, S.; Klaunig, J.E. Protective effects of antioxidants on acrylonitrile-induced oxidative stress in female f344 rats. *Environ. Toxicol.* **2015**. [CrossRef] [PubMed]
32. Olteanu, E.D.; Filip, A.; Clichici, S.; Daicoviciu, D.; Achim, M.; Postescu, I.D.; Bolfa, P.; Bolojan, L.; Vlase, L.; Muresan, A. Photochemoprotective effect of calluna vulgaris extract on skin exposed to multiple doses of ultraviolet b in skh-1 hairless mice. *J. Environ. Pathol. Toxicol. Oncol.* **2012**, *31*, 233–243. [CrossRef] [PubMed]
33. Chaudhary, P.; Shukla, S.K.; Sharma, R.K. Rec-2006-a fractionated extract of podophyllum hexandrum protects cellular DNA from radiation-induced damage by reducing the initial damage and enhancing its repair in vivo. *Evid.-Based Complement. Altern. Med.* **2011**, *2011*, 473953. [CrossRef] [PubMed]
34. Matic, S.; Stanic, S.; Bogojevic, D.; Vidakovic, M.; Grdovic, N.; Dinic, S.; Solujic, S.; Mladenovic, M.; Stankovic, N.; Mihailovic, M. Methanol extract from the stem of cotinus coggygria scop., and its major bioactive phytochemical constituent myricetin modulate pyrogallol-induced DNA damage and liver injury. *Mutat. Res.* **2013**, *755*, 81–89. [CrossRef] [PubMed]
35. Prasad, R.; Katiyar, S.K. Polyphenols from green tea inhibit the growth of melanoma cells through inhibition of class i histone deacetylases and induction of DNA damage. *Genes Cancer* **2015**, *6*, 49–61. [PubMed]
36. Durgo, K.; Kostic, S.; Gradiski, K.; Komes, D.; Osmak, M.; Franekic, J. Genotoxic effects of green tea extract on human laryngeal carcinoma cells in vitro. *Arch. Hig. Rada Toksikol.* **2011**, *62*, 139–146. [CrossRef] [PubMed]
37. Perez-Sanchez, A.; Barrajon-Catalan, E.; Caturla, N.; Castillo, J.; Benavente-Garcia, O.; Alcaraz, M.; Micol, V. Protective effects of citrus and rosemary extracts on uv-induced damage in skin cell model and human volunteers. *J. Photochem. Photobiol. B Biol.* **2014**, *136*, 12–18. [CrossRef] [PubMed]
38. Cornaghi, L.; Arnaboldi, F.; Calo, R.; Landoni, F.; Baruffaldi Preis, W.F.; Marabini, L.; Donetti, E. Effects of uv rays and thymol/thymus vulgaris l. Extract in an ex vivo human skin model: Morphological and genotoxicological assessment. *Cells Tissues Organs* **2016**, *201*, 180–192. [CrossRef] [PubMed]
39. Calo, R.; Visone, C.M.; Marabini, L. Thymol and thymus vulgaris L. Activity against uva- and uvb-induced damage in nctc 2544 cell line. *Mutat. Res. Genet. Toxicol. Environ. Mutagen.* **2015**, *791*, 30–37. [CrossRef] [PubMed]
40. Perez-Sanchez, A.; Barrajon-Catalan, E.; Herranz-Lopez, M.; Castillo, J.; Micol, V. Lemon balm extract (*Melissa officinalis* L.) promotes melanogenesis and prevents uvb-induced oxidative stress and DNA damage in a skin cell model. *J. Dermatol. Sci.* **2016**, *84*, 169–177. [CrossRef] [PubMed]
41. Venuprasad, M.P.; Hemanth Kumar, K.; Khanum, F. Neuroprotective effects of hydroalcoholic extract of ocimum sanctum against h2o2 induced neuronal cell damage in sh-sy5y cells via its antioxidative defence mechanism. *Neurochem. Res.* **2013**, *38*, 2190–2200. [CrossRef] [PubMed]
42. Thirugnanasampandan, R.; Jayakumar, R. Protection of cadmium chloride induced DNA damage by lamiaceae plants. *Asian Pac. J. Trop. Biomed.* **2011**, *1*, 391–394. [CrossRef]
43. Giampieri, F.; Alvarez-Suarez, J.M.; Tulipani, S.; Gonzales-Paramas, A.M.; Santos-Buelga, C.; Bompadre, S.; Quiles, J.L.; Mezzetti, B.; Battino, M. Photoprotective potential of strawberry (fragaria x ananassa) extract against uv-a irradiation damage on human fibroblasts. *J. Agric. Food Chem.* **2012**, *60*, 2322–2327. [CrossRef] [PubMed]
44. Giampieri, F.; Alvarez-Suarez, J.M.; Mazzoni, L.; Forbes-Hernandez, T.Y.; Gasparrini, M.; Gonzalez-Paramas, A.M.; Santos-Buelga, C.; Quiles, J.L.; Bompadre, S.; Mezzetti, B.; et al. Polyphenol-rich strawberry extract protects human dermal fibroblasts against hydrogen peroxide oxidative damage and improves mitochondrial functionality. *Molecules* **2014**, *19*, 7798–7816. [CrossRef] [PubMed]
45. Braga, P.C.; Antonacci, R.; Wang, Y.Y.; Lattuada, N.; Dal Sasso, M.; Marabini, L.; Fibiani, M.; Lo Scalzo, R. Comparative antioxidant activity of cultivated and wild vaccinium species investigated by epr, human neutrophil burst and comet assay. *Eur. Rev. Med. Pharmacol. Sci.* **2013**, *17*, 1987–1999. [PubMed]
46. Yamamoto, A.; Nakashima, K.; Kawamorita, S.; Sugiyama, A.; Miura, M.; Kamitai, Y.; Kato, Y. Protective effects of raw and cooked blackcurrant extract on DNA damage induced by hydrogen peroxide in human lymphoblastoid cells. *Pharm. Biol.* **2014**, *52*, 782–788. [CrossRef] [PubMed]

47. Bellion, P.; Digles, J.; Will, F.; Dietrich, H.; Baum, M.; Eisenbrand, G.; Janzowski, C. Polyphenolic apple extracts: Effects of raw material and production method on antioxidant effectiveness and reduction of DNA damage in caco-2 cells. *J. Agric. Food Chem.* **2010**, *58*, 6636–6642. [CrossRef] [PubMed]
48. Tan, A.C.; Konczak, I.; Ramzan, I.; Sze, D.M. Native australian fruit polyphenols inhibit cell viability and induce apoptosis in human cancer cell lines. *Nutr. Cancer* **2011**, *63*, 444–455. [CrossRef] [PubMed]
49. Botden, I.P.; Oeseburg, H.; Durik, M.; Leijten, F.P.; Van Vark-Van Der Zee, L.C.; Musterd-Bhaggoe, U.M.; Garrelds, I.M.; Seynhaeve, A.L.; Langendonk, J.G.; Sijbrands, E.J.; et al. Red wine extract protects against oxidative-stress-induced endothelial senescence. *Clin. Sci.* **2012**, *123*, 499–507. [CrossRef] [PubMed]
50. Yalcin, C.O.; Aliyazicioglu, Y.; Demir, S.; Turan, I.; Bahat, Z.; Misir, S.; Deger, O. Evaluation of the radioprotective effect of turkish propolis on foreskin fibroblast cells. *J. Cancer Res. Ther.* **2016**, *12*, 990–994. [PubMed]
51. Tsai, Y.C.; Wang, Y.H.; Liou, C.C.; Lin, Y.C.; Huang, H.; Liu, Y.C. Induction of oxidative DNA damage by flavonoids of propolis: Its mechanism and implication about antioxidant capacity. *Chem. Res. Toxicol.* **2012**, *25*, 191–196. [CrossRef] [PubMed]
52. Nguyen, M.M.; Ahmann, F.R.; Nagle, R.B.; Hsu, C.H.; Tangrea, J.A.; Parnes, H.L.; Sokoloff, M.H.; Gretzer, M.B.; Chow, H.H. Randomized, double-blind, placebo-controlled trial of polyphenon e in prostate cancer patients before prostatectomy: Evaluation of potential chemopreventive activities. *Cancer Prev. Res.* **2012**, *5*, 290–298. [CrossRef] [PubMed]
53. Ferk, F.; Misik, M.; Nersesyan, A.; Pichler, C.; Jager, W.; Szekeres, T.; Marculescu, R.; Poulsen, H.E.; Henriksen, T.; Bono, R.; et al. Impact of xanthohumol (a prenylated flavonoid from hops) on DNA stability and other health-related biochemical parameters: Results of human intervention trials. *Mol. Nutr. Food Res.* **2016**, *60*, 773–786. [CrossRef] [PubMed]
54. Cariddi, L.N.; Sabini, M.C.; Escobar, F.M.; Montironi, I.; Manas, F.; Iglesias, D.; Comini, L.R.; Sabini, L.I.; Dalcero, A.M. Polyphenols as possible bioprotectors against cytotoxicity and DNA damage induced by ochratoxin A. *Environ. Toxicol. Pharmacol.* **2015**, *39*, 1008–1018. [CrossRef] [PubMed]
55. Papiez, M.A. The influence of curcumin and (−)-epicatechin on the genotoxicity and myelosuppression induced by etoposide in bone marrow cells of male rats. *Drug Chem. Toxicol.* **2013**, *36*, 93–101. [CrossRef] [PubMed]
56. Rehman, M.U.; Tahir, M.; Ali, F.; Qamar, W.; Lateef, A.; Khan, R.; Quaiyoom, A.; Oday, O.H.; Sultana, S. Cyclophosphamide-induced nephrotoxicity, genotoxicity, and damage in kidney genomic DNA of swiss albino mice: The protective effect of ellagic acid. *Mol. Cell. Biochem.* **2012**, *365*, 119–127. [CrossRef] [PubMed]
57. Srivastava, A.K.; Bhatnagar, P.; Singh, M.; Mishra, S.; Kumar, P.; Shukla, Y.; Gupta, K.C. Synthesis of plga nanoparticles of tea polyphenols and their strong in vivo protective effect against chemically induced DNA damage. *Int. J. Nanomed.* **2013**, *8*, 1451–1462.
58. Li, G.X.; Chen, Y.K.; Hou, Z.; Xiao, H.; Jin, H.; Lu, G.; Lee, M.J.; Liu, B.; Guan, F.; Yang, Z.; et al. Pro-oxidative activities and dose-response relationship of (−)-epigallocatechin-3-gallate in the inhibition of lung cancer cell growth: A comparative study in vivo and in vitro. *Carcinogenesis* **2010**, *31*, 902–910. [CrossRef] [PubMed]
59. Marrazzo, G.; Bosco, P.; La Delia, F.; Scapagnini, G.; Di Giacomo, C.; Malaguarnera, M.; Galvano, F.; Nicolosi, A.; Li Volti, G. Neuroprotective effect of silibinin in diabetic mice. *Neurosci. Lett.* **2011**, *504*, 252–256. [CrossRef] [PubMed]
60. Rocha de Oliveira, C.; Ceolin, J.; Rocha de Oliveira, R.; Goncalves Schemitt, E.; Raskopf Colares, J.; De Freitas Bauermann, L.; Hilda Costabeber, I.; Morgan-Martins, M.I.; Mauriz, J.L.; Da Silva, J.; et al. Effects of quercetin on polychlorinated biphenyls-induced liver injury in rats. *Nutr. Hosp.* **2014**, *29*, 1141–1148. [PubMed]
61. Patil, S.L.; Rao, N.B.; Somashekarappa, H.M.; Rajashekhar, K.P. Antigenotoxic potential of rutin and quercetin in swiss mice exposed to gamma radiation. *Biomed. J.* **2014**, *37*, 305–313. [CrossRef] [PubMed]
62. Manzolli, E.S.; Serpeloni, J.M.; Grotto, D. Protective effects of the flavonoid chrysin against methylmercury-induced genotoxicity and alterations of antioxidant status, in vivo. *Oxidative Med. Cell. Longev.* **2015**, *2015*, 602360. [CrossRef] [PubMed]
63. Ma, J.Q.; Ding, J.; Xiao, Z.H.; Liu, C.M. Puerarin ameliorates carbon tetrachloride-induced oxidative DNA damage and inflammation in mouse kidney through erk/nrf2/are pathway. *Food Chem. Toxicol.* **2014**, *71*, 264–271. [CrossRef] [PubMed]
64. Liu, C.M.; Ma, J.Q.; Sun, Y.Z. Quercetin protects the rat kidney against oxidative stress-mediated DNA damage and apoptosis induced by lead. *Environ. Toxicol. Pharmacol.* **2010**, *30*, 264–271. [CrossRef] [PubMed]

65. Hobbs, C.A.; Swartz, C.; Maronpot, R.; Davis, J.; Recio, L.; Koyanagi, M.; Hayashi, S.M. Genotoxicity evaluation of the flavonoid, myricitrin, and its aglycone, myricetin. *Food Chem. Toxicol.* **2015**, *83*, 283–292. [CrossRef] [PubMed]
66. Gupta, C.; Vikram, A.; Tripathi, D.N.; Ramarao, P.; Jena, G.B. Antioxidant and antimutagenic effect of quercetin against den induced hepatotoxicity in rat. *Phytother. Res.* **2010**, *24*, 119–128. [CrossRef] [PubMed]
67. Ansar, S.; Siddiqi, N.J.; Zargar, S.; Ganaie, M.A.; Abudawood, M. Hepatoprotective effect of quercetin supplementation against acrylamide-induced DNA damage in wistar rats. *BMC Complement. Altern. Med.* **2016**, *16*, 327. [CrossRef] [PubMed]
68. Carino-Cortes, R.; Alvarez-Gonzalez, I.; Martino-Roaro, L.; Madrigal-Bujaidar, E. Effect of naringin on the DNA damage induced by daunorubicin in mouse hepatocytes and cardiocytes. *Biol. Pharm. Bull.* **2010**, *33*, 697–701. [CrossRef] [PubMed]
69. Das, S.; Das, J.; Paul, A.; Samadder, A.; Khuda-Bukhsh, A.R. Apigenin, a bioactive flavonoid from lycopodium clavatum, stimulates nucleotide excision repair genes to protect skin keratinocytes from ultraviolet b-induced reactive oxygen species and DNA damage. *J. Acupunct. Meridian Stud.* **2013**, *6*, 252–262. [CrossRef] [PubMed]
70. Cha, J.W.; Piao, M.J.; Kim, K.C.; Yao, C.W.; Zheng, J.; Kim, S.M.; Hyun, C.L.; Ahn, Y.S.; Hyun, J.W. The polyphenol chlorogenic acid attenuates uvb-mediated oxidative stress in human hacat keratinocytes. *Biomol. Ther.* **2014**, *22*, 136–142. [CrossRef] [PubMed]
71. Burgos-Moron, E.; Calderon-Montano, J.M.; Orta, M.L.; Pastor, N.; Perez-Guerrero, C.; Austin, C.; Mateos, S.; Lopez-Lazaro, M. The coffee constituent chlorogenic acid induces cellular DNA damage and formation of topoisomerase i- and ii-DNA complexes in cells. *J. Agric. Food Chem.* **2012**, *60*, 7384–7391. [CrossRef] [PubMed]
72. Hasegawa, T.; Shimada, S.; Ishida, H.; Nakashima, M. Chafuroside b, an oolong tea polyphenol, ameliorates uvb-induced DNA damage and generation of photo-immunosuppression related mediators in human keratinocytes. *PLoS ONE* **2013**, *8*, e77308. [CrossRef] [PubMed]
73. Vanella, L.; Barbagallo, I.; Acquaviva, R.; Di Giacomo, C.; Cardile, V.; Abraham, N.G.; Sorrenti, V. Ellagic acid: Cytodifferentiating and antiproliferative effects in human prostatic cancer cell lines. *Curr. Pharm. Des.* **2013**, *19*, 2728–2736. [CrossRef] [PubMed]
74. Abib, R.T.; Quincozes-Santos, A.; Zanotto, C.; Zeidan-Chulia, F.; Lunardi, P.S.; Goncalves, C.A.; Gottfried, C. Genoprotective effects of the green tea-derived polyphenol/epicatechin gallate in c6 astroglial cells. *J. Med. Food* **2010**, *13*, 1111–1115. [CrossRef] [PubMed]
75. Miene, C.; Weise, A.; Glei, M. Impact of polyphenol metabolites produced by colonic microbiota on expression of cox-2 and gstt2 in human colon cells (lt97). *Nutr. Cancer* **2011**, *63*, 653–662. [CrossRef] [PubMed]
76. Hossain, M.Z.; Patel, K.; Kern, S.E. Salivary alpha-amylase, serum albumin, and myoglobin protect against DNA-damaging activities of ingested dietary agents in vitro. *Food Chem. Toxicol.* **2014**, *70*, 114–119. [CrossRef] [PubMed]
77. Mohan, S.; Thiagarajan, K.; Chandrasekaran, R. In vitro evaluation of antiproliferative effect of ethyl gallate against human oral squamous carcinoma cell line kb. *Nat. Prod. Res.* **2015**, *29*, 366–369. [CrossRef] [PubMed]
78. Zielinska-Przyjemska, M.; Ignatowicz, E.; Krajka-Kuzniak, V.; Baer-Dubowska, W. Effect of tannic acid, resveratrol and its derivatives, on oxidative damage and apoptosis in human neutrophils. *Food Chem. Toxicol.* **2015**, *84*, 37–46. [CrossRef] [PubMed]
79. Kumar, D.; Basu, S.; Parija, L.; Rout, D.; Manna, S.; Dandapat, J.; Debata, P.R. Curcumin and ellagic acid synergistically induce ros generation, DNA damage, p53 accumulation and apoptosis in hela cervical carcinoma cells. *Biomed. Pharmacother.* **2016**, *81*, 31–37. [CrossRef] [PubMed]
80. Sebastia, N.; Montoro, A.; Hervas, D.; Pantelias, G.; Hatzi, V.I.; Soriano, J.M.; Villaescusa, J.I.; Terzoudi, G.I. Curcumin and trans-resveratrol exert cell cycle-dependent radioprotective or radiosensitizing effects as elucidated by the pcc and g2-assay. *Mutat. Res.* **2014**, *766–767*, 49–55. [CrossRef] [PubMed]
81. Lewinska, A.; Wnuk, M.; Grabowska, W.; Zabek, T.; Semik, E.; Sikora, E.; Bielak-Zmijewska, A. Curcumin induces oxidation-dependent cell cycle arrest mediated by sirt7 inhibition of rdna transcription in human aortic smooth muscle cells. *Toxicol. Lett.* **2015**, *233*, 227–238. [CrossRef] [PubMed]
82. Sun, B.; Ross, S.M.; Trask, O.J.; Carmichael, P.L.; Dent, M.; White, A.; Andersen, M.E.; Clewell, R.A. Assessing dose-dependent differences in DNA-damage, p53 response and genotoxicity for quercetin and curcumin. *Toxicol. In Vitro* **2013**, *27*, 1877–1887. [CrossRef] [PubMed]

83. Ide, H.; Yu, J.; Lu, Y.; China, T.; Kumamoto, T.; Koseki, T.; Muto, S.; Horie, S. Testosterone augments polyphenol-induced DNA damage response in prostate cancer cell line, LNCaP. *Cancer Sci.* **2011**, *102*, 468–471. [CrossRef] [PubMed]
84. Seo, Y.N.; Lee, M.Y. Inhibitory effect of antioxidants on the benz[a]anthracene-induced oxidative DNA damage in lymphocyte. *J. Environ. Biol./Acad. Environ. Biol. India* **2011**, *32*, 7–10.
85. Lu, J.J.; Cai, Y.J.; Ding, J. Curcumin induces DNA damage and caffeine-insensitive cell cycle arrest in colorectal carcinoma hct116 cells. *Mol. Cell. Biochem.* **2011**, *354*, 247–252. [CrossRef] [PubMed]
86. Lu, J.J.; Cai, Y.J.; Ding, J. The short-time treatment with curcumin sufficiently decreases cell viability, induces apoptosis and copper enhances these effects in multidrug-resistant k562/a02 cells. *Mol. Cell. Biochem.* **2012**, *360*, 253–260. [CrossRef] [PubMed]
87. Turkez, H.; Sisman, T. The genoprotective activity of resveratrol on aflatoxin b(1)-induced DNA damage in human lymphocytes in vitro. *Toxicol. Ind. Health* **2012**, *28*, 474–480. [CrossRef] [PubMed]
88. Chen, C.; Jiang, X.; Hu, Y.; Zhang, Z. The protective role of resveratrol in the sodium arsenite-induced oxidative damage via modulation of intracellular gsh homeostasis. *Biol. Trace Element Res.* **2013**, *155*, 119–131. [CrossRef] [PubMed]
89. Demoulin, B.; Hermant, M.; Castrogiovanni, C.; Staudt, C.; Dumont, P. Resveratrol induces DNA damage in colon cancer cells by poisoning topoisomerase ii and activates the atm kinase to trigger p53-dependent apoptosis. *Toxicol. In Vitro* **2015**, *29*, 1156–1165. [CrossRef] [PubMed]
90. Rashid, A.; Liu, C.; Sanli, T.; Tsiani, E.; Singh, G.; Bristow, R.G.; Dayes, I.; Lukka, H.; Wright, J.; Tsakiridis, T. Resveratrol enhances prostate cancer cell response to ionizing radiation. Modulation of the ampk, akt and mtor pathways. *Radiat. Oncol.* **2011**, *6*, 669–672. [CrossRef] [PubMed]
91. Gonthier, B.; Allibe, N.; Cottet-Rousselle, C.; Lamarche, F.; Nuiry, L.; Barret, L. Specific conditions for resveratrol neuroprotection against ethanol-induced toxicity. *J. Toxicol.* **2012**, *2012*, 973134. [CrossRef] [PubMed]
92. Yilmaz, D.; Aydemir, N.C.; Vatan, O.; Tuzun, E.; Bilaloglu, R. Influence of naringin on cadmium-induced genomic damage in human lymphocytes in vitro. *Toxicol. Ind. Health* **2012**, *28*, 114–121. [CrossRef] [PubMed]
93. Cristina Marcarini, J.; Ferreira Tsuboy, M.S.; Cabral Luiz, R.; Regina Ribeiro, L.; Beatriz Hoffmann-Campo, C.; Segio Mantovani, M. Investigation of cytotoxic, apoptosis-inducing, genotoxic and protective effects of the flavonoid rutin in htc hepatic cells. *Exp. Toxicol. Pathol.* **2011**, *63*, 459–465. [CrossRef] [PubMed]
94. Maeda, J.; Roybal, E.J.; Brents, C.A.; Uesaka, M.; Aizawa, Y.; Kato, T.A. Natural and glucosyl flavonoids inhibit poly(adp-ribose) polymerase activity and induce synthetic lethality in brca mutant cells. *Oncol. Rep.* **2014**, *31*, 551–556. [PubMed]
95. Wu, L.Y.; Lu, H.F.; Chou, Y.C.; Shih, Y.L.; Bau, D.T.; Chen, J.C.; Hsu, S.C.; Chung, J.G. Kaempferol induces DNA damage and inhibits DNA repair associated protein expressions in human promyelocytic leukemia hl-60 cells. *Am. J. Chin. Med.* **2015**, *43*, 365–382. [CrossRef] [PubMed]
96. Kurzawa-Zegota, M.; Najafzadeh, M.; Baumgartner, A.; Anderson, D. The protective effect of the flavonoids on food-mutagen-induced DNA damage in peripheral blood lymphocytes from colon cancer patients. *Food Chem. Toxicol.* **2012**, *50*, 124–129. [CrossRef] [PubMed]
97. Kozics, K.; Valovicova, Z.; Slamenova, D. Structure of flavonoids influences the degree inhibition of benzo(a)pyrene—Induced DNA damage and micronuclei in hepg2 cells. *Neoplasma* **2011**, *58*, 516–524. [CrossRef] [PubMed]
98. Kim, J.Y.; Jeon, Y.K.; Jeon, W.; Nam, M.J. Fisetin induces apoptosis in huh-7 cells via downregulation of birc8 and bcl2l2. *Food Chem. Toxicol.* **2010**, *48*, 2259–2264. [CrossRef] [PubMed]
99. Huang, W.W.; Chiu, Y.J.; Fan, M.J.; Lu, H.F.; Yeh, H.F.; Li, K.H.; Chen, P.Y.; Chung, J.G.; Yang, J.S. Kaempferol induced apoptosis via endoplasmic reticulum stress and mitochondria-dependent pathway in human osteosarcoma u-2 os cells. *Mol. Nutr. Food Res.* **2010**, *54*, 1585–1595. [CrossRef] [PubMed]
100. Barcelos, G.R.; Grotto, D.; Angeli, J.P.; Serpeloni, J.M.; Rocha, B.A.; Bastos, J.K.; Barbosa, F., Jr. Evaluation of antigenotoxic effects of plant flavonoids quercetin and rutin on hepg2 cells. *Phytother. Res.* **2011**, *25*, 1381–1388. [CrossRef] [PubMed]
101. Barcelos, G.R.; Angeli, J.P.; Serpeloni, J.M.; Grotto, D.; Rocha, B.A.; Bastos, J.K.; Knasmuller, S.; Junior, F.B. Quercetin protects human-derived liver cells against mercury-induced DNA-damage and alterations of the redox status. *Mutat. Res.* **2011**, *726*, 109–115. [CrossRef] [PubMed]

102. Ding, M.; Zhao, J.; Bowman, L.; Lu, Y.; Shi, X. Inhibition of ap-1 and mapk signaling and activation of nrf2/are pathway by quercitrin. *Int. J. Oncol.* **2010**, *36*, 59–67. [CrossRef] [PubMed]
103. Duthie, S.J.; Johnson, W.; Dobson, V.L. The effect of dietary flavonoids on DNA damage (strand breaks and oxidised pyrimdines) and growth in human cells. *Mutat. Res.* **1997**, *390*, 141–151. [CrossRef]
104. Duthie, S.J.; Collins, A.R.; Duthie, G.G.; Dobson, V.L. Quercetin and myricetin protect against hydrogen peroxide-induced DNA damage (strand breaks and oxidised pyrimidines) in human lymphocytes. *Mutat. Res.* **1997**, *393*, 223–231. [CrossRef]

2

Molecular Targets Underlying the Anticancer Effects of Quercetin

Fazlullah Khan [1,2], Kamal Niaz [1,2], Faheem Maqbool [1,2], Fatima Ismail Hassan [1,2], Mohammad Abdollahi [1,2,*], Kalyan C. Nagulapalli Venkata [3], Seyed Mohammad Nabavi [4] and Anupam Bishayee [3,*]

1 Pharmaceutical Sciences Research Center, International Campus, Tehran University of Medical Sciences, Tehran 1417614411, Iran; fazlullahdr@gmail.com (F.K.); kamalniaz1989@gmail.com (K.N.); faheemthepharmacist@gmail.com (F.M.) pharm.fatee@yahoo.com (F.I.H.)
2 Department of Toxicology and Pharmacology, Faculty of Pharmacy, Tehran University of Medical Sciences, Tehran 1417614411, Iran
3 Department of Pharmaceutical Sciences, College of Pharmacy, Larkin Health Sciences Institute, Miami, FL 33169, USA; kvenkata@Ularkin.org
4 Applied Biotechnology Research Center, Baqiyatallah University of Medical Sciences, Tehran 1435916471, Iran; nabavi208@gmail.com
* Correspondence: Mohammad.Abdollahi@UToronto.Ca or Mohammad@TUMS.Ac.Ir (M.A.); abishayee@Ularkin.org or abishayee@gmail.com (A.B.)

Abstract: Quercetin, a medicinally important member of the flavonoid family, is one of the most prominent dietary antioxidants. It is present in a variety of foods—including fruits, vegetables, tea, wine, as well as other dietary supplements—and is responsible for various health benefits. Numerous pharmacological effects of quercetin include protection against diseases, such as osteoporosis, certain forms of malignant tumors, and pulmonary and cardiovascular disorders. Quercetin has the special ability of scavenging highly reactive species, such as hydrogen peroxide, superoxide anion, and hydroxyl radicals. These oxygen radicals are called reactive oxygen species, which can cause oxidative damage to cellular components, such as proteins, lipids, and deoxyribonucleic acid. Various oxygen radicals play important roles in pathophysiological and degenerative processes, such as aging. Subsequently, several studies have been performed to evaluate possible advantageous health effects of quercetin and to collect scientific evidence for these beneficial health claims. These studies also gather data in order to evaluate the exact mechanism(s) of action and toxicological effects of quercetin. The purpose of this review is to present and critically analyze molecular pathways underlying the anticancer effects of quercetin. Current limitations and future directions of research on this bioactive dietary polyphenol are also critically discussed.

Keywords: quercetin; cancer prevention; diet; bioavailability; DNA damage; polyphenols

1. Introduction

During the last decade, the proportion of scientific studies based on non-nutritive components of diet has increased. Such components are present in diet and have the ability to protect the body from the harmful effects of degenerative diseases, cancer, and cardiovascular ailments. Carotenoids and flavonoids, two distinct groups of phytochemicals, represent valuable constituents of food. Other dietary agents—such as phytoalexins, phenolic acids, indole-3-carbinol, and organosulfur compounds—are also important phytochemicals with interesting biological activities [1,2]. Phytochemicals are generally present in a variety of foods, fruits, vegetables, beverages, and many other food products and medicinally important herbal preparations. The important point that brings the attention of the scientists towards the naturally occurring compounds for the purpose of testing is the presence of numerous phytochemicals existing in plant-derived foods. There are a wide variety of biological activities which are still unknown for the majority of these compounds [3]. Plant-derived phytochemicals activate various cell signaling pathways that play key roles in the prevention of physiological disorders in the body, which are mainly responsible for the development of cancers, neurodegenerative and cardiovascular diseases [4,5]. Various scientific studies conducted on experimental animal models for the assessment of the exact mechanisms through which phytochemicals exert their actions provide a good and valuable description of how food supplements containing abundant amounts of phytochemicals exhibit protective roles against degenerative disorders [6]. It is noteworthy to find out that such plant-derived medicinally important constituents have the ability to demonstrate preventive and protective measures against pathological disorders.

Flavonoids are mostly present in nature in the form of benzo-γ-pyrone derivatives. These compounds are mostly present in a variety of plants, vegetables, and flowers. Flavonoids have diverse structural frameworks and play important roles in the body's defense system. The beneficial effects of flavonoid-rich foods have been demonstrated by various studies [7]. Data collected from different clinical trials have tried to underscore the exact mode of action exerted by flavonoids. There is a need to evaluate new possible ways to understand the beneficial activities associated with the consumption of flavonoid-rich food in order to advance our knowledge about the possible beneficial action of plant extracts. There are 4000 types of different flavonoids found in nature with diverse subcategories, such as flavones, isoflavones, flavonones, and chalcones. Flavonoids possess important biological activities, such as anti-inflammatory, antioxidant, hepatoprotective, and antimicrobial properties [8].

Quercetin is a key member of the polyphenol family and is largely found in various vegetables and fruits, such as capers, lovage, dill, cilantro, onions, various berries (e.g., chokeberries, cranberries, and lingonberries), and apples. Quercetin is well known for its anticarcinogenic potential. The anticancer property of quercetin is due to various cell signaling mechanisms and its ability to inhibit enzymes responsible for the activation of carcinogens. Moreover, quercetin exerts anticancer effect by binding to cellular receptors and proteins [9,10].

Several previous publications [11–16] present an excellent overview of research related to the therapeutic application of quercetin in cancer prevention and treatment. Nevertheless, there exists a need for a systematic, up-to-date, and critical evaluation of literature to understand biochemical and molecular mechanisms of the anticancer action of quercetin. In this review article, first we focused on chemical reactivity of quercetin and related analogs. Secondly, we discussed the molecular targets as well as signaling pathways implicated in anticancer and cancer preventive potential of quercetin. Thirdly, we presented epidemiological evidences regarding quercetin consumption and cancer occurrence. Finally, we discussed future directions of research to understand the full potential of quercetin in cancer prevention and treatment.

2. Bibliographic Search

The scientific information gathered in this review was collected by widespread search of several electronic databases, including PubMed, Scopus, Medline, Web of Science, EBASE, and Google Scholar. The criteria for the exclusion of articles was the language of reports being other than English, reports with unavailable abstracts, studies related to quercetin effects apart from its anticancer profile, and studies which showed the linkage between cancer and cancer risk factors, such as tobacco smoking and alcohol consumption. Various appropriate articles not indexed by PubMed were also considered, and 27 such reports which fulfilled the criteria for inclusion were further recovered from Google Scholar. Therefore, the total number of included articles in this review is 127 (Figure 1).

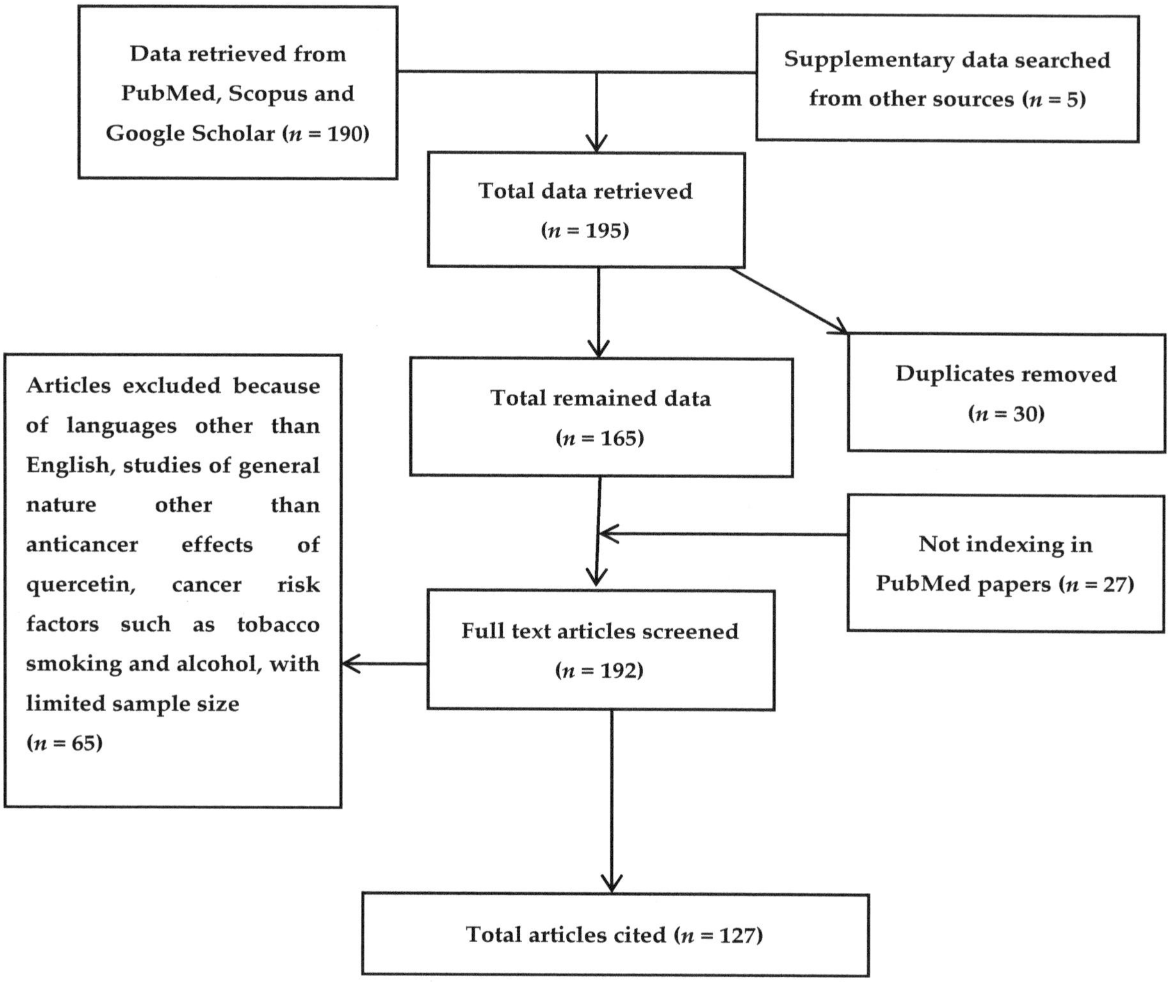

Figure 1. Flow diagram of included studies. The number of citations and resource materials that have been screened, excluded and/or included in this review is indicated in parenthesis.

3. Chemistry of Quercetin and Its Analogs

Quercetin is a polyphenolic secondary metabolite that belongs to the flavonol class of flavonoids. It is characterized by a benzo-(γ)-pyrone skeletal structure with C6-C3-C6 carbon framework, consisting of two benzene rings, A and B, linked by a three-carbon pyrone ring C as shown in Figure 2 [17]. Quercetin is referred to as pentahydroxyflavonol due to the presence of five hydroxyl groups on its flavonol skeletal framework at 3, 3′, 4′, 5, and 7 carbons [12]. The wide range of biochemical and pharmacological activities of quercetin and its metabolites is due to the relative substitution of various functional groups on the flavonol molecule [18].

Phytochemical investigations of various plant extracts have revealed that quercetin can exist in a free state as an aglycone, or as its derivative by conjugating with: (1) carbohydrates as quercetin glycosides, (2) lipids as prenylated quercetin, (3) alcohols as quercetin ethers, and (4) a sulfate group as quercetin sulfate [19].

Quercetin glycosides are formed through the *O*-glycosidic bond between a sugar and the hydroxyl group of quercetin molecule, and the general glycosylation site on the quercetin molecule is at the 3-hydroxyl position. However, glycosylation of other hydroxyl groups has also been reported [20]. The sugar moieties can be monosaccharides, disaccharides, or polysaccharides, and the most common carbohydrate substituents are glucose, galactose, rhamnose, and xylose. Isoquercetin, hyperoside, quercitrin, and rutin are a few of the most abundant and well-studied quercetin glycosides (Figure 2) [21].

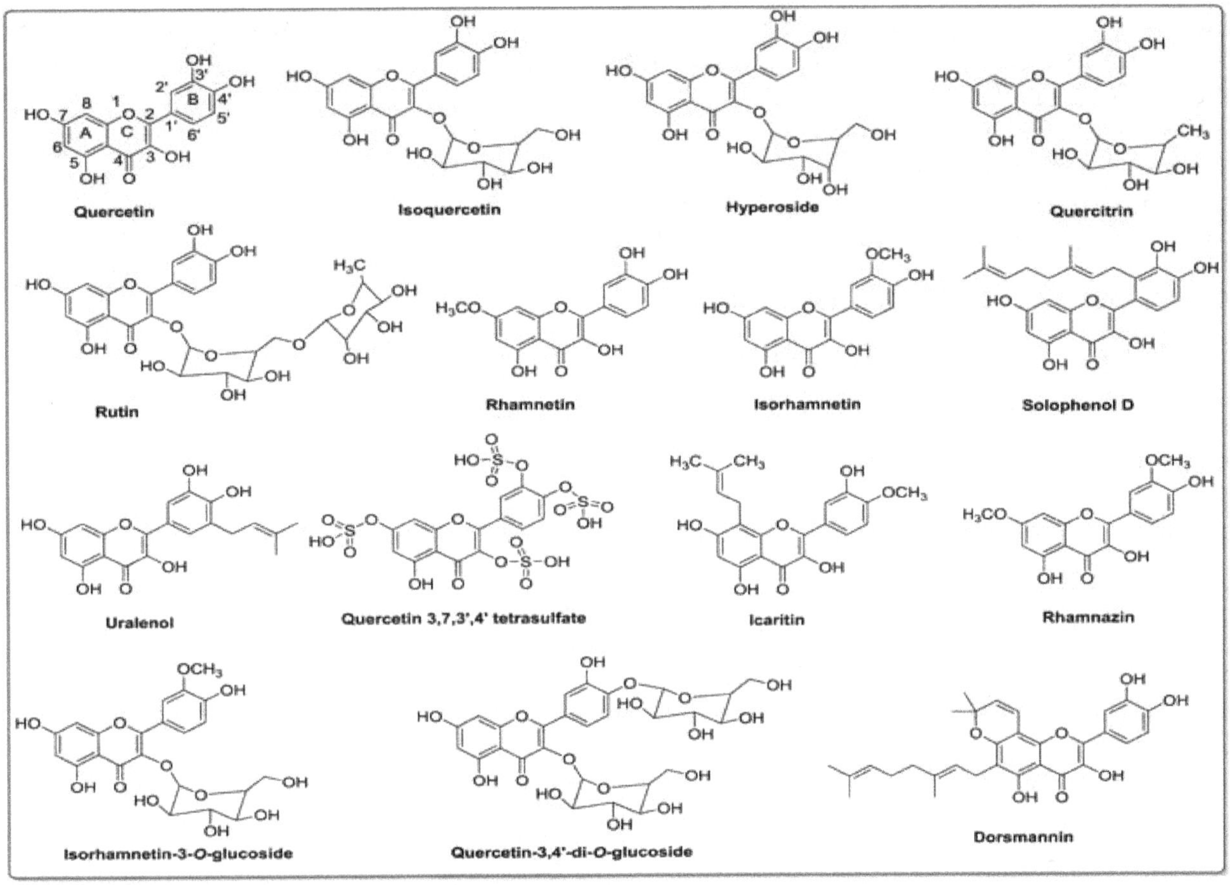

Figure 2. Structures of quercetin and its derivatives [19–24].

Quercetin methyl ethers are one of the most widely studied natural pigments, and they are formed through the conjugation of the quercetin hydroxyl group with alcohol, generally methanol. Quercetin ethers can exist in various configurations, from mono-ethers to penta-ethers, with substitution on all the hydroxyl groups of quercetin molecule. Rhamnetin, isorhamnetin, and rhamnazin are a few representatives of quercetin ether analogs [19].

Prenylflavonols are an important group of molecules belonging to the flavonol subclass. They are well-known for their wide range of biological activities, such as antioxidant, antibacterial, anti-inflammatory, and anticancer properties [22]. Structurally, in C-prenylflavonols, prenyl groups are attached to the carbon atom of the flavonol skeleton. In the past few years, prenylated quercetin analogs, such as solophenol D and uralenol, have gained a lot of attention due to their antibacterial properties. It has been reported that prenylation may enhance the biological functions of quercetin by increasing its hydrophobicity and bioavailability [23,24].

In addition to the sugar, lipid, and alcohol derivatives, quercetin also exists as sulfate conjugate in nature. Quercetin 3,7,3′,4′-tetrasulfate, isolated from the leaves *Flaveria bidentis*, has shown remarkable anticoagulant properties [25]. The multisubstituted derivatives, such as icaritin, isorhamnetin 3-*O*-glucoside, quercetin-3,4′-di-*O*-glucoside, and dorsmannin, can form from the combination of same or different functional groups. The number and nature of these functional group substitutions have profound effects on the physicochemical properties and biological effects of quercetin analogs [26].

The best described biochemical property of quercetin is its ability to act as an antioxidant. The antioxidant activity and free radical scavenging properties of quercetin are attributed to its chemical structure [27]. There are three important structural features: (1) catechol functionality (ortho-dihydroxyl) on B ring, (2) a Δ^2 double bond adjacent to a 4-oxo group in pyrone C ring, and (3) hydroxyl groups at C-3 and C-5 carbons in the benzopyrone AC ring [28]. The structural variables—such as configuration, substitution, and number of hydroxyl groups—greatly influence the mechanisms involved in antioxidant activity, like their ability to scavenge radical species and their ability to chelate metals [29].

Quercetin also inhibits the lipid peroxidation process, a common consequence of oxidative stress, and consequently protects against lipid membrane damage [30]. Due to its lower redox potential, quercetin is able to reduce highly oxidizing free radicals, such as superoxide and peroxide radicals. Because of its ability to chelate metal ions, quercetin can inhibit the generation of free radicals [28].

4. Bioavailability and Metabolism of Quercetin

In order to estimate the efficacy of quercetin in terms of its anticarcinogenic effect, it is important to understand the bioavailability of quercetin as well as its intestinal absorption and metabolism conversion rate. When quercetin was administered intravenously to rodents, it immediately disappeared from the plasma. It was evident from this experiment that quercetin was rapidly metabolized and eliminated from the body through urine and no evidence was observed regarding the storage of quercetin inside the tissues and body fluids. Previously, there was a common belief about the excretion of quercetin into feces without being absorbed by the intestine, but it is evident from recent studies that an excessive amount of quercetin found in foods is likely to be absorbed from the intestine and subsequently converted to its respective metabolites [31]. In the transportation of the metabolites of quercetin, the body's lymphatic system is also involved [32]. Repeated intake of onion resulted in accumulation of quercetin metabolites in various tissues and blood, which reached a total plasma concentration of 0.6 μM after 1 week. Hence, it is important to keep the plasma quercetin metabolite concentration at an acceptable and significant level [33].

It is evident from studies conducted recently that the metabolites of quercetin were rapidly distributed among various organs at low levels after intake of dietary quercetin for a long time [34]. It is also evident that regular consumption of dietary quercetin results in the storage of metabolites throughout the body [35]. Generally, the conversion of quercetin to its metabolic derivatives decreases its free radical scavenging activity, but there are some metabolic derivatives of quercetin, which are capable of removing the reactive species from the body. Moreover, during the process of inflammation, quercetin-3-glucuronide is metabolized, resulting in the accumulation of quercetin aglycone [36]. Recent studies showed that glucuronide, a more active form of aglycone metabolite of quercetin, was used for the incorporation into macrophages [34]. This study showed those actions of quercetin metabolites which are mostly site-specific in nature and are recommended for inflammatory conditions. The modified forms of quercetin are present in human blood and stored in inactive forms, which are further converted into active residues and ultimately converted into the active constituents to exert their actions at specific target sites.

5. Protective Effects of Quercetin

Quercetin and its metabolites are crucial due to their physiological functions as well as their role in the elimination of cancerous cells. Therefore, it is important to further investigate this specialized aspect of quercetin in terms of protection against cancer and other degenerative disorders, as these ailments are the leading causes of death throughout the world.

It was investigated recently that by influencing the pentose phosphate pathway with the production of CYP450, the preventive environment for cytochrome c-mediated apoptosis can be maintained. This cytochrome is an important part of the electron transport chain and is released from mitochondria during the apoptosis process. Therefore, the cancerous cells keep constant control over cell death through the release of cytochrome c [37]. These metabolic changes are important for the survival of cells for a longer time and also for the spreading of cancer cells [38]. Various studies have been performed to evaluate the pharmacological actions of quercetin in biological systems in order to investigate the precise mode of action of quercetin [39,40]. Therefore, it is evident from these studies that quercetin and its metabolites, which are present in various plants, play crucial roles in the protection against cancer and oxidative stress. When PC-12 cells were treated with nerve growth factor (NGF), the cells ceased to multiply and began to extend branching varicose processes similar to those produced by sympathetic neurons in primary cell culture [41]. Quercetin exhibited NGF-like action when it came in contact with PC-12 cells. Quercetin also causes cell differentiation similar to that caused by NGF [42]. Although the exact mechanism is still unclear, the well-characterized NGF-inducing capacity is more likely related to the differentiation-inducing effects of quercetin [43]. The protective effects of quercetin have also been observed in primary cultures [39]. Quercetin increased the rate of survival of cells when it was administered 24 h before the oxidative stress. In a cell culture model, it was reported that quercetin internalization into neurons happened rapidly, and a neuroprotective pathway involved Nrf2-dependent variation of the GSH redox system was observed [44].

When the aqueous quercetin was administered in experimental animals, there was a significant reduction in brain ischemic lesions [45]. Quercetin has been used in a variety of studies to evaluate its protective effects. In one study, the anticancer effects of quercetin were studied in animal models. The investigators examined the physiological changes after they administered colchicine by intracerebroventricular route [46].

In a similar study, quercetin was administered to mice for a period of seven days through intraperitoneal (i.p.) route. After administration of quercetin, memory improvement was observed in mice [47]. In this study the developmental changes were linked with the inhibition of cyclooxygenase 2 enzyme. It was observed that there was a noteworthy improvement in the learning ability of mice in comparison with the control group of mice [48]. Quercetin also increased the activity of superoxide dismutase (SOD) and lowered the level of malondialdehyde. Quercetin and other flavonoids acted as prodrugs and were metabolized into active hydroxyphenyl acetic acid metabolites by microflora in the intestine [49]. The protective effects of quercetin were observed in rats with known evidence of cerebral ischemia [50]. By administering two consecutive doses of quercetin, the memory problem in rats—which was induced by repeated cerebral ischemia—was improved and the level of cell death was reduced in the region I of hippocampus proper area (CA1). In another study, when quercetin was administered through i.p. route to rats with spinal cord injuries for a period of 10 days, half of the rats started walking [51].

In a study evaluating the penetration of quercetin across the blood–brain barrier, it was observed that quercetin induced various changes within different brain regions based on an in situ brain perfusion model in rats [52].

6. Molecular Mechanisms of Quercetin

Quercetin is used for therapeutic purposes in various disorders due to its antioxidant capability The reactive oxygen species (ROS) scavenging activity is attributed to a change in OH^- ions, which has a relation to electron exchange [53]. Catechol oxidative agents, such as semiquinones and quinones formed due to quercetin, alter redox homeostasis and inhibit primary positive effects [27]. In vitro study predicted that due to this special feature quercetin has a protective role in the nervous system. In the current scenario, the neuroprotective activity of quercetin cannot be ignored and additional in vivo studies should be investigated with different humanized animal models to translate the efficacy. Quercetin exerts its antioxidant activity by competitively inhibiting the xanthine oxidase enzyme and noncompetitively blocking the xanthine dehydrogenase enzyme. The inhibitory capabilities are due to its flavonoid structure rather than to its antioxidant potential [54].

6.1. HMGB1 Signaling Pathway

High-mobility group box protein 1 (HMGB1) is a nuclear protein which is highly preserved. It is secreted by the action of macrophages previously activated and it works as a crucial "late" facilitator of fatal endotoxemia and sepsis formation [55]. The HMGB1 protein, which is present outside the cell, can motivate the release of tumor necrosis factor-α (TNF-α), interleukin-1β (IL-1β), and other inflammatory mediators from monocytes [55,56]. Quercetin stimulates the inhibition of HMGB1-induced TNF-α and IL-1β mRNA expression, which suggests that quercetin modulates cell signaling that in turn regulates the action of proinflammatory cytokines. The activation of mitogen-activated protein kinase (MAPK) signaling pathway is a significant step in the HMGB1-induced gene expression process, which causes the release of inflammatory cytokines—such as TNF-α, and IL-1β—inside macrophages, neutrophils, and endothelial cells. HMGB1-induced cytokine release partially interferes with MAPK pathways. HMGB1 or lipopolysaccharides (LPS) time-dependently induce phosphorylation of p38, c-Jun *N*–terminal kinase, and extracellular signal-regulated kinase in macrophages. Quercetin considerably inhibits HMGB1- or LPS-induced phosphorylation of each kinase [57]. Apart from MAPK activation, the nuclear factor-κB (NF-κB) signal transduction pathway is also involved in HMGB1-induced cellular activation, and NF-κB-dependent transcriptional activity is very important for cytokine expression [58,59]. In cells, NF-κB subunits (p50 and p65) exist as inactive trimers in the cytosol through the interaction with IκBα, which is the most important member of the IκB family [60]. Quercetin significantly inhibits IκBα degradation and nuclear translocation of NF-κB p65. Therefore, after stimulation with HMGB1 or LPS, p65, the key activator of NF-κB-regulated transcription, becomes available to NF-κB-regulated genes in the nucleus and nuclear localization is most effectively inhibited by quercetin.

6.2. *Thymic Stromal Lymphopoietin (TSLP) Activation*

The level of TSLP, which is an epithelial-derived cytokine with a role in T helper (Th) cells' Type-2 immunity, is considerably increased in human skin as well as blood. The TSLP signaling process is initiated through proteins, including 1L-7 chain of receptor, which has potential to enhance the B lymphocyte activation and dendritic cells [61]. Primary skin keratinocytes are mostly responsible for expressing the TSLP in smooth muscle and lung connective tissues. TSLP contributes its main biological role by influencing various cells [62]. It is evident that TSLP has the potential to activate both $CD4^+$ T and $CD8^+$ cells along with other B lymphocytes' differentiation, which in turn promotes the release and activation of chemokines. Additionally, it can enhance the secretory mechanism of the Th2 cytokines from mast cells. During the binding of TSLP with respective receptors, various signaling pathways are activated [63]. It has been reported in a recent study that due to the activation of these receptors, there is a marked promotion in the phosphorylation process of Janus kinase-signal transducers and activators of transcription (JAK-STAT) signaling, which further causes skin inflammation [64]. Thus, targeting the above signaling pathway is a viable approach to design a treatment plan for various inflammatory diseases, including cancer.

6.3. *JAK-STAT Signaling Pathway*

JAK-STAT signaling pathway is a typical signal transduction pathway for various types of inflammatory cytokines and growth regulatory factors. The binding of ligands to their respective receptors leads to the activation of JAK, which further increases the phosphorylation process and hence leads to the activation of STAT. The STATs, which are already activated, enter the nucleus, where they start the regulation of gene expression [65]. Studies have shown that the activated mast cells stimulate the formation of the Th2 cytokines and decrease the secretory mechanism of Th1 cytokines. JAK-STAT signaling is activated by mast cells, which in turn activate the IL-13 production in the Th2 cell line [66].

Quercetin has the ability to actively inhibit the JAK-STAT signaling pathway in various inflammatory disorders. Furthermore, treatment of activated T cells with quercetin in vitro inhibited the interleukin-12 (IL-12)-induced phosphorylation of JAK2, tyrosine kinase-2 (TYK2), STAT3, and STAT4, which result in decreased levels of T cell propagation and Th1 variation [67]. Therefore, these anti-inflammatory and antiapoptotic properties of quercetin have a key role in the reduction of cancer by controlling the toll-like receptor-2 (TLR2) and JAK2/STAT3 pathway and causing the inhibition of STAT3 tyrosine phosphorylation within inflammatory cells [68]. Pretreatment of cholangiocarcinoma cells with quercetin inhibited the cytokine-mediated upregulation of inducible nitric oxide synthase (iNOS) and expression of intercellular adhesion molecule-1 (ICAM-1) in the

JAK/STAT cascade pathway. Also, quercetin blocked the activation of inflammatory cytokine interleukin-6 and interferon-γ [69]. It was reported that LPS-induced STAT1 activation was inhibited by quercetin in combination with its profound inhibitory effects on iNOS and NF-κB expression, which are persistently involved in activation of interleukin-2 (IL-2) as shown in Figure 3 [70].

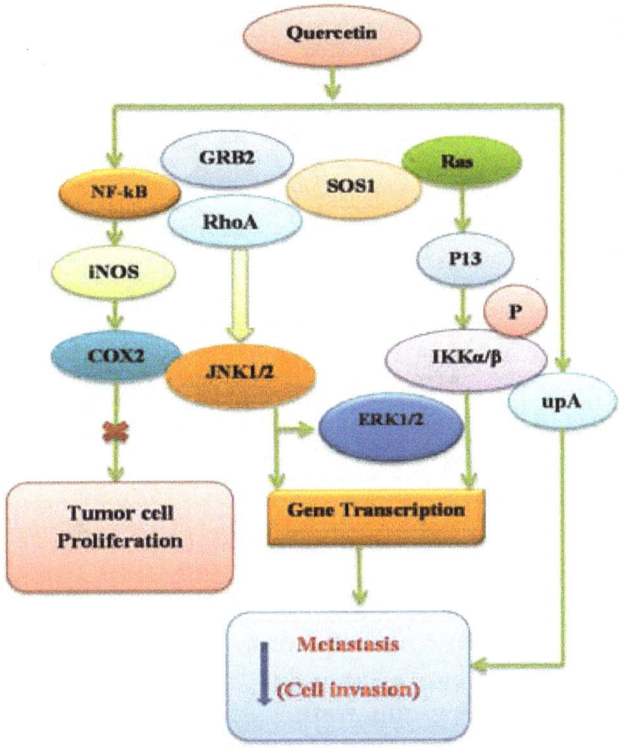

Figure 3. Anticancer pathways and mechanisms of quercetin.

7. Anticancer Effects of Quercetin

Vegetables and fruits are rich sources of phytochemicals with significant potential to prevent cancer due to the presence of abundant antioxidants. Among polyphenols, quercetin is the most important and naturally occurring cancer-preventing agent. The importance of dietary quercetin is due to its antioxidant potential and anti-inflammatory effects [47]. The cancer preventive and therapeutic effects of quercetin have been demonstrated through in vitro (Table 1) as well as in vivo (Table 2) experimental findings.

Table 1. In vitro anticancer effects of quercetin and its analogs.

Compound tested	Cell lines	Effects	Mechanisms	References
Quercetin	MCF-7, HCC1937, SK-Br3, 4T1, MDA-MB-231	Induced apoptosis	↑Bcl-2,↓Bax expression,↓Her-2, inhibition of PI3K-Akt pathway	[71]
Quercetin	MIA PaCa-2, BxPC-3	Inhibited proliferation	↓Her-2, regulation of Wnt/β-catenin	[72]
Quercetin	CX-1, SW480, HT-29, HCT116	Inhibited proliferation	↓HIF-1κ, regulation of Wnt/β-catenin	[73]
Quercetin	LNCaP, PC-3	Inhibited proliferation	↓VEGF secretion, ↓mRNA levels	[74]
Quercetin	HepG2	Inhibited proliferation	↓PI3K,↓PKC	[75]

Table 1. *Cont.*

Compound tested	Cell lines	Effects	Mechanisms	References
Rutin	ACC	Inhibited proliferation	↓PI3K,↓Akt,↓IKK-α,↓NF-κB	[76]
Rutin	SKOV3	Inhibited cell growth	↓Cyclin D1	[77]
Rutin	HeLa	Inhibited cell growth	↑p53,↓NF-κB	[78]
Quercetin	A549	Inhibited cell growth	↓cdk1,↓cyclin B	[79]
Quercetin	JB6 P+	Inhibited cell migration	Regulation of p13K/Akt	[5]
Quercetin	U373MG	Inhibited cell migration	↑caspase-7,↑JNK,↑p53	[80]

Quercetin, when used in pharmacologically safe doses, inhibits the phosphatidylinositol 3-kinase (PI3K)-Akt/PKB (protein kinase B) pathway in cancer cells [81]. Both Raf and MAPK/extracellular signal-regulated kinase (ERK) kinase (MEK) act as direct targets for quercetin, leading to the potential to decrease MEK1 activity more powerfully when compared to PD098059, which is a specific MEK inhibitor. Quercetin donates a hydrogen bond to the main amide group of Ser-212, which is known to stabilize the inactive conformation of the activated loop of MEK1 [82]. When a dose of 10 g quercetin/kg was administered to rats for 11 weeks, physiological changes were observed inside the rats' colons. This study indicated that quercetin extensively downregulated the potential oncogenic MAPK signaling in vivo [83]. Various in vitro studies have demonstrated that quercetin plays a key role in cancer prevention and tumor suppression in different cell lines [84]. The doses of quercetin that showed anticancer effects in vitro were ranging from 3 to 50 μM [85]. The cancer prevention properties of quercetin in vivo studies have been confirmed in colon cancer [11]. Furthermore, quercetin has been shown to exhibit anticancer effects in melanoma [86]. The inhibition of tumor growth by quercetin was evaluated when it was administered as a food supplement to experimental models. However, contradictory results have been reported in the literature [87].

Table 2. In vivo anticancer effects of quercetin and its analogs.

Compound tested	Animal models	Effects	Mechanisms	Dose	Duration	References
Quercetin	FemaleCF1 mice	Retarded tumor growth	↓PCNA; ↑mmu-miR-205-5P	8 g/kg/day (diet)	42 days	[88]
Quercetin	Male F344 rats	Inhibited tumor growth	↓EphA2;↓PI3K; ↓MMP-2;↓MMP-9	100 mg/kg (i.p.)	18 days	[89]
Rutin	Male F344 rats	Suppressed tumor growth	↓ACF	25 mg/kg (i.p.)	28 days	[89]
Quercetin	Female CD-1 mice	Inhibited tumor nodule formation	↓papilloma	3–6 mg/kg (p.o.)	14 days	[90]
Quercetin	Male Swiss mice	Inhibited tumor nodule formation	↓AD	6 mg/kg (i.p.)	2 times/ week 21 days	[91]
Quercetin	Female Sprague-Dawley rats	Reduced tumor volume	↓ADC	17.5 mg/kg (i.v.)	2 times/ week for 24 days	[92]

i.p., intraperitoneal; i.v., intravenous; p.o., per os.

7.1. Binding Ability of Quercetin to SEK1–JNK1/2 and MEK1–ERK1/2

Studies have shown that various pathways are the possible molecular targets of quercetin to inhibit inflammatory responses as shown in Figure 3. Quercetin chemically binds to protein kinase as evidenced by the bead-bound pull-down assay, which has been recognized as a potent screening tool. Quercetin binds with SAPK/ERK kinase 1 (SEK1), c-Jun *N*-terminal kinase 1/2 (JNK1/2), MEK1 and ERK1/2 [93].

Several studies have provided useful evidences that there are many hydrogen bonds between different hydroxyl groups of quercetin and amino acid residues of SEK1–JNK1/2 and MEK1–ERK1/2. The ERK1/2 is part of a MAPK cascade, which consists of consecutively functioning kinases, such as Raf, MEK, and ERK1/2 [94]. The active ERK1/2 induces reprogramming events related to gene expression by actively phosphorylating diverse intracellular molecular target proteins and other transcription factors, and hence potentiates cellular growth, spreading, and antiapoptotic properties.

7.2. Cellular Senescence Induction and Telomerase Inhibition

It is a process of irreversible cell aging that occurs in most of the normal cells in response to the restriction of telomerase enzymes or due to changes in the three-dimensional structure of telomerase. The cellular death activity is also associated with oncogenic activation or stress caused by oxidation [95]. The process of senescence induction by phytochemicals is a new alternative approach to chemoprevention. In a recent study, it was confirmed that both quercetin and resveratrol induced the cell death process even in very low doses in cells which showed resistance to glioma formation [96]. Despite the fact that there was no proper identification of a molecular target, there was a marked decrease in Akt phosphorylation. In the senescence induction process, quercetin also targeted the telomerase induction in eluding the replicate immortality.

Telomerases are specialized DNA polymerases having the ability to join the repeating parts of the telomerase enzymes with the ends of the DNA strands. The enzyme telomerase is significantly expressed at certain intervals in the majority of the cells, including the excessively proliferating human cells. The presence of telomerase activity is closely related to cell death resistance [95]. Quercetin and other polyphenols, including epigallocatechin-3-gallate (EGCG), inhibit the activity of telomerase in a cell-free system. The telomerase inhibitory effect was confirmed using adenocarcinoma and breast carcinoma patients [97].

7.3. Cell Death Induction Activity

Programmed cell death is an important mechanism which is activated to eliminate cancer cells in the body [95]. There are extrinsic and intrinsic pathways which control the cell death activity in the body, and these pathways are under the influence of cytokines, which act by binding with tumor necrosis factor receptors (TNF-R). The cytokines are large molecules which are mostly involved in the development of immunity [98].

Quercetin bypasses the cell damage resistance through various mechanisms. One example of quercetin action is evident in lymphocytic leukemia cell line. Quercetin is introduced to the body with minimum toxic concentrations to induce the apoptotic process. From this study, it is evident that quercetin induces the apoptotic process when combined with antibodies for the enhancement of immunity [99].

At molecular levels, quercetin acts by lowering the ROS inside the cell. This property of scavenging free radical species is a unique function of quercetin among flavonoid derivatives [100]. Apoptosis-inducing activity of quercetin has been confirmed in leukemia and also in cells which are resistant to TNF-related apoptosis-inducing ligand (TRAIL)-induced apoptosis [101].

7.4. Interactions of Quercetin with Cellular Receptors

Quercetin binds with different receptors present throughout the body and shows its anticancer properties. In a recent study, it was concluded that both Raf and MEK are molecular targets of quercetin in the prevention and treatment of cancer [102]. Whether quercetin has direct interactions with cell receptors is still unclear, but there are reports that aryl hydrocarbon receptor (AhR) is a known molecular target receptor for the majority of flavonoids, including quercetin. The AhR receptor is a ligand-gated transcription factor which is activated by the interaction with synthetic and natural chemicals [45,103]. Similarly, AhR is responsible for the regulation and expression of cytochrome P-450 (CYP) 1 family, and this family is fully capable of activating procarcinogens. In the biotransformation of polycyclic aromatic hydrocarbons (PAHs) to metabolites, which are carcinogenic in nature, the CYP1 family members are actively involved [104]. The process of biotransformation is closely associated with cancer development in the lung. Also, a high level of CYP1 is responsible for colon cancer, a major cause of cancer-related death [105].

Quercetin inhibits the transformation of AhR and protects the cells from the toxicity induced by dioxins [106]. The IC_{50} values of quercetin 3-*O*-β-D-glucuronide and quercetin 4′-*O*-β-D-glucuronide were 42.6 and 181 μM, respectively. It is indicated from this result that aglycones have stronger antagonistic activity than glucuronides and other metabolites. Quercetin also blocks the biotransformation of AhR in rat hepatocytes. It is noteworthy that the inhibitory effect of quercetin is much stronger than the effects of α-naphthoflavone, a well-known antagonist for AhR [107]. It is evident from these results that quercetin is a strong antagonist for AhR and hence exerts its pharmacological effects against carcinogenicity developed by PAHs. Quercetin also interacts with other receptors, which are involved in the prevention of cancer, but the exact mechanism is still unclear [108]. Quercetin has no role in the increase or decrease and distribution of estrogen receptors-beta isoforms in breast cancer [109]. Quercetin has been shown to possess inhibitory effects in human prostate cancer, and this effect is linked to the expression of androgen receptors [110]. It has been suggested in a recent report that a transcription factor is involved in quercetin-mediated inhibition of androgenic receptor [111].

7.5. Signal Transduction Modification

There are various reports which document modulatory effects of quercetin and other flavonoids on signal transduction pathways. The use of quercetin enhances the cell death process in HepG2 human hepatoma cells. There are two mechanisms involved in this process; one is the activation of caspase-3 and caspase-9, but not caspase-8. The other mechanism involves an increase in the translocation of proapoptotic Bax to the membrane of mitochondria [112]. In a similar study, it has been shown that quercetin causes the cleavage of polymerase and also potentiates the upregulation of Bax (Figure 4). Quercetin decreases the levels of key oncogenic protein Ras in cancer cells and blocks the cell proliferation and survival [113].

Quercetin has been shown to cause changes in apoptosis in mesangial cells by inhibiting the activation of JNK and other ERKs pathways. It is also clear that there is no significant effect on the level of p38 MAPK [114]. In a similar study, it is reported that quercetin caused the inhibition of phosphorylation of p38 and Bcl2. This property of quercetin is useful as it may stop the apoptotic process [115]. The action of quercetin may be considered as short-term or long-term. The short-term effect causes scavenging of free radicals and it is mostly antioxidative and antiapoptotic in nature, while the long term effect is pro-oxidative [116]. The proapoptotic action of quercetin is linked mostly to a decreased level of glutamate-stimulating hormones (GSH). It is evident that GSH plays an important role in determining the antioxidant nature of flavonoids. The action of quercetin may depend upon the concentrations of quercetin in cell culture medium [117].

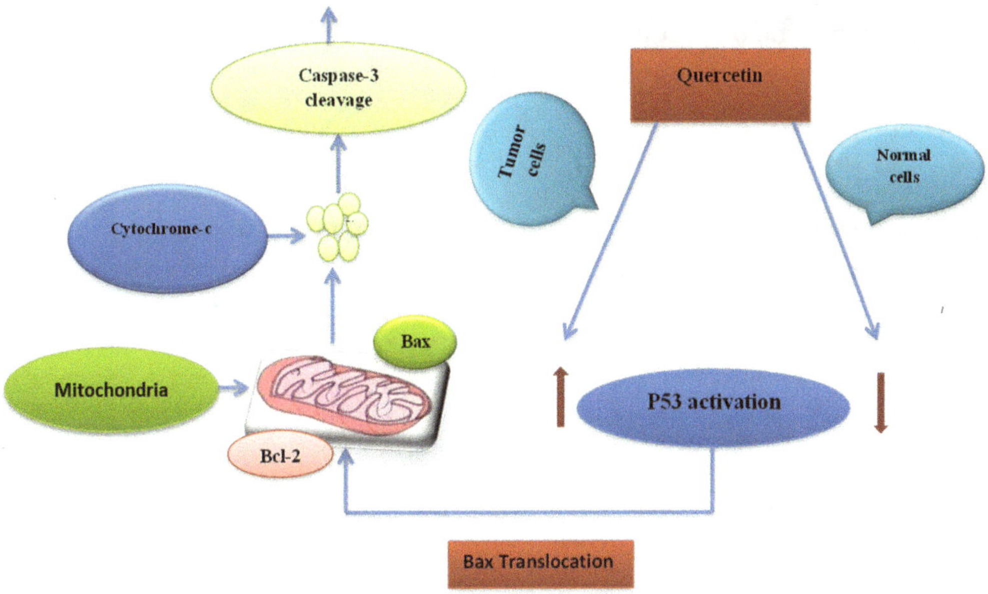

Figure 4. Modulation of mitochondrial apoptotic signaling pathways by quercetin. Quercetin induces p53 activation resulting in upregulation of Bax and downregulation of Bcl-2 in tumor cells. This leads to caspase activation and ultimately apoptotic cell death.

How to determine the accurate mechanism through which quercetin exerts its effect in controlling the signal transduction pathway is still unclear. There are few studies on the mechanisms of action of quercetin, and the specific targets of quercetin are not well known [118]. Apart from the findings mentioned above, it has been reported that the MEK/ERK pathway is activated by quercetin during the process of programmed cell death in human lung cancer. This contradiction may be because of the basic difference in investigational conditions, including the use of various cell lines [119]. Quercetin is important in the regulation of signal transduction pathways, and such pathways are crucial in the production of inflammatory mediators. Quercetin also decreases the LPS formation of cytokinase, and this enzyme causes the inhibition of iNOS by further suppressing ERK and p38 MAPK [120]. Moreover, quercetin significantly reduces the half-life of Ras protein, which is oncogenic in nature, but no significant action was reported when the cells were treated with proteasome inhibitor [113].

8. Epidemiological Studies about Quercetin

Emerging studies suggest that intake of fruits and vegetables decrease the risk of human carcinomas, including colon, breast, bladder, stomach, and lung cancer [121]. A plethora of phytochemicals present in plant-based food products are consumed by humans on a daily basis. However, it is still unknown which one among these phytoconstituents is responsible for protective action against cancer. The most studied phytochemicals for anticancer potential are flavonoids [122]. A few studies indicate an opposite relation among the dietary consumption of polyphenols and cancer risk [123]. However, Hertog and his coworkers [124] assert that there is no association between the intake of flavonol or flavone derivatives and cancer-related mortality rates.

Regarding quercetin, an opposite co-relation exists between the consumption of quercetin found in foods and the development of lung cancer caused by smoking [125]. A recent multiethnic clinical study has provided evidence about the cancer preventive effects of quercetin in the progression of pancreatic cancer in individuals who were chain smokers and nonsmokers. However, the effect was more pronounced in smokers compared to nonsmokers, as quercetin imparted its antioxidant activity in smokers who had increased oxidative stress relative to nonsmokers [126]. It is evident from many studies that quercetin has beneficial effects against cancer risks. In a study, Gates and coworkers [127] evaluated the relationship between the intake of quercetin and the incidence rate of the ovarian cancer among the nursing staff. The data collected from these results revealed that quercetin intake had a nonsignificant 29% decrease in ovarian cancer risk compared to women with the lowest intake of quercetin.

9. Conclusion and Future Perspectives

The studies presented here suggest the potential effects of quercetin in cancer therapy. Numerous in vitro and in vivo experiments have shown various mechanisms of action that could suppress multiple oncogenic signaling pathways. Quercetin is safe with no reported toxicity when applied for the treatment of human cancer. Since quercetin and its derivatives have great benefits, it is the need of the hour to investigate further the effects of these molecules in the prevention and intervention of cancer. However, there is still no conclusive evidence regarding its exact mode of action in order to enhance its clinical application in the treatment of human cancer. Therefore, the future perspective of research should concentrate on the evaluation of quercetin's precise mechanisms of action. Similarly, it is necessary to perform more clinical studies on the efficacy and bioavailability of quercetin in biological systems for the future use in human population, especially in the treatment of cancer. Moreover, the conversions of quercetin to its metabolites must be considered while assessing the efficacy and bioavailability of quercetin for further pharmacological use. The conjugation of xenobiotics with quercetin alters the reactivity of quercetin, but there are some metabolites of quercetin in conjugated form which showed beneficial biological activities. It is important to investigate further mechanisms of action of quercetin, especially in terms of suppressing carcinogenicity in rodents. The results obtained from the current epidemiological studies shows that there is shortage of evidence of quercetin intake for the prevention of human cancer. There is a need to conduct further epidemiological studies to evaluate the role of quercetin in human cancer prevention. Updating the database related to dietary flavonoids will deliver significant information for future epidemiological studies. The use of quercetin in the field of pharmaceuticals is limited because of its poor water solubility and oral bioavailability. In order to enhance the solubility and bioavailability of quercetin inside human body, various scientific approaches have been taken into consideration, including the application of novel drug delivery systems such as nanoparticles and liposomes. These and additional approaches may help us to understand the full potential of quercetin in cancer prevention and therapy.

Acknowledgments: This article is the outcome of an in-house financially non-supported study.

Author Contributions: All authors have directly participated in the planning or drafting of the manuscript and read and approved the final version.

References

1. Surh, Y.J. Cancer chemoprevention with dietary phytochemicals. *Nat. Rev. Cancer* **2003**, *3*, 768–780. [CrossRef] [PubMed]
2. Russo, G.L. Ins and outs of dietary phytochemicals in cancer chemoprevention. *Biochem. Pharmacol.* **2007**, *74*, 533–544. [CrossRef] [PubMed]
3. Kris-Etherton, P.; Lefevre, M.; Beecher, G.; Gross, M.; Keen, C.; Etherton, T. Bioactive compounds in nutrition and health-research methodologies for establishing biological function: The antioxidant and anti-inflammatory effects of flavonoids on atherosclerosis. *Annu. Rev. Nutr.* **2004**, *24*, 511–538. [CrossRef] [PubMed]
4. Kim, J.; Lee, H.J.; Lee, K.W. Naturally occurring phytochemicals for the prevention of Alzheimer's disease. *J. Neurochem.* **2010**, *112*, 1415–1430. [CrossRef] [PubMed]
5. Lee, K.W.; Bode, A.M.; Dong, Z. Molecular targets of phytochemicals for cancer prevention. *Nat. Rev. Cancer* **2011**, *11*, 211–218. [CrossRef] [PubMed]
6. Crowe, F.L.; Roddam, A.W.; Key, T.J.; Appleby, P.N.; Overvad, K.; Jakobsen, M.U.; Tjønneland, A.; Hansen, L.; Boeing, H.; Weikert, C. Fruit and vegetable intake and mortality from ischaemic heart disease: Results from

the European Prospective Investigation into Cancer and Nutrition (EPIC)-Heart study. *Eur. Heart J.* **2011**, *32*, 1235–1243. [CrossRef] [PubMed]

7. Benavente-Garcia, O.; Castillo, J. Update on uses and properties of citrus flavonoids: New findings in anticancer, cardiovascular, and anti-inflammatory activity. *J. Agric. Food. Chem.* **2008**, *56*, 6185–6205. [CrossRef] [PubMed]
8. Kanadaswami, C.; Lee, L.T.; Lee, P.P.; Hwang, J.J.; Ke, F.C.; Huang, Y.T.; Lee, M.T. The antitumor activities of flavonoids. *In Vivo* **2005**, *19*, 895–909.
9. Canivenc-Lavier, M.C.; Vernevaut, M.F.; Totis, M.; Siess, M.H.; Magdalou, J.; Suschetet, M. Comparative effects of flavonoids and model inducers on drug-metabolizing enzymes in rat liver. *Toxicology* **1996**, *114*, 19–27. [CrossRef]
10. Shih, H.; Pickwell, G.V.; Quattrochi, L.C. Differential effects of flavonoid compounds on tumor promoter-induced activation of the human CYP1A2 enhancer. *Arch. Biochem.* **2000**, *373*, 287–294. [CrossRef] [PubMed]
11. Murakami, A.; Ashida, H.; Terao, J. Multitargeted cancer prevention by quercetin. *Cancer Lett.* **2008**, *269*, 315–325. [CrossRef] [PubMed]
12. Mendoza-Wilson, A.M.; Glossman-Mitnik, D. CHIH-DFT determination of the molecular structure, infrared and ultraviolet spectra of the flavonoid quercetin. *J. Mol. Struc. Theochem.* **2004**, *681*, 71–76. [CrossRef]
13. Mendoza, E.; Burd, R. Quercetin as a systemic chemopreventative agent: Structural and functional mechanisms. *Mini. Rev. Med. Chem.* **2011**, *11*, 1216–1221. [CrossRef] [PubMed]
14. Russo, G.L.; Russo, M.; Spagnuolo, C.; Tedesco, I.; Bilotto, S.; Iannitti, R.; Palumbo, R. Quercetin: A pleiotropic kinase inhibitor against cancer. In *Advances in Nutrition and Cancer*; Springer: Berlin/Heidelberg, Geramny, 2014; pp. 185–205.
15. Sak, K. Site-specific anticancer effects of dietary flavonoid quercetin. *Nutr. Cancer* **2014**, *66*, 177–193. [CrossRef] [PubMed]
16. Brito, A.F.; Ribeiro, M.; Abrantes, A.M.; Pires, A.S.; Teixo, R.J.; Tralhao, G.J.; Botelho, M.F. Quercetin in Cancer Treatment, Alone or in Combination with Conventional Therapeutics? *Curr. Med. Chem.* **2015**, *22*, 3025–3039. [CrossRef] [PubMed]
17. Cook, N.; Samman, S. Flavonoids, chemistry, metabolism, cardioprotective effects, and dietary sources. *J. Nutr. Biochem.* **1996**, *7*, 66–76. [CrossRef]
18. Materska, M. Quercetin and its derivatives: Chemical structure and bioactivity—A review. *Pol. J. Food Nutr. Sci.* **2008**, *58*, 407–413.
19. Williams, C.A.; Grayer, R.J. Anthocyanins and other flavonoids. *Nat. Prod. Rep.* **2004**, *21*, 539–573. [CrossRef] [PubMed]
20. Biesaga, M.; Pyrzynska, K. Analytical procedures for determination of quercetin and its glycosides in plant material. *Crit. Rev. Chem.* **2009**, *39*, 95–107. [CrossRef]
21. Hollman, P.C.; Bijsman, M.N.; van Gameren, Y.; Cnossen, E.P.; de Vries, J.H.; Katan, M.B. The sugar moiety is a major determinant of the absorption of dietary flavonoid glycosides in man. *Free Radic. Res.* **1999**, *31*, 569–573. [CrossRef] [PubMed]
22. Chen, X.; Mukwaya, E.; Wong, M.; Zhang, Y. A systematic review on biological activities of prenylated flavonoids. *Pharm. Biol.* **2014**, *52*, 655–660. [CrossRef] [PubMed]
23. Inui, S.; Hosoya, T.; Shimamura, Y.; Masuda, S.; Ogawa, T.; Kobayashi, H.; Shirafuji, K.; Moli, R.T.; Kozone, I.; Shin-ya, K.; et al. Solophenols B–D and Solomonin: New Prenylated Polyphenols Isolated from Propolis Collected from The Solomon Islands and Their Antibacterial Activity. *J. Agric. Food Chem.* **2012**, *60*, 11765–11770. [CrossRef] [PubMed]
24. Jia, S.; Ma, C.; Wang, J. Studies on flavonoid constituents isolated from the leaves of *Glycyrrhiza uralensis* Fisch. *Acta Pharm. Sin.* **1989**, *25*, 758–762.
25. De Santiago, O.P.; Juliani, H. Isolation of quercetin 3,7,3′,4′-tetrasulphate from *Flaveria bidentis* L. Otto Kuntze. *Experientia* **1972**, *28*, 380–381. [CrossRef]
26. Dastagir, G.; Hussain, F.; Khan, A.A. Antibacterial activity of some selected plants of family Zygophyllaceae and Euphorbiaceae. *J. Med. Plants Res.* **2012**, *6*, 5360–5368.
27. Boots, A.W.; Haenen, G.R.; Bast, A. Health effects of quercetin: From antioxidant to nutraceutical. *Eur. J. Pharmacol.* **2008**, *585*, 325–337. [CrossRef] [PubMed]

28. Heim, K.E.; Tagliaferro, A.R.; Bobilya, D.J. Flavonoid antioxidants: Chemistry, metabolism and structure-activity relationships. *J. Nutr. Biochem.* **2002**, *13*, 572–584. [CrossRef]
29. Dangles, O.; Dufoura, C.; Fargeixa, G. Inhibition of lipid peroxidation by quercetin and quercetin derivatives: Antioxidant and prooxidant effects. *J. Chem. Soc. Perkin Trans.* **2000**, *2*, 1215–1222. [CrossRef]
30. Heijnen, C.G.; Haenen, G.R.; Minou Oostveen, R.; Stalpers, E.M.; Bast, A. Protection of flavonoids against lipid peroxidation: The structure activity relationship revisited. *Free Radic. Res.* **2002**, *36*, 575–581. [CrossRef] [PubMed]
31. Murota, K.; Shimizu, S.; Miyamoto, S.; Izumi, T.; Obata, A.; Kikuchi, M.; Terao, J. Unique uptake and transport of isoflavone aglycones by human intestinal Caco-2 cells: Comparison of isoflavonoids and flavonoids. *J. Nutr.* **2002**, *132*, 1956–1961. [PubMed]
32. Terao, J.; Kawai, Y.; Murota, K. Vegetable flavonoids and cardiovascular disease. *Asia Pac. J. Clin. Nutr.* **2008**, *17*, 291–293. [PubMed]
33. Moon, J.-H.; Nakata, R.; Oshima, S.; Inakuma, T.; Terao, J. Accumulation of quercetin conjugates in blood plasma after the short-term ingestion of onion by women. *Am. J. Physiol. Regul. Integr. Comp. Physiol.* **2000**, *279*, 461–467.
34. Shimoi, K.; Saka, N.; Nozawa, R.; Sato, M.; Amano, I.; Nakayama, T.; Kinae, N. Deglucuronidation of a flavonoid, luteolin monoglucuronide, during inflammation. *Drug Metab. Dispos.* **2001**, *29*, 1521–1524. [PubMed]
35. De Boer, V.C.; Dihal, A.A.; van der Woude, H.; Arts, I.C.; Wolffram, S.; Alink, G.M.; Rietjens, I.M.C.M.; Keijer, J.; Hollman, P.C.H. Tissue distribution of quercetin in rats and pigs. *J. Nutr.* **2005**, *135*, 1718–1725. [PubMed]
36. Kawai, Y.; Nishikawa, T.; Shiba, Y.; Saito, S.; Murota, K.; Shibata, N.; Kobayashi, M.; Kanayama, M.; Uchida, K.; Terao, J. Macrophage as a target of quercetin glucuronides in human atherosclerotic arteries implication in the anti-atherosclerotic mechanism of dietary flavonoids. *J. Biol. Chem.* **2008**, *283*, 9424–9434. [CrossRef] [PubMed]
37. Ahangarpour, A.; Eskandari, M.; Vaezlari, A. Effect of aqueous and hydroalcoholic extract of Beberis vulgaris on insulin secretion from islets of langerhans isolated from male mice. *Armaghane Danesh* **2012**, *17*, 289–298.
38. Ruckenstuhl, C.; Büttner, S.; Carmona-Gutierrez, D.; Eisenberg, T.; Kroemer, G.; Sigrist, S.J.; Fröhlich, K.U.; Madeo, F. The Warburg effect suppresses oxidative stress induced apoptosis in a yeast model for cancer. *PLoS ONE* **2009**, *4*, 4592. [CrossRef]
39. Dajas, F.; Arredondo, F.; Echeverry, C.; Ferreira, M.; Morquio, A.; Rivera, F. Flavonoids and the brain: Evidences and putative mechanisms for a protective capacity. *Curr. Neuropharmacol.* **2005**, *3*, 193–205. [CrossRef]
40. Ossola, B.; Kääriäinen, T.M.; Männistö, P.T. The multiple faces of quercetin in neuroprotection. *Expert Opin. Drug Saf.* **2009**, *8*, 397–409. [CrossRef] [PubMed]
41. Greene, L.A.; Tischler, A.S. Establishment of a noradrenergic clonal line of rat adrenal pheochromocytoma cells which respond to nerve growth factor. *Proc. Natl. Acad. Sci. USA* **1976**, *73*, 2424–2428. [CrossRef] [PubMed]
42. Blasina, M.; Vaamonde, L.; Morquio, A.; Echeverry, C.; Arredondo, F.; Dajas, F. Differentiation induced by *Achyrocline satureioides* (Lam) infusion in PC12 cells. *Phytother. Res.* **2009**, *23*, 1263–1269. [CrossRef] [PubMed]
43. Rydén, M.; Hempstead, B.; Ibáñez, C.F. Differential modulation of neuron survival during development by nerve growth factor binding to the p75 neurotrophin receptor. *J. Biol. Chem.* **1997**, *272*, 16322–16328. [CrossRef] [PubMed]
44. Arredondo, F.; Echeverry, C.; Abin-Carriquiry, J.A.; Blasina, F.; Antúnez, K.; Jones, D.P.; Go, Y.M.; Liang, Y.L.; Dajas, F. After cellular internalization, quercetin causes Nrf2 nuclear translocation, increases glutathione levels, and prevents neuronal death against an oxidative insult. *Free Radic. Biol. Med.* **2010**, *49*, 738–747. [CrossRef] [PubMed]
45. Dajas, F.; Rivera, F.; Blasina, F.; Arredondo, F.; Echeverry, C.; Lafon, L.; Morquio, A.; Heizen, H. Cell culture protection and in vivo neuroprotective capacity of flavonoids. *Neurotox. Res.* **2003**, *5*, 425–432. [CrossRef] [PubMed]
46. Kumar, A.; Sehgal, N.; Kumar, P.; Padi, S.; Naidu, P. Protective effect of quercetin against ICV colchicine-induced cognitive dysfunctions and oxidative damage in rats. *Phytother. Res.* **2008**, *22*, 1563–1569. [CrossRef] [PubMed]

47. Patil, C.S.; Singh, V.P.; Satyanarayan, P.; Jain, N.K.; Singh, A.; Kulkarni, S.K. Protective effect of flavonoids against aging-and lipopolysaccharide-induced cognitive impairment in mice. *Pharmacology* **2003**, *69*, 59–67. [CrossRef] [PubMed]
48. Lu, J.; Zheng, Y.L.; Luo, L.; Wu, D.M.; Sun, D.X.; Feng, Y.J. Quercetin reverses D-galactose induced neurotoxicity in mouse brain. *Behav. Brain Res.* **2006**, *171*, 251–260. [CrossRef] [PubMed]
49. Vissiennon, C.; Nieber, K.; Kelber, O.; Butterweck, V. Route of administration determines the anxiolytic activity of the flavonols kaempferol, quercetin and myricetin—Are they prodrugs? *J. Nutr. Biochem.* **2012**, *23*, 733–740. [CrossRef] [PubMed]
50. Pu, F.; Mishima, K.; Irie, K.; Motohashi, K.; Tanaka, Y.; Orito, K.; Egawa, T.; Kitamura, Y.; Egashira, N.; Iwasaki, K. Neuroprotective effects of quercetin and rutin on spatial memory impairment in an 8-arm radial maze task and neuronal death induced by repeated cerebral ischemia in rats. *J. Pharmacol. Sci.* **2007**, *104*, 329–334. [CrossRef] [PubMed]
51. Schültke, E.; Kamencic, H.; Skihar, V.; Griebel, R.; Juurlink, B. Quercetin in an animal model of spinal cord compression injury: Correlation of treatment duration with recovery of motor function. *Spinal Cord* **2010**, *48*, 112–117. [CrossRef] [PubMed]
52. Youdim, K.A.; Shukitt-Hale, B.; Joseph, J.A. Flavonoids and the brain: Interactions at the blood-brain barrier and their physiological effects on the central nervous system. *Free Radic. Biol. Med.* **2004**, *37*, 1683–1693. [CrossRef] [PubMed]
53. Boots, A.W.; Haenen, G.R.; den Hartog, G.J.; Bast, A. Oxidative damage shifts from lipid peroxidation to thiol arylation by catechol-containing antioxidants. *Biochim. Biophys. Acta* **2002**, *1583*, 279–284. [CrossRef]
54. Bindoli, A.; Valente, M.; Cavallini, L. Inhibitory action of quercetin on xanthine oxidase and xanthine dehydrogenase activity. *Pharmacol. Res. Commun.* **1985**, *17*, 831–839. [CrossRef]
55. Rendon-Mitchell, B.; Ochani, M.; Li, J.; Han, J.; Wang, H.; Yang, H.; Susarla, S.; Czura, C.; Mitchell, R.A.; Chen, G. IFN-γ induces high mobility group box 1 protein release partly through a TNF-dependent mechanism. *J. Immunol.* **2003**, *170*, 3890–3897. [CrossRef] [PubMed]
56. Andersson, U.; Wang, H.; Palmblad, K.; Aveberger, A.C.; Bloom, O.; Erlandsson-Harris, H.; Janson, A.; Kokkola, R.; Zhang, M.; Yang, H.; et al. High mobility group 1 protein (HMG-1) stimulates proinflammatory cytokine synthesis in human monocytes. *J. Exp. Med.* **2000**, *192*, 565–570. [CrossRef] [PubMed]
57. Degryse, B.; Bonaldi, T.; Scaffidi, P.; Müller, S.; Resnati, M.; Sanvito, F.; Arrigoni, G.; Bianchi, M.E. The high mobility group (HMG) boxes of the nuclear protein HMG1 induce chemotaxis and cytoskeleton reorganization in rat smooth muscle cells. *J. Cell Biol.* **2001**, *152*, 1197–1206. [CrossRef] [PubMed]
58. Park, J.S.; Svetkauskaite, D.; He, Q.; Kim, J.Y.; Strassheim, D.; Ishizaka, A.; Abraham, E. Involvement of toll-like receptors 2 and 4 in cellular activation by high mobility group box 1 protein. *J. Biol. Chem.* **2004**, *279*, 7370–7377. [CrossRef] [PubMed]
59. Kokkola, R.; Andersson, A.; Mullins, G.; Östberg, T.; Treutiger, C.J.; Arnold, B.; Nawroth, P.; Andersson, U.; Harris, R.A.; Harris, H.E. RAGE is the major receptor for the proinflammatory activity of HMGB1 in rodent macrophages. *Scand. J. Immunol.* **2005**, *61*, 1–9. [CrossRef] [PubMed]
60. Luo, J.L.; Kamata, H.; Karin, M. IKK/NF-κB signaling: Balancing life and death—A new approach to cancer therapy. *J. Clin. Investig.* **2005**, *115*, 2625–2632. [CrossRef] [PubMed]
61. Briot, A.; Deraison, C.; Lacroix, M.; Bonnart, C.; Robin, A.; Besson, C.; Dubus, P.; Hovnanian, A. Kallikrein 5 induces atopic dermatitis-like lesions through PAR2-mediated thymic stromal lymphopoietin expression in Netherton syndrome. *J. Exp. Med.* **2009**, *206*, 1135–1147. [CrossRef] [PubMed]
62. Wilson, S.R.; Thé, L.; Batia, L.M.; Beattie, K.; Katibah, G.E.; McClain, S.P.; Pellegrino, M.; Estandian, D.; Bautista, D. The epithelial cell-derived atopic dermatitis cytokine TSLP activates neurons to induce itch. *Cell* **2013**, *155*, 285–295. [CrossRef] [PubMed]
63. Zhong, J.; Sharma, J.; Raju, R.; Palapetta, S.M.; Prasad, T.K.; Huang, T.C.; Yoda, A.; Tyner, J.W.; Bodegom, D.V.; Weinstock, D.M. TSLP signaling pathway map: A platform for analysis of TSLP-mediated signaling. *Database* **2014**, *2014*. [CrossRef] [PubMed]
64. Arima, K.; Watanabe, N.; Hanabuchi, S.; Chang, M.; Sun, S.C.; Liu, Y.J. Distinct signal codes generate dendritic cell functional plasticity. *Sci. Signal.* **2010**, *3*, 165. [CrossRef] [PubMed]
65. Bao, L.; Zhang, H.; Chan, L.S. The involvement of the JAK-STAT signaling pathway in chronic inflammatory skin disease atopic dermatitis. *JAK-STAT* **2013**, *2*, 24137. [CrossRef] [PubMed]

66. Horr, B.; Borck, H.; Thurmond, R.; Grösch, S.; Diel, F. STAT1 phosphorylation and cleavage is regulated by the histamine (H4) receptor in human atopic and non-atopic lymphocytes. *Int. Immunopharmacol.* **2006**, *6*, 1577–1585. [CrossRef] [PubMed]
67. Muthian, G.; Bright, J.J. Quercetin, a flavonoid phytoestrogen, ameliorates experimental allergic encephalomyelitis by blocking IL-12 signaling through JAK-STAT pathway in T lymphocyte. *J. Clin. Immunol.* **2004**, *24*, 542–552. [CrossRef] [PubMed]
68. Liao, Y.R.; Lin, J.Y. Quercetin, but not its metabolite quercetin-3-glucuronide, exerts prophylactic immunostimulatory activity and therapeutic antiinflammatory effects on lipopolysaccharide-treated mouse peritoneal macrophages ex vivo. *J. Agric. Food Chem.* **2014**, *62*, 2872–2880. [CrossRef] [PubMed]
69. Senggunprai, L.; Kukongviriyapan, V.; Prawan, A.; Kukongviriyapan, U. Quercetin and EGCG exhibit chemopreventive effects in cholangiocarcinoma cells via suppression of JAK/STAT signaling pathway. *Phytother. Res.* **2014**, *28*, 841–848. [CrossRef] [PubMed]
70. Hämäläinen, M.; Nieminen, R.; Vuorela, P.; Heinonen, M.; Moilanen, E. Anti-inflammatory effects of flavonoids: Genistein, kaempferol, quercetin, and daidzein inhibit STAT-1 and NF-κB activations, whereas flavone, isorhamnetin, naringenin, and pelargonidin inhibit only NF-κB activation along with their inhibitory effect on iNOS expression and NO production in activated macrophages. *Mediators Inflamm.* **2007**, *2007*, 45673. [PubMed]
71. Duo, J.; Ying, G.; Wang, G.W.; Zhang, L. Quercetin inhibits human breast cancer cell proliferation and induces apoptosis via Bcl-2 and Bax regulation. *Mol. Med. Rep.* **2012**, *5*, 1453–1456. [PubMed]
72. Kim, H.; Seo, E.M.; Sharma, A.R.; Ganbold, B.; Park, J.; Sharma, G.; Kang, Y.H.; Song, D.K.; Lee, S.S.; Nam, J.S. Regulation of Wnt signaling activity for growth suppression induced by quercetin in 4T1 murine mammary cancer cells. *Int. J. Oncol.* **2013**, *43*, 1319–1325. [PubMed]
73. Shan, B.E.; Wang, M.X.; Li, R.Q. Quercetin inhibit human SW480 colon cancer growth in association with inhibition of cyclin D1 and survivin expression through Wnt/β-catenin signaling pathway. *Cancer Investig.* **2009**, *27*, 604–612. [CrossRef] [PubMed]
74. Bhat, F.A.; Sharmila, G.; Balakrishnan, S.; Arunkumar, R.; Elumalai, P.; Suganya, S.; Raja, S.P.; Srinivasan, N.; Arunakaran, J. Quercetin reverses EGF-induced epithelial to mesenchymal transition and invasiveness in prostate cancer (PC-3) cell line via EGFR/PI3K/Akt pathway. *J. Nutr. Biochem.* **2014**, *25*, 1132–1139. [CrossRef] [PubMed]
75. Maurya, A.K.; Vinayak, M. Anticarcinogenic action of quercetin by downregulation of phosphatidylinositol 3-kinase (PI3K) and protein kinase C (PKC) via induction of p53 in hepatocellular carcinoma (HepG2) cell line. *Mol. Biol. Rep.* **2015**, *42*, 1419–1429. [CrossRef] [PubMed]
76. Sun, Z.J.; Chen, G.; Hu, X.; Zhang, W.; Liu, Y.; Zhu, L.X.; Zhou, Q.; Zhao, Y.F. Activation of PI3K/Akt/IKK-α/NF-κB signaling pathway is required for the apoptosis-evasion in human salivary adenoid cystic carcinoma: Its inhibition by quercetin. *Apoptosis* **2010**, *15*, 850–863. [CrossRef] [PubMed]
77. Catanzaro, D.; Ragazzi, E.; Vianello, C.; Caparrotta, L.; Montopoli, M. Effect of Quercetin on Cell Cycle and Cyclin Expression in Ovarian Carcinoma and Osteosarcoma Cell Lines. *Nat. Prod. Commun.* **2015**, *10*, 1365–1368. [PubMed]
78. Priyadarsini, R.V.; Murugan, R.S.; Maitreyi, S.; Ramalingam, K.; Karunagaran, D.; Nagini, S. The flavonoid quercetin induces cell cycle arrest and mitochondria-mediated apoptosis in human cervical cancer (HeLa) cells through p53 induction and NF-κB inhibition. *Eur. J. Pharmacol.* **2010**, *649*, 84–91. [CrossRef] [PubMed]
79. Yeh, S.L.; Yeh, C.L.; Chan, S.T.; Chuang, C.H. Plasma rich in quercetin metabolites induces G2/M arrest by upregulating PPAR-γ expression in human A549 lung cancer cells. *Planta Med.* **2011**, *77*, 992–998. [CrossRef] [PubMed]
80. Kim, H.; Moon, J.Y.; Ahn, K.S.; Cho, S.K. Quercetin induces mitochondrial mediated apoptosis and protective autophagy in human glioblastoma U373MG cells. *Oxid. Med. Cell Longev.* **2013**, *2013*, 596496. [CrossRef] [PubMed]
81. Gulati, N.; Laudet, B.; Zohrabian, V.M.; Murali, R.; Jhanwar, M.U. The antiproliferative effect of Quercetin in cancer cells is mediated via inhibition of the PI3K-Akt/PKB pathway. *Anticancer Res.* **2006**, *26*, 1177–1181. [PubMed]
82. Lee, D.H.; Lee, Y.J. Quercetin suppresses hypoxia-induced accumulation of hypoxia-inducible factor-1α (HIF-1α) through inhibiting protein synthesis. *J. Cell. Biochem.* **2008**, *105*, 546–553. [CrossRef] [PubMed]

83. Dihal, A.A.; van der Woude, H.; Hendriksen, P.J.; Charif, H.; Dekker, L.J.; IJsselstijn, L.; De Boer, V.C.J.; Alink, G.M.; Burgers, P.C.; Rietjens, I.M.C.M. Transcriptome and proteome profiling of colon mucosa from quercetin fed F344 rats point to tumor preventive mechanisms, increased mitochondrial fatty acid degradation and decreased glycolysis. *Proteomics* **2008**, *8*, 45–61. [CrossRef] [PubMed]
84. Braganhol, E.; Zamin, L.L.; Canedo, A.D.; Horn, F.; Tamajusuku, A.S.; Wink, M.R.; Salbego, C.; Battastini, A.M. Antiproliferative effect of quercetin in the human U138MG glioma cell line. *Anticancer Drugs* **2006**, *17*, 663–671. [CrossRef] [PubMed]
85. Lamson, D.W.; Brignall, M.S. Antioxidants and cancer, part 3: Quercetin. *Altern. Med. Rev. J. Clin. Ther.* **2000**, *5*, 196–208.
86. Caltagirone, S.; Rossi, C.; Poggi, A.; Ranelletti, F.O.; Natali, P.G.; Brunetti, M.; Aiello, F.B.; Piantelli, M. Flavonoids apigenin and quercetin inhibit melanoma growth and metastatic potential. *Int. J. Cancer* **2000**, *87*, 595–600. [CrossRef]
87. Yang, C.S.; Landau, J.M.; Huang, M.T.; Newmark, H.L. Inhibition of carcinogenesis by dietary polyphenolic compounds. *Annu. Rev. Nutr.* **2001**, *21*, 381–406. [CrossRef] [PubMed]
88. Deschner, E.E.; Ruperto, J.; Wong, G.; Newmark, H.L. Quercetin and rutin as inhibitors of azoxymethanol-induced colonic neoplasia. *Carcinogenesis* **1991**, *12*, 1193–1196. [CrossRef] [PubMed]
89. Dihal, A.A.; de Boer, V.C.; van der Woude, H.; Tilburgs, C.; Bruijntjes, J.P.; Alink, G.M.; Rietjens, I.M.; Woutersen, R.A.; Stierum, R.H. Quercetin, but not its glycosidated conjugate rutin, inhibits azoxymethane-induced colorectal carcinogenesis in F344 rats. *J. Nutr.* **2006**, *136*, 2862–2867. [PubMed]
90. Kato, R.; Nakadate, T.; Yamamoto, S.; Sugimura, T. Inhibition of 12-*O*-tetradecanoylphorbol-13-acetate-induced tumor promotion and ornithine decarboxylase activity by quercetin: Possible involvement of lipoxygenase inhibition. *Carcinogenesis* **1983**, *4*, 1301–1305. [CrossRef] [PubMed]
91. Khanduja, K.; Gandhi, R.; Pathania, V.; Syal, N. Prevention of *N*-nitrosodiethylamine-induced lung tumorigenesis by ellagic acid and quercetin in mice. *Food Chem. Toxicol.* **1999**, *37*, 313–318. [CrossRef]
92. Verma, A.K.; Johnson, J.A.; Gould, M.N.; Tanner, M.A. Inhibition of 7, 12-dimethylbenz (a) anthracene-and *N*-nitrosomethylurea-induced rat mammary cancer by dietary flavonol quercetin. *Cancer Res.* **1988**, *48*, 5754–5758. [PubMed]
93. Kumamoto, T.; Fujii, M.; Hou, D.X. Akt is a direct target for myricetin to inhibit cell transformation. *Mol. Cell. Biochem.* **2009**, *332*, 33–41. [CrossRef] [PubMed]
94. Raman, M.; Chen, W.; Cobb, M. Differential regulation and properties of MAPKs. *Oncogene* **2007**, *26*, 3100–3112. [CrossRef] [PubMed]
95. Hanahan, D.; Weinberg, R.A. Hallmarks of cancer: The next generation. *Cell* **2011**, *144*, 646–674. [CrossRef] [PubMed]
96. Zamin, L.L.; Filippi-Chiela, E.C.; Dillenburg-Pilla, P.; Horn, F.; Salbego, C.; Lenz, G. Resveratrol and quercetin cooperate to induce senescence-like growth arrest in C6 rat glioma cells. *Cancer Sci.* **2009**, *100*, 1655–1662. [CrossRef] [PubMed]
97. Cosan, D.T.; Soyocak, A.; Basaran, A.; Degirmenci, İ.; Gunes, H.V.; Sahin, F.M. Effects of various agents on DNA fragmentation and telomerase enzyme activities in adenocarcinoma cell lines. *Mol. Biol. Rep.* **2011**, *38*, 2463–2469. [CrossRef] [PubMed]
98. Russo, M.; Mupo, A.; Spagnuolo, C.; Russo, G.L. Exploring death receptor pathways as selective targets in cancer therapy. *Biochem. Pharmacol.* **2010**, *80*, 674–682. [CrossRef] [PubMed]
99. Russo, M.; Palumbo, R.; Mupo, A.; Tosto, M.; Iacomino, G.; Scognamiglio, A.; Tedesco, I.; Galano, G.; Russo, G.L. Flavonoid quercetin sensitizes a CD95-resistant cell line to apoptosis by activating protein kinase Cα. *Oncogene* **2003**, *22*, 3330–3342. [CrossRef] [PubMed]
100. Russo, M.; Palumbo, R.; Tedesco, I.; Mazzarella, G.; Russo, P.; Iacomino, G.; Russo, G.L. Quercetin and anti-CD95 (Fas/Apo1) enhance apoptosis in HPB-ALL cell line. *FEBS Lett.* **1999**, *462*, 322–328. [CrossRef]
101. Russo, M.; Nigro, P.; Rosiello, R.; D'Arienzo, R.; Russo, G. Quercetin enhances CD95-and TRAIL-induced apoptosis in leukemia cell lines. *Leukemia* **2007**, *21*, 1130–1133. [CrossRef] [PubMed]
102. Lee, K.W.; Kang, N.J.; Heo, Y.S.; Rogozin, E.A.; Pugliese, A.; Hwang, M.K.; Bowden, G.T.; Bode, A.M.; Lee, H.J.; Dong, Z. Raf and MEK protein kinases are direct molecular targets for the chemopreventive effect of quercetin, a major flavonol in red wine. *Cancer Res.* **2008**, *68*, 946–955. [CrossRef] [PubMed]
103. Denison, M.S.; Pandini, A.; Nagy, S.R.; Baldwin, E.P.; Bonati, L. Ligand binding and activation of the Ah receptor. *Chem. Biol. Interact.* **2002**, *141*, 3–24. [CrossRef]

104. Guengerich, F.P.; Shimada, T. Oxidation of toxic and carcinogenic chemicals by human cytochrome P-450 enzymes. *Chem. Res. Toxicol.* **1991**, *4*, 391–407. [CrossRef] [PubMed]
105. Moon, Y.J.; Wang, X.; Morris, M.E. Dietary flavonoids: Effects on xenobiotic and carcinogen metabolism. *Toxicol. in Vitro* **2006**, *20*, 187–210. [CrossRef] [PubMed]
106. Ashida, H.; Fukuda, I.; Yamashita, T.; Kanazawa, K. Flavones and flavonols at dietary levels inhibit a transformation of aryl hydrocarbon receptor induced by dioxin. *FEBS Lett.* **2000**, *476*, 213–217. [CrossRef]
107. Fukuda, I.; Ashida, H. Suppressive effects of flavonoids on activation of the aryl hydrocarbon receptor induced by dioxins. In *ACS Symposium Series*; Oxford University Press: Cary, NC, USA, 2008; Volume 993, pp. 369–374.
108. Van Der Woude, H.; Ter Veld, M.G.; Jacobs, N.; Van Der Saag, P.T.; Murk, A.J.; Rietjens, I.M. The stimulation of cell proliferation by quercetin is mediated by the estrogen receptor. *Mol. Nutr. Food Res.* **2005**, *49*, 763–771. [CrossRef] [PubMed]
109. Cappelletti, V.; Miodini, P.; Di Fronzo, G.; Daidone, M.G. Modulation of estrogen receptor-β isoforms by phytoestrogens in breast cancer cells. *Int. J. Oncol.* **2006**, *28*, 1185–1191. [CrossRef] [PubMed]
110. Xing, N.; Chen, Y.; Mitchell, S.H.; Young, C.Y. Quercetin inhibits the expression and function of the androgen receptor in LNCaP prostate cancer cells. *Carcinogenesis* **2001**, *22*, 409–414. [CrossRef] [PubMed]
111. Yuan, H.; Gong, A.; Young, C.Y. Involvement of transcription factor Sp1 in quercetin-mediated inhibitory effect on the androgen receptor in human prostate cancer cells. *Carcinogenesis* **2005**, *26*, 793–801. [CrossRef] [PubMed]
112. Duraj, J.; Zazrivcova, K.; Bodo, J.; Sulikova, M.; Sedlak, J. Flavonoid quercetin, but not apigenin or luteolin, induced apoptosis in human myeloid leukemia cells and their resistant variants. *Neoplasma* **2004**, *52*, 273–279.
113. Psahoulia, F.H.; Moumtzi, S.; Roberts, M.L.; Sasazuki, T.; Shirasawa, S.; Pintzas, A. Quercetin mediates preferential degradation of oncogenic Ras and causes autophagy in Ha-RAS-transformed human colon cells. *Carcinogenesis* **2007**, *28*, 1021–1031. [CrossRef] [PubMed]
114. Ishikawa, Y.; Kitamura, M. Anti-apoptotic effect of quercetin: Intervention in the JNK-and ERK-mediated apoptotic pathways. *Kidney Int.* **2000**, *58*, 1078–1087. [CrossRef] [PubMed]
115. Marone, M.; D'Andrilli, G.; Das, N.; Ferlini, C.; Chatterjee, S.; Scambia, G. Quercetin abrogates taxol-mediated signaling by inhibiting multiple kinases. *Exp. Cell Res.* **2001**, *270*, 1–12. [CrossRef] [PubMed]
116. Ferraresi, R.; Troiano, L.; Roat, E.; Lugli, E.; Nemes, E.; Nasi, M.; Pinti, M.; Fernandez, M.I.; Cooper, E.L.; Cossarizza, A. Essential requirement of reduced glutathione (GSH) for the anti-oxidant effect of the flavonoid quercetin. *Free Radic. Res.* **2005**, *39*, 1249–1258. [CrossRef] [PubMed]
117. Robaszkiewicz, A.; Balcerczyk, A.; Bartosz, G. Antioxidative and prooxidative effects of quercetin on A549 cells. *Cell Biol. Int.* **2007**, *31*, 1245–1250. [CrossRef] [PubMed]
118. Zebisch, A.; Czernilofsky, A.P.; Keri, G.; Smigelskaite, J.; Sill, H.; Troppmair, J. Signaling through RAS-RAF-MEK-ERK: From basics to bedside. *Curr. Med. Chem.* **2007**, *14*, 601–623. [CrossRef] [PubMed]
119. Nguyen, T.; Tran, E.; Nguyen, T.; Do, P.; Huynh, T.; Huynh, H. The role of activated MEK-ERK pathway in quercetin-induced growth inhibition and apoptosis in A549 lung cancer cells. *Carcinogenesis* **2004**, *25*, 647–659. [CrossRef] [PubMed]
120. Cho, S.Y.; Park, S.J.; Kwon, M.J.; Jeong, T.S.; Bok, S.H.; Choi, W.Y.; Jeong, W.I.; Ryu, S.Y.; Do, S.H.; Lee, C.S. Quercetin suppresses proinflammatory cytokines production through MAP kinases and NF-κB pathway in lipopolysaccharide-stimulated macrophage. *Mol. Cell. Biochem.* **2003**, *243*, 153–160. [CrossRef] [PubMed]
121. Ross, J.A.; Kasum, C.M. Dietary flavonoids: Bioavailability, metabolic effects, and safety. *Annu. Rev. Nutr.* **2002**, *22*, 19–34. [CrossRef] [PubMed]
122. Neuhouser, M.L. Review: Dietary flavonoids and cancer risk: Evidence from human population studies. *Nutr. Cancer* **2004**, *50*, 1–7. [CrossRef] [PubMed]
123. Hirvonen, T.; Virtamo, J.; Korhonen, P.; Albanes, D.; Pietinen, P. Flavonol and flavone intake and the risk of cancer in male smokers (Finland). *Cancer Causes Control* **2001**, *12*, 797–802. [CrossRef]
124. Hertog, M.G.; Hollman, P.C.; Katan, M.B.; Kromhout, D. Intake of potentially anticarcinogenic flavonoids and their determinants in adults in The Netherlands. *Nutr. Cancer* **1993**, *20*, 21–29. [CrossRef] [PubMed]
125. Stefani, E.D.; Boffetta, P.; Deneo-Pellegrini, H.; Mendilaharsu, M.; Carzoglio, J.C.; Ronco, A.; Olivera, L. Dietary antioxidants and lung cancer risk: A case-control study in Uruguay. *Nutr. Cancer* **1999**, *34*, 100–110. [CrossRef] [PubMed]

126. Nöthlings, U.; Murphy, S.P.; Wilkens, L.R.; Henderson, B.E.; Kolonel, L.N. Flavonols and pancreatic cancer risk the multiethnic cohort study. *Am. J. Epidemiol.* **2007**, *166*, 924–931. [CrossRef] [PubMed]
127. Gates, M.A.; Tworoger, S.S.; Hecht, J.L.; De Vivo, I.; Rosner, B.; Hankinson, S.E. A prospective study of dietary flavonoid intake and incidence of epithelial ovarian cancer. *Int. J. Cancer* **2007**, *121*, 2225–2232. [CrossRef] [PubMed]

3

The Anti-Cancer Effect of Polyphenols against Breast Cancer and Cancer Stem Cells: Molecular Mechanisms

Ahmed Abdal Dayem, Hye Yeon Choi, Gwang-Mo Yang, Kyeongseok Kim, Subbroto Kumar Saha and Ssang-Goo Cho *

Department of Stem Cell & Regenerative Biotechnology, Incurable Disease Animal Model and Stem Cell Institute (IDASI), Konkuk University, Gwangjin-gu, Seoul 05029, Korea; ahmed_morsy86@yahoo.com (A.A.D.); hyeon.choi24@gmail.com (H.Y.C.); slayersgod@nate.com (G.-M.Y.); proproggs@naver.com (K.K.); subbroto@konkuk.ac.kr (S.K.S.)

* Correspondence: ssangoo@konkuk.ac.kr

Abstract: The high incidence of breast cancer in developed and developing countries, and its correlation to cancer-related deaths, has prompted concerned scientists to discover novel alternatives to deal with this challenge. In this review, we will provide a brief overview of polyphenol structures and classifications, as well as on the carcinogenic process. The biology of breast cancer cells will also be discussed. The molecular mechanisms involved in the anti-cancer activities of numerous polyphenols, against a wide range of breast cancer cells, in vitro and in vivo, will be explained in detail. The interplay between autophagy and apoptosis in the anti-cancer activity of polyphenols will also be highlighted. In addition, the potential of polyphenols to target cancer stem cells (CSCs) via various mechanisms will be explained. Recently, the use of natural products as chemotherapeutics and chemopreventive drugs to overcome the side effects and resistance that arise from using chemical-based agents has garnered the attention of the scientific community. Polyphenol research is considered a promising field in the treatment and prevention of breast cancer.

Keywords: polyphenols; breast cancer; anti-cancer activity; autophagy; apoptosis; cancer stem cells

---

1. Introduction

Currently, cancer is one of the most common life-threatening diseases worldwide, and breast cancer has the highest rate of diagnosis amongst women. There are three main strategies to block and postpone the stages of carcinogenesis [1–3]. The primary strategy considered is a preventive approach, which blocks the toxic, as well as the mutagenic, effects, which consequently inhibits tumor initiation and promotion. The secondary strategy presents anti-cancer potential during the early stages of carcinogenesis via various mechanisms, such as control of signal transduction, blocking angiogenesis, antioxidant mechanisms, hormones, and modulation of immunity, which finally result in the blockage of cancer progression. The third strategy for cancer treatment and prevention involves blocking the invasiveness and metastatic properties of a tumor via regulation of cell-adhesion molecules, protection of the extracellular matrix (ECM) from degradation, and up-regulation of genes that block metastasis [1,2].

The link between a diet that is rich in fruits and vegetables, and the prevention, as well as the reduction, of the occurrence of health-daunting diseases has been evidenced, and is partially ascribed to polyphenols [4–6]. The term polyphenol was first given to natural compounds bearing multiple (poly) phenol rings, which are widespread in various fruits, vegetables, wine, nuts, tea, coffee, and in many foods that are consumed daily by humans [7]. Polyphenols possess a broad spectrum of structural variations, which lead to a wide range of biological functions; among them, anti-cancer functions. Polyphenols possess a broad spectrum of structural variations in the carbon backbone chains, as well as alterations to primary and secondary structures due to methylation, glycosylation, and hydroxylation [6,8]. These structural variations may be responsible for their various health benefits, including antioxidant [9,10], anti-inflammatory, anti-angiogenic [11,12], and anti-proliferative mechanisms, as well as regulation of key signaling protein and enzyme functions [13].

2. Carcinogenesis: Overview and Molecular Basis

The tumorigenic process is complicated and occurs through a multistep procedure, including initiation, promotion, and progression, as illustrated in Figure 1 [14,15]. Initiation includes the entrance and distribution of cancer-causing agents in the cell, in particular, the nucleus, and interaction with DNA that finally results in the mutagenesis and emergence of the toxic effect [16]. This stage is irreversible, but can be prevented by phase I and phase II metabolizing enzymes, which transform the carcinogens into less toxic and soluble products [17,18].

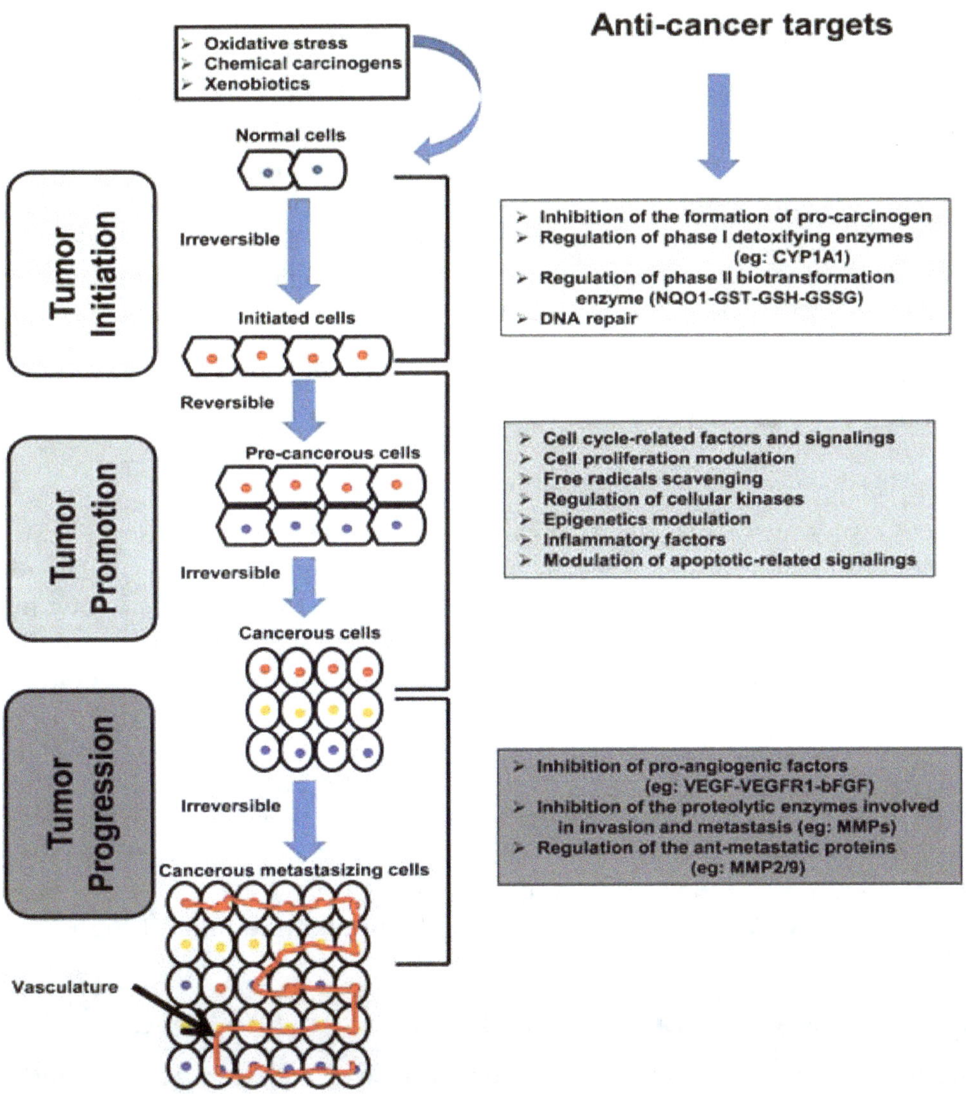

Figure 1. Schematic representation depicting the multistage process, including initiation, promotion, and progression, of carcinogenesis, and the biological targets of polyphenols at each step.

Polyphenols present preventive effects against tumor initiation via numerous mechanisms, such as prevention of the formation of genotoxic molecules and blocking the activity of the mutagens-transforming enzymes [19,20]; regulation of heme-containing phase I enzymes, such as cytochrome P450s (CYPs) [21,22]; regulation of carcinogen-detoxifying phase II enzymes, such as NADPH-quinone oxidoreductase-1 (NQO1), quinone reductase (QR), glutathione *S*-transferase (GST), and uridine diphospho (UDP) glucuronosyl transferase (UGT) [23,24]; and prevention of the formation of DNA adducts [25].

The promotion stage, which takes time, is related to the proliferation of tumor-initiating cells. It is considered a reversible stage of tumorigenesis, and gives rise to pre-cancerous cells. The main features of this stage are cell proliferation and apoptosis. The tumor progression stage is the stage in which cells gradually transform to the malignant state. Metastasis and invasiveness also emerge during this stage, via the angiogenesis process, with the growth of new blood capillaries in the tumor, which is enhanced by the secretion of specific growth factors and growth factor receptors, such as platelet-derived growth factor (PDGF), PDGF receptor (PDGFR), vascular endothelial growth factor (VEGF), and VEGF receptor (VEGFR), leading to overgrowth and spread of the tumor [26].

Cathepsins, which belong to the lysosomal proteases superfamily, are implicated in tumor progression [27]. Cathepsin D, an aspartic protease, is considered to be a candidate as a clinical marker for breast cancer, and is involved in the activation of the inactive form of cathepsin B (procathepsin B) [28]. Cathepsin B is essential for the growth of breast cancer [29] and its down-regulation leads to a reduction of tumor progression [30]. The up-regulation of cathepsin B is an indicator of cancer progression and is a poor prognosis [31].

The urokinase plasminogen activator (uPA) system consists of serine protease uPA and various serine protease inhibitors, such as plasminogen activator inhibitors 1 and 2 (PAI-1 and PAI-2). Upon binding of uPA to urokinase plasminogen activator anchored receptor (uPAR), the activation of plasminogen takes place and leads to the production of the broad spectrum protease, plasmin [32]. Plasmin directly degrades the ECM, or indirectly via the activation of the zymogens of metalloproteinases (MMPs) [33].

There are numerous polyphenols that show potent inhibitory effects on the invasiveness and metastatic properties of cancer, which will be explained in detail in the following sections.

3. Overview on Breast Cancer and Cancer Stem Cells (CSCs)

Breast cancer represents about 25.2% of cancer cases in women, and commonly occurs in US women at a rate of one in eight cases [34,35]. In 2012, approximately 522,000 deaths were due to breast cancer [36]. Despite the success of emergent breast cancer therapeutics in decreasing mortality cases, the prognosis, in particular for the stage IV cancer, remains poor and needs further improvement [37]. The presence of small populations of cells with unique tumor recurrence and metastases represents a serious challenge during cancer therapy, and may be ascribed to the presence of a small population of specialized malignant cells, which are believed to be cancer stem cells (CSCs) [38,39].

In 2003, Al-Hajj et al. discovered the presence of CSCs in breast cancer [40]. They carried out fluorescence-activated cell sorting (FACS) analyses of primary breast cancer cells for the expression of the following markers, cluster of differentiation 44 (CD44), cluster of differentiation 24 (CD24), and epithelial specific antigen (ESA). They confirmed that $CD44^{+}$ $CD24^{-/low}$ cells possess the same characteristic features of CSCs, including self-renewal, differentiation, and high tumor induction properties [40].

4. Therapeutic Approaches to Breast Cancer and Development of Resistance

The main approaches for the treatment of breast cancer are surgical intervention, hormonal therapy, immunotherapy, chemotherapy, and radiotherapy. However, the recovery rate after application of these conventional methods is about 60%–80% for primary cancers and about 50% for metastatic ones [41,42].

Previously, the heterogenic features of cancer were calibrated, based on the following parameters: histological analysis, tumor grading, condition of lymph nodes, and specific markers, such as estrogen receptor (ER), progesterone receptor (PR), and, recently, human epidermal growth factor receptor 2 (HER2) [43]. Furthermore, tumor heterogeneity was verified using gene expression analysis and cDNA microarrays analysis [44].

There are four fundamental groups of patients with metastatic breast cancer that are subjected to treatment, including hormone receptor (HR)-positive patients, who are classified into two classes: luminal A type, with the highest invasiveness and the best prognosis, which is characterized by ER^+, PR^+, $HER2^-$, and low ki67, and luminal B, which is characterized by ER^+, PR^+, $HER2^+$ or $HER2^-$, and high ki67 [45,46]. HR^+ breast cancers have the best prognosis and can be treated with tamoxifen, an ER antagonist, fulvestrant, which directly hampers ER synthesis, and aromatase inhibitors, namely, anastrozole, exemestane, and letrozole [47].

$HER2^+$, another subtype of metastatic breast cancer, is an ER^- breast cancer, and, therefore, is considered to be from the worst aggressive type of breast cancer [48,49]. To eliminate this type of cancer, various therapeutic strategies have been developed, such as a drug targeting HER2 receptor using humanized monoclonal antibodies, including trastuzumab (herceptin), pertuzumab, and lapatinib [49].

Triple-negative breast cancer (TNBC), voided of ER, PR, and HER2, is considered the worst type of metastatic breast cancer and has highly invasive properties, a large tumor size, poor prognosis, a high chance to relapse, is not responsive to hormonal therapy, and has lymph node involvement. There are several approaches to counteract TNBC, such as neoadjuvant chemotherapy, anthracyclines, taxanes, poly (ADP-ribose) polymerase protein (PARP) inhibitors, epidermal growth factor receptor (EGFR) inhibitors, and platinum-containing chemotherapeutic agents [50–52].

Chemotherapy remains a crucial approach for cancer management in all patient groups. However, HER2-positive tumor patients, and patients with TNBC, need endocrine therapy in addition to chemotherapy [53]. Taken together, new, alternative therapeutics, in particular, natural products, need to be explored using mammosphere culture in order to overcome this problem.

5. Overview on Polyphenols

Polyphenols, a broad category of natural compounds and plant metabolites, possess one, or numerous, benzene rings that bear one, or several, hydroxyl groups. They are considered to be complicated antioxidants that are abundantly present in our daily diet, in particular, they can be found in fruits, legumes, spices, cocoa, vegetable, coffee, nuts, beer, wine, and olive oil [54]. Average daily consumption of polyphenols is estimated to be around one gram [55]. In nature, polyphenols generally exist conjugated with organic acids and sugars, and, accordingly, can be classified into two main categories; flavonoids and non-flavonoids, as shown in Figure 2.

The flavonoid category consists of two benzene rings, linked by a heterocyclic pyrone C-ring, and the non-flavonoid category contains more complicated molecules (benzoic acid, hydroxycinnamates, stilbenes, lignans, gallic acids tannins, and gallotannins) [56,57].

Polyphenols have been reported to possess special activities that are beneficial for human health, such as anti-oxidant [58], anti-infection [59–61], anti-cancer [62,63], neuroprotective [64], and anti-inflammatory [65] effects. Their broad activity could be attributed to several mechanisms, including interaction with, as well as modulation of, a wide range of proteins, enzymes, and membrane receptors, regulation of gene expression, apoptosis induction, vasodilatation, and modulation of cell signaling pathways [66–70].

There are similarities between some groups of flavonoids, such as isoflavones and lignans, and the estrogens, and, accordingly, they are considered as a phytoestrogen. Their anti-estrogenic activity has been exploited and applied in a wide range of studies [71]. Especially, the potent anti-cancer activity of polyphenols can be ascribed to their targeting of aromatase, antioxidant mechanisms, anti-inflammatory mechanisms, and anti-estrogenic mechanisms [72–76].

Flavonoids are considered to be the largest category of the polyphenols, and are characterized by their low molecular weight [77,78]. The structural characteristics of flavonoids can determine their functions and bioavailability, and can be used for classification into various groups.

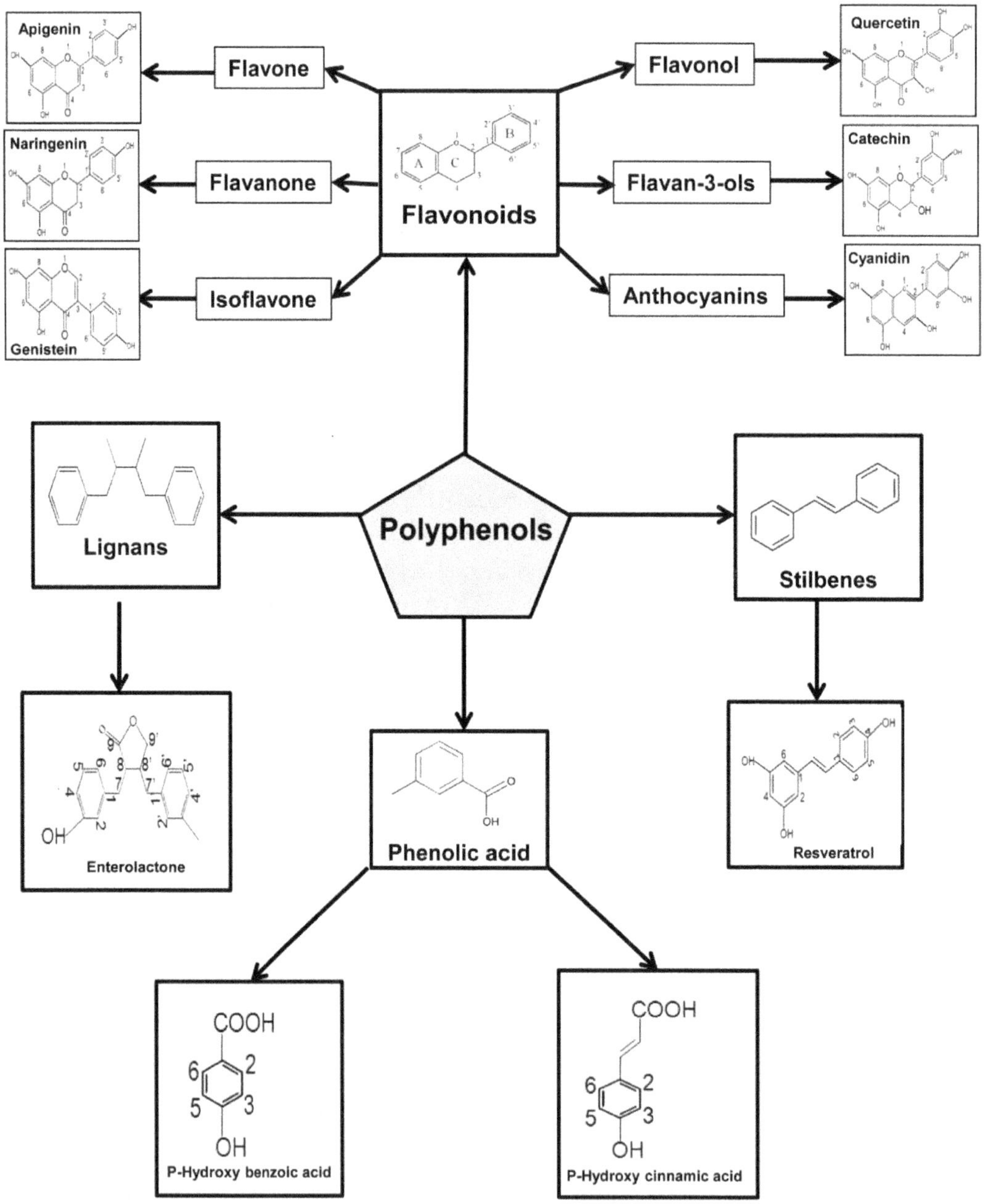

Figure 2. Diagram summarizing the classes of polyphenols and their basic chemical structures. Polyphenols can be separated into two main classes: flavonoids and non-flavonoids. The flavonoid class consists of two benzene rings, linked by a heterocyclic pyrone C-ring. The non-flavonoids class contains more intricate molecules, namely, benzoic acid, hydroxycinnamates, stilbenes, lignans, gallic acids tannins, and gallotannins.

The basic structure of flavonoids consists of a flavan nucleus (2-phenylchroman) containing 15 atoms that constitute three rings (A-ring (C6), B-ring (C6), and C-ring (C3)). The variation among flavonoids depends on the following: changes in the C-ring (presence of the 3-hydroxyl group, and double bond or 4-oxo group) and changes in the A- and B-rings, such as the difference in the number and the position of the hydroxyl and methoxyl groups. If one or more sugar group binds to the flavonoid structure, they are called "flavonoid glycosides", whereas flavonoids without a sugar group are described as "aglycones".

Dietary flavonoids are mainly "flavonoids glycosides", except for flavanols. Moreover, our research group revealed various aspects of the biological activities and health benefits of numerous flavonoids, such as antioxidant, antiviral, and anti-cancer properties, which were evidenced in vitro and in vivo [79–84].

Polyphenols are considered the main natural antioxidant component in fruits, vegetables, tea, oils, and cereals. The wide range of health benefits of dietary polyphenols is ascribed to their potential in reducing the risk, as well as preventing, serious diseases, such as cancer, metabolic diseases, neurodegenerative diseases, and heart diseases, which threaten human life and negatively affect quality of life, as summarized in Figure 3 [85].

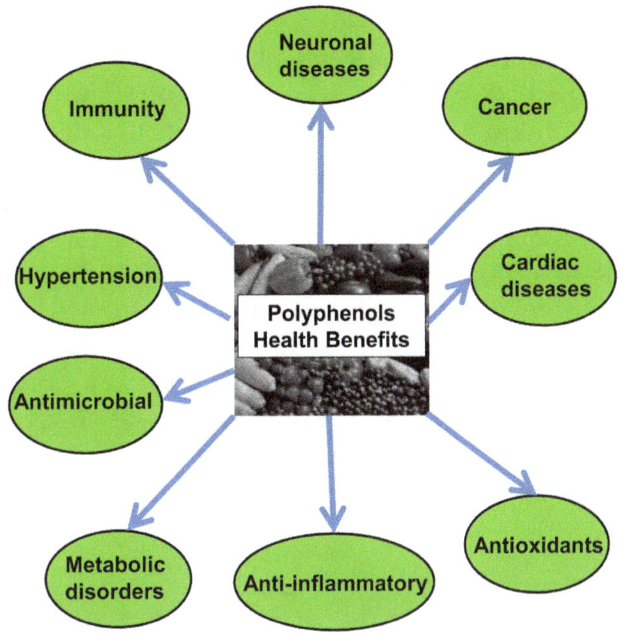

Figure 3. Overview summarizing the main health benefits of polyphenols. Polyphenols play key roles in the prevention of serious diseases that threaten human life and negatively affect quality of life, such as cancer, metabolic diseases, neurodegenerative diseases, hypertension, and cardiac diseases.

There is a large body of literature that describes the impact of polyphenols on human health and disease prevention [86,87]. Polyphenols are present in foods as intricate combinations of various chemical formulations of several polyphenol compounds, such as oligomers, chlorogenic acid, hydroxycinnamic acids, and epicatechin (in apples) [88]. Moreover, these dietary polyphenols are present in combination with sugar residues that conjugate with hydroxyl groups and aromatic carbons, can be combined with organic and carboxylic acids, and with amines [89]. In cereals, polyphenols are conjugated with polysaccharides of the cell wall [90], and in fruits, the amount of conjugated polyphenols is much higher than the amount of free polyphenols [91].

The absorption rate and site of polyphenols are modulated by their structures [92]. For instance, glycosides can be absorbed in the small intestine, except for glycosides that link to the rhamnose group metabolized by the enzyme, α-rhamnosidase, which is secreted by microflora in the colon [93]. Glycosides can be metabolized by several enzymes, including cytosolic β-glucosidase and the membrane-located lactase phlorizin hydrolase [94,95].

On the other hand, the acylated polyphenol compounds, flavan-3-ols (epicatechin), are absorbed directly into the enterocyte without hydrolysis [96]. Hydroxycinnamic acids, which are esterified with organic acids, lipids, and sugar, are partially absorbed in the small intestine, and a major portion is metabolized by colonic microflora. The colon is considered a suitable site for the absorption of polymeric proanthocyanidins.

6. Correlation between Polyphenols' Anti-Cancer Activity and Autophagy

Autophagy is a cellular phenomenon that occurs as a response reaction against stress factors, such as starvation, oxidative stress, and toxicity [97]. During the autophagy process, catabolic lysosomal degradation takes place in order to maintain cellular homeostasis.

Autophagy-related genes (ATG) and their proteins are essential for the formation of the double-membrane vesicles needed for the engulfment of damaged cellular organelles in the cytosol. Beclin-1 (Atg6 in yeast), which is located on human chromosome 17q21, is considered one of the key components of ATG proteins. It exhibits haploinsufficiency, and its identification may have unveiled a crosslink between autophagy and human cancer. Its monoallelic deletion has been detected in breast, ovary, and prostate cancers [98,99].

The crosslink between diet and autophagy is well-known, and dietary restriction or starvation are related to autophagy induction and influence on health [100,101]. Autophagy induction is modulated by the level of cellular ATP and energy, which are detected by the cellular energy sensor, adenosine monophosphate kinase (AMPK). AMPK activation is enhanced as a response to the low ratio of ATP/AMP and nutrient deprivation via its upstream kinase, liver kinase BQ (LKB1 kinase). AMPK inhibits the activity of the mammalian target of rapamycin 1 (mTORC1) directly via phosphorylation of RAPTOR, or indirectly through activation of TSC1/2, which enhance the activity of GTP-Rheb [102,103]. Inactivated mTOR is involved in autophagy induction via activation of complexes, including ULK1, Atg13, and the FAK-family interacting protein of 200 kDa (FIP200) [104].

Below, we will discuss examples of polyphenols, and how autophagy signaling pathways and transcription factors are involved in their anti-cancer potentials, as summarized in Figure 4.

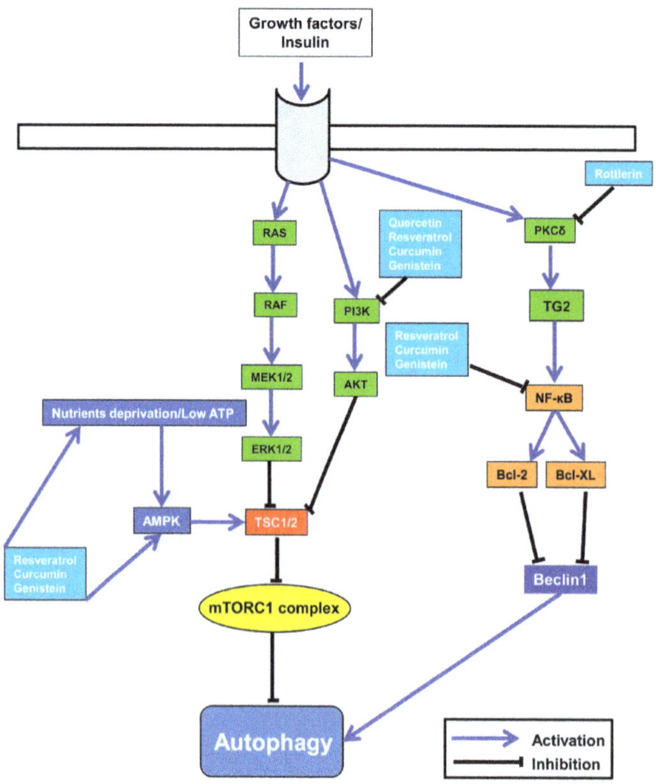

Figure 4. Role of polyphenols in the modulation of autophagy in breast cancer. Polyphenols modulate the autophagy process by regulating various signaling pathways, such as the PI3K/AKT, RAS/RAF/ERK, PKCδ, and AMPK signaling pathways.

6.1. Resveratrol

Resveratrol (3,4′,5-trihydroxy-trans-stilbene), the main polyphenol in grapes and peanuts, exists in red wine at a concentration of about 0.1–1.8 g per 100 mL. In mice, resveratrol potently mitigates the harmful consequences of a high-fat diet that influences longevity and lifespan [105]. This lifespan-increasing effect is attributed to the activation of sirtuin (SIRT1) via an autophagy-mediated mechanism [106]. The crosslink between SIRT1 and autophagy is attributed to the potency of SIRT1 to deacetylate the core elements, such as Atg5, Atg7, and Atg8, of autophagy induction [107]. Resveratrol is a well-known polyphenol modulating SIRT1 [108]. The anti-cancer activity of resveratrol has been proven in vitro and in vivo [109–111], and is mediated by numerous mechanisms, such as apoptosis, cell cycle arrest, kinase signaling pathways, and autophagy [109,112].

The implication of resveratrol in the induction of autophagy via the accumulation of autophagosomes has been proved in various cell lines [109,113,114]; however, resveratrol treatment induces non-canonical autophagy, which is independent of Beclin-1, vacuolar protein sorting 34 (Vps34), and Atg-dependent autophagy in breast cancer cells [115].

Apoptosis-resistant cell lines, such as breast cancer MCF-7 cells, which are deficient in caspase-3, showed sensitivity to resveratrol treatment, and, interestingly, activation of caspase-9, as well as chromatin condensation, were detected in resveratrol-treated MCF-7 cells [116].

Recently, FoxO transcription factors have been shown to play an important role in apoptosis and autophagy induced by resveratrol treatment [117]. In human colorectal cancer, resveratrol-induced cell death was abolished upon genetic inhibition of the function of autophagy-related proteins, including PI3K, Lamp2b, and Beclin1 [113]. In human epidermoid carcinoma cells, exposure to resveratrol led to a decrease in the expression level of Rictor protein, and of mTORC2, and ultimately a reduction of RhoA-GTPase [118].

Reactive oxygen species (ROS) mediate the significant up-regulation of AMPK upon resveratrol treatment in etoposide-resistant HT-29 colon cancer cells, and, in turn, augment the potential of etoposide to induce apoptosis [119]. In addition, resveratrol exposure increased ROS generation and cleavage of caspase-8 and caspase-9, and ultimately induced autophagy via up-regulation of microtubule-associated protein 1 light chain 3-II (LC3-II) expression in colon cancer [120].

Resveratrol leads to autophagy induction via the up-regulation of p62/sequestome-1 (SQSTM1), and AMPK/mTOR-mediated, by JNK in imatinib-sensitive and imatinib-resistant chronic myelogenous leukemia cells (CML) K562 [121].

6.2. Silibinin

Silibinin, which is a flavonolignan extracted from milk thistle (*Silybum marianum*), possesses protective effects for the liver [122] and neurons [123,124]. Recently, the anti-cancer activity of silibinin has been demonstrated in vitro and in vivo [125–127]. In human colon cancer cells, silibinin treatment led to activation of the extrinsic (receptor-related) and intrinsic (mitochondria-related) apoptosis pathways, as well as activation of the autophagic process [128]. Pharmacological inhibition of autophagy with treatment of bafilomycin-A1 (Baf-A1) in silibinin-exposed human colon cancer cells resulted in autophagy inhibition, which is accompanied by activation of cell death. Accordingly, silibinin treatment of human cancer cells induced cytoprotective autophagy, and ROS was a mediator in silibinin-induced apoptosis and autophagy in tumor cells [129,130]. On the other hand, the ROS-scavenging activity of silibinin was also shown in vitro and in vivo [123,131].

An interesting study demonstrated the potential of silibinin to induce autophagic cell death in breast cancer cells. This effect was confirmed by high expression of LC3-II, increase of Beclin-1, high Atg-12-Atg-5, and down-regulation of Bcl-2 [132]. Upon treatment with pharmacological inhibitors of autophagy, 3-methyladenine (3-MA) and Baf-A1, silibinin-induced breast cancer cell death was mitigated. Silibinin treatment led to ROS generation, which was correlated with the disruption of mitochondrial membrane potential and ATP depletion, which were further blocked by treatment of *N*-acetyl cysteine (NAC) and ascorbic acid [132].

Of note, silibinin-exposed breast cancer cells showed up-regulation of Bcl-2 adenovirus E1B 19-kDa-interacting protein 3 (BNIP3). Small interfering RNA (siRNA) targeting BNIP3 abrogated silibinin-induced cell death, ROS generation, ATP depletion, and the disruption of mitochondrial membrane potential [132].

Silibinin-induced autophagy and apoptosis in MCF-7 cells are concomitant with the down-regulation of AKT, mTOR, and ERK [133]. Co-treatment of ERα antagonist, methyl-piperidinopyrazole (MPP) dihydrochloride, with silibinin led to the aggravation of the apoptosis and autophagy induced by silibinin treatment. These results indicate that ERα inhibition by silibinin mediates the down-regulation of AKT, mTOR, and ERK, and the final induction of apoptosis and autophagy in MCF-7 cells [133].

6.3. Quercetin

Quercetin (3,3′,4′,5,7-pentahydroxyflavanone), a flavonol, exists in a wide range of fruits and vegetables, such as onions, apples, and berries, and is considered one of the most common antioxidants in the human diet [134]. The application of quercetin to inhibit tyrosine kinase has been approved for clinical trials [135]. The anti-cancer potential of quercetin has been shown in various in vitro and in vivo studies [136–139]. Down-regulation of mTOR activity, and the subsequent formation of autophagosomes by quercetin treatment, have been evidenced [140].

In gastric cancer cells, quercetin induced cytoprotective autophagy that was abrogated upon treatment with the lysosomal inhibitor, chloroquine, or silencing of Atg5 or Beclin-1 using siRNA, and led to apoptotic cell death [141].

Hypoxia-induced factor 1α (HIF-1α) and Akt-mTOR signaling pathways are mediators of quercetin-induced cytoprotective autophagy. The components of the mTOR signaling pathway, in particular, mTORC1, play key roles in the maintenance of cellular homeostasis via modulation of protein synthesis through p70S6 kinase, which activates the ribosomal S6 subunit, and phosphorylation of 4E-BP1 (eIF4E binding protein 1) that inhibits the sequestration of the eukaryotic initiation factor of protein biosynthesis (eIF4). In various cancer cell lines, quercetin modulates the mTOR signaling pathway through down-regulation of the phosphorylation level of the ribosomal S6 subunit via p70S6 kinase, as well as via activation of 4E-BP1 [140].

6.4. Genistein

Genistein (4′,5,7-trihydroxyisoflavone), an isoflavone, is widely distributed in soybean and presents a broad spectrum of in vitro and in vivo anti-cancer potential in numerous cancer cells, through cell cycle arrest, induction of apoptosis, blocking of angiogenesis, inhibition of telomerase activity, and blocking inhibition of DNA topoisomerase II [142–145].

In ovarian cancer cells, genistein treatment led to cell death, which is independent of caspase signaling pathways and induced autophagy [146]. The autophagy induced by genistein treatment can be recovered upon treatment with methyl pyruvate, the substrate for oxidative phosphorylation and fatty acid synthesis.

Genistein-exposed ovarian cancer cells showed a marked reduction in glucose uptake that may be attributed to the inactivation of AKT signaling [146]. Inhibition of the aggregate that is formed by the interaction between cyclic AMP phosphodiesterase-4A4 (PDE4A4) and SQSTM1 protein (p62) is essential for the induction of autophagy. This can be explained by the role of SQSTM1 protein in interacting with LC3, which has a pivotal role in vesicle formation in autophagosomes [147]. Genistein-treated ovarian cancer cells showed marked autophagy due to inhibition of the formation of PDE4A4 and SQSTM1 aggregates, activated by ERK and PKC inhibitors [148].

6.5. Curcumin

Curcumin, diferuloylmethane extracted from *Curcuma longa*, is the key constituent of turmeric, and possesses various biological functions with minimal toxicity, such as antioxidant, anti-inflammatory, and anti-cancer functions [149,150]. In malignant glioma cells, curcumin exposure led to cell cycle arrest and autophagy induction through up-regulation of the ERK1/2 signaling pathways and down-regulation of the Akt/mTOR/p70S6K signaling pathways [151]. In bladder cancer cells, curcumin dephosphorylated AKT, and, in turn, activated LC3-II [152].

The autophagy-inducing capacity of curcumin was exploited in cellular protection against oxidative stress-induced cell death in human umbilical vein endothelial cells. This was mediated by modulation of the autophagy machinery, including activation of LC3-II, inhibition of PI3K/Akt/mTOR core signaling, and promotion of FOXO1 (autophagy mediator) [153]. In curcumin-exposed human colon cancer cells, there was a significant increase in the conversion of LC3-I to LC3-II, as well as degradation of SQSTM1 [154]. These effects were markedly abrogated after treatment with an ROS scavenging compound, NAC, indicating that ROS is a mediator of curcumin-induced autophagosome formation and cell death [154].

In malignant glioma cells, curcumin treatment induced autophagy that is attributed to the up-regulation of ERK signaling, which is concomitant with the down-regulation of the Akt/mTOR/p70 ribosomal protein S6 kinase (p70S6K) pathway [155]. Moreover, SIRT1 was modulated by curcumin in the regulation of autophagy and other cellular events [108].

Curcumin remarkably enhanced the expression of AMPK, accompanied by p38 signaling-mediated cell death in ovarian cancer cells [156]. Similarly, curcumin induced ROS generation at the beginning of apoptosis and autophagy in oral squamous cell carcinoma, and NAC treatment abolished curcumin-mediated autophagosome formation [157]. In addition to the induction of autophagy, curcumin exposure led to apoptosis via inactivation of Bcl-2 protein and down-regulation of NF-κB in cancer cells [158,159].

6.6. Rottlerin

Rottlerin, also called mallotoxin, is one of the active components of the Kamala tree (*Mallotus philippensis*), which grows widely in Southeast Asia. In 1994, the pharmacological effects of rottlerin were revealed, after its potential to specifically inhibit the activity of protein kinase C delta (PKCδ) was demonstrated [160]. Therefore, the potency of rottlerin to block PKCδ activity has been exploited in various biological functions related to PKCδ [161].

Recently, rottlerin was shown to exhibit various biological activities, including human T-cell response inhibition [162], potassium channel activation [163], in vitro and in vivo neuroprotection [164], antioxidant activity [165], antihistaminic activity [166], and anti-cancer activity [167]. The crosslink between tissue transglutaminase (TG2) and NF-κB was evidenced [168]. Moreover, implication of NF-κB in the autophagy process was proven [169].

In pancreatic cancer cells, rottlerin, as well as PKCδ siRNA treatment, led to a drastic decrease in cell proliferation, which was accompanied by a significant reduction in mRNA and protein levels of TG2, without showing any apoptotic changes [170]. However, rottlerin-treated pancreatic cancer cells showed significant autophagy, which was evidenced by cytoplasmic acidic vacuoles and the up-regulation of LC3-II, similar to that of TG2-specific siRNA-treated cells. Belin-1 knockdown abrogated the potential of rottlerin and TG2 siRNA to induce autophagy in pancreatic cancer cells.

In human pancreatic CSCs, rottlerin treatment led to early autophagy, evidenced by the formation of autophagosomes, LC3-II formation, up-regulation of Atg7 and Beclin-1, as well as down-regulation of the pro-apoptotic proteins, Bcl-2 and Bcl-X_L [171]. Treatment of 3-MA or genetic inhibition of autophagy via silencing of the autophagy-specific genes, Atg7 and Beclin-1, blocked the potential of rottlerin to induce autophagy and enhanced rottlerin-induced apoptosis [171].

In human breast cancer cells, rottlerin treatment showed TSC2-dependent inhibition of the mTORC1 signaling pathway and the accumulation of autophagosomes as a consequence [172]. Taken together, we described the mechanisms of polyphenols in autophagy modulation in terms of their anti-cancer functions. However, these findings need to be scrutinized in depth with respect to breast cancer and in vivo using animal models that possess genetic modifications of autophagy-related genes.

7. Anti-Cancer Activity of Polyphenols against Breast Cancer: Molecular Mechanisms

The anti-cancer activities of polyphenols against a wide range of cancers, such as breast cancer [173], prostate cancer [174], colorectal cancer [175], pancreatic cancer, lung cancer, colorectal fibrosarcoma, and leukemia, have been proven [176]. The possible mechanisms underlying the anticancer activity of polyphenols against breast cancer are summarized in Figure 5, and the possible molecular mechanisms by which polyphenols kill breast cancer are described below.

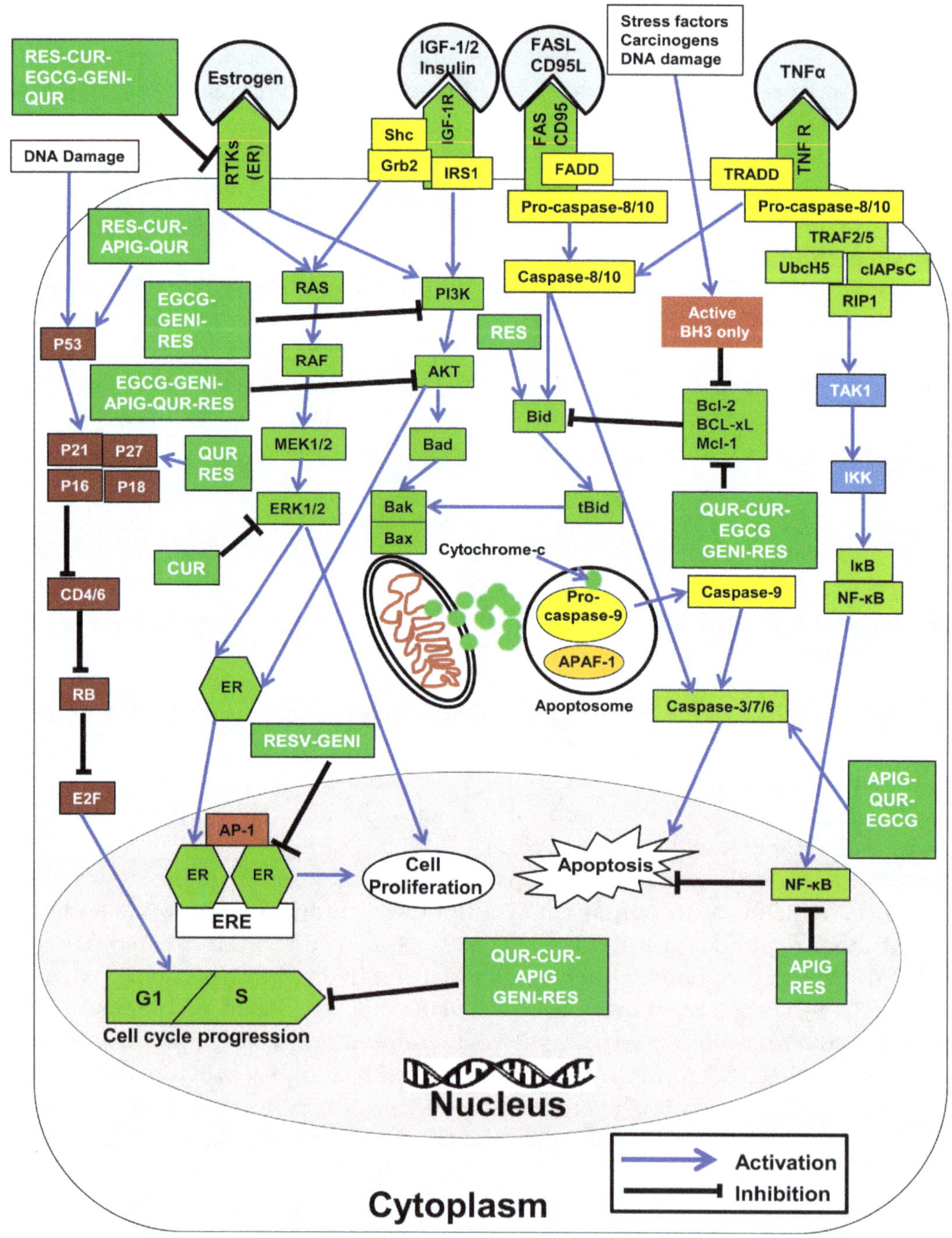

Figure 5. Comprehensive representation summarizing the possible mechanisms of action of polyphenols against breast cancer. The anti-cancer activity of polyphenols is mediated via the regulation of various signaling pathways, such as intrinsic and extrinsic apoptotic pathways, estrogen-related signaling pathways, cell cycle arrest, and inflammation-related signaling pathways. RES, resveratrol; CUR, curcumin; GENI, genistein; QUR, quercetin; APIG, apigenin.

7.1. Modulation of ROS

In fruits, polyphenols represent a major portion of the antioxidants compared to vitamin C [177]. Antioxidant activity is one of the key mechanisms that contribute to the protective effect of polyphenols against oxidative damage.

Cellular redox balance can be maintained by cellular antioxidant enzymes, including superoxide dismutase (SOD), peroxiredoxins (PRXs), catalase (CAT), glutathione peroxidase (GPx), and glutathione reductase (GR) [178]. However, mitigation of excessive generation of ROS by the cellular antioxidant enzymes is difficult [179].

Polyphenols are directly involved in the reduction of the Fenton reaction, via chelation of iron, thereby protecting cells from oxidation from highly reactive hydroxyl radicals [180–182]. The potent antioxidant activity of polyphenols is attributed to their ability to scavenge a broad spectrum of highly reactive species, such as ROS, reactive nitrogen species (NOS), chlorine species, peroxynitrous acid (ONOOH), and hypochlorous acid (HOCl) [183]; they also block the chain reactions of lipid peroxidation (chain breakers) as a consequence [180,184]. The antioxidant activity of flavonoid compounds is also mediated by targeting NFκB- and MAPK-related signaling pathways [185]. Polyphenols can work as co-antioxidants, as they show synergistic activity with other antioxidants, such as α-tocopherol (vitamin E), leading to the regeneration of vitamin E [186].

The polyphenols structures, such as the hydroxyl group's number and position, hydroxylation degree, and distance between the aromatic ring and the carbonyl group, play a pivotal role in its antioxidant activity and metal chelating property. For instance, within the flavonol group, quercetin showed the most potent antioxidant activity due to its 3-hydroxy group [187]. Additionally, polyphenol potential for metal chelation and scavenging of free radicals could be elevated with a B-ring bearing catechol moiety, C-ring bearing 4-oxo group, and the presence of a double bond [188].

Cinnamic acid and its derivatives showed relatively better antioxidant properties compared to benzoic acid, due to the longer distance between the aromatic ring and the carbonyl group. Additionally, the presence of the hydroxyl group at the para and/or ortho position on the benzoic ring enhances antioxidant potential compared to the presence of the hydroxyl group at other positions [189].

Biochanin A, an isoflavonoid purified from red clover (*Trifolium pratense*) showed preventive activity against the incidence of mammary gland cancer, after exposure to carcinogenic agents in prepubertal rat [190]. It potentially counteracted oxidative stress through a significant up-regulation of SOD, CAT, GPx, GST, and DT-diaphorase (DTD), as well as a remarkable reduction of lactate dehydrogenase (LDH) and lipid peroxidation (LPO) activities.

The protective action of resveratrol against 17β-estradiol (E2)-induced carcinogenesis was evidenced in vitro and in vivo, and was mediated by a significant increase in the expression of nuclear factor erythroid-related factor-2 (Nrf-2), which consequently up-regulated the expression of antioxidant genes, including NQO1, SOD3, and 8-oxoguanine DNA glycosylase 1 (OGG1) [191].

Green tea is composed of four main catechins, (−)-epicatechin (EC), (−)-epicatechin gallate (ECG), (−)-epigallocatechin (EGC), and (−)-epigallocatechin-3-gallate (EGCG). EGCG, the most abundant polyphenolic catechin, is considered the most active catechin, possessing various biological functions in vitro and in vivo [15,192]. Low concentrations of EGCG resulted in significant reduction in ROS generation, which was induced on exposure to environmental carcinogens [193]. However, it had no significant effect on the regulation of the antioxidant enzymes (SOD and CAT) in MCF-7 breast cancer cell lines, but showed up-regulated expression of NQO1, the main detoxification enzyme of phase II [193].

Genistein showed significant antioxidant action and better mitochondrial function in T47D with low ERα/ERβ ratios, whereas no significant antioxidant effect was shown in MCF-7 cells with high ERα/ERβ ratios [194]. Therefore, ERβ is essential for the antioxidant potential of genistein [194].

Curcumin-treated breast cancer cells showed a significant decrease in cell proliferation, mediated by Nrf-2 nuclear translocation, associated with the down-regulation of Flap endonuclease 1

(Fen1), which is a nuclease involved in DNA repair [195]. It also showed ROS scavenging actions in MCF-7 breast cancer cells exposed to nickel oxide nanoparticles [196].

On the other hand, polyphenols presented a pro-oxidant action that was determined by the application of high concentrations, or the presence of, metal ions that mediate the formation of chelates and the oxidation of polyphenols [197–199]. The pro-oxidant effects of polyphenols are involved in their anti-cancer activity. For example, the pro-oxidant activity of polyphenols was correlated with mitochondrial dysfunction and DNA damage mediated by high oxidative stress, and, in turn, resulted in apoptosis [200,201]. In breast cancer cells, 50 μM of soy isoflavone, genistein, showed a pro-oxidant action via mobilization of copper ions that led to DNA damage, an increase in ROS generation, and apoptosis [202]. The pro-oxidant effect of curcumin via ROS generation, in a time-dependent manner, in MCF-7 and MDA-MB-231 breast cancer cell lines, was demonstrated [203]. Additionally, high concentration of EGCG showed a marked increase in ROS generation in Hs578T breast cancer cells [204]. In vivo studies are needed to confirm, as well as explain, the contradictory findings of the antioxidant and the pro-oxidant effects of polyphenols.

7.2. Modulation of Inflammation-Related Factors

Cancer occurs at sites of chronic inflammation, and is proved by the presence of inflammatory cells in cancer [205]. For instance, inflammatory responses from microbial infection represent 15%–20% of cancer death cases worldwide [205], and, therefore, non-steroidal, anti-inflammatory drugs are one option to mitigate cancer deaths arising from inflammatory responses [206,207]. Chronic inflammation can give rise to an aggressive type of breast cancer, inflammatory breast cancer (IBC), which represents 5% of breast cancers and is associated with 8%–10% of breast cancer deaths [208,209].

Polyphenols from blueberry powder present potent in vitro and in vivo inhibitory properties against breast cancer proliferation and metastasis by regulation of interlukin-6 (IL-6) [210]. Polyphenol-enriched blueberry preparation (PEBP) potently inhibited breast cancer proliferation, cell movement, and migration, by targeting inflammatory signaling cascades, including the ERK, AKT, and STAT3 pathways [211]. In this regard, the anti-inflammatory activity of polyphenols may be important mechanisms underlying their anti-cancer and chemopreventive potentials. The anti-inflammatory activity of polyphenols is attributed to their ability to block properties against NF-κB [212], cyclooxygenase (COX-2) [213], and lipoxygenase (LOX) [214] activities.

NF-κB plays a pivotal role in the control of the expression level of inflammation-related cytokines, TNFα and IL-1 [215], as well as up-regulation of COX-2, which is an inducible prostaglandin G/H synthase that is highly expressed in numerous tumor cells [216]. The possible mechanisms by which dietary polyphenols block the up-regulation of NF-κB involve the inhibition of phosphorylation and/or proteasomal degradation of IκBs, inhibition of the liberation of NF-κB dimers from the cytoplasm into the nucleus, and hampering the interaction between NF-κB and target DNA [217,218]. Curcumin [219], green tea rich polyphenols [220], quercetin [221], and resveratrol [222] showed potent anti-cancer activities by blocking the expression level of NF-κB.

The potential of curcumin to inhibit cancer metastasis has been confirmed in vitro using breast cancer cells, as well as in vivo, using immunodeficient mice. In this study, the authors showed the crosslink between curcumin and the inhibition of the expression level of MMPs via down-regulation of the expression level of NF-κB and transcription factor AP-1, as well as inhibition of the phosphorylation of NF-κB, in turn, reducing the phosphorylation of IκB and p65 [223]. The anti-metastatic action of curcumin in breast cancer cells is explained by its inhibition of the nuclear translocation of NF-κB via dephosphorylation of IκB, resulting in the down-regulation of inflammation-related cytokines, such as CXCL1/2 [224].

Green tea catechin, EGCG, stimulated apoptosis in γ-radiation-exposed breast cancer cells, and was associated with the inactivation of NF-κB [225]. Combined treatment with EGCG and curcumin potently reduced the expression of the BCSC marker, CD44, via dephosphorylation of

STAT3, and, in turn, prevented its nuclear translocation and its interaction with NF-κB for activation of target transcription factors [226].

The activation of STAT3 is essential for the proliferation and metastasis of a wide range of cancer, and its high expression is indicative of a poor prognosis. Targeting the STAT3 pathway is considered one of the key therapeutic approaches to block cancer proliferation and metastasis [227,228]. The inhibitory activity of silibinin against the phosphorylation of STAT3 has been demonstrated in preclinical studies in various cancers [229]; however, further clinical trials are needed to fully characterize silibinin activity as a STAT3 inhibitor.

In nude mice inoculated with MCF-7 cells, oral administration of xanthohumol, a prenylated flavonoid that was purified from hops (*Humulus lupulus* L.), resulted in a significant reduction in infiltration of mononuclear and polymorphonuclear inflammatory cells, an increase in the percentage of apoptosis, a reduction in the density of microvessels, and a decrease in nuclear and cytoplasmic NF-κβ expression and cytoplasmic staining of Pi-Iκβα, compared to tumors in untreated control mice [230].

7.3. Modulation of the Estrogen Receptor

Estrogens are a commonly-listed human carcinogen, and high exposure to estrogen is highly related to the incidence of breast cancer, via increased cell proliferation through interaction with ER [231]. Patients with breast cancer show a high level of estrogen in the circulating blood [232]. Simply, breast cancer could be treated by inhibition of this action, as well as the production of estrogens, or interference, in the binding to ER [233,234]. ER targeting can be performed using classical drugs, such as raloxifene and tamoxifen, which are collectively called selective estrogen receptor modulators (SERMs) and are effectively applied in pre-and post-menopausal women [235].

Two types of ER, ERα and ERβ, are differentially expressed in organs, and ERα is highly expressed in the uterus and is involved in the proliferation of the endometrium, whereas ERβ is abundant in mammary glands, ovary, and the hypothalamus [236]. ERβ was involved in the induction of various transcription factors that are related to the modulation of cell proliferation and death, the cell cycle, and differentiation [237,238].

Owing to the similarity in the structure of non-steroidal compounds or phytoestrogens and E2, several phytoestrogens were shown to bind to ERα and ERβ. The binding affinity of genistein to ERβ is about 7–48-fold higher than to ERα [239–241]. In contrast, a flavonoid, xanthohumol, showed potent anti-cancer activity against luminal-type breast cancer by inhibiting the interaction between the growth of luminal-type guanine nucleotide-exchange protein 3 (BIG3) and tumor suppressor prohibitin 2 (PHB2) [242]. The released PHB2 binds to the nuclear and cytoplasmic ERα, and blocks E2-associated signaling pathways, thereby inhibiting the proliferation of ERα-positive breast cancer cells in vitro and in vivo.

The flavonoid compound, ellagic acid, which is widely distributed in berries, grapes, and nuts, possesses phenolic rings and ortho-dihydroxyl groups involved in the recognition of ER receptors [243]. Ellagic acid significantly reduced cancer size and occurrence in ACI rats exposed to estrogen with decreased CYP1A1 activity [244].

Similar to most flavones, including fisetin, apigenin, and kaempferol, morin (3,5,7,2′,4′-pentahydroxyflavone), a flavonol compound that is found in copious amounts in onion, mill (*Prunus dulcis*), and fig (*Chlorophora tinctoria*), showed strong inhibitory effects against oxidative stress [245]. Morin possesses hydroxyl groups in the 7- and 4′-positions, parallel to the 3- and 4′-positions, on synthetic estrogen diethylstilbestrol (DES), and is therefore considered a phytoestrogen [246].

Luteolin (3′,4′,5,7-tetrahydroxyflavone) potentially decreased the expression of insulin-like growth factor-1 (IGF-1), which correlated with MCF-7 proliferation. This effect was attributed to the capacity of luteolin to down-regulate ERα expression [247]. Knockdown of ERα led to the abolishment of the potency of luteolin to inhibit MCF-7 cell proliferation.

The chemical structure (2 hydroxyl groups and phenolic ring) of quercetin is akin to the structure of estrogen and it is considered a phytoestrogen that potentially binds to ER and modulates cell cycle progression. It also presents anti-cancer actions via estrogen-related pathways [248,249].

Resveratrol inhibits the growth of various breast cancer cells (MCF-7 and MBA-MB-231) via modulation of the expression level of various transcription factors associated with cell cycle regulation, apoptosis, metastasis, and angiogenesis. These actions were more pronounced in ER^+ cells than in ER^- cells, assuring the importance of the binding to ER in the enhancement of the anti-cancer activity of resveratrol against breast cancer [250].

In ERα-positive MCF-7 cell lines, the physiological dose of EGCG induced a significant reduction in cell growth, which was correlated with the reduction in the protein levels of ERα and IGF-1 receptor (IGF-1R), as well as the up-regulation of p53 and p21 [251]. Whereas, in ERα-positive T47D cell lines expressing mutated p53, EGCG treatment had no significant inhibitory effects on cell growth; however, EGCG treatment enhanced the expression of ERα, and increased the sensitivity of cells to treatment with an ERα antagonist, tamoxifen. Moreover, EGCG-exposed ERα-negative MDA-MB-231 cell lines, expressing mutated p53, showed a marked decrease in cell growth and up-regulation of ERα and IGF-1R, which resulted in an increased responsiveness of the cell to tamoxifen treatment [251].

There are paradoxical findings on the effect of genistein on the proliferation of ER^+ and ER^- breast cancer cells that are associated with concentration of genistein [252,253]. For instance, ER^+ and ER^- breast cancer cells treated with a high concentration of genistein showed a significant reduction in growth rate, while lower concentrations enhanced their growth rate. Similarly, tamoxifen and SERMs showed controversial effects, which correlated with the applied concentration and the type of tissue [254].

Taken together, the application of phytoestrogens is intricate, due to the controversial effects attributed to variations in doses [255]. Therefore, further comprehensive research is needed to characterize the side effects of using these phytoestrogens, which may be beneficial for endocrine disorder-related public health in the future.

7.4. Modulation of the Aromatase Activity

Aromatase, an estrogen synthase, belongs to the cytochrome P450 enzyme family [256,257]. It is highly expressed in breast cancer tissue compared to normal breast tissue [232]. Aromatase inhibitors showed a better capacity for the treatment of breast cancer when compared to tamoxifen [258]. Aromatase stimulation is correlated with ER-independent malignancy [259]. The efficiency of various synthetic aromatase inhibitors in the clinical application of breast cancer treatment, in ER^+ patients at the postmenopausal stage, was demonstrated [260].

Owing to the similarity between the A and C rings of flavonoids with D and C rings of androstenedione, which is the substrate of aromatase, as well as to the potential of the C4 position's oxo-group to interact with the heme group of the aromatase, flavonoid compounds potently inhibit aromatase activity [261]. Flavones and isoflavones were reported to bind to estrogen receptors and to the active sites of the aromatase [262]. The potential of flavonoids to influence the promoter activity of aromatase was demonstrated [263,264], additionally their role in the regulation of breast cancer's aromatase expression has been proven [265].

Aromatase activity is markedly inhibited by luteolin [266], but is up-regulated by hesperetin (3′,5,7-trihydroxy-4-methoxyflavanone) [265]. The imidazolyl quinoline derivative of flavonoids, XHN27, a potent aromatase inhibitor, significantly suppresses the proliferation of breast cancer T47D cells, determined after screening a library of 7000 compounds [267].

7.5. Modulation of the Cell Cycle

During carcinogenesis, there is an imbalance between the action of cell cycle progression proteins and cell cycle arrest proteins, resulting in marked cell division and proliferation. Cell cycle progression can be mediated by cyclins and cyclin-dependent kinases (CDK), and its arrest is mediated by CDK inhibitors (CDKi), such as p15, p16, p21, p27, p53, and retinoblastoma tumor suppressor protein (RB). Loss of function of RB, a tumor suppressor gene, is involved in resistance to chemotherapeutic drugs, such as tamoxifen.

Numerous polyphenol-treated cancer cells showed down-regulation of CDK, as well as modulation of CDKi, consequently leading to cell cycle arrest and apoptosis at the G2/M phase [268,269]. In breast cancer cells, the synergy between E2 and IGF-1 is essential for cell cycle progression via up-regulation of Cdk2, Cdk4, and cyclin D1 [270].

In breast and colon cancer cells, ginnalins A–C polyphenols isolated from *Acer saccharum* Marsh. sugar and red maple (*Acer rubrum* L.) species showed remarkable anti-cancer activities via induction of cell cycle arrest, in particular, in the S- and G_2/M-phases, as well as down-regulation of cyclins A and D1 proteins [268].

The potency of quercetin-3-methyl ether was exploited to induce cell cycle arrest in the G2/M phase, and up-regulation of the phosphorylation level of cyclin B1 (Ser 147) to potently block the growth of breast cancer cells that are resistant or sensitive to lapatinib, a reversible inhibitor of EGFR and HER2 [271]. Therefore, quercetin-3-methyl ether is considered a naturally occurring polyphenol that overcomes the resistance against the common anti-breast-cancer drug, lapatinib. In addition, quercetin-exposed MDA-MB-453 breast cancer cells showed a marked increase in the number of cells in the G2/M phase and a reduction in cell populations in the G1 phase [138].

Quercetin led to down-regulation of cyclin A and cyclin B, and a significant up-regulation of CDK inhibitors, including p53, p21CIP1/waf1, and p27Kip1 [272,273]. As a part of its anti-cancer activities, resveratrol also resulted in the modulation of cell cycle and apoptosis [274].

Curcumin possesses anti-cancer activities via the modulation of apoptosis and the cell cycle [275]. Curcumin-treated human MCF-7 breast cancer cells showed a drastic reduction in proliferation, mediated by cell-cycle arrest in the G_2/M phase [275]. Curcumin treatment led to apoptotic cell death, which was confirmed by the detection of a high fraction of cells accumulated in the G_0/G_1 phase, as well as by the up-regulation of Bax through a p53-dependent mechanism [276]. It was evidenced that curcumin can induce the monopolar spindle formation, accumulation of mitotic arrest deficient 2 (Mad2), and Mad3/BubR1, thereby activating the mitotic checkpoint [277].

Apigenin (4′,5,7-trihydroxyflavone), a flavone, significantly inhibited the proliferation of SK-BR-3 breast cancer cells through inhibition of cell cycle progression at the G2M phase, with the up-regulation of $p21^{Cip1}$, as well as down-regulation of CDK1 and cyclin A and B [278].

EGCG inhibited the division and growth of cancer cells via dephosphorylation of the myosin II regulatory light chain (MRLC), which is essential for contractile ring formation [279]. Consequently, EGCG-treated cells showed high percentages of cell population in the G2/M phase and a decrease in cell growth and division. Of note, EGCG-induced dephosphorylation of MRLC was attributed to its interaction with metastasis-associated 67 kDa laminin receptor (67LR) [279].

7.6. Modulation of Apoptosis

Apoptosis is a type of programmed cell death, which is essential for various physiological processes, such as homeostasis and development. Intrinsic or mitochondrial type apoptosis is modulated by the B cell lymphoma (Bcl-2) family proteins [280]. The extrinsic apoptotic pathway is activated by binding of death receptors with their ligands, such as binding of tumor necrosis factor receptor 1 (TNFR1) and tumor necrosis factor (TNF), and the recruitment of receptor-interacting protein (RIP), TNFR1-associated death domain protein (TRADD), and TNFR-associated factor (TRAF), or binding of death-inducing signaling complexes [280].

Apoptosis plays important roles in the potential of quercetin to inhibit the proliferation of human MDA-MB-453 breast cancer cells that are mediated by up-regulation of BAX and down-regulation of Bcl-2 expression, as well as cleavage of caspase-3 and PARP proteins [138]. Quercetin-exposed MCF-7 breast cancer cells showed apoptotic cell death with a reduction in mitochondrial membrane potential, down-regulation of Bcl-2 protein, and activation of the initiator caspases, caspase-8 and caspase-9, and the effector caspase, caspase-6, which were attributed to the binding of quercetin to the Fas/CD95 receptor [273]. Moreover, quercetin significantly inhibited MD-MBA-231 breast cancer cells through the activation of caspase-3/-8/-9 [281].

Apigenin-treated SK-BR-3 breast cancer cells showed apoptotic cell death, evidenced by the up-regulation of p53 and its downstream effectors, BAX and cytochrome c [278]. A recent study detected a dramatic decrease in cell proliferation, as well as significant stimulation of apoptosis signaling pathways, such as PARP cleavage and caspase-8 and -9 cleavages in apigenin-treated SKBR3 breast cancer cells [282]. This study concluded that STAT3 inhibition mediated apigenin-enhanced apoptosis signaling pathways in SKBR3 cells.

On treatment with green tea polyphenols and EGCG, a significant reduction in cell growth associated with apoptotic changes, such as stimulation of BAX, cleavage of PARP, and down-regulation of Bcl-2, was observed in MD-MB-231 human breast cancer cells [283].

Resveratrol treatment led to apoptotic cell death in T47D breast cancer cells via activation of CD95L, which is involved in the extrinsic apoptotic pathway [284], as well as activation of p53 [285]. PARP cleavage was significantly induced in resveratrol-treated MDA-MB-231 cells, and was correlated with the activation of caspase-3 [286]. Moreover, resveratrol induced apoptosis in various malignant cells (including MDA-MB-231 and MDA-MB-468 cell lines), via inhibition of Src tyrosine kinase activity and blockage of STAT3 activation [287]. In estrogen-positive breast cancer cells, resveratrol markedly reduced growth rate by stimulating apoptosis through reduction of the ratio of Bcl2/BAX, which was independent of the presence of E2 [288]. Therefore, resveratrol is considered a potential and safe chemopreventive alternative to hormone replacement therapy (HRT), in particular, in postmenopausal women, and against hormone-dependent breast cancer.

Genistein-exposed MCF-7 cells showed up-regulation of BAX and reduction of Bcl-2 at the protein and mRNA levels, resulting in a reduction in the Bcl-2/BAX ratio [289]. This effect is mediated by blocking the activation of the IGF receptor (IGFR), as well as the phosphorylation of AKT.

Fisetin (3,3′,4′,7-tetrahydroxyflavone), a flavonoid, which is widely distributed in fruits and vegetables, induced an uncommon form of apoptosis in caspase-voided MCF-7 cells characterized by the activation of caspase-7/-8/-9, cleaved PARP, mitochondrial membrane depolarization, up-regulation of p53, and break in the plasma membrane, while no change was detected in DNA or phosphatidylserine (PS) [290]. These apoptotic changes were abolished upon treatment with a pan-caspase inhibitor, z-VAD-fmk.

7.7. Modulation of the Multidrug Resistance (MDR)

Despite the potency of anti-cancer drugs in decreasing cancer size, a few populations of CSCs potently resist chemotherapy and lead to tumor recurrence and MDR [291]. The crosslink between the virulence of CSCs and MDR is correlated with reduction of intracellular concentrations of anti-cancer drugs, continual growth, and cancer relapse [292].

The emergence of MDR is linked to over-expression of the ATP-binding cassette (ABC) transporters family, which is composed of energy-dependent transporter proteins, which act as pumps. ABC transporters are involved in drug efflux, thereby decreasing in intracellular concentrations [293]. Transporter proteins include various proteins, such as multidrug resistant-associated proteins (MRPs), mitoxantrone resistance protein (MXR or ABCG2), and P-glycoprotein (P-gp) or ABCB1.

EGCG treatment leads to the accumulation of rhodamine-123 dye in MDR cell lines and an increase in the intracellular concentration of anti-cancer drugs [294]. Moreover, a group of six common polyphenols (naringenin, silymarin, daidzein, quercetin, resveratrol, and hesperetin) potently inhibit the activity of MRP family proteins, thereby inhibiting efflux [295].

Curcumin treatment leads to down-regulation of MDR-1b expression by its interaction with PI3K/AKT/NF-κB signaling [296]. Moreover, it enhances the sensitivity of MDR cell lines to chemotherapeutic agents, such as cisplatin, vincristine, doxorubicin, tamoxifen, and mitoxantrone [297].

7.8. Modulation of Signaling Pathways Related to Self-Renewal Capacity and Transformation of CSCs

$CD44^{+}/CD24^{low}$ BCSCs showed a high degree of tumorigenicity with enhanced sphere formation and self-renewal capacities [298,299]. Embryonic development-related signaling pathways, such as Notch, Wnt/β-catenin, and Hedgehog, were significantly implicated in the self-renewal property of BCSCs [300]. We will discuss the potential of polyphenols to interfere with the stemness-related signaling pathways below.

7.8.1. Hedgehog (Hh) Signaling Pathway

Hh, encoding secreted proteins, modulates cellular differentiation, proliferation, and development processes via autocrine- and paracrine-mediated signaling pathways [301]. There are three main mammalian homologs of the Hh gene, namely Sonic hedgehog (Shh), Indian hedgehog, and Desert hedgehog [302]. The interaction of the Hh proteins with the transmembrane protein, patched (PTC), leads to activation or phosphorylation of another transmembrane protein, smoothened (SMO) [303]. The Hh pathway is correlated with the development and maintenance of CSCs in breast cancer, myeloid leukaemia, glioma, gastric cancer, and multiple myeloma [304–307]. Therefore, the discovery of new inhibitors targeting the Hh signaling pathway is a potent anti-cancer strategy and is under clinical trials (phases I and II) [308].

Cyclopamine, extracted from *Veratrum californicum* or corn lily, was the first discovered phytochemical that inhibits Hh signaling pathways by inactivation of SMO [306,309]. Cyclopamine inhibits breast CSC proliferation and mammosphere formation [304].

Genistein potently inhibits the growth of $CD44^{+}/CD24^{-}$ BCSCs by the notable down-regulation of mRNA levels and the protein levels of SMO and Gli1, which are key factors for modulation of Hedgehog-Gli1 signaling [310].

7.8.2. Notch Signaling Pathway

Notch proteins are composed of four transmembrane glycoproteins, namely, Notch1, Notch2, Notch3, and Notch4, and also have five ligands, Delta-like1, Delta-like3, Delta-like4, Jagged1, and Jagged2 [311]. The Notch signaling pathway is involved in cellular proliferation and differentiation [312]. Its activation is mediated by the interaction between the extracellular domains of receptors with ligands and the release of the Notch intracellular domain (NICD) into the nucleus through proteolytic cleavage.

Resveratrol leads to down-regulation of Notch proteins only at the post-translational level, a decrease in mRNA levels of pre-TCRα and HES1, an increase in p53, and a reduction of PI3K/AKT signaling in MOLT-4 acute lymphoblastic leukemia cells [313].

7.8.3. Wingless/Integration 1 (Wnt) and the β-Catenin Signaling Pathway

The Wnt/β-Catenin signaling pathway is considered one of the essential signaling pathways for the self-renewal of BCSCs [314]. β-Catenin is an integral effector of the Wnt signaling pathway in the nucleus. In response to Wnt activation, stabilized β-catenin moves to the nucleus and activates target genes by its interaction with the TC/LEF transcription factor [314,315]. Glycogen synthase kinase3β (GSK3β), axin, casein kinase1α, and adenomatous polyposis coli (APC) protein complex are linked to regulation of the intracellular level of β-Catenin.

EGCG significantly inhibits the formation and invasiveness of breast cancer by suppressing the Wnt signaling pathway and reducing c-myc expression [316]; additionally, it potently reduces nuclear β-Catenin [317]. Curcumin also targets β-Catenin in the caspase-mediated mechanism in colon cancer [318]. Sulforaphane, a product of the conversion of glucoraphanin, which is the main glucosinolate in broccoli and its sprouts, has potent chemoprevention activity against a wide range of cancers [319–321].

Sulforaphane-exposed human cervical carcinoma and hepatocarcinoma cell lines show a significant increase in apoptosis by degradation of the β-Catenin protein [322]. Sulforaphane potently eliminates BCSCs in vitro and in vivo by targeting the Wnt/β-Catenin-mediated self-renewal property of BCSCs [321].

Piperine, an alkaloid isolated from black pepper (*Piper nigrum*) and long pepper (*Piper longum*), shows potent in vivo reduction of lung metastasis [323]; in addition, it inhibits the self-renewal property of BCSCs through down-regulation of the Wnt signaling pathway [324].

Oxymatrine, an alkaloid isolated from *Sophora japonica*, markedly decreases the proliferation of breast cancer and its drastic reduction of the growth of the sorted side population (SP) of CSCs was demonstrated [325]. In addition, it significantly reduced the activity of the Wnt/β-catenin signaling pathway.

7.9. Modulation of Autophagy

Autophagy plays a pivotal role in maintaining stem cell characteristics. Conditional deletion of Atg7 leads to a loss in properties, and disturbance in hematopoietic stem cell function [326]. In BCSCs, a high basal level of autophagy was detected in ALDH1+ cell populations [327]. Autophagy is essential for the enhancement of the invasiveness and metastatic properties of glioblastoma stem cells, which are mediated by DRAM1 and p62 [328].

Rottlerin significantly inhibits the growth of human BCSCs and induces autophagy via up-regulation of Atg12 and Beclin-1, and conversion of LC3-I into LC3-II [329]. Up-regulation of BAX, reduction in phosphorylation of AKT, mTOR, and AMPK, and a significant decrease in the expression of anti-apoptotic factors, were demonstrated over a long period of time of rottlerin treatment. shRNAs targeting Atg7 and Beclin-1 abrogated the capacity of rottlerin to induce autophagy. Autophagy inhibitors, 3-MA, Baf-A1, and cycloheximide, alleviate rottlerin-induced apoptosis and phosphorylation of AMPK. Inactivation of AMPK was concomitant with the down-regulation of Beclin-1, Atg12, and LC3.

Resveratrol blocks the growth of BCSCs and number of mammospheres [330]. It showed significant up-regulation of LC3-II, Atg7, and Beclin1, which is concomitant with cell toxicity.

7.10. Modulation of the Epithelial Mesenchymal Transition (EMT)

EMT is an intricate developmental process, in which special differentiated polarized epithelial cells undergo morphogenesis via loss of their differentiation characteristics, such as cell–cell adhesion, cell polarity, immotile status, and the transformation into mesenchymal cells with invasive and migratory properties [331,332].

During EMT, there is a decrease in the expression of epithelial markers, such as γ-catenin and E-cadherin, and up-regulation of mesenchymal markers, including vimentin, N-cadherin, fibronectin, and MMP-2/9. In contrast, mesenchymal-epithelial transition (MET) takes place after the migration and invasion of cells to their designated sites [333]. E-cadherin, encoded by CDH1, plays a pivotal role in the inhibition of tumor invasiveness and malignancy, as well as suppression of EMT.

There are various transcription factors, the Snail superfamily of zinc-finger transcriptional repressors, such as Snail 1 and Snail 2 (also known as slug); the ZEB family, such as ZEB1 (also known as TCF8 and δEF1) and ZEB2 (also known as Smad-interacting protein 1 (SIP1); and basic helix-loop-helix (bHLH), such as E47 (also known as TCF3), TCF4 (also known as E2-2), and TWIST1 [331], which represent transcription repressors of the CDH1 gene, and, thereby, inhibit tumor malignancy and invasiveness.

Up-regulation of the EMT transcription repressor is induced by a complicated signaling network that is enhanced by receptor tyrosine kinases (RTKs) and transforming growth factor β (TGFβ) [334]. The NF-κB signaling pathway is involved in the activation of Snail, Slug, ZEB-1/2, and Twist, as well as the up-regulation of mesenchymal markers, including MMPs, fibronectin, and vimentin [335].

Resveratrol treatment triggers apoptosis and recovers the expression of γ-catenin and E-cadherin in tamoxifen-resistant breast cancer cells (MCF-7/TR) via targeting of TGFβ and its downstream effector, Smad [336]. Moreover, resveratrol recovered epithelial characteristics in EGF-transformed breast cancer cell lines via repression of the ERK1/2 signaling pathways [337].

Baicalin and baicalein, the main flavones isolated from *Scutellaria baicalensis*, potently inhibit EMT by targeting TGF-β1, and the inactivation of NF-κB-induced activation of Slug [338]. Furthermore, Chrysin (5,7-dihydroxyflavone), a flavone isolated from passion flower (*Passiflora caerulea*) and honeycomb of *Apis mellifera*, significantly inhibits the metastatic and invasive characteristics of TNBC through down-regulation of Slug, Snail, and Vimentin, and inhibition of MMP-10 via blocking of the PI3K-AKT signaling pathway [339].

Honokiol, isolated from seed cones from *Magnolia grandiflora* led to inhibition of EMT, which was mediated by inactivation of STAT3 and, in turn, blocked off the repressive action of ZEB1 on E-cadherin [340].

To sum up, several interesting studies have showed the capacity of polyphenols to potently restore epithelial characteristics in transformed breast cancer cells, and prevented the emergence of CSC phenotype and drug resistance.

8. Conclusions and Perspectives

In this review, we provide detailed information on the broad spectrum of mechanistic actions of polyphenols against breast cancer and CSCs. Many studies revealed that apoptosis- and/or autophagy-related signaling pathways are modulated by polyphenol treatment. Pharmacological inhibition of autophagy plays a pivotal role in polyphenol-induced cell death. We also explained the potential of polyphenols to target breast cancer and CSCs via modulation of various stemness-related signaling pathways and transcription factors.

This review provides useful information that will guide future research, which will provide strategies for efficient, polyphenol-based prevention, or treatment, of breast cancer. Further efforts are needed to resolve several remaining hurdles, such as the variations in applied dose, the large discrepancy between the in vitro and in vivo doses, and exposure time. Moreover, a better understanding of the interconnection between apoptosis and autophagy in the polyphenol-mediated treatment of breast cancer is needed to characterize the key factors involved in the actions of polyphenols. However, the progress in technology continues to provide answers to unresolved questions. To determine the potential of polyphenols in curing breast cancer in clinical trials, discovered polyphenols need to be elucidated. Chemotherapy remains.

In fact, there is a paucity of information related to the application of polyphenols as chemopreventive compounds. What lies ahead is the application of previously-discovered polyphenols in the treatment of breast cancer in clinical trials. Collectively, the therapeutic applications of polyphenols in breast cancer are promising, as these compounds present various mechanistic actions and their clinical applications need to be tested.

Acknowledgments: This work was supported by grants from the National Research Foundation (NRF) funded by the Korean government (2013M3A9D3045880 and 2015R1A5A1009701), by a grant (No. 312062-05) from the Bio-industry Technology Development Program, Ministry of Agriculture, Food and Rural Affairs, Republic of Korea, and by the 2016 KU Brain Pool of Konkuk University.

Author Contributions: Ahmed Abdal Dayem designed this work, collected the data, and co-wrote the manuscript, Hye Yeon Choi, Gwang-Mo Yang, Kyeongseok Kim, and Subbroto Kumar Saha collected the data and helped edit the manuscript. Ssang-Goo Cho designed the work, collected and reorganized the data, and wrote and edited the manuscript.

References

1. De Flora, S.; Ferguson, L.R. Overview of mechanisms of cancer chemopreventive agents. *Mutat. Res. Fundam. Mol. Mech. Mutagen.* **2005**, *591*, 8–15. [CrossRef] [PubMed]

2. De Flora, S.; Izzotti, A.; D'Agostini, F.; Balansky, R.M.; Noonan, D.; Albini, A. Multiple points of intervention in the prevention of cancer and other mutation-related diseases. *Mutat. Res. Fundam. Mol. Mech. Mutagen.* **2001**, *480*, 9–22. [CrossRef]
3. Mocanu, M.M.; Nagy, P.; Szöllősi, J. Chemoprevention of breast cancer by dietary polyphenols. *Molecules* **2015**, *20*, 22578–22620. [CrossRef] [PubMed]
4. Ui, A.; Kuriyama, S.; Kakizaki, M.; Sone, T.; Nakaya, N.; Ohmori-Matsuda, K.; Hozawa, A.; Nishino, Y.; Tsuji, I. Green tea consumption and the risk of liver cancer in Japan: The Ohsaki Cohort study. *Cancer Causes Control* **2009**, *20*, 1939–1945. [CrossRef] [PubMed]
5. Wu, Y.; Zhang, L.; Na, R.; Xu, J.; Xiong, Z.; Zhang, N.; Dai, W.; Jiang, H.; Ding, Q. Plasma genistein and risk of prostate cancer in Chinese population. *Int. Urol. Nephrol.* **2015**, *47*, 965–970. [CrossRef] [PubMed]
6. Crozier, A.; Jaganath, I.B.; Clifford, M.N. Dietary phenolics: Chemistry, bioavailability and effects on health. *Natl. Prod. Rep.* **2009**, *26*, 1001–1043. [CrossRef] [PubMed]
7. Sharma, R. Polyphenols in health and disease: Practice and mechanisms of benefits. *Polyphen. Hum. Health Dis. Acad. San Diego* **2014**, 757–778.
8. Halbwirth, H. The creation and physiological relevance of divergent hydroxylation patterns in the flavonoid pathway. *Int. J. Mol. Sci.* **2010**, *11*, 595–621. [CrossRef] [PubMed]
9. Danesi, F.; Kroon, P.A.; Saha, S.; de Biase, D.; D'Antuono, L.F.; Bordoni, A. Mixed pro-and anti-oxidative effects of pomegranate polyphenols in cultured cells. *Int. J. Mol. Sci.* **2014**, *15*, 19458–19471. [CrossRef] [PubMed]
10. Hsieh, S.R.; Cheng, W.C.; Su, Y.M.; Chiu, C.H.; Liou, Y.M. Molecular targets for anti-oxidative protection of green tea polyphenols against myocardial ischemic injury. *BioMedicine* **2014**, *4*, 23. [CrossRef] [PubMed]
11. Lewandowska, U.; Szewczyk, K.; Owczarek, K.; Hrabec, Z.; Podsędek, A.; Sosnowska, D.; Hrabec, E. Procyanidins from evening primrose (oenothera paradoxa) defatted seeds inhibit invasiveness of breast cancer cells and modulate the expression of selected genes involved in angiogenesis, metastasis, and apoptosis. *Nutr. Cancer* **2013**, *65*, 1219–1231. [CrossRef] [PubMed]
12. Duluc, L.; Jacques, C.; Soleti, R.; Andriantsitohaina, R.; Simard, G. Delphinidin inhibits VEGF induced-mitochondrial biogenesis and Akt activation in endothelial cells. *Int. J. Biochem. Cell Biol.* **2014**, *53*, 9–14. [CrossRef] [PubMed]
13. Symonds, E.L.; Konczak, I.; Fenech, M. The Australian fruit Illawarra plum (*Podocarpus elatus* Endl., Podocarpaceae) inhibits telomerase, increases histone deacetylase activity and decreases proliferation of colon cancer cells. *Br. J. Nutr.* **2013**, *109*, 2117–2125. [CrossRef] [PubMed]
14. Steward, W.; Brown, K. Cancer chemoprevention: A rapidly evolving field. *Br. J. Cancer* **2013**, *109*, 1–7. [CrossRef] [PubMed]
15. Surh, Y.J. Cancer chemoprevention with dietary phytochemicals. *Nat. Rev. Cancer* **2003**, *3*, 768–780. [CrossRef] [PubMed]
16. Minamoto, T.; Mai, M.; Ronai, Z.E. Environmental factors as regulators and effectors of multistep carcinogenesis. *Carcinogenesis* **1999**, *20*, 519–527. [CrossRef] [PubMed]
17. Galati, G.; Teng, S.; Moridani, M.Y.; Chan, T.S.; O'Brien, P.J. Cancer chemoprevention and apoptosis mechanisms induced by dietary polyphenolics. *Drug Metab. Drug Interact.* **2000**, *17*, 311–350. [CrossRef]
18. Guengerich, F.P. Metabolism of chemical carcinogens. *Carcinogenesis* **2000**, *21*, 345–351. [CrossRef] [PubMed]
19. Frassinetti, S.; Della Croce, C.M.; Caltavuturo, L.; Longo, V. Antimutagenic and antioxidant activity of *Lisosan G* in *Saccharomyces cerevisiae*. *Food Chem.* **2012**, *135*, 2029–2034. [CrossRef] [PubMed]
20. Słoczyńska, K.; Powroźnik, B.; Pękala, E.; Waszkielewicz, A.M. Antimutagenic compounds and their possible mechanisms of action. *J. Appl. Genet.* **2014**, *55*, 273–285. [CrossRef] [PubMed]
21. Rodeiro, I.; Donato, M.T.; Jimenez, N.; Garrido, G.; Molina-Torres, J.; Menendez, R.; Castell, J.V.; Gómez-Lechón, M.J. Inhibition of human p450 enzymes by natural extracts used in traditional medicine. *Phytother. Res.* **2009**, *23*, 279–282. [CrossRef] [PubMed]
22. Basheer, L.; Kerem, Z. Interactions between cyp3a4 and dietary polyphenols. *Oxid. Med. Cell. Longev.* **2015**, *2015*, 854015. [CrossRef] [PubMed]
23. Munday, R.; Munday, C.M. Induction of phase ii detoxification enzymes in rats by plant-derived isothiocyanates: Comparison of allyl isothiocyanate with sulforaphane and related compounds. *J. Agric. Food Chem.* **2004**, *52*, 1867–1871. [CrossRef] [PubMed]

24. Kou, X.; Kirberger, M.; Yang, Y.; Chen, N. Natural products for cancer prevention associated with nrf2-ARE pathway. *Food Sci. Hum. Wellness* **2013**, *2*, 22–28. [CrossRef]
25. Lu, F.; Zahid, M.; Wang, C.; Saeed, M.; Cavalieri, E.L.; Rogan, E.G. Resveratrol prevents estrogen-DNA adduct formation and neoplastic transformation in MCF-10F cells. *Cancer Prev. Res.* **2008**, *1*, 135–145. [CrossRef] [PubMed]
26. Niu, G.; Chen, X. Vascular endothelial growth factor as an anti-angiogenic target for cancer therapy. *Curr. Drug Targets* **2010**, *11*, 1000–1017. [CrossRef] [PubMed]
27. Wu, S.; Huang, Y.; Yeh, C.; Tsai, M.; Liao, C.; Cheng, W.; Chen, W.; Lin, K. Cathepsin H regulated by the thyroid hormone receptors associate with tumor invasion in human hepatoma cells. *Oncogene* **2011**, *30*, 2057–2069. [CrossRef] [PubMed]
28. Van Der Stappen, J.W.; Williams, A.C.; Maciewicz, R.A.; Paraskeva, C. Activation of cathepsin B, secreted by a colorectal cancer cell line requires low pH and is mediated by cathepsin D. *Int. J. Cancer* **1996**, *67*, 547–554. [CrossRef]
29. Nouh, M.A.; Mohamed, M.M.; El-Shinawi, M.; Shaalan, M.A.; Cavallo-Medved, D.; Khaled, H.M.; Sloane, B.F. Cathepsin B: A potential prognostic marker for inflammatory breast cancer. *J. Transl. Med.* **2011**, *9*, 1. [CrossRef] [PubMed]
30. Zhang, C.; Sun, J.B.; Liu, D.C.; Cui, Y.Q.; Liu, S.; Sun, H.C. Preliminary research on the pathological role of cathepsin-B in subcutaneous heteroplastic pancreatic carcinoma in nude mice. *Chin. Med. J.* **2009**, *122*, 2489. [PubMed]
31. Sevenich, L.; Werner, F.; Gajda, M.; Schurigt, U.; Sieber, C.; Müller, S.; Follo, M.; Peters, C.; Reinheckel, T. Transgenic expression of human cathepsin B promotes progression and metastasis of polyoma-middle-t-induced breast cancer in mice. *Oncogene* **2011**, *30*, 54–64. [CrossRef] [PubMed]
32. Ellis, V.; Behrendt, N.; Danø, K. Plasminogen activation by receptor-bound urokinase. A kinetic study with both cell-associated and isolated receptor. *J. Biol. Chem.* **1991**, *266*, 12752–12758. [PubMed]
33. Curran, S.; Murray, G.I. Matrix metalloproteinases in tumour invasion and metastasis. *J. Pathol.* **1999**, *189*, 300–308. [CrossRef]
34. Van Pham, P. *Breast Cancer Stem Cells & Therapy Resistance*; Springer: Berlin, Germany, 2015.
35. Stewart, B.; Wild, C. World Cancer Report 2014. In *International Agency for Research on Cancer*; World Health Organization: Geneva, Swizerland, 2014.
36. IARC; World Heath Organization. *Globocan: Estimated Cancer Incidence, Mortality, Prevalence Worldwide in 2012*; IARC: Lyon, France, 2014.
37. Torre, L.A.; Bray, F.; Siegel, R.L.; Ferlay, J.; Lortet-Tieulent, J.; Jemal, A. Global cancer statistics, 2012. *CA Cancer J. Clin.* **2015**, *65*, 87–108. [CrossRef] [PubMed]
38. Visvader, J.E.; Lindeman, G.J. Cancer stem cells in solid tumours: Accumulating evidence and unresolved questions. *Nat. Rev. Cancer* **2008**, *8*, 755–768. [CrossRef] [PubMed]
39. Eyler, C.E.; Rich, J.N. Survival of the fittest: Cancer stem cells in therapeutic resistance and angiogenesis. *J. Clin. Oncol.* **2008**, *26*, 2839–2845. [CrossRef] [PubMed]
40. Al-Hajj, M.; Wicha, M.S.; Benito-Hernandez, A.; Morrison, S.J.; Clarke, M.F. Prospective identification of tumorigenic breast cancer cells. *Proc. Natl. Acad. Sci. USA* **2003**, *100*, 3983–3988. [CrossRef] [PubMed]
41. Bartsch, R.; Wenzel, C.; Steger, G.G. Trastuzumab in the management of early and advanced stage breast cancer. *Biologics* **2007**, *1*, 19–31. [PubMed]
42. Vici, P.; Colucci, G.; Gebbia, V.; Amodio, A.; Giotta, F.; Belli, F.; Conti, F.; Gebbia, N.; Pezzella, G.; Valerio, M.R. First-line treatment with epirubicin and vinorelbine in metastatic breast cancer. *J. Clin. Oncol.* **2002**, *20*, 2689–2694. [CrossRef] [PubMed]
43. Holliday, D.L.; Speirs, V. Choosing the right cell line for breast cancer research. *Breast Cancer Res.* **2011**, *13*, 215. [CrossRef] [PubMed]
44. Eisen, M.B.; Brown, P.O. DNA arrays for analysis of gene expression. *Methods Enzymol.* **1999**, *303*, 179–205. [PubMed]
45. Brenton, J.D.; Carey, L.A.; Ahmed, A.A.; Caldas, C. Molecular classification and molecular forecasting of breast cancer: Ready for clinical application? *J. Clin. Oncol.* **2005**, *23*, 7350–7360. [CrossRef] [PubMed]
46. Parker, J.S.; Mullins, M.; Cheang, M.C.; Leung, S.; Voduc, D.; Vickery, T.; Davies, S.; Fauron, C.; He, X.; Hu, Z. Supervised risk predictor of breast cancer based on intrinsic subtypes. *J. Clin. Oncol.* **2009**, *27*, 1160–1167. [CrossRef] [PubMed]

47. Tang, Y.; Wang, Y.; Kiani, M.F.; Wang, B. Classification, treatment strategy, and associated drug resistance in breast cancer. *Clin. Breast Cancer* **2016**. [CrossRef] [PubMed]
48. Sotiriou, C.; Pusztai, L. Gene-expression signatures in breast cancer. *N. Engl. J. Med.* **2009**, *360*, 790–800. [CrossRef] [PubMed]
49. Mitri, Z.; Constantine, T.; O'Regan, R. The HER2 receptor in breast cancer: Pathophysiology, clinical use, and new advances in therapy. *Chemother. Res. Pract.* **2012**, *2012*, 743193. [CrossRef] [PubMed]
50. Carey, L.A.; Dees, E.C.; Sawyer, L.; Gatti, L.; Moore, D.T.; Collichio, F.; Ollila, D.W.; Sartor, C.I.; Graham, M.L.; Perou, C.M. The triple negative paradox: Primary tumor chemosensitivity of breast cancer subtypes. *Clin. Cancer Res.* **2007**, *13*, 2329–2334. [CrossRef] [PubMed]
51. Sirohi, B.; Arnedos, M.; Popat, S.; Ashley, S.; Nerurkar, A.; Walsh, G.; Johnston, S.; Smith, I. Platinum-based chemotherapy in triple-negative breast cancer. *Ann. Oncol.* **2008**, *19*, 1847–1852. [CrossRef] [PubMed]
52. Anders, C.; Carey, L.A. Understanding and treating triple-negative breast cancer. *Oncology* **2008**, *22*, 1233. [PubMed]
53. Fedele, P.; Calvani, N.; Marino, A.; Orlando, L.; Schiavone, P.; Quaranta, A.; Cinieri, S. Targeted agents to reverse resistance to endocrine therapy in metastatic breast cancer: Where are we now and where are we going? *Crit. Rev. Oncol. Hematol.* **2012**, *84*, 243–251. [CrossRef] [PubMed]
54. Vinson, J.A.; Su, X.; Zubik, L.; Bose, P. Phenol antioxidant quantity and quality in foods: Fruits. *J. Agric. Food Chem.* **2001**, *49*, 5315–5321. [CrossRef] [PubMed]
55. Scalbert, A.; Williamson, G. Dietary intake and bioavailability of polyphenols. *J. Nutr.* **2000**, *130*, 2073S–2085S. [PubMed]
56. Parisi, O.; Puoci, F.; Restuccia, D.; Farina, G.; Iemma, F.; Picci, N. Polyphenols and their formulations: Different strategies to overcome the drawbacks associated with their poor stability and bioavailability. *Polyphen. Hum. Health Dis.* **2014**, *4*, 29–45.
57. Yang, C.S.; Lee, M.J.; Chen, L.; Yang, G.Y. Polyphenols as inhibitors of carcinogenesis. *Environ. Health Perspect.* **1997**, *105*, 971. [CrossRef] [PubMed]
58. Dehkharghanian, M.; Lacroix, M.; Vijayalakshmi, M.A. Antioxidant properties of green tea polyphenols encapsulated in caseinate beads. *Dairy Sci. Technol.* **2009**, *89*, 485–499. [CrossRef]
59. Baydar, N.G.; Sagdic, O.; Ozkan, G.; Cetin, S. Determination of antibacterial effects and total phenolic contents of grape (*Vitis vinifera* L.) seed extracts. *Int. J. Food Sci. Technol.* **2006**, *41*, 799–804. [CrossRef]
60. Jung, H.J.; Hwang, I.A.; Sung, W.S.; Kang, H.; Kang, B.S.; Seu, Y.B.; Lee, D.G. Fungicidal effect of resveratrol on human infectious fungi. *Arch. Pharm. Res.* **2005**, *28*, 557–560. [CrossRef] [PubMed]
61. Chávez, J.H.; Leal, P.C.; Yunes, R.A.; Nunes, R.J.; Barardi, C.R.; Pinto, A.R.; Simões, C.M.; Zanetti, C.R. Evaluation of antiviral activity of phenolic compounds and derivatives against rabies virus. *Vet. Microbiol.* **2006**, *116*, 53–59. [CrossRef] [PubMed]
62. Hudson, T.S.; Hartle, D.K.; Hursting, S.D.; Nunez, N.P.; Wang, T.T.; Young, H.A.; Arany, P.; Green, J.E. Inhibition of prostate cancer growth by muscadine grape skin extract and resveratrol through distinct mechanisms. *Cancer Res.* **2007**, *67*, 8396–8405. [CrossRef] [PubMed]
63. Lazzè, M.C.; Pizzala, R.; Gutiérrez Pecharromán, F.J.; Gatòn Garnica, P.; Antolín Rodríguez, J.M.; Fabris, N.; Bianchi, L. Grape waste extract obtained by supercritical fluid extraction contains bioactive antioxidant molecules and induces antiproliferative effects in human colon adenocarcinoma cells. *J. Med. Food* **2009**, *12*, 561–568. [CrossRef] [PubMed]
64. Aquilano, K.; Baldelli, S.; Rotilio, G.; Ciriolo, M.R. Role of nitric oxide synthases in parkinson's disease: A review on the antioxidant and anti-inflammatory activity of polyphenols. *Neurochem. Res.* **2008**, *33*, 2416–2426. [CrossRef] [PubMed]
65. Nichols, J.A.; Katiyar, S.K. Skin photoprotection by natural polyphenols: Anti-inflammatory, antioxidant and DNA repair mechanisms. *Arch. Dermatol. Res.* **2010**, *302*, 71–83. [CrossRef] [PubMed]
66. Gamet-Payrastre, L.; Manenti, S.; Gratacap, M.P.; Tulliez, J.; Chap, H.; Payrastre, B. Flavonoids and the inhibition of PKC and PI 3-kinase. *Gen. Pharmacol. Vasc. Syst.* **1999**, *32*, 279–286. [CrossRef]
67. Richard, T.; Lefeuvre, D.; Descendit, A.; Quideau, S.; Monti, J. Recognition characters in peptide-polyphenol complex formation. *Biochim. Biophys. Acta Gen. Subj.* **2006**, *1760*, 951–958. [CrossRef] [PubMed]
68. Duthie, G.G.; Duthie, S.J.; Kyle, J.A. Plant polyphenols in cancer and heart disease: Implications as nutritional antioxidants. *Nutr. Res. Rev.* **2000**, *13*, 79–106. [CrossRef] [PubMed]

69. Andrade, R.G.; Ginani, J.S.; Lopes, G.K.; Dutra, F.; Alonso, A.; Hermes-Lima, M. Tannic acid inhibits in vitro iron-dependent free radical formation. *Biochimie* **2006**, *88*, 1287–1296. [CrossRef] [PubMed]
70. Baechler, B.J.; Nita, F.; Jones, L.; Frestedt, J.L. A novel liquid multi-phytonutrient supplement demonstrates DNA-protective effects. *Plant Foods Hum. Nutr.* **2009**, *64*, 81–85. [CrossRef] [PubMed]
71. Adlercreutz, H. Phyto-oestrogens and cancer. *Lancet Oncol.* **2002**, *3*, 364–373. [CrossRef]
72. Quideau, S.; Deffieux, D.; Douat-Casassus, C.; Pouységu, L. Plant polyphenols: Chemical properties, biological activities, and synthesis. *Angew. Chem. Int. Ed.* **2011**, *50*, 586–621. [CrossRef] [PubMed]
73. Scalbert, A.; Manach, C.; Morand, C.; Rémésy, C.; Jiménez, L. Dietary polyphenols and the prevention of diseases. *Crit. Rev. Food Sci. Nutr.* **2005**, *45*, 287–306. [CrossRef] [PubMed]
74. García-Lafuente, A.; Guillamón, E.; Villares, A.; Rostagno, M.A.; Martínez, J.A. Flavonoids as anti-inflammatory agents: Implications in cancer and cardiovascular disease. *Inflamm. Res.* **2009**, *58*, 537–552. [CrossRef] [PubMed]
75. Thomasset, S.C.; Berry, D.P.; Garcea, G.; Marczylo, T.; Steward, W.P.; Gescher, A.J. Dietary polyphenolic phytochemicals—Promising cancer chemopreventive agents in humans? A review of their clinical properties. *Int. J. Cancer* **2007**, *120*, 451–458. [CrossRef] [PubMed]
76. Barnes, S.; Prasain, J.; D'Alessandro, T.; Arabshahi, A.; Botting, N.; Lila, M.A.; Jackson, G.; Janle, E.M.; Weaver, C.M. The metabolism and analysis of isoflavones and other dietary polyphenols in foods and biological systems. *Food Funct.* **2011**, *2*, 235–244. [CrossRef] [PubMed]
77. Erdman, J.W.; Balentine, D.; Arab, L.; Beecher, G.; Dwyer, J.T.; Folts, J.; Harnly, J.; Hollman, P.; Keen, C.L.; Mazza, G. Flavonoids and heart health: Proceedings of the ILSI North America Flavonoids Workshop, May 31–June 1, 2005, Washington, DC. *J. Nutr.* **2007**, *137*, 718S–737S. [PubMed]
78. Maru, G.; Kumar, G.; Ghantasala, S.; Tajpara, P. *Polyphenol-Mediated in Vivo Cellular Responses during Carcinogenesis Polyphenols in Human Health and Disease*; Academic Press: Cambridge, MA, USA, 2014.
79. Lee, E.R.; Kang, Y.J.; Choi, H.Y.; Kang, G.H.; Kim, J.H.; Kim, B.W.; Han, Y.S.; Nah, S.Y.; Paik, H.D.; Park, Y.S. Induction of apoptotic cell death by synthetic naringenin derivatives in human lung epithelial carcinoma a549 cells. *Biol. Pharm. Bull.* **2007**, *30*, 2394–2398. [CrossRef] [PubMed]
80. Lee, E.R.; Kang, G.H.; Cho, S.G. Effect of flavonoids on human health: Old subjects but new challenges. *Recent Pat. Biotechnol.* **2007**, *1*, 139–150. [CrossRef] [PubMed]
81. Kim, B.W.; Lee, E.R.; Min, H.M.; Jeong, H.S.; Ahn, J.Y.; Kim, J.H.; Choi, H.Y.; Choi, H.; Kim, E.Y.; Park, S.P. Sustained ERK activation is involved in the kaempferol-induced apoptosis of breast cancer cells and is more evident under 3-D culture condition. *Cancer Biol. Ther.* **2008**, *7*, 1080–1089. [CrossRef] [PubMed]
82. Kim, J.H.; Song, M.; Kang, G.H.; Lee, E.R.; Choi, H.Y.; Lee, C.; Kim, J.H.; Kim, Y.; Koo, B.N.; Cho, S.G. Combined treatment of 3-hydroxyflavone and imatinib mesylate increases apoptotic cell death of imatinib mesylate-resistant leukemia cells. *Leuk. Res.* **2012**, *36*, 1157–1164. [CrossRef] [PubMed]
83. Lee, E.R.; Kim, J.H.; Choi, H.Y.; Jeon, K.; Cho, S.G. Cytoprotective effect of eriodictyol in UV-irradiated keratinocytes via phosphatase-dependent modulation of both the p38 MAPK and Akt signaling pathways. *Cell. Physiol. Biochem.* **2011**, *27*, 513–524. [CrossRef] [PubMed]
84. Dayem, A.A.; Choi, H.Y.; Kim, Y.B.; Cho, S.G. Antiviral effect of methylated flavonol isorhamnetin against influenza. *PLoS ONE* **2015**, *10*, e0121610. [CrossRef] [PubMed]
85. Scalbert, A.; Johnson, I.T.; Saltmarsh, M. Polyphenols: Antioxidants and beyond. *Am. J. Clin. Nutr.* **2005**, *81*, 215S–217S. [PubMed]
86. Birt, D.F.; Hendrich, S.; Wang, W. Dietary agents in cancer prevention: Flavonoids and isoflavonoids. *Pharmacol. Ther.* **2001**, *90*, 157–177. [CrossRef]
87. Kris-Etherton, P.M.; Keen, C.L. Evidence that the antioxidant flavonoids in tea and cocoa are beneficial for cardiovascular health. *Curr. Opin. Lipidol.* **2002**, *13*, 41–49. [CrossRef] [PubMed]
88. Kalinowska, M.; Bielawska, A.; Lewandowska-Siwkiewicz, H.; Priebe, W.; Lewandowski, W. Apples: Content of phenolic compounds vs. Variety, part of apple and cultivation model, extraction of phenolic compounds, biological properties. *Plant Physiol. Biochem.* **2014**, *84*, 169–188. [CrossRef] [PubMed]
89. Kondratyuk, T.P.; Pezzuto, J.M. Natural product polyphenols of relevance to human health. *Pharm. Biol.* **2004**, *42*, 46–63. [CrossRef]
90. Vitaglione, P.; Napolitano, A.; Fogliano, V. Cereal dietary fibre: A natural functional ingredient to deliver phenolic compounds into the gut. *Trends Food Sci. Technol.* **2008**, *19*, 451–463. [CrossRef]

91. Fogliano, V.; Corollaro, M.L.; Vitaglione, P.; Napolitano, A.; Ferracane, R.; Travaglia, F.; Arlorio, M.; Costabile, A.; Klinder, A.; Gibson, G. In vitro bioaccessibility and gut biotransformation of polyphenols present in the water-insoluble cocoa fraction. *Med. Nutr. Food Res.* **2011**, *55*, S44–S55. [CrossRef] [PubMed]
92. Marín, L.; Miguélez, E.M.; Villar, C.J.; Lombó, F. Bioavailability of dietary polyphenols and gut microbiota metabolism: Antimicrobial properties. *BioMed Res. Int.* **2015**, *2015*, 905215. [CrossRef] [PubMed]
93. Bang, S.H.; Hyun, Y.J.; Shim, J.; Hong, S.W.; Kim, D.H. Metabolism of rutin and poncirin by human intestinal microbiota and cloning of their metabolizing α-l-rhamnosidase from bifidobacterium dentium. *J. Microbiol. Biotechnol.* **2015**, *25*, 18–25. [CrossRef] [PubMed]
94. Day, A.J.; Cañada, F.J.; Díaz, J.C.; Kroon, P.A.; Mclauchlan, R.; Faulds, C.B.; Plumb, G.W.; Morgan, M.R.; Williamson, G. Dietary flavonoid and isoflavone glycosides are hydrolysed by the lactase site of lactase phlorizin hydrolase. *FEBS Lett.* **2000**, *468*, 166–170. [CrossRef]
95. Gee, J.M.; DuPont, M.S.; Day, A.J.; Plumb, G.W.; Williamson, G.; Johnson, I.T. Intestinal transport of quercetin glycosides in rats involves both deglycosylation and interaction with the hexose transport pathway. *J. Nutr.* **2000**, *130*, 2765–2771. [PubMed]
96. Nakagawa, K.; Okuda, S.; Miyazawa, T. Dose-dependent incorporation of tea catechins, (–)-epigallocatechin-3-gallate and (–)-epigallocatechin, into human plasma. *Biosci. Biotechnol. Biochem.* **1997**, *61*, 1981–1985. [CrossRef] [PubMed]
97. Filomeni, G.; De Zio, D.; Cecconi, F. Oxidative stress and autophagy: The clash between damage and metabolic needs. *Cell Death Differ.* **2015**, *22*, 377–388. [CrossRef] [PubMed]
98. Liang, X.H.; Jackson, S.; Seaman, M.; Brown, K.; Kempkes, B.; Hibshoosh, H.; Levine, B. Induction of autophagy and inhibition of tumorigenesis by beclin 1. *Nature* **1999**, *402*, 672–676. [PubMed]
99. Aita, V.M.; Liang, X.H.; Murty, V.; Pincus, D.L.; Yu, W.; Cayanis, E.; Kalachikov, S.; Gilliam, T.C.; Levine, B. Cloning and genomic organization of beclin 1, a candidate tumor suppressor gene on chromosome 17q21. *Genomics* **1999**, *59*, 59–65. [CrossRef] [PubMed]
100. Dilova, I.; Easlon, E.; Lin, S.J. Calorie restriction and the nutrient sensing signaling pathways. *Cell. Med. Life Sci.* **2007**, *64*, 752–767. [CrossRef] [PubMed]
101. Trepanowski, J.F.; Canale, R.E.; Marshall, K.E.; Kabir, M.M.; Bloomer, R.J. Impact of caloric and dietary restriction regimens on markers of health and longevity in humans and animals: A summary of available findings. *Nutr. J.* **2011**, *10*, 1. [CrossRef] [PubMed]
102. Inoki, K.; Zhu, T.; Guan, K.L. TSC2 mediates cellular energy response to control cell growth and survival. *Cell* **2003**, *115*, 577–590. [CrossRef]
103. Gwinn, D.M.; Shackelford, D.B.; Egan, D.F.; Mihaylova, M.M.; Mery, A.; Vasquez, D.S.; Turk, B.E.; Shaw, R.J. AMPK phosphorylation of raptor mediates a metabolic checkpoint. *Med. Cell* **2008**, *30*, 214–226. [CrossRef] [PubMed]
104. Jung, C.H.; Jun, C.B.; Ro, S.H.; Kim, Y.M.; Otto, N.M.; Cao, J.; Kundu, M.; Kim, D.H. ULK-Atg13-FIP200 complexes mediate mtor signaling to the autophagy machinery. *Med. Biol. Cell* **2009**, *20*, 1992–2003. [CrossRef] [PubMed]
105. Baur, J.A.; Pearson, K.J.; Price, N.L.; Jamieson, H.A.; Lerin, C.; Kalra, A.; Prabhu, V.V.; Allard, J.S.; Lopez-Lluch, G.; Lewis, K. Resveratrol improves health and survival of mice on a high-calorie diet. *Nature* **2006**, *444*, 337–342. [CrossRef] [PubMed]
106. Morselli, E.; Maiuri, M.C.; Markaki, M.; Megalou, E.; Pasparaki, A.; Palikaras, K.; Criollo, A.; Galluzzi, L.; Malik, S.A.; Vitale, I. The life span-prolonging effect of sirtuin-1 is mediated by autophagy. *Autophagy* **2010**, *6*, 186–188. [CrossRef] [PubMed]
107. Ng, F.; Tang, B.L. Sirtuins' modulation of autophagy. *J. Cell. Physiol.* **2013**, *228*, 2262–2270. [CrossRef] [PubMed]
108. Chung, S.; Yao, H.; Caito, S.; Hwang, J.W.; Arunachalam, G.; Rahman, I. Regulation of sirt1 in cellular functions: Role of polyphenols. *Arch. Biochem. Biophys.* **2010**, *501*, 79–90. [CrossRef] [PubMed]
109. Opipari, A.W.; Tan, L.; Boitano, A.E.; Sorenson, D.R.; Aurora, A.; Liu, J.R. Resveratrol-induced autophagocytosis in ovarian cancer cells. *Cancer Res.* **2004**, *64*, 696–703. [CrossRef] [PubMed]
110. Carbó, N.; Costelli, P.; Baccino, F.M.; López-Soriano, F.J.; Argilés, J.M. Resveratrol, a natural product present in wine, decreases tumour growth in a rat tumour model. *Biochem. Biophys. Res. Commun.* **1999**, *254*, 739–743. [CrossRef] [PubMed]

111. Baur, J.A.; Sinclair, D.A. Therapeutic potential of resveratrol: The in vivo evidence. *Nat. Rev. Drug Discov.* **2006**, *5*, 493–506. [CrossRef] [PubMed]
112. Signorelli, P.; Ghidoni, R. Resveratrol as an anticancer nutrient: Molecular basis, open questions and promises. *J. Nutr. Biochem.* **2005**, *16*, 449–466. [CrossRef] [PubMed]
113. Trincheri, N.F.; Follo, C.; Nicotra, G.; Peracchio, C.; Castino, R.; Isidoro, C. Resveratrol-induced apoptosis depends on the lipid kinase activity of vps34 and on the formation of autophagolysosomes. *Carcinogenesis* **2008**, *29*, 381–389. [CrossRef] [PubMed]
114. Armour, S.M.; Baur, J.A.; Hsieh, S.N.; Land-Bracha, A.; Thomas, S.M.; Sinclair, D.A. Inhibition of mammalian s6 kinase by resveratrol suppresses autophagy. *Aging* **2009**, *1*, 515–528. [CrossRef] [PubMed]
115. Scarlatti, F.; Maffei, R.; Beau, I.; Codogno, P.; Ghidoni, R. Role of non-canonical beclin 1-independent autophagy in cell death induced by resveratrol in human breast cancer cells. *Cell Death Differ.* **2008**, *15*, 1318–1329. [CrossRef] [PubMed]
116. Kim, Y.; Choi, B.T.; Lee, Y.T.; Park, D.I.; Rhee, S.H.; Park, K.Y.; Choi, Y.H. Resveratrol inhibits cell proliferation and induces apoptosis of human breast carcinoma MCF-7 cells. *Oncol. Rep.* **2004**, *11*, 441–446. [CrossRef] [PubMed]
117. Roy, S.K.; Chen, Q.; Fu, J.; Shankar, S.; Srivastava, R.K. Resveratrol inhibits growth of orthotopic pancreatic tumors through activation of foxo transcription factors. *PLoS ONE* **2011**, *6*, e25166. [CrossRef] [PubMed]
118. Back, J.H.; Zhu, Y.; Calabro, A.; Queenan, C.; Kim, A.S.; Arbesman, J.; Kim, A.L. Resveratrol-mediated downregulation of rictor attenuates autophagic process and suppresses UV-induced skin carcinogenesis. *Photochem. Photobiol.* **2012**, *88*, 1165–1172. [CrossRef] [PubMed]
119. Hwang, J.T.; Kwak, D.W.; Lin, S.K.; Kim, H.M.; Kim, Y.M.; Park, O.J. Resveratrol induces apoptosis in chemoresistant cancer cells via modulation of AMPK signaling pathway. *Ann. N. Y. Acad. Sci.* **2007**, *1095*, 441–448. [CrossRef] [PubMed]
120. Miki, H.; Uehara, N.; Kimura, A.; Sasaki, T.; Yuri, T.; Yoshizawa, K.; Tsubura, A. Resveratrol induces apoptosis via ros-triggered autophagy in human colon cancer cells. *Int. J. Oncol.* **2012**, *40*, 1020–1028. [PubMed]
121. Puissant, A.; Auberger, P. AMPK-and p62/SQSTM1-dependent autophagy mediate resveratrol-induced cell death in chronic myelogenous leukemia. *Autophagy* **2010**, *6*, 655–657. [CrossRef] [PubMed]
122. Saller, R.; Brignoli, R.; Melzer, J.; Meier, R. An updated systematic review with meta-analysis for the clinical evidence of silymarin. *Forsch. Komplement. Res. Complement. Med.* **2008**, *15*, 9–20. [CrossRef] [PubMed]
123. Lu, P.; Mamiya, T.; Lu, L.; Mouri, A.; Zou, L.; Nagai, T.; Hiramatsu, M.; Ikejima, T.; Nabeshima, T. Silibinin prevents amyloid β peptide-induced memory impairment and oxidative stress in mice. *Br. J. Pharmacol.* **2009**, *157*, 1270–1277. [CrossRef] [PubMed]
124. Marrazzo, G.; Bosco, P.; La Delia, F.; Scapagnini, G.; Di Giacomo, C.; Malaguarnera, M.; Galvano, F.; Nicolosi, A.; Volti, G.L. Neuroprotective effect of silibinin in diabetic mice. *Neurosci. Lett.* **2011**, *504*, 252–256. [CrossRef] [PubMed]
125. Singh, R.P.; Agarwal, R. Mechanisms and preclinical efficacy of silibinin in preventing skin cancer. *Eur. J. Cancer* **2005**, *41*, 1969–1979. [CrossRef] [PubMed]
126. Singh, R.P.; Agarwal, R. Prostate cancer chemoprevention by silibinin: Bench to bedside. *Mol. Carcinogen.* **2006**, *45*, 436–442. [CrossRef] [PubMed]
127. Tyagi, A.; Singh, R.P.; Ramasamy, K.; Raina, K.; Redente, E.F.; Dwyer-Nield, L.D.; Radcliffe, R.A.; Malkinson, A.M.; Agarwal, R. Growth inhibition and regression of lung tumors by silibinin: Modulation of angiogenesis by macrophage-associated cytokines and nuclear factor-κb and signal transducers and activators of transcription 3. *Cancer Prev. Res.* **2009**, *2*, 74–83. [CrossRef] [PubMed]
128. Kauntz, H.; Bousserouel, S.; Gossé, F.; Raul, F. Silibinin triggers apoptotic signaling pathways and autophagic survival response in human colon adenocarcinoma cells and their derived metastatic cells. *Apoptosis* **2011**, *16*, 1042–1053. [CrossRef] [PubMed]
129. Duan, W.; Jin, X.; Li, Q.; Tashiro, S.I.; Onodera, S.; Ikejima, T. Silibinin induced autophagic and apoptotic cell death in HT1080 cells through a reactive oxygen species pathway. *J. Pharmacol. Sci.* **2010**, *113*, 48–56. [CrossRef] [PubMed]
130. Fan, S.; Li, L.; Chen, S.; Yu, Y.; Qi, M.; Tashiro, S.I.; Onodera, S.; Ikejima, T. Silibinin induced-autophagic and apoptotic death is associated with an increase in reactive oxygen and nitrogen species in hela cells. *Free Radic. Res.* **2011**, *45*, 1307–1324. [CrossRef] [PubMed]

131. Mira, L.; Silva, M.; Manso, C. Scavenging of reactive oxygen species by silibinin dihemisuccinate. *Biochem. Pharmacol.* **1994**, *48*, 753–759. [CrossRef]
132. Jiang, K.; Wang, W.; Jin, X.; Wang, Z.; Ji, Z.; Meng, G. Silibinin, a natural flavonoid, induces autophagy via ROS-dependent mitochondrial dysfunction and loss of ATP involving BNIP3 in human MCF7 breast cancer cells. *Oncol. Rep.* **2015**, *33*, 2711–2718. [CrossRef] [PubMed]
133. Zheng, N.; Zhang, P.; Huang, H.; Liu, W.; Hayashi, T.; Zang, L.; Zhang, Y.; Liu, L.; Xia, M.; Tashiro, S.I. Erα down-regulation plays a key role in silibinin-induced autophagy and apoptosis in human breast cancer MCF-7 cells. *J. Pharmacol. Sci.* **2015**, *128*, 97–107. [CrossRef] [PubMed]
134. Boots, A.W.; Haenen, G.R.; Bast, A. Health effects of quercetin: From antioxidant to nutraceutical. *Eur. J. Pharmacol.* **2008**, *585*, 325–337. [CrossRef] [PubMed]
135. Ferry, D.R.; Smith, A.; Malkhandi, J.; Fyfe, D.W.; Anderson, D.; Baker, J.; Kerr, D. Phase I clinical trial of the flavonoid quercetin: Pharmacokinetics and evidence for in vivo tyrosine kinase inhibition. *Clin. Cancer Res.* **1996**, *2*, 659–668. [PubMed]
136. Aalinkeel, R.; Bindukumar, B.; Reynolds, J.L.; Sykes, D.E.; Mahajan, S.D.; Chadha, K.C.; Schwartz, S.A. The dietary bioflavonoid, quercetin, selectively induces apoptosis of prostate cancer cells by down-regulating the expression of heat shock protein 90. *Prostate* **2008**, *68*, 1773–1789. [CrossRef] [PubMed]
137. Borska, S.; Drag-Zalesinska, M.; Wysocka, T.; Sopel, M.; Dumanska, M.; Zabel, M.; Dziegiel, P. Antiproliferative and pro-apoptotic effects of quercetin on human pancreatic carcinoma cell lines EPP85–181P and EPP85–181RDB. *Folia Histochem. Cytobiol.* **2010**, *48*, 222–229. [CrossRef] [PubMed]
138. Choi, E.J.; Bae, S.M.; Ahn, W.S. Antiproliferative effects of quercetin through cell cycle arrest and apoptosis in human breast cancer MDA-MB-453 cells. *Arch. Pharm. Res.* **2008**, *31*, 1281–1285. [CrossRef] [PubMed]
139. Conklin, C.M.; Bechberger, J.F.; MacFabe, D.; Guthrie, N.; Kurowska, E.M.; Naus, C.C. Genistein and quercetin increase connexin43 and suppress growth of breast cancer cells. *Carcinogenesis* **2006**, *28*, 93–100. [CrossRef] [PubMed]
140. Klappan, A.K.; Hones, S.; Mylonas, I.; Brüning, A. Proteasome inhibition by quercetin triggers macroautophagy and blocks mtor activity. *Histochem. Cell Biol.* **2012**, *137*, 25–36. [CrossRef] [PubMed]
141. Wang, K.; Liu, R.; Li, J.; Mao, J.; Lei, Y.; Wu, J.; Zeng, J.; Zhang, T.; Wu, H.; Chen, L. Quercetin induces protective autophagy in gastric cancer cells: Involvement of Akt-mTOR-and hypoxia-induced factor 1α-mediated signaling. *Autophagy* **2011**, *7*, 966–978. [CrossRef] [PubMed]
142. Polkowski, K.; Popiołkiewicz, J.; Krzeczyński, P.; Ramza, J.; Pucko, W.; Zegrocka-Stendel, O.; Boryski, J.; Skierski, J.S.; Mazurek, A.P.; Grynkiewicz, G. Cytostatic and cytotoxic activity of synthetic genistein glycosides against human cancer cell lines. *Cancer Lett.* **2004**, *203*, 59–69. [CrossRef] [PubMed]
143. Yu, Z.; Li, W.; Liu, F. Inhibition of proliferation and induction of apoptosis by genistein in colon cancer HT-29 cells. *Cancer Lett.* **2004**, *215*, 159–166. [CrossRef] [PubMed]
144. Ouchi, H.; Ishiguro, H.; Ikeda, N.; Hori, M.; Kubota, Y.; Uemura, H. Genistein induces cell growth inhibition in prostate cancer through the suppression of telomerase activity. *Int. J. Urol.* **2005**, *12*, 73–80. [CrossRef] [PubMed]
145. Li, Y.; Upadhyay, S.; Bhuiyan, M.; Sarkar, F.H. Induction of apoptosis in breast cancer cells MDA-MB-231 by genistein. *Oncogene* **1999**, *18*, 3166–3172. [CrossRef] [PubMed]
146. Gossner, G.; Choi, M.; Tan, L.; Fogoros, S.; Griffith, K.A.; Kuenker, M.; Liu, J.R. Genistein-induced apoptosis and autophagocytosis in ovarian cancer cells. *Gynecol. Oncol.* **2007**, *105*, 23–30. [CrossRef] [PubMed]
147. Houslay, M.D.; Christian, F. P62 (SQSTM1) forms part of a novel, reversible aggregate containing a specific conformer of the camp degrading phosphodiesterase, PDE4A4. *Autophagy* **2010**, *6*, 1198–1200. [CrossRef] [PubMed]
148. Christian, F.; Anthony, D.F.; Vadrevu, S.; Riddell, T.; Day, J.P.; McLeod, R.; Adams, D.R.; Baillie, G.S.; Houslay, M.D. P62 (SQSTM1) and cyclic amp phosphodiesterase-4A4 (PDE4A4) locate to a novel, reversible protein aggregate with links to autophagy and proteasome degradation pathways. *Cell Signal.* **2010**, *22*, 1576–1596. [CrossRef] [PubMed]
149. Dhillon, N.; Aggarwal, B.B.; Newman, R.A.; Wolff, R.A.; Kunnumakkara, A.B.; Abbruzzese, J.L.; Ng, C.S.; Badmaev, V.; Kurzrock, R. Phase ii trial of curcumin in patients with advanced pancreatic cancer. *Clin. Cancer Res.* **2008**, *14*, 4491–4499. [CrossRef] [PubMed]

150. Sharma, R.A.; Euden, S.A.; Platton, S.L.; Cooke, D.N.; Shafayat, A.; Hewitt, H.R.; Marczylo, T.H.; Morgan, B.; Hemingway, D.; Plummer, S.M. Phase i clinical trial of oral curcumin biomarkers of systemic activity and compliance. *Clin. Cancer Res.* **2004**, *10*, 6847–6854. [CrossRef] [PubMed]
151. Zhuang, W.; Long, L.; Zheng, B.; Ji, W.; Yang, N.; Zhang, Q.; Liang, Z. Curcumin promotes differentiation of glioma-initiating cells by inducing autophagy. *Cancer Sci.* **2012**, *103*, 684–690. [CrossRef] [PubMed]
152. Chadalapaka, G.; Jutooru, I.; Burghardt, R.; Safe, S. Drugs that target specificity proteins downregulate epidermal growth factor receptor in bladder cancer cells. *Mol. Cancer Res.* **2010**, *8*, 739–750. [CrossRef] [PubMed]
153. Han, J.; Pan, X.Y.; Xu, Y.; Xiao, Y.; An, Y.; Tie, L.; Pan, Y.; Li, X.J. Curcumin induces autophagy to protect vascular endothelial cell survival from oxidative stress damage. *Autophagy* **2012**, *8*, 812–825. [CrossRef] [PubMed]
154. Lee, Y.J.; Kim, N.Y.; Suh, Y.A.; Lee, C. Involvement of ROS in curcumin-induced autophagic cell death. *Korean J. Physiol. Pharmacol.* **2011**, *15*, 1–7. [CrossRef] [PubMed]
155. Aoki, H.; Takada, Y.; Kondo, S.; Sawaya, R.; Aggarwal, B.B.; Kondo, Y. Evidence that curcumin suppresses the growth of malignant gliomas in vitro and in vivo through induction of autophagy: Role of Akt and extracellular signal-regulated kinase signaling pathways. *Med. Pharmacol.* **2007**, *72*, 29–39. [CrossRef] [PubMed]
156. Pan, W.; Yang, H.; Cao, C.; Song, X.; Wallin, B.; Kivlin, R.; Lu, S.; Hu, G.; Di, W.; Wan, Y. AMPK mediates curcumin-induced cell death in CaOV3 ovarian cancer cells. *Oncol. Rep.* **2008**, *20*, 1553–1559. [PubMed]
157. Kim, J.Y.; Cho, T.J.; Woo, B.H.; Choi, K.U.; Lee, C.H.; Ryu, M.H.; Park, H.R. Curcumin-induced autophagy contributes to the decreased survival of oral cancer cells. *Arch. Oral Biol.* **2012**, *57*, 1018–1025. [CrossRef] [PubMed]
158. Shinojima, N.; Yokoyama, T.; Kondo, Y.; Kondo, S. Roles of the Akt/mTOR/p70S6K and ERK1/2 signaling pathways in curcumin-induced autophagy. *Autophagy* **2007**, *3*, 635–637. [CrossRef] [PubMed]
159. Jia, Y.L.; Li, J.; Qin, Z.H.; Liang, Z.Q. Autophagic and apoptotic mechanisms of curcumin-induced death in K562 cells. *J. Asian Natl. Prod. Res.* **2009**, *11*, 918–928. [CrossRef] [PubMed]
160. Gschwendt, M.; Muller, H.; Kielbassa, K.; Zang, R.; Kittstein, W.; Rincke, G.; Marks, F. Rottlerin, a novel protein kinase inhibitor. *Biochem. Biophys. Res. Commun.* **1994**, *199*, 93–98. [CrossRef] [PubMed]
161. Soltoff, S.P. Rottlerin: An inappropriate and ineffective inhibitor of PKCδ. *Trends Pharmacol. Sci.* **2007**, *28*, 453–458. [CrossRef] [PubMed]
162. Springael, C.; Thomas, S.; Rahmouni, S.; Vandamme, A.; Goldman, M.; Willems, F.; Vosters, O. Rottlerin inhibits human T cell responses. *Biochem. Pharmacol.* **2007**, *73*, 515–525. [CrossRef] [PubMed]
163. Zeng, H.; Lozinskaya, I.M.; Lin, Z.; Willette, R.N.; Brooks, D.P.; Xu, X. Mallotoxin is a novel human ether-a-go-go-related gene (hERG) potassium channel activator. *J. Pharmacol. Exp. Ther.* **2006**, *319*, 957–962. [CrossRef] [PubMed]
164. Zhang, D.; Anantharam, V.; Kanthasamy, A.; Kanthasamy, A.G. Neuroprotective effect of protein kinase cδ inhibitor rottlerin in cell culture and animal models of parkinson's disease. *J. Pharmacol. Exp. Ther.* **2007**, *322*, 913–922. [CrossRef] [PubMed]
165. Guimarães, E.L.; Empsen, C.; Geerts, A.; van Grunsven, L.A. Advanced glycation end products induce production of reactive oxygen species via the activation of NADPH oxidase in murine hepatic stellate cells. *J. Hepatol.* **2010**, *52*, 389–397. [CrossRef] [PubMed]
166. Mizuguchi, H.; Terao, T.; Kitai, M.; Ikeda, M.; Yoshimura, Y.; Das, A.K.; Kitamura, Y.; Takeda, N.; Fukui, H. Involvement of protein kinase Cdelta/extracellular signal-regulated kinase/poly (ADP-ribose) polymerase-1 (PARP-1) signaling pathway in histamine-induced up-regulation of histamine H_1 receptor gene expression in Hela cells. *J. Biol. Chem.* **2011**, *286*, 30542–30551. [CrossRef] [PubMed]
167. Sharma, V. A polyphenolic compound rottlerin demonstrates significant in vitro cytotoxicity against human cancer cell lines: Isolation and characterization from the fruits of *Mallotus philippinensis*. *J. Plant Biochem. Biotechnol.* **2011**, *20*, 190–195. [CrossRef]
168. Mann, A.P.; Verma, A.; Sethi, G.; Manavathi, B.; Wang, H.; Fok, J.Y.; Kunnumakkara, A.B.; Kumar, R.; Aggarwal, B.B.; Mehta, K. Overexpression of tissue transglutaminase leads to constitutive activation of nuclear factor-kappaB in cancer cells: Delineation of a novel pathway. *Cancer Res.* **2006**, *66*, 8788–8795. [CrossRef] [PubMed]

169. Fabre, C.; Carvalho, G.; Tasdemir, E.; Braun, T.; Ades, L.; Grosjean, J.; Boehrer, S.; Metivier, D.; Souquere, S.; Pierron, G. NF-kappaB inhibition sensitizes to starvation-induced cell death in high-risk myelodysplastic syndrome and acute myeloid leukemia. *Oncogene* **2007**, *26*, 4071–4083. [CrossRef] [PubMed]
170. Akar, U.; Ozpolat, B.; Mehta, K.; Fok, J.; Kondo, Y.; Lopez-Berestein, G. Tissue transglutaminase inhibits autophagy in pancreatic cancer cells. *Mol. Cancer Res.* **2007**, *5*, 241–249. [CrossRef] [PubMed]
171. Singh, B.N.; Kumar, D.; Shankar, S.; Srivastava, R.K. Rottlerin induces autophagy which leads to apoptotic cell death through inhibition of PI3K/Akt/mTOR pathway in human pancreatic cancer stem cells. *Biochem. Pharmacol.* **2012**, *84*, 1154–1163. [CrossRef] [PubMed]
172. Balgi, A.D.; Fonseca, B.D.; Donohue, E.; Tsang, T.C.; Lajoie, P.; Proud, C.G.; Nabi, I.R.; Roberge, M. Screen for chemical modulators of autophagy reveals novel therapeutic inhibitors of mTORC1 signaling. *PLoS ONE* **2009**, *4*, e7124. [CrossRef] [PubMed]
173. Li, M.J.; Yin, Y.C.; Wang, J.; Jiang, Y.F. Green tea compounds in breast cancer prevention and treatment. *World J. Clin. Oncol.* **2014**, *5*, 520–528. [CrossRef] [PubMed]
174. Harper, C.E.; Patel, B.B.; Wang, J.; Arabshahi, A.; Eltoum, I.A.; Lamartiniere, C.A. Resveratrol suppresses prostate cancer progression in transgenic mice. *Carcinogenesis* **2007**, *28*, 1946–1953. [CrossRef] [PubMed]
175. Trincheri, N.F.; Nicotra, G.; Follo, C.; Castino, R.; Isidoro, C. Resveratrol induces cell death in colorectal cancer cells by a novel pathway involving lysosomal cathepsin D. *Carcinogenesis* **2007**, *28*, 922–931. [CrossRef] [PubMed]
176. Rodrigo, R.; Gil-Becerra, D. Implications of polyphenols on endogenous antioxidant defense systems in human diseases. In *Polyphenols in Human Health Disease*; Elsevier: Amsterdam, The Netherlands, 2014; pp. 201–207.
177. Wang, H.; Cao, G.; Prior, R.L. Total antioxidant capacity of fruits. *J. Agric. Food Chem.* **1996**, *44*, 701–705. [CrossRef]
178. Bhattacharyya, A.; Chattopadhyay, R.; Mitra, S.; Crowe, S.E. Oxidative stress: An essential factor in the pathogenesis of gastrointestinal mucosal diseases. *Physiol. Rev.* **2014**, *94*, 329–354. [CrossRef] [PubMed]
179. Pham-Huy, L.A.; He, H.; Pham-Huy, C. Free radicals, antioxidants in disease and health. *Int. J. Biomed. Sci.* **2008**, *4*, 89–96. [PubMed]
180. Perron, N.R.; Brumaghim, J.L. A review of the antioxidant mechanisms of polyphenol compounds related to iron binding. *Cell Biochem. Biophys.* **2009**, *53*, 75–100. [CrossRef] [PubMed]
181. Guo, J.J.; Hsieh, H.Y.; Hu, C.H. Chain-breaking activity of carotenes in lipid peroxidation: A theoretical study. *J. Phys. Chem. B* **2009**, *113*, 15699–15708. [CrossRef] [PubMed]
182. Pietta, P.G. Flavonoids as antioxidants. *J. Natl. Prod.* **2000**, *63*, 1035–1042. [CrossRef]
183. Tsao, R.; Li, H. Antioxidant properties in vitro and in vivo: Realistic assessments of efficacy of plant extracts. *CAB Rev.* **2012**, *7*, 9.
184. Rice-Evans, C.A.; Miller, N.J.; Paganga, G. Structure-antioxidant activity relationships of flavonoids and phenolic acids. *Free Radic. Biol. Med.* **1996**, *20*, 933–956. [CrossRef]
185. Chuang, C.C.; McIntosh, M.K. Potential mechanisms by which polyphenol-rich grapes prevent obesity-mediated inflammation and metabolic diseases. *Annu. Rev. Nutr.* **2011**, *31*, 155–176. [CrossRef] [PubMed]
186. Zhou, B.; Wu, L.M.; Yang, L.; Liu, Z.L. Evidence for α-tocopherol regeneration reaction of green tea polyphenols in SDS micelles. *Free Radic. Biol. Med.* **2005**, *38*, 78–84. [CrossRef] [PubMed]
187. Tsao, R. Chemistry and biochemistry of dietary polyphenols. *Nutrients* **2010**, *2*, 1231–1246. [CrossRef] [PubMed]
188. Van Acker, S.A.; van den Berg, D.J.; Tromp, M.N.; Griffioen, D.H.; van Bennekom, W.P.; van der Vijgh, W.J.; Bast, A. Structural aspects of antioxidant activity of flavonoids. *Free Radic. Biol. Med.* **1996**, *20*, 331–342. [CrossRef]
189. Göçer, H.; Gülçin, İ. Caffeic acid phenethyl ester (CAPE): Correlation of structure and antioxidant properties. *Int. J. Food Sci. Nutr.* **2011**, *62*, 821–825. [CrossRef] [PubMed]
190. Mishra, P.; Kale, R.; Kar, A. Chemoprevention of mammary tumorigenesis and chemomodulation of the antioxidative enzymes and peroxidative damage in prepubertal Sprague Dawley rats by Biochanin A. *Mol. Cell. Biochem.* **2008**, *312*, 1–9. [CrossRef] [PubMed]
191. Singh, B.; Shoulson, R.; Chatterjee, A.; Ronghe, A.; Bhat, N.K.; Dim, D.C.; Bhat, H.K. Resveratrol inhibits estrogen-induced breast carcinogenesis through induction of NRF2-mediated protective pathways. *Carcinogenesis* **2014**, *35*, 1872–1880. [CrossRef] [PubMed]

192. Yang, C.S.; Li, G.; Yang, Z.; Guan, F.; Chen, A.; Ju, J. Cancer prevention by tocopherols and tea polyphenols. *Cancer Lett.* **2013**, *334*, 79–85. [CrossRef] [PubMed]
193. Hsieh, T.C.; Wu, J.M. Suppression of cell proliferation and gene expression by combinatorial synergy of EGCG, resveratrol and γ-tocotrienol in estrogen receptor-positive MCF-7 breast cancer cells. *Int. J. Oncol.* **2008**, *33*, 851–859. [PubMed]
194. Nadal-Serrano, M.; Pons, D.G.; Sastre-Serra, J.; del Mar Blanquer-Rosselló, M.; Roca, P.; Oliver, J. Genistein modulates oxidative stress in breast cancer cell lines according to ERA/ERB ratio: Effects on mitochondrial functionality, sirtuins, uncoupling protein 2 and antioxidant enzymes. *Int. J. Biochem. Cell Biol.* **2013**, *45*, 2045–2051. [CrossRef] [PubMed]
195. Chen, B.; Zhang, Y.; Wang, Y.; Rao, J.; Jiang, X.; Xu, Z. Curcumin inhibits proliferation of breast cancer cells through Nrf2-mediated down-regulation of Fen1 expression. *J. Steroid Biochem. Mol. Biol.* **2014**, *143*, 11–18. [CrossRef] [PubMed]
196. Siddiqui, M.A.; Ahamed, M.; Ahmad, J.; Khan, M.M.; Musarrat, J.; Al-Khedhairy, A.A.; Alrokayan, S.A. Nickel oxide nanoparticles induce cytotoxicity, oxidative stress and apoptosis in cultured human cells that is abrogated by the dietary antioxidant curcumin. *Food Chem. Toxicol.* **2012**, *50*, 641–647. [CrossRef] [PubMed]
197. Azam, S.; Hadi, N.; Khan, N.U.; Hadi, S.M. Prooxidant property of green tea polyphenols epicatechin and epigallocatechin-3-gallate: Implications for anticancer properties. *Toxicol. in Vitro* **2004**, *18*, 555–561. [CrossRef] [PubMed]
198. Bouayed, J.; Bohn, T. Exogenous antioxidants—Double-edged swords in cellular redox state: Health beneficial effects at physiologic doses versus deleterious effects at high doses. *Oxid. Med. Cell. Longev.* **2010**, *3*, 228–237. [CrossRef] [PubMed]
199. Wätjen, W.; Michels, G.; Steffan, B.; Niering, P.; Chovolou, Y.; Kampkötter, A.; Tran-Thi, Q.H.; Proksch, P.; Kahl, R. Low concentrations of flavonoids are protective in rat H4IIE cells whereas high concentrations cause DNA damage and apoptosis. *J. Nutr.* **2005**, *135*, 525–531. [PubMed]
200. Sandoval-Acuña, C.; Ferreira, J.; Speisky, H. Polyphenols and mitochondria: An update on their increasingly emerging ROS-scavenging independent actions. *Arch. Biochem. Biophys.* **2014**, *559*, 75–90. [CrossRef] [PubMed]
201. Perron, N.R.; García, C.R.; Pinzón, J.R.; Chaur, M.N.; Brumaghim, J.L. Antioxidant and prooxidant effects of polyphenol compounds on copper-mediated DNA damage. *J. Inorg. Biochem.* **2011**, *105*, 745–753. [CrossRef] [PubMed]
202. Ullah, M.F.; Ahmad, A.; Zubair, H.; Khan, H.Y.; Wang, Z.; Sarkar, F.H.; Hadi, S.M. Soy isoflavone genistein induces cell death in breast cancer cells through mobilization of endogenous copper ions and generation of reactive oxygen species. *Mol. Nutr. Food Res.* **2011**, *55*, 553–559. [CrossRef] [PubMed]
203. Singh, D.V.; Agarwal, S.; Singh, P.; Godbole, M.M.; Misra, K. Curcumin conjugates induce apoptosis via a mitochondrion dependent pathway in MCF-7 and MDA-MB-231 cell lines. *Asian Pac. J. Cancer Prev.* **2013**, *14*, 5797–5804. [CrossRef] [PubMed]
204. Braicu, C.; Pilecki, V.; Balacescu, O.; Irimie, A.; Berindan Neagoe, I. The relationships between biological activities and structure of flavan-3-ols. *Int. J. Mol. Sci.* **2011**, *12*, 9342–9353. [CrossRef] [PubMed]
205. Balkwill, F.; Mantovani, A. Inflammation and cancer: Back to virchow? *Lancet* **2001**, *357*, 539–545. [CrossRef]
206. Flossmann, E.; Rothwell, P.M. Effect of aspirin on long-term risk of colorectal cancer: Consistent evidence from randomised and observational studies. *Lancet* **2007**, *369*, 1603–1613. [CrossRef]
207. Chan, A.T.; Ogino, S.; Fuchs, C.S. Aspirin and the risk of colorectal cancer in relation to the expression of COX-2. *N. Engl. J. Med.* **2007**, *356*, 2131–2142. [CrossRef] [PubMed]
208. Anderson, W.F.; Schairer, C.; Chen, B.E.; Hance, K.W.; Levine, P.H. Epidemiology of inflammatory breast cancer (IBC). *Breast Dis.* **2005**, *22*, 9–23. [CrossRef] [PubMed]
209. Hance, K.W.; Anderson, W.F.; Devesa, S.S.; Young, H.A.; Levine, P.H. Trends in inflammatory breast carcinoma incidence and survival: The surveillance, epidemiology, and end results program at the national cancer institute. *J. Natl. Cancer Inst.* **2005**, *97*, 966–975. [CrossRef] [PubMed]
210. Kanaya, N.; Adams, L.; Takasaki, A.; Chen, S. Whole blueberry powder inhibits metastasis of triple negative breast cancer in a xenograft mouse model through modulation of inflammatory cytokines. *Nutr. Cancer* **2014**, *66*, 242–248. [CrossRef] [PubMed]

211. Vuong, T.; Mallet, J.F.; Ouzounova, M.; Rahbar, S.; Hernandez-Vargas, H.; Herceg, Z.; Matar, C. Role of a polyphenol-enriched preparation on chemoprevention of mammary carcinoma through cancer stem cells and inflammatory pathways modulation. *J. Transl. Med.* **2016**, *14*, 13. [CrossRef] [PubMed]
212. Biswas, S.K.; McClure, D.; Jimenez, L.A.; Megson, I.L.; Rahman, I. Curcumin induces glutathione biosynthesis and inhibits NF-κB activation and interleukin-8 release in alveolar epithelial cells: Mechanism of free radical scavenging activity. *Antioxid. Redox Signal.* **2005**, *7*, 32–41. [CrossRef] [PubMed]
213. Gerhäuser, C.; Klimo, K.; Heiss, E.; Neumann, I.; Gamal-Eldeen, A.; Knauft, J.; Liu, G.Y.; Sitthimonchai, S.; Frank, N. Mechanism-based in vitro screening of potential cancer chemopreventive agents. *Mutat. Res.* **2003**, *523–524*, 163–172. [CrossRef]
214. Wadsworth, T.L.; Koop, D.R. Effects of the wine polyphenolics quercetin and resveratrol on pro-inflammatory cytokine expression in raw 264.7 macrophages. *Biochem. Pharmacol.* **1999**, *57*, 941–949. [CrossRef]
215. Lawrence, T. The nuclear factor NF-κB pathway in inflammation. *Cold Spring Harb. Perspect. Biol.* **2009**, *1*, a001651. [CrossRef] [PubMed]
216. Dannenberg, A.J.; Subbaramaiah, K. Targeting cyclooxygenase-2 in human neoplasia: Rationale and promise. *Cancer Cell* **2003**, *4*, 431–436. [CrossRef]
217. Mackenzie, G.G.; Oteiza, P.I. Modulation of transcription factor NF-κB in Hodgkin's lymphoma cell lines: Effect of (−)-epicatechin. *Free Radic. Res.* **2006**, *40*, 1086–1094. [CrossRef] [PubMed]
218. Mackenzie, G.G.; Carrasquedo, F.; Delfino, J.M.; Keen, C.L.; Fraga, C.G.; Oteiza, P.I. Epicatechin, catechin, and dimeric procyanidins inhibit PMA-induced NF-κB activation at multiple steps in Jurkat T cells. *FASEB J.* **2004**, *18*, 167–169. [PubMed]
219. Divya, C.S.; Pillai, M.R. Antitumor action of curcumin in human papillomavirus associated cells involves downregulation of viral oncogenes, prevention of NFkB and AP-1 translocation, and modulation of apoptosis. *Mol. Carcinogen.* **2006**, *45*, 320–332. [CrossRef] [PubMed]
220. Wahyudi, S.; Sargowo, D. Green tea polyphenols inhibit oxidized LDL-induced NF-kB activation in human umbilical vein endothelial cells. *Acta Med. Indones.* **2007**, *39*, 66–70. [PubMed]
221. Granado-Serrano, A.B.; Martín, M.Á.; Bravo, L.; Goya, L.; Ramos, S. Quercetin attenuates TNF-induced inflammation in hepatic cells by inhibiting the NF-κB pathway. *Nutr. Cancer* **2012**, *64*, 588–598. [CrossRef] [PubMed]
222. Estrov, Z.; Shishodia, S.; Faderl, S.; Harris, D.; Van, Q.; Kantarjian, H.M.; Talpaz, M.; Aggarwal, B.B. Resveratrol blocks interleukin-1β–induced activation of the nuclear transcription factor NF-κB, inhibits proliferation, causes S-phase arrest, and induces apoptosis of acute myeloid leukemia cells. *Blood* **2003**, *102*, 987–995. [CrossRef] [PubMed]
223. Bachmeier, B.E.; Nerlich, A.G.; Iancu, C.M.; Cilli, M.; Schleicher, E.; Vené, R.; Dell'Eva, R.; Jochum, M.; Albini, A.; Pfeffer, U. The chemopreventive polyphenol curcumin prevents hematogenous breast cancer metastases in immunodeficient mice. *Cell. Physiol. Biochem.* **2007**, *19*, 137–152. [CrossRef] [PubMed]
224. Bachmeier, B.E.; Mohrenz, I.V.; Mirisola, V.; Schleicher, E.; Romeo, F.; Höhneke, C.; Jochum, M.; Nerlich, A.G.; Pfeffer, U. Curcumin downregulates the inflammatory cytokines CXCL1 and-2 in breast cancer cells via NFκB. *Carcinogenesis* **2008**, *29*, 779–789. [CrossRef] [PubMed]
225. Singh, B.N.; Shankar, S.; Srivastava, R.K. Green tea catechin, epigallocatechin-3-gallate (EGCG): Mechanisms, perspectives and clinical applications. *Biochem. Pharmacol.* **2011**, *82*, 1807–1821. [CrossRef] [PubMed]
226. Chung, S.S.; Vadgama, J.V. Curcumin and epigallocatechin gallate inhibit the cancer stem cell phenotype via down-regulation of STAT3–NFκB signaling. *Anticancer Res.* **2015**, *35*, 39–46. [PubMed]
227. Lamy, S.; Akla, N.; Ouanouki, A.; Lord-Dufour, S.; Béliveau, R. Diet-derived polyphenols inhibit angiogenesis by modulating the interleukin-6/STAT3 pathway. *Exp. Cell Res.* **2012**, *318*, 1586–1596. [CrossRef] [PubMed]
228. Zhao, X.; Sun, X.; Li, X.L. Expression and clinical significance of STAT3, P-STAT3, and VEGF-C in small cell lung cancer. *Asian Pac. J. Cancer Prev.* **2012**, *13*, 2873–2877. [CrossRef] [PubMed]
229. Bosch-Barrera, J.; Menendez, J.A. Silibinin and STAT3: A natural way of targeting transcription factors for cancer therapy. *Cancer Treat. Rev.* **2015**, *41*, 540–546. [CrossRef] [PubMed]
230. Monteiro, R.; Calhau, C.; Pinheiro-Silva, S.; Guerreiro, S.; Gärtner, F.; Azevedo, I.; Soares, R. Xanthohumol inhibits inflammatory factor production and angiogenesis in breast cancer xenografts. *J. Cell. Biochem.* **2008**, *104*, 1699–1707. [CrossRef] [PubMed]

231. Schneider, H.; Mueck, A.; Kuhl, H. IARC monographs program on carcinogenicity of combined hormonal contraceptives and menopausal therapy. *Climacteric* **2005**, *8*, 311–316. [CrossRef] [PubMed]
232. Miller, W.; Dixon, J. Local endocrine effects of aromatase inhibitors within the breast. *J. Steroid Biochem. Mol. Biol.* **2001**, *79*, 93–102. [CrossRef]
233. Czajka-Oraniec, I.; Simpson, E.R. Aromatase research and its clinical significance. *Endokrynol. Pol.* **2010**, *61*, 126–134. [PubMed]
234. Jiao, J.; Xiang, H.; Liao, Q. Recent advancement in nonsteroidal aromatase inhibitors for treatment of estrogen-dependent breast cancer. *Curr. Med. Chem.* **2010**, *17*, 3476–3487. [CrossRef] [PubMed]
235. Wang, T.; You, Q.; Huang, F.S.-G.; Xiang, H. Recent advances in selective estrogen receptor modulators for breast cancer. *Mini Rev. Med. Chem.* **2009**, *9*, 1191–1201. [CrossRef] [PubMed]
236. Jefferson, W.N.; Padilla-Banks, E.; Newbold, R.R. Adverse effects on female development and reproduction in CD-1 mice following neonatal exposure to the phytoestrogen genistein at environmentally relevant doses. *Biol. Reprod.* **2005**, *73*, 798–806. [CrossRef]
237. Pearce, S.T.; Jordan, V.C. The biological role of estrogen receptors α and β in cancer. *Crit. Rev. Oncol. Hematol.* **2004**, *50*, 3–22. [CrossRef] [PubMed]
238. Nemenoff, R.A.; Winn, R.A. Role of nuclear receptors in lung tumourigenesis. *Eur. J. Cancer* **2005**, *41*, 2561–2568. [CrossRef] [PubMed]
239. Hsieh, R.W.; Rajan, S.S.; Sharma, S.K.; Guo, Y.; DeSombre, E.R.; Mrksich, M.; Greene, G.L. Identification of ligands with bicyclic scaffolds provides insights into mechanisms of estrogen receptor subtype selectivity. *J. Biol. Chem.* **2006**, *281*, 17909–17919. [CrossRef] [PubMed]
240. Barnes, S. Effect of genistein on in vitro and in vivo models of cancer. *J. Nutr.* **1995**, *125*, 7778–7838.
241. Kuiper, G.G.; Lemmen, J.G.; Carlsson, B.; Corton, J.C.; Safe, S.H.; van Der Saag, P.T.; van Der Burg, B.; Gustafsson, J.A. Interaction of estrogenic chemicals and phytoestrogens with estrogen receptor β. *Endocrinology* **1998**, *139*, 4252–4263. [PubMed]
242. Yoshimaru, T.; Komatsu, M.; Tashiro, E.; Imoto, M.; Osada, H.; Miyoshi, Y.; Honda, J.; Sasa, M.; Katagiri, T. Xanthohumol suppresses oestrogen-signalling in breast cancer through the inhibition of BIG3-PHB2 interactions. *Sci. Rep.* **2014**, *4*, 7355. [CrossRef] [PubMed]
243. Papoutsi, Z.; Kassi, E.; Tsiapara, A.; Fokialakis, N.; Chrousos, G.P.; Moutsatsou, P. Evaluation of estrogenic/antiestrogenic activity of ellagic acid via the estrogen receptor subtypes ERα and ERβ. *J. Agric. Food Chem.* **2005**, *53*, 7715–7720. [CrossRef] [PubMed]
244. Aiyer, H.S.; Gupta, R.C. Berries and ellagic acid prevent estrogen-induced mammary tumorigenesis by modulating enzymes of estrogen metabolism. *Cancer Prev. Res.* **2010**, *3*, 727–737. [CrossRef] [PubMed]
245. Nandhakumar, R.; Salini, K.; Devaraj, S.N. Morin augments anticarcinogenic and antiproliferative efficacy against 7, 12-dimethylbenz (a)-anthracene induced experimental mammary carcinogenesis. *Med. Cell. Biochem.* **2012**, *364*, 79–92. [CrossRef] [PubMed]
246. Fang, H.; Tong, W.; Shi, L.M.; Blair, R.; Perkins, R.; Branham, W.; Hass, B.S.; Xie, Q.; Dial, S.L.; Moland, C.L. Structure-activity relationships for a large diverse set of natural, synthetic, and environmental estrogens. *Chem. Res. Toxicol.* **2001**, *14*, 280–294. [CrossRef] [PubMed]
247. Wang, L.M.; Xie, K.P.; Huo, H.N.; Shang, F.; Zou, W.; Xie, M.J. Luteolin inhibits proliferation induced by IGF-1 pathway dependent ERα in human breast cancer MCF-7 cells. *Asian Pac. J. Cancer Prev.* **2012**, *13*, 1431–1437. [CrossRef] [PubMed]
248. Chen, F.P.; Chien, M.H. Phytoestrogens induce apoptosis through a mitochondria/caspase pathway in human breast cancer cells. *Climacteric* **2014**, *17*, 385–392. [CrossRef] [PubMed]
249. Huang, C.; Lee, S.Y.; Lin, C.L.; Tu, T.H.; Chen, L.H.; Chen, Y.J.; Huang, H.C. Co-treatment with quercetin and 1, 2, 3, 4, 6-penta-O-galloyl-β-d-glucose causes cell cycle arrest and apoptosis in human breast cancer MDA-MB-231 and AU565 cells. *J. Agric. Food Chem.* **2013**, *61*, 6430–6445. [CrossRef] [PubMed]
250. Le Corre, L.; Chalabi, N.; Delort, L.; Bignon, Y.J.; Bernard-Gallon, D.J. Differential expression of genes induced by resveratrol in human breast cancer cell lines. *Nutr. Cancer* **2006**, *56*, 193–203. [CrossRef] [PubMed]
251. Zeng, L.; Holly, J.M.; Perks, C.M. Effects of physiological levels of the green tea extract epigallocatechin-3-gallate on breast cancer cells. *Front. Endocrinol.* **2014**, *5*, 61. [CrossRef] [PubMed]
252. Messina, M.; Nagata, C.; Wu, A.H. Estimated asian adult soy protein and isoflavone intakes. *Nutr. Cancer* **2006**, *55*, 1–12. [CrossRef] [PubMed]
253. Wang, T.T.; Sathyamoorthy, N.; Phang, J.M. Molecular effects of genistein on estrogen receptor mediated pathways. *Carcinogenesis* **1996** *17*, 271–275. [CrossRef] [PubMed]

254. Oseni, T.; Patel, R.; Pyle, J.; Jordan, V.C. Selective estrogen receptor modulators and phytoestrogens. *Planta Med.* **2008**, *74*, 1656–1665. [CrossRef] [PubMed]
255. Patisaul, H.B.; Jefferson, W. The pros and cons of phytoestrogens. *Front. Neuroendocrinol.* **2010**, *31*, 400–419. [CrossRef] [PubMed]
256. Simpson, E.R. Aromatase: Biologic Relevance of Tissue-Specific Expression. *Semin. Reprod. Med.* **2004**, *22*, 11–23. [PubMed]
257. Ghosh, D.; Griswold, J.; Erman, M.; Pangborn, W. Structural basis for androgen specificity and oestrogen synthesis in human aromatase. *Nature* **2009**, *457*, 219–223. [CrossRef] [PubMed]
258. Kudachadkar, R.; O'Regan, R.M. Aromatase inhibitors as adjuvant therapy for postmenopausal patients with early stage breast cancer. *CA Cancer J. Clin.* **2005**, *55*, 145–163. [CrossRef] [PubMed]
259. Kim, M.J.; Woo, S.J.; Yoon, C.H.; Lee, J.S.; An, S.; Choi, Y.H.; Hwang, S.G.; Yoon, G.; Lee, S.J. Involvement of autophagy in oncogenic K-Ras-induced malignant cell transformation. *J. Biol. Chem.* **2011**, *286*, 12924–12932. [CrossRef] [PubMed]
260. Balunas, M.J.; Su, B.; Brueggemeier, R.W.; Kinghorn, A.D. Natural products as aromatase inhibitors. *Anti-Cancer Agents Med. Chem.* **2008**, *8*, 646–682. [CrossRef] [PubMed]
261. Brueggemeier, R.W.; Hackett, J.C.; Diaz-Cruz, E.S. Aromatase inhibitors in the treatment of breast cancer. *Endocr. Rev.* **2005**, *26*, 331–345. [CrossRef] [PubMed]
262. Kao, Y.C.; Zhou, C.; Sherman, M.; Laughton, C.A.; Chen, S. Molecular basis of the inhibition of human aromatase (estrogen synthetase) by flavone and isoflavone phytoestrogens: A site-directed mutagenesis study. *Environ. Health Perspect.* **1998**, *106*, 85–92. [CrossRef] [PubMed]
263. Wang, Y.; Gho, W.M.; Chan, F.L.; Chen, S.; Leung, L.K. The red clover (*Trifolium pratense*) isoflavone biochanin a inhibits aromatase activity and expression. *Br. J. Nutr.* **2008**, *99*, 303–310. [CrossRef] [PubMed]
264. Ye, L.; Gho, W.M.; Chan, F.L.; Chen, S.; Leung, L.K. Dietary administration of the licorice flavonoid isoliquiritigenin deters the growth of MCF-7 cells overexpressing aromatase. *Int. J. Cancer* **2009**, *124*, 1028–1036. [CrossRef] [PubMed]
265. Li, F.; Ye, L.; Lin, S.M.; Leung, L.K. Dietary flavones and flavonones display differential effects on aromatase (CYP19) transcription in the breast cancer cells MCF-7. *Mol. Cell. Endocrinol.* **2011**, *344*, 51–58. [CrossRef] [PubMed]
266. Li, F.; Wong, T.Y.; Lin, S.M.; Chow, S.; Cheung, W.H.; Chan, F.L.; Chen, S.; Leung, L.K. Coadministrating luteolin minimizes the side effects of the aromatase inhibitor letrozole. *J. Pharmacol. Exp. Ther.* **2014**, *351*, 270–277. [CrossRef] [PubMed]
267. Ji, J.Z.; Lao, K.J.; Hu, J.; Pang, T.; Jiang, Z.Z.; Yuan, H.L.; Miao, J.S.; Chen, X.; Ning, S.S.; Xiang, H. Discovery of novel aromatase inhibitors using a homogeneous time-resolved fluorescence assay. *Acta Pharmacol. Sin.* **2014**, *35*, 1082–1092. [CrossRef] [PubMed]
268. González-Sarrías, A.; Ma, H.; Edmonds, M.E.; Seeram, N.P. Maple polyphenols, ginnalins A–C, induce S-and G2/M-cell cycle arrest in colon and breast cancer cells mediated by decreasing cyclins A and D1 levels. *Food Chem.* **2013**, *136*, 636–642. [CrossRef] [PubMed]
269. Liang, Y.C.; Lin-Shiau, S.Y.; Chen, C.F.; Lin, J.K. Inhibition of cyclin-dependent kinases 2 and 4 activities as well as induction of cdk inhibitors p21 and p27 during growth arrest of human breast carcinoma cells by (−)-epigallocatechin-3-gallate. *J. Cell. Biochem.* **1999**, *75*, 1–12. [CrossRef]
270. Mawson, A.; Lai, A.; Carroll, J.S.; Sergio, C.M.; Mitchell, C.J.; Sarcevic, B. Estrogen and insulin/IGF-1 cooperatively stimulate cell cycle progression in MCF-7 breast cancer cells through differential regulation of c-Myc and cyclin D1. *Mol. Cell. Endocrinol.* **2005**, *229*, 161–173. [CrossRef] [PubMed]
271. Li, J.; Zhu, F.; Lubet, R.A.; De Luca, A.; Grubbs, C.; Ericson, M.E.; D'Alessio, A.; Normanno, N.; Dong, Z.; Bode, A.M. Quercetin-3-methyl ether inhibits lapatinib-sensitive and-resistant breast cancer cell growth by inducing G2/M arrest and apoptosis. *Mol. Carcinogen.* **2013**, *52*, 134–143. [CrossRef] [PubMed]
272. Choi, J.A.; Kim, J.Y.; Lee, J.Y.; Kang, C.M.; Kwon, H.J.; Yoo, Y.D.; Kim, T.W.; Lee, Y.S.; Lee, S.J. Induction of cell cycle arrest and apoptosis in human breast cancer cells by quercetin. *Int. J. Oncol.* **2001**, *19*, 837–844. [CrossRef] [PubMed]

273. Chou, C.C.; Yang, J.S.; Lu, H.F.; Ip, S.W.; Lo, C.; Wu, C.C.; Lin, J.P.; Tang, N.Y.; Chung, J.G.; Chou, M.J. Quercetin-mediated cell cycle arrest and apoptosis involving activation of a caspase cascade through the mitochondrial pathway in human breast cancer MCF-7 cells. *Arch. Pharm. Res.* **2010**, *33*, 1181–1191. [CrossRef] [PubMed]
274. Hsieh, T.C.; Wong, C.; John Bennett, D.; Wu, J.M. Regulation of p53 and cell proliferation by resveratrol and its derivatives in breast cancer cells: An in silico and biochemical approach targeting integrin αvβ3. *Int. J. Cancer* **2011**, *129*, 2732–2743. [CrossRef] [PubMed]
275. Simon, A.; Allais, D.; Duroux, J.; Basly, J.; Durand-Fontanier, S.; Delage, C. Inhibitory effect of curcuminoids on MCF-7 cell proliferation and structure–activity relationships. *Cancer Lett.* **1998**, *129*, 111–116. [CrossRef]
276. Choudhuri, T.; Pal, S.; Agwarwal, M.L.; Das, T.; Sa, G. Curcumin induces apoptosis in human breast cancer cells through p53-dependent bax induction. *FEBS Lett.* **2002**, *512*, 334–340. [CrossRef]
277. Banerjee, M.; Singh, P.; Panda, D. Curcumin suppresses the dynamic instability of microtubules, activates the mitotic checkpoint and induces apoptosis in MCF-7 cells. *FEBS J.* **2010**, *277*, 3437–3448. [CrossRef] [PubMed]
278. Choi, E.J.; Kim, G.H. Apigenin causes G(2)/m arrest associated with the modulation of p21(Cip1) and Cdc2 and activates p53-dependent apoptosis pathway in human breast cancer SK-BR-3 cells. *J. Nutr. Biochem.* **2009**, *20*, 285–290. [CrossRef] [PubMed]
279. Umeda, D.; Tachibana, H.; Yamada, K. Epigallocatechin-3-*O*-gallate disrupts stress fibers and the contractile ring by reducing myosin regulatory light chain phosphorylation mediated through the target molecule 67kDa laminin receptor. *Biochem. Biophys. Res. Commun.* **2005**, *333*, 628–635. [CrossRef] [PubMed]
280. Elmore, S. Apoptosis: A review of programmed cell death. *Toxicol. Pathol.* **2007**, *35*, 495–516. [CrossRef] [PubMed]
281. Chien, S.Y.; Wu, Y.C.; Chung, J.G.; Yang, J.S.; Lu, H.F.; Tsou, M.F.; Wood, W.; Kuo, S.J.; Chen, D.R. Quercetin-induced apoptosis acts through mitochondrial-and caspase-3-dependent pathways in human breast cancer MDA-MB-231 cells. *Hum. Exp. Toxicol.* **2009**, *28*, 493–503. [CrossRef] [PubMed]
282. Seo, H.S.; Ku, J.M.; Choi, H.S.; Woo, J.K.; Jang, B.H.; Go, H.; Shin, Y.C.; Ko, S.G. Apigenin induces caspase-dependent apoptosis by inhibiting signal transducer and activator of transcription 3 signaling in HER2-overexpressing SKBR3 breast cancer cells. *Mol. Med. Rep.* **2015**, *12*, 2977–2984. [PubMed]
283. Thangapazham, R.L.; Passi, N.; Maheshwari, R.K. Green tea polyphenol and epigallocatechin gallate induce apoptosis and inhibit invasion in human breast cancer cells. *Cancer Biol. Ther.* **2007**, *6*, 1938–1943. [CrossRef] [PubMed]
284. Clément, M.V.; Hirpara, J.L.; Chawdhury, S.H.; Pervaiz, S. Chemopreventive agent resveratrol, a natural product derived from grapes, triggers CD95 signaling-dependent apoptosis in human tumor cells. *Blood* **1998**, *92*, 996–1002. [PubMed]
285. Alkhalaf, M. Resveratrol-induced apoptosis is associated with activation of p53 and inhibition of protein translation in T47D human breast cancer cells. *Pharmacology* **2007**, *80*, 134–143. [CrossRef] [PubMed]
286. Alkhalaf, M.; El-Mowafy, A.; Renno, W.; Rachid, O.; Ali, A.; Al-Attyiah, R. Resveratrol-induced apoptosis in human breast cancer cells is mediated primarily through the caspase-3-dependent pathway. *Arch. Med. Res.* **2008**, *39*, 162–168. [CrossRef] [PubMed]
287. Kotha, A.; Sekharam, M.; Cilenti, L.; Siddiquee, K.; Khaled, A.; Zervos, A.S.; Carter, B.; Turkson, J.; Jove, R. Resveratrol inhibits Src and Stat3 signaling and induces the apoptosis of malignant cells containing activated Stat3 protein. *Mol. Cancer Ther.* **2006**, *5*, 621–629. [CrossRef] [PubMed]
288. Sakamoto, T.; Horiguchi, H.; Oguma, E.; Kayama, F. Effects of diverse dietary phytoestrogens on cell growth, cell cycle and apoptosis in estrogen-receptor-positive breast cancer cells. *J. Nutr. Biochem.* **2010**, *21*, 856–864. [CrossRef] [PubMed]
289. Chen, J.; Duan, Y.; Zhang, X.; Ye, Y.; Ge, B.; Chen, J. Genistein induces apoptosis by the inactivation of the IGF-1R/p-Akt signaling pathway in MCF-7 human breast cancer cells. *Food Funct.* **2015**, *6*, 995–1000. [CrossRef] [PubMed]
290. Yang, P.M.; Tseng, H.H.; Peng, C.W.; Chen, W.S.; Chiu, S.J. Dietary flavonoid fisetin targets caspase-3-deficient human breast cancer MCF-7 cells by induction of caspase-7-associated apoptosis and inhibition of autophagy. *Int. J. Oncol.* **2012**, *40*, 469. [PubMed]

291. Gottesman, M.M. Mechanisms of cancer drug resistance. *Annu. Rev. Med.* **2002**, *53*, 615–627. [CrossRef] [PubMed]
292. Dean, M.; Fojo, T.; Bates, S. Tumour stem cells and drug resistance. *Nat. Rev. Cancer* **2005**, *5*, 275–284. [CrossRef] [PubMed]
293. Gottesman, M.M.; Fojo, T.; Bates, S.E. Multidrug resistance in cancer: Role of ATP–dependent transporters. *Nat. Rev. Cancer* **2002**, *2*, 48–58. [CrossRef] [PubMed]
294. Jodoin, J.; Demeule, M.; Béliveau, R. Inhibition of the multidrug resistance P-glycoprotein activity by green tea polyphenols. *Biochim. Biophys. Acta* **2002**, *1542*, 149–159. [CrossRef]
295. Wu, C.P.; Calcagno, A.M.; Hladky, S.B.; Ambudkar, S.V.; Barrand, M.A. Modulatory effects of plant phenols on human multidrug-resistance proteins 1, 4 and 5 (ABCC1, 4 and 5). *FEBS J.* **2005**, *272*, 4725–4740. [CrossRef] [PubMed]
296. Choi, B.H.; Kim, C.G.; Lim, Y.; Shin, S.Y.; Lee, Y.H. Curcumin down-regulates the multidrug-resistance *mdr1b* gene by inhibiting the PI3K/Akt/NFκB pathway. *Cancer Lett.* **2008**, *259*, 111–118. [CrossRef] [PubMed]
297. Harbottle, A.; Daly, A.K.; Atherton, K.; Campbell, F.C. Role of glutathione S-transferase p1, P-glycoprotein and multidrug resistance-associated protein 1 in acquired doxorubicin resistance. *Int. J. Cancer* **2001**, *92*, 777–783. [CrossRef] [PubMed]
298. O'Connor, M.L.; Xiang, D.; Shigdar, S.; Macdonald, J.; Li, Y.; Wang, T.; Pu, C.; Wang, Z.; Qiao, L.; Duan, W. Cancer stem cells: A contentious hypothesis now moving forward. *Cancer Lett.* **2014**, *344*, 180–187. [CrossRef] [PubMed]
299. Camerlingo, R.; Ferraro, G.A.; De Francesco, F.; Romano, M.; Nicoletti, G.; Di Bonito, M.; Rinaldo, M.; D'Andrea, F.; Pirozzi, G. The role of CD44+/CD24-/low biomarker for screening, diagnosis and monitoring of breast cancer. *Oncol. Rep.* **2014**, *31*, 1127–1132. [PubMed]
300. Valkenburg, K.C.; Graveel, C.R.; Zylstra-Diegel, C.R.; Zhong, Z.; Williams, B.O. Wnt/β-catenin signaling in normal and cancer stem cells. *Cancers* **2011**, *3*, 2050–2079. [CrossRef] [PubMed]
301. Ingham, P.W.; McMahon, A.P. Hedgehog signaling in animal development: Paradigms and principles. *Genes Dev.* **2001**, *15*, 3059–3087. [CrossRef] [PubMed]
302. McMahon, A.P.; Ingham, P.W.; Tabin, C.J. 1 Developmental roles and clinical significance of hedgehog signaling. *Curr. Top. Dev. Biol.* **2003**, *53*, 1–114. [PubMed]
303. Murone, M.; Rosenthal, A.; de Sauvage, F.J. Sonic hedgehog signaling by the patched-smoothened receptor complex. *Curr. Biol.* **1999**, *9*, 76–84. [CrossRef]
304. Liu, S.; Dontu, G.; Mantle, I.D.; Patel, S.; Ahn, N.S.; Jackson, K.W.; Suri, P.; Wicha, M.S. Hedgehog signaling and Bmi-1 regulate self-renewal of normal and malignant human mammary stem cells. *Cancer Res.* **2006**, *66*, 6063–6071. [CrossRef] [PubMed]
305. Ehtesham, M.; Sarangi, A.; Valadez, J.; Chanthaphaychith, S.; Becher, M.; Abel, T.; Thompson, R.; Cooper, M. Ligand-dependent activation of the hedgehog pathway in glioma progenitor cells. *Oncogene* **2007**, *26*, 5752–5761. [CrossRef] [PubMed]
306. Peacock, C.D.; Wang, Q.; Gesell, G.S.; Corcoran-Schwartz, I.M.; Jones, E.; Kim, J.; Devereux, W.L.; Rhodes, J.T.; Huff, C.A.; Beachy, P.A. Hedgehog signaling maintains a tumor stem cell compartment in multiple myeloma. *Proc. Natl. Acad. Sci. USA* **2007**, *104*, 4048–4053. [CrossRef] [PubMed]
307. Zhang, C.; Li, C.; He, F.; Cai, Y.; Yang, H. Identification of CD44+ CD24+ gastric cancer stem cells. *J. Cancer Res. Clin. Oncol.* **2011**, *137*, 1679–1686. [CrossRef] [PubMed]
308. Ng, J.M.; Curran, T. The hedgehog's tale: Developing strategies for targeting cancer. *Nat. Rev. Cancer* **2011**, *11*, 493–501. [CrossRef] [PubMed]
309. Feldmann, G.; Dhara, S.; Fendrich, V.; Bedja, D.; Beaty, R.; Mullendore, M.; Karikari, C.; Alvarez, H.; Iacobuzio-Donahue, C.; Jimeno, A. Blockade of hedgehog signaling inhibits pancreatic cancer invasion and metastases: A new paradigm for combination therapy in solid cancers. *Cancer Res.* **2007**, *67*, 2187–2196. [CrossRef] [PubMed]
310. Fan, P.; Fan, S.; Wang, H.; Mao, J.; Shi, Y.; Ibrahim, M.M.; Ma, W.; Yu, X.; Hou, Z.; Wang, B.; et al. Genistein decreases the breast cancer stem-like cell population through hedgehog pathway. *Stem Cell Res. Ther.* **2013**, *4*, 146. [CrossRef] [PubMed]
311. Bray, S.J. Notch signalling: A simple pathway becomes complex. *Nat. Rev. Mol. Cell Biol.* **2006**, *7*, 678–689. [CrossRef] [PubMed]

312. Ishii, H.; Iwatsuki, M.; Ieta, K.; Ohta, D.; Haraguchi, N.; Mimori, K.; Mori, M. Cancer stem cells and chemoradiation resistance. *Cancer Sci.* **2008**, *99*, 1871–1877. [CrossRef] [PubMed]
313. Cecchinato, V.; Chiaramonte, R.; Nizzardo, M.; Cristofaro, B.; Basile, A.; Sherbet, G.V.; Comi, P. Resveratrol-induced apoptosis in human T-cell acute lymphoblastic leukaemia MOLT-4 cells. *Biochem. Pharmacol.* **2007**, *74*, 1568–1574. [CrossRef] [PubMed]
314. Liu, S.; Dontu, G.; Wicha, M.S. Mammary stem cells, self-renewal pathways, and carcinogenesis. *Breast Cancer Res.* **2005**, *7*, 86–95. [CrossRef] [PubMed]
315. Clevers, H. Wnt/β-catenin signaling in development and disease. *Cell* **2006**, *127*, 469–480. [CrossRef] [PubMed]
316. Kim, J.; Zhang, X.; Rieger-Christ, K.M.; Summerhayes, I.C.; Wazer, D.E.; Paulson, K.E.; Yee, A.S. Suppression of Wnt signaling by the green tea compound (–)-epigallocatechin 3-gallate (EGCG) in invasive breast cancer cells. Requirement of the transcriptional repressor HBP1. *J. Biol. Chem.* **2006**, *281*, 10865–10875. [CrossRef] [PubMed]
317. Ju, J.; Hong, J.; Zhou, J.N.; Pan, Z.; Bose, M.; Liao, J.; Yang, G.Y.; Liu, Y.Y.; Hou, Z.; Lin, Y. Inhibition of intestinal tumorigenesis in Apcmin/+ mice by (−)-epigallocatechin-3-gallate, the major catechin in green tea. *Cancer Res.* **2005**, *65*, 10623–10631. [CrossRef] [PubMed]
318. Jaiswal, A.S.; Marlow, B.P.; Gupta, N.; Narayan, S. Beta-catenin-mediated transactivation and cell–cell adhesion pathways are important in curcumin (diferuylmethane)-induced growth arrest and apoptosis in colon cancer cells. *Oncogene* **2002**, *21*, 8414–8427. [CrossRef] [PubMed]
319. Clarke, J.D.; Dashwood, R.H.; Ho, E. Multi-targeted prevention of cancer by sulforaphane. *Cancer Lett.* **2008**, *269*, 291–304. [CrossRef] [PubMed]
320. Kallifatidis, G.; Rausch, V.; Baumann, B.; Apel, A.; Beckermann, B.M.; Groth, A.; Mattern, J.; Li, Z.; Kolb, A.; Moldenhauer, G. Sulforaphane targets pancreatic tumour-initiating cells by NF-κB-induced antiapoptotic signalling. *Gut* **2009**, *58*, 949–963. [CrossRef] [PubMed]
321. Li, Y.; Zhang, T.; Korkaya, H.; Liu, S.; Lee, H.F.; Newman, B.; Yu, Y.; Clouthier, S.G.; Schwartz, S.J.; Wicha, M.S. Sulforaphane, a dietary component of broccoli/broccoli sprouts, inhibits breast cancer stem cells. *Clin. Cancer Res.* **2010**, *16*, 2580–2590. [CrossRef] [PubMed]
322. Park, S.Y.; Kim, G.Y.; Bae, S.J.; Yoo, Y.H.; Choi, Y.H. Induction of apoptosis by isothiocyanate sulforaphane in human cervical carcinoma HeLa and hepatocarcinoma HepG2 cells through activation of caspase-3. *Oncol. Rep.* **2007**, *18*, 181–187. [CrossRef] [PubMed]
323. Pradeep, C.; Kuttan, G. Effect of piperine on the inhibition of lung metastasis induced B16F-10 melanoma cells in mice. *Clin. Exp. Metastasis* **2002**, *19*, 703–708. [CrossRef] [PubMed]
324. Kakarala, M.; Brenner, D.E.; Korkaya, H.; Cheng, C.; Tazi, K.; Ginestier, C.; Liu, S.; Dontu, G.; Wicha, M.S. Targeting breast stem cells with the cancer preventive compounds curcumin and piperine. *Breast Cancer Res. Treat.* **2010**, *122*, 777–785. [CrossRef] [PubMed]
325. Zhang, Y.; Piao, B.; Zhang, Y.; Hua, B.; Hou, W.; Xu, W.; Qi, X.; Zhu, X.; Pei, Y.; Lin, H. Oxymatrine diminishes the side population and inhibits the expression of β-catenin in MCF-7 breast cancer cells. *Med. Oncol.* **2011**, *28* (Suppl. 1), S99–S107. [CrossRef] [PubMed]
326. Mortensen, M.; Soilleux, E.J.; Djordjevic, G.; Tripp, R.; Lutteropp, M.; Sadighi-Akha, E.; Stranks, A.J.; Glanville, J.; Knight, S.; Jacobsen, S.-E.W. The autophagy protein Atg7 is essential for hematopoietic stem cell maintenance. *J. Exp. Med.* **2011**, *208*, 455–467. [CrossRef] [PubMed]
327. Gong, C.; Song, E.; Codogno, P.; Mehrpour, M. The roles of BECN1 and autophagy in cancer are context dependent. *Autophagy* **2012**, *8*, 1853–1855. [CrossRef] [PubMed]
328. Galavotti, S.; Bartesaghi, S.; Faccenda, D.; Shaked-Rabi, M.; Sanzone, S.; McEvoy, A.; Dinsdale, D.; Condorelli, F.; Brandner, S.; Campanella, M. The autophagy-associated factors DRAM1 and p62 regulate cell migration and invasion in glioblastoma stem cells. *Oncogene* **2013**, *32*, 699–712. [CrossRef] [PubMed]
329. Kumar, D.; Shankar, S.; Srivastava, R.K. Rottlerin-induced autophagy leads to the apoptosis in breast cancer stem cells: Molecular mechanisms. *Mol. Cancer* **2013**, *12*, 171. [CrossRef] [PubMed]
330. Fu, Y.; Chang, H.; Peng, X.; Bai, Q.; Yi, L.; Zhou, Y.; Zhu, J.; Mi, M. Resveratrol inhibits breast cancer stem-like cells and induces autophagy via suppressing Wnt/β-catenin signaling pathway. *PLoS ONE* **2014**, *9*, e102535. [CrossRef] [PubMed]
331. Singh, A.; Settleman, J. EMT, cancer stem cells and drug resistance: An emerging axis of evil in the war on cancer. *Oncogene* **2010**, *29*, 4741–4751. [CrossRef] [PubMed]

332. Polyak, K.; Weinberg, R.A. Transitions between epithelial and mesenchymal states: Acquisition of malignant and stem cell traits. *Nat. Rev. Cancer* **2009**, *9*, 265–273. [CrossRef] [PubMed]
333. Hugo, H.; Ackland, M.L.; Blick, T.; Lawrence, M.G.; Clements, J.A.; Williams, E.D.; Thompson, E.W. Epithelial-mesenchymal and mesenchymal-epithelial transitions in carcinoma progression. *J. Cell. Physiol.* **2007**, *213*, 374–383. [CrossRef] [PubMed]
334. Thiery, J.P.; Sleeman, J.P. Complex networks orchestrate epithelial–mesenchymal transitions. *Nat. Rev. Mol. Cell Biol.* **2006**, *7*, 131–142. [CrossRef] [PubMed]
335. Min, C.; Eddy, S.F.; Sherr, D.H.; Sonenshein, G.E. NF-κB and epithelial to mesenchymal transition of cancer. *J. Cell. Biochem.* **2008**, *104*, 733–744. [CrossRef] [PubMed]
336. Shi, X.P.; Miao, S.; Wu, Y.; Zhang, W.; Zhang, X.F.; Ma, H.Z.; Xin, H.L.; Feng, J.; Wen, A.D.; Li, Y. Resveratrol sensitizes tamoxifen in antiestrogen-resistant breast cancer cells with epithelial-mesenchymal transition features. *Int. J. Mol. Sci.* **2013**, *14*, 15655–15668. [CrossRef] [PubMed]
337. Vergara, D.; Valente, C.M.; Tinelli, A.; Siciliano, C.; Lorusso, V.; Acierno, R.; Giovinazzo, G.; Santino, A.; Storelli, C.; Maffia, M. Resveratrol inhibits the epidermal growth factor-induced epithelial mesenchymal transition in MCF-7 cells. *Cancer Lett.* **2011**, *310*, 1–8. [CrossRef] [PubMed]
338. Chung, H.; Choi, H.S.; Seo, E.K.; Kang, D.H.; Oh, E.S. Baicalin and baicalein inhibit transforming growth factor-β1-mediated epithelial-mesenchymal transition in human breast epithelial cells. *Biochem. Biophys. Res. Commun.* **2015**, *458*, 707–713. [CrossRef] [PubMed]
339. Yang, B.; Huang, J.; Xiang, T.; Yin, X.; Luo, X.; Huang, J.; Luo, F.; Li, H.; Li, H.; Ren, G. Chrysin inhibits metastatic potential of human triple-negative breast cancer cells by modulating matrix metalloproteinase-10, epithelial to mesenchymal transition, and PI3K/Akt signaling pathway. *J. Appl. Toxicol.* **2014**, *34*, 105–112. [CrossRef] [PubMed]
340. Nagaraj, G.; Ellis, M.J.; Ma, C.X. The natural history of hormone receptor-positive breast cancer: Attempting to decipher an intriguing concept. *Oncology* **2012**, *26*, 696–697, 700. [PubMed]

4

Evidence to Support the Anti-Cancer Effect of Olive Leaf Extract and Future Directions

Anna Boss [1,*], Karen S. Bishop [2], Gareth Marlow [1], Matthew P. G. Barnett [3] and Lynnette R. Ferguson [1,2]

1 Discipline of Nutrition, FM & HS, University of Auckland Medical School, Private Bag 92019, Auckland 1142, New Zealand; MarlowG@cardiff.ac.uk (G.M.); l.ferguson@auckland.ac.nz (L.R.F.)
2 Auckland Cancer Society Research Centre, FM & HS, University of Auckland Medical School, Private Bag 92019, Auckland 1142, New Zealand; k.bishop@auckland.ac.nz
3 Food Nutrition & Health Team, Food & Bio-based Products Group, AgResearch Limited, Grasslands Research Centre, Tennent Drive, Palmerston North 4442, New Zealand; matthew.barnett@agresearch.co.nz
* Correspondence: abos517@aucklanduni.ac.nz

Abstract: The traditional Mediterranean diet (MD) is associated with long life and lower prevalence of cardiovascular disease and cancers. The main components of this diet include high intake of fruit, vegetables, red wine, extra virgin olive oil (EVOO) and fish, low intake of dairy and red meat. Olive oil has gained support as a key effector of health benefits and there is evidence that this relates to the polyphenol content. Olive leaf extract (OLE) contains a higher quantity and variety of polyphenols than those found in EVOO. There are also important structural differences between polyphenols from olive leaf and those from olive fruit that may improve the capacity of OLE to enhance health outcomes. Olive polyphenols have been claimed to play an important protective role in cancer and other inflammation-related diseases. Both inflammatory and cancer cell models have shown that olive leaf polyphenols are anti-inflammatory and protect against DNA damage initiated by free radicals. The various bioactive properties of olive leaf polyphenols are a plausible explanation for the inhibition of progression and development of cancers. The pathways and signaling cascades manipulated include the NF-κB inflammatory response and the oxidative stress response, but the effects of these bioactive components may also result from their action as a phytoestrogen. Due to the similar structure of the olive polyphenols to oestrogens, these have been hypothesized to interact with oestrogen receptors, thereby reducing the prevalence and progression of hormone related cancers. Evidence for the protective effect of olive polyphenols for cancer in humans remains anecdotal and clinical trials are required to substantiate these claims idea. This review aims to amalgamate the current literature regarding bioavailability and mechanisms involved in the potential anti-cancer action of olive leaf polyphenols.

Keywords: olive leaf; oleuropein; oxidative stress; inflammation; Mediterranean diet; Cyclooxygenase-2

---

1. Introduction

Cancer is a group of diseases involving proliferation of mutated cells [1]. In 2012, over 14 million new cases of cancer were reported [2], triggering a push to further develop treatments and preventative strategies. Cancer is predominantly an age-related disease, therefore with better conditions of life and increased longevity it is likely to continue increasing in prevalence. However, there are clearly factors other than age that contribute to its development. The traditional Mediterranean diet (MD) has gained robust scientific support for providing protection against some cancers [3,4]. The MD has shown an ability to influence the inflammatory response, which plays a pivotal role in aging and in reducing its age-associated non-communicable diseases such as cancer. However, the mechanisms of action behind the effects of the MD on inflammation are not entirely clear [5–7]. It has been suggested that the NF-κB inflammatory response, eicosanoid pathways and oxidative stress via free radical formation, have been suggested to play a role in MD related health benefits [5,8,9]. The diet, as a whole, has shown a protective role in cancer, however, the distribution of people still consuming it is gradually receding due to the spread of the western-type urban society, globalization and consumption [10]. Because of this, it is important to understand whether any beneficial effects ascribed to the MD are due to a particular component of the diet, rather than the whole diet. As one example, polyphenol bioactive components have shown particular promise and have therefore been a research focus.

Extra virgin olive oil (EVOO) is typically used as a traditional component of the MD and has also been correlated with improved cardiovascular disease and cancer outcomes [11,12]. EVOO is manufactured by pressing olives to create a paste, which is churned to amalgamate oil droplets which are then extracted. There is a considerable variation in EVOO characteristics that can be attributed to the olive variety, the geographical location the olives were derived from [13] and the method of oil extraction [14]. Intake of both MD and EVOO has been shown to correlate with a reduced overall risk of cancer and is more specifically associated with reduced risk of cancers of the digestive system, prostate and breast [12].

EVOO is primarily a monounsaturated fatty acid (MUFA) in the form of oleic acid, with minor components including various phenolics [15]. It has been recognised that the polyphenol content plays an important role in health benefits. The European Food Safety Authority (EFSA) have approved the use of the general claim "olive oil polyphenols contribute to the protection of blood lipids from oxidative stress" when oil contains no less than 5 mg of hydroxytyrosol (HT) and its derivatives (such as tyrosol and oleuropein) per 20 mL OO [16] (Figure 1). There are several studies that have shown that EVOO with higher phenolic content provides stronger anti-inflammatory and antioxidant effects than OO with a lower phenolic content [17,18]. This suggests the phenolic component, rather than the fat in the oil, is the effector.

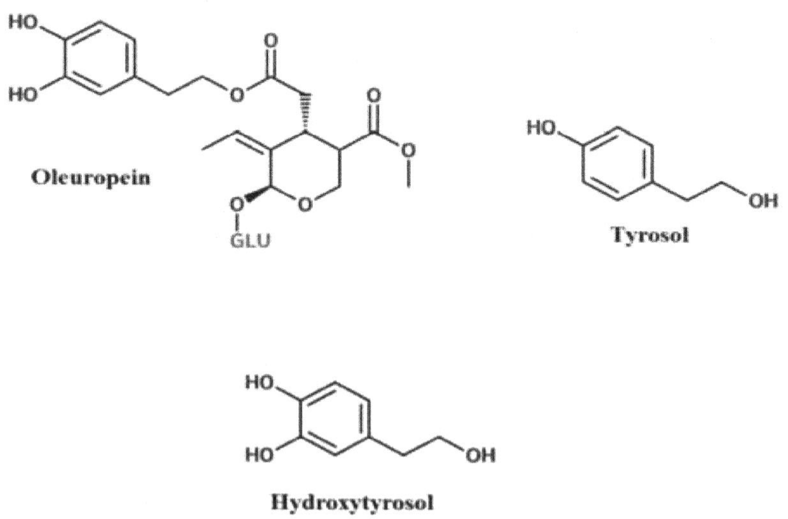

Figure 1. The olive polyphenol hydroxytyrosol and its derivatives, oleuropein and tyrosol (adapted from [19]).

Olive tree leaves (*Olea europaea*) are widely used in traditional medicine in the Mediterranean region [20]. In the Bible, the olive plant is referenced numerous times for its medicinal use [21]. The bioactive properties of the leaf have created a foundation for use as an antioxidant, anti-hypertensive, anti-atherogenic, anti-inflammatory, hypoglycemic, and hypocholesterolemic treatment [20]. Olive tree leaves contain similar polyphenols to those found in EVOO or the fruit itself, albeit at a much higher concentration [20,22]. Consequently, olive leaf extract (OLE) may hold an even greater potential than EVOO for improving health outcomes. During EVOO processing leaves can unintentionally be left in the mixture if the separation methods are inadequate, alternately leaves can also be added to EVOO mixtures to provide health benefits and improve flavor [23]. The addition of leaves increase the phenolic and chlorophyll content of the oil but also the organoleptic traits as measured in volunteer taste tests [24]. Components of OLE that are not detected in the oil from the fruit include several flavonoids, namely luteolin and apigenin, which have demonstrated anti-cancer properties [25–29]. In addition, the structure of phenolics differs between the olive fruit and leaf, with OLE containing a higher proportion with a glycoside moiety (Figure 2 and Table 1) [19]. The presence of a glucose molecule could play an important role in respect to both bioavailability and bioactive potential of the polyphenols, thereby impacting the health benefits for humans.

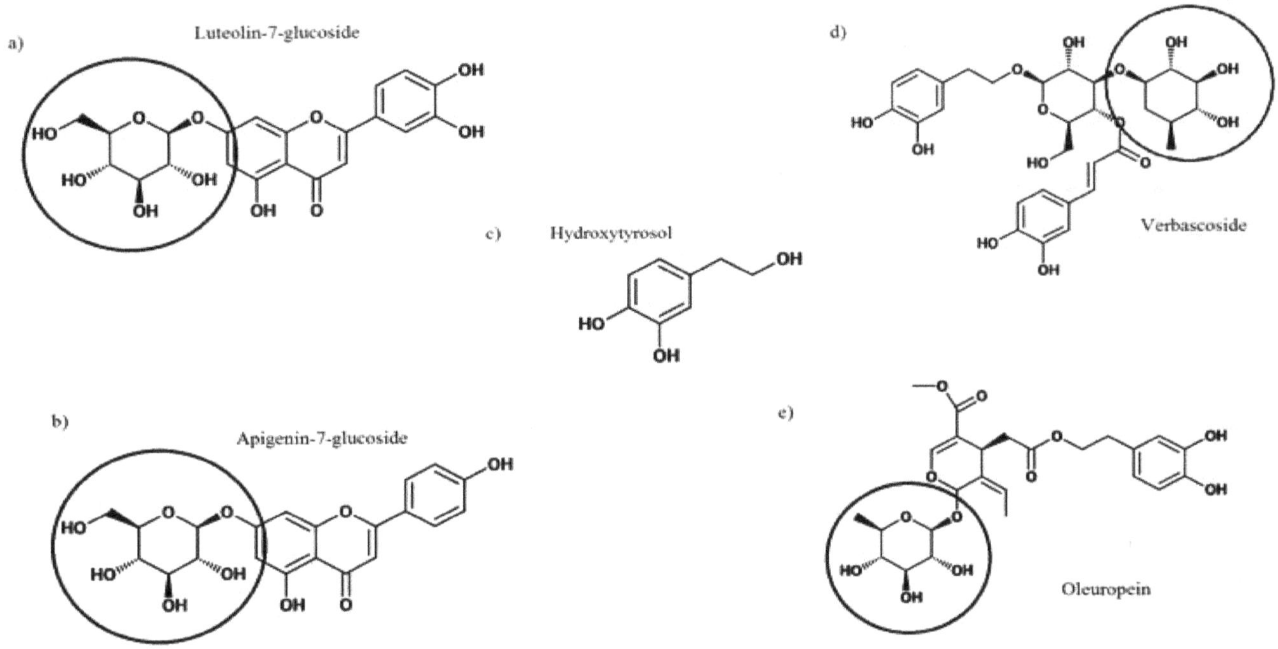

Figure 2. Most abundant phenolics present in OLE. Structures (**a**) and (**b**) are flavonoids. Structures (**d**) and (**e**) are esters of (**c**) which is a simple phenolic. The glucoside moieties are circled. This figure is adapted from [19].

Table 1. Comparison of phenolic compounds found in olive leaf extract and olive oil, with values reported in mg/kg [30]. Luteolin, apigenin, verbascoside and oleuropein all have a glucoside moiety. Values are an estimated range generated from a comprehensive review of the published literature.

	Hydroxytyrosol	Oleuropein	Luteolin-7-Glucoside	Apigenin-7-Glucoside	Verbascoside	Oleuropein Aglycone	Reference
Olive oil mg/Kg	131.77 ± 32	ND	ND	ND	ND	17.24 ± 1.15	[30]
	3.0 ± 0.2	ND	ND	ND	0.08 ± 0.02	NM	[31]
	12.5	ND	NM	NM	NM	NM	[32]
	4.3–9.9	ND	4.0–7.6	1.5–2.6	ND	67.7–136.4	[33]
	0.15–1.53	ND	ND	ND	ND	0.35–6.43	[34]
Olive leaf mg/Kg	NM	26,471.4 ± 1760.2	4208.9 ± 97.8	2333.1 ± 74.7	966.1 ± 18.1	NM	[35]
	ND	19,050 ± 880	155 ± 10	207 ± 10	1428 ± 46	NM	[31]
	NM	19,860 ± 54	NM	NM	200 ± 40	NM	[36]
	NM	22,610 ± 632	970 ± 43	1072 ± 38	488 ± 21	NM	[37]
	NM	5173–12,921	219–444	192–488	213–501	NM	[38]

Abbreviations: not detected: ND; not measured: NM.

Although there is a large body of research that has investigated the phenolic components of olive products and the benefits they provide to human health [39–42], there are currently no approved claims in regard to OLE. OLE not only contains a higher quantity and variety of polyphenols than those found in EVOO, but many of the polyphenols also contain a glucose moiety. This structural difference in the polyphenols may have important consequences by altering their capacity to improve health outcomes [43,44]. In previous work, OLE polyphenols have demonstrated the ability to inhibit proliferation of several cancer cell lines including pancreatic [45], leukaemia [46] and breast [28,47]. Cellular models for breast and prostate cancers have been inhibited by the olive polyphenols oleuropein and HT [48–51]. Importantly, oleuropein and HT have consistently been reported to discriminate between cancer and normal cells; inhibiting proliferation and inducing apoptosis only in cancer cells. The intake of polyphenols in observational studies is difficult to quantify and therefore assign effect and intervention studies in regards to cancer have not been carried out, therefore the relationship between polyphenols and cancer outcomes in humans has not been substantiated.

Research into the anti-cancer properties of olive polyphenols is abundant with a focus on the health effects of EVOO. Evidence suggests that the bioactive components of OLE, although similar to EVOO, may be more potent and therefore show more potential for improving health outcomes. This review aims to amalgamate the current literature regarding bioavailability and anti-cancer mechanisms involved in OLE polyphenol action. The literature identified for this review was found using the search engines PubMed-NCBI, Scopus and ScienceDirect with a combination of block searching and pearl-growing. Key words used for the search were olive leaf extract, polyphenols, cancer, oleuropein, hydroxytyrosol, Mediterranean diet, inflammation, and bioavailability. The key components from the research articles pivotal to this review have been summarized in Supplementary Table S1.

2. Olive Leaf Polyphenols

The Mediterranean region, where olive trees are predominantly grown, is characterized by extended periods of sunlight and high rates of pathogen and insect attack. To combat these stressors, olive trees synthesize high volumes of polyphenols which are largely stored in their thick leaves [52]. The concentration and variety of polyphenols present in the leaves will be influenced by many factors such as geographical location, cultivar of tree, and the age of the tree [49]. Polyphenols comprise multiple phenolic groups, each consisting of an aromatic ring with a varying number of hydroxyl groups [19]. The polyphenols predominantly occur in a conjugated form, with one or several sugars attached to the hydroxyl group [53]. The number and structure of phenol rings in a polyphenol are used for classification and will determine its bioactive properties. The main phenolic compounds are the secoiridoids (namely oleuropein) and flavonoids (Figure 2), these have shown the ability to influence human and animal inflammatory and metabolic biomarkers [41,54–56].

Secoiridoids are a group of compounds found exclusively in plants of the *Olearaceae* family, and make up the majority of olive polyphenols (~85% of olive leaf polyphenols) [57]. In OLE the secoiridoid, oleuropein is the most abundant polyphenol (Figure 2), while its derivatives oleuropein aglycone, oleoside, and ligstroside aglycone are also present at varying concentrations [19]. The research surrounding oleuropein is abundant. It has been associated with numerous health benefits including the ability to: lower blood pressure in rats [58], decrease plasma glucose concentrations in rats [55], inhibit the growth of microbes grown on agar plates [59], inhibit cultured parasitic protozoans [60] and has also shown the ability to induce apoptosis in cancer cell models: colorectal [61], breast ([61–63] and prostate [48]. Human trials looking into the effect of OLE on cancer do not yet exist.

Hydrolysis of oleuropein gives rise to oleuropein aglycone, elenolic acid, HT and a glucose molecule (Figure 3) [64]. HT is a phenolic alcohol and the second most abundant phenolic acid in olive leaf. Tyrosol is another phenolic acid derived from oleuropein, but is found in low concentrations in the leaf (Table 1). Other related compounds include verbascoside, which also has demonstrated anti-inflammatory, anti-oxidant and antineoplastic properties similar to the other olive leaf bioactives [65], as well as caffeic acid (220.5 ± 23.3 mg/kg) [35] and p-coumaric acid.

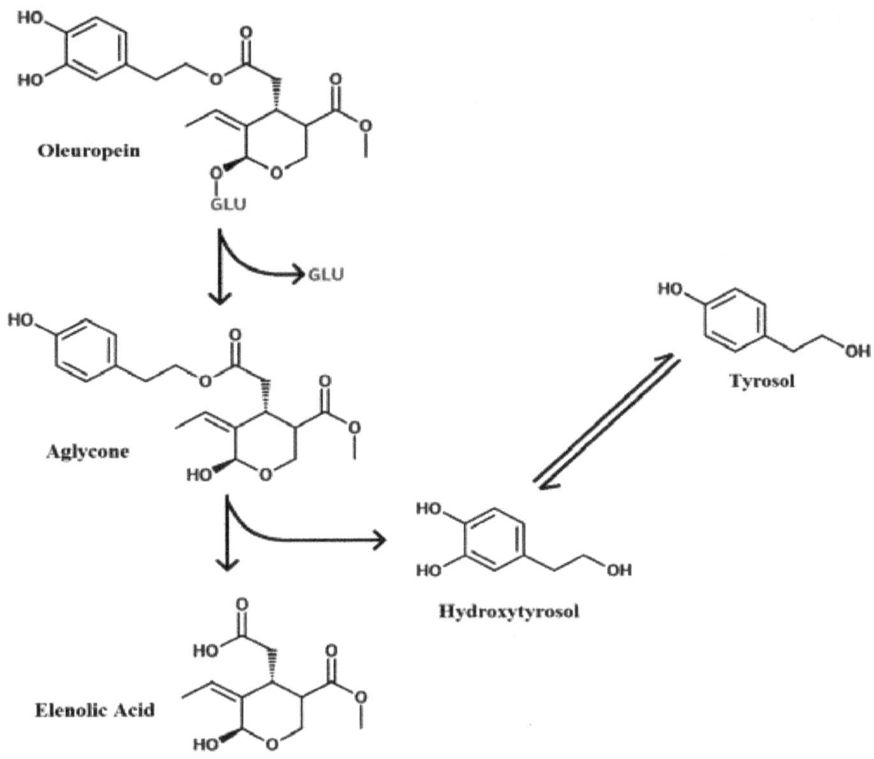

Figure 3. Glycosylation of oleuropein to its aglycone this gives rise to elenolic acid and hydroxytyrosol. Tyrosol in turn is hydrolysed from hydroxytyrosol (modified from Granados-Principal et al., 2010 [64]).

OLE consists of a number of flavonoids (~2% of olive leaf polyphenols) including luteolin, apigenin (Table 1), rutin (495.9 ± 12.2 mg/kg) [35], catechin (19.3–32.6 mg/g dried extract) [66] and diosmetin (8.70 mg/g dried extract) [22]. Luteolin is able to suppress inflammatory expression in macrophages and adipocytes [67]. Apigenin is present at relatively low concentrations within olive leaf, but it has also been linked to anti-inflammatory, anti-cancer and anti-oxidising properties [68].

Other components of OLE that occur in smaller concentrations include oleanolic acid [69], vanillin and vanillic acid, [59], as well as tocopherols and β carotene [70]. In human studies, α tocopherols have been correlated to lower prostate cancer mortality, but β carotene at high concentrations, has been correlated to increased mortality of lung cancer patients [71].

Thousands of phytochemicals with differing attributes have been identified and isolated, but a point which is often overlooked is that it can be a combination of compounds that induce health benefits [72–74]. Within plants, polyphenols are present in mixtures and not as independent compounds; the polyphenols have evolved together, generally for the purpose of deterring insect feeding and the levels of the different bioactives with these mixtures need to be considered when looking at bioactive properties for human health. While the evolutionary purpose for the polyphenol mixtures it not for human benefit, the nature of the mixtures may nevertheless be important for human health. Several studies have demonstrated that the phenolic compounds from OLE may display a synergistic effect when in the same proportions as occurring naturally in the olive leaf. The secoiridoids, flavonoids and other phenols in OLE provide a stronger anti-microbial and antioxidant effect when working together, as opposed to the phenolics independently [59,75,76]. Through the use of different antioxidant assays it was determined that OLE flavonoids, simple phenols and secoiridoids utilize different mechanisms to exert an anti-oxidant effect [75], which at least in part explains their additive effect.

3. Bioavailability of Olive Leaf Polyphenols

In nutrition, bioavailability refers to the amount of compound/nutrient extracted from a food or supplement that is capable of being absorbed and made available for physiological use by the body [77]. There are many factors that will influence the bioavailability of a compound including the vector, time taken for absorption, structure of compound/bioactive target or the individual person [78]. The matrix that the olive leaf is consumed and maintained may also have an impact on the bioavailability of the active components. The leaves can be consumed in tea, as a powder or in an extract form As an example, De Bock and co-authors demonstrated that the polyphenol derivatives measured in plasma differed when the OLE was administered as a safflower oil compared to a glycerol matrix [79].

The ability to produce health benefits in different organs throughout the body requires that the bioactive olive leaf polyphenols, or their metabolites, are able to infiltrate these areas. After an acute load of olive phenolic (3 g phenolic extract from olive cake/kg of body weight) extract in mice, samples demonstrated that phenolic derivatives and conjugates (oleuropein, tyrosol, HT and luteolin) were absorbed, metabolised and present in the plasma (oleuropein derivative: max 4 h: 24 nmol/L and HT: max 2 h: 5.2 nmol/L), the heart (luteolin derivative at 1 h: 0.47 nmol/g), kidney (luteolin derivative 1 h: 0.04 nmol/g, HT max 4 h: 3.8 nmol/g), testicles (olueropein derivative Cmax 2 h: 0.07 nmol/g and HT max 2 h: 2.7 nmol/g) and had even passed the blood brain barrier (olueropein derivative at 2 h: 2.8 nmol/g) [80].

The research looking into bioavailability of polyphenols from OLE in commercial glycerol formulations consistently show that oleuropein is bioavailable in humans but there is differing evidence regarding the metabolites found in plasma [79,81]. De Bock reported the primary metabolite recovered to be glucoronidated and sulphated HT [79]. In contrast, Kendall's group reported that no HT was detected in urine samples, but glucuronic acid conjugates, derived from oleuropein aglycone were detected [81]. In rats fed oleuropein, liquid chromatography-mass spectrometry (LC-MS) detected oleuropein, oleuropein aglycone, elenolic acid and HT both within faeces and urine at 24 h [82]. This demonstrates the stability of these compounds and therefore the potential ability to reach other parts of the body intact and in an active form.

Corona et al. (2006) reported HT and tyrosol traversed the perfused small intestine membrane of rats but oleuropein did not, and would therefore likely reach the large intestine intact [83]. Incubating with anaerobic human microbiota with olueropein resulted in rapid and extensive microbiota degradation of oleuropein to HT and other metabolites [83]. Specifically the gastrointestinal bacterium *Lactobacillus planatarum* has the ability to metabolize oleuropein to HT [84]. The microbiota acting to break down oleuropein to HT would have an important impact on bioavailability if oleuropein cannot traverse membranes, but HT and other metabolites can, as reported by Corona et al. 2006. Another study has since found that oleuropein orally administered to rats resulted in the production of oleuropein metabolites from the gastrointestinal tract as well as metabolites in the blood [82]. The most recent research looking into the metabolism of oleuropein verses oleuropein aglycone in rodents (5 mg phenol/kg/day) found that oleuropein resulted in the greatest bioavailabilty (measured by the highest content of HT excreted in urine) and a greater diversity of microbial metabolites due to its superior ability to reach the colon intact [44].

Glycosylation of Polyphenols

The glucose moiety that is present on many of the olive leaf polyphenols could have an important impact on their bioactive properties. The glucose molecule significantly increases the molar mass of the polyphenol; oleuropein is 540.51 g/mol, where the oleuropein aglycone is 394 g/mol. The glucose molecule may improve stability and bioavailability, and facilitate cell entry but it also may impede bioactive properties.

Through collection and processing methods of olives and leaves, different glycosylation enzymes are activated [85]. The transformation of oleuropein is dependent on the type of glycosylation enzyme acting (β-glucosidase, hemicellulase, tannase, neutral protease, cellulase, glucoamylase, papain, alkaline protease, amylase, β-glucanase) and this will result in varied concentrations and ratios of HT, oleuropein aglycone, elonolic acid and total phenolics [86,87]. The combination of polyphenols may improve the OLE biostability, insuring polyphenols are still present in the olive leaf extract when consumed by humans but also improving the polyphenols ability to reach different areas of the body intact. For example oxidoreductase enzymes reduce the abundance of oleuropein in OLE, but the presence of HT is able to inhibit their action [86].

Olive leaf polyphenols containing a glucose moiety have been suggested to play an important role in relation to cancer cell treatment. A study looking at oleuropein found removal of the glucose moiety reduced its ability to inhibit proliferation of cancer cells [43]. This indicated that the hydrophilic glucose may be enabling oleuropein to enter cells via GLUT transporters to create the anti-cancer affect. GLUT mRNA expression is often increased in cancer cells and is correlated to cancer progression [88]. The glucose moiety in oleuropein may facilitate its diffusion into these cells in precedence to normal cells and therefore result in a greater inhibitory effect on cancer versus normal cells. Another study has indicated that the olive flavonoid apigenin is able to reduce the expression of GLUT1 in prostate cancer cell lines thereby inhibiting proliferation of the cancer [29].

Another study looking at the effect of oleuropein (dissolved in water) verses oleuropein aglycone (dissolved in ethanol 100%) (6 to 100 μM) in MCF-7 found the aglycone to be more effective at reducing cell viability [89]. This would suggest that the glycoside is essential for anti-cancer effects.

Protective effects of the MD and EVOO against cancers, as discussed in the introduction, are primarily associated with cancers of the digestive system. This could be due to the bioavailability of the polyphenols, with the polyphenol constituents creating the anti-cancer effects not being able to reach other parts of the body to have an impact. Consequently if the glucose moiety, a prominent characteristic of olive leaf polyphenols improves bioavailability it may also improve protective effects for different cancers.

4. OLE and Evidence of the Ability of Olive Leaf Polyphenols to Scavenge Nitric Oxide and Quench Reactive Oxygen Species

Reactive oxygen species (ROS) and nitrogen species (NOS) are essential for cell function. They are involved in energy supply, detoxification, chemical signaling and immune response. However, when overproduced they can create stress by damaging DNA, lipids and proteins and they are widely accepted to play an important role in pathologies and aging [20,90]. Chronic disease is associated with oxidative stress, therefore an increased antioxidant intake or intake of compounds that enhance the body's own antioxidant system is expected to reduce the risk of these diseases. It was this hypothesis that has led to an increased interest in antioxidants and their bioactive properties. Phenolics are one group for which there is robust evidence supporting the health promoting effects of antioxidants. There is a general consensus that olive leaf phenolics have a strong ability to scavenge nitric oxide (NO) and quench ROS [91,92].

Antioxidant properties have been an important focus of research into polyphenols and are a widely accepted mechanism for their health benefits. However, it has been suggested that several constraints impede polyphenol in vivo scavenging of radicals, and that they would be inefficient at mounting an antioxidant defense [93]. Concerns that have been highlighted include bioavailability (the anti-oxidizing agent must reach these radicals in an active form to quench them) and kinetic constraints for antioxidant scavenging (radicals may actually react with other biological molecules such as DNA and lipids in the cell at the same rate as the antioxidants) [93]. This could mean that a very high concentration of polyphenols would need to be ingested to perceive any effect in humans. Instead it is suggested that antioxidant compounds, such as polyphenols, are able to activate transcription factors such as nuclear factor (erythroid-derived 2)-like 2 (Nrf2) that bind to the Electrophile Response Element (EpRE) and thereby transcribe genes for protective enzymes that provide the health benefits (Forman et al., 2014 and Figure 4). Several in vitro studies using humans cells and animal in vivo studies investigating olive polyphenols have supported Nrf2 activation and its consequential expression of protective genes [72,94]. Conversely, a recent human intervention study has shown no evidence of altered phase II enzyme expression (the downstream product of Nrf2 activation) in peripheral blood mononuclear cells following consumption of HT (5 mg and 25 mg per day in olive mill waste water) [95]. The olive mill waste water was tested to confirm oleuropein was not present.

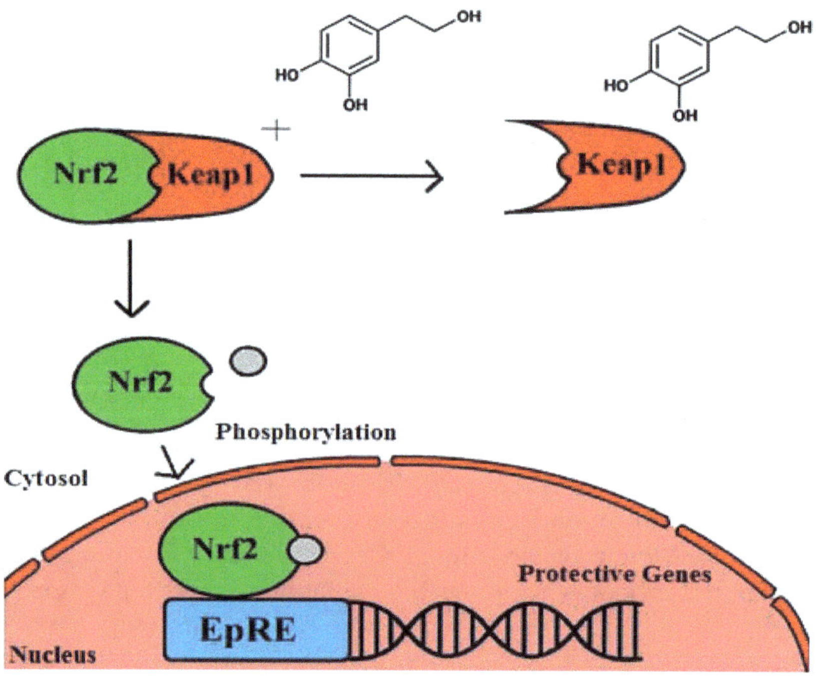

Figure 4. Polyphenol interaction with Nrf2 and activation of *EpRE* genes. The polyphenol (HT) reacts with Keap1 permitting Nrf2 to escape. Nrf2 requires phosphorylation before it is able to enter the nucleus. This schematic is modified from [93].

The Xenohormesis hypothesis suggests the stress-induced secondary metabolite production in plants is recognized by humans upon consumption, and these signals initiate stress response pathways [72,73]. Similarities in the human and plant extracellular signal-regulated kinase (ERK) pathways (these are able to activate many transcription factors and play an important role in cell regulation functions) show that polyphenols are able to activate pathways, such as AMP-activated protein kinase (AMPK) and hold the potential to modulate redox and mitochondrial signaling [96,97]. During eukaryotic evolution, glucose was the preferred carbon source. Rapid cell growth was the best way to utilize glucose, and AMPK activation provided the off switch mechanism in this process [72]. Therefore, AMPK activation (or similar pathways) could result in decreased ATP and increases in mitochondrial free radicals, implicating protection from chronic disease and aging [72]. Evidence for this theory was provided by microarray analysis of gene expression after EVOO treatment of breast cancer cells. These results demonstrated up-regulation of AMPK, and the top Canonical pathway regulated was the Nrf2 Mediated Oxidative stress pathway [72].

HT in vitro studies using human cell lines has been shown to up-regulate the expression of endogenous antioxidant genes (Heme Oxygenase 1 (HO-1), NAD(P)H-quinone oxidoreductase (NQO1), Glutathione (GSH)) via Nrf2 overexpression. The c-Jun N-terminal kinase (JNK) pathway plays an important role in inflammatory signaling. The JNK pathway was up-regulated following treatment with HT and inhibiting this pathway established its requirement for GSH and *p62* regulation. However, *HO-1* or *NQ-1* were unaffected [94]. p62 inactivates *Keap1*, increasing Nrf2 in the nucleus and consequently increasing the expression of oxidation defense enzyme genes [98]. Oleuropein in a human in vitro model has also been shown to activate Nrf2 and HO-1 expression [99]. However, in vivo human trials with HT have failed to find an up-regulation of phase 2 enzymes which are the by-product of EpRE and Nrf2 stimulation [95].

5. Olive Leaf Properties That Protect against Development and Progression of Cancer

Genetic changes are involved in the prevalence of cancers, however it is environmental and lifestyle factors such as obesity [100], unbalanced diet, tobacco, lack of exercise and alcohol consumption that account for the majority of the attributing cause [101]. Olive leaf contains strong anti-oxidants, it would be logical to conclude that these would help in mitigating the effect of genetic lesions that give rise to cancer. However, olive leaf has also attracted attention as a potential cancer treatment [28,46,102,103]. In previous work, olive leaf polyphenols have demonstrated the ability to inhibit the proliferation of several cancer cell lines including pancreatic [45], leukaemia [46], breast [28,47,49], prostate [48] and colorectal [61]. Importantly, oleuropein and HT have consistently been reported to discriminate between cancer and normal cells; inhibiting proliferation and inducing apoptosis only in cancer cells [48,49]. The challenge with relating the anti-cancer effects in cell models to in vivo arises when considering bioavailability of the polyphenols. This could explain why OO protective effects in humans show a strong association with cancers of the digestive system [12]. In other cancers OO phenolics has been suggested to act as phytoestrogens and anti-inflammatory agents, thus producing a protective effect.

A higher risk of breast cancer is linked to over-exposure to oestrogen [104,105] and growth of breast cancer can be stimulated by estradiol, which binds to the oestrogen receptor (ER). This receptor is an important biomarker and target for breast cancer prevention and treatment [106]. Work with breast cancer cell lines and OLE polyphenols have indicated potential mechanisms of action that include action as a phytoestrogen. Oleuropein and HT both possess an aromatic ring that is similar to that in estradiol, therefore these compounds are hypothesized to compete with oestrogens for receptor binding sites [50,107]. In the MCF-7 breast cancer cell line, HT and oleuropein (at doses between 10 and 75 μM) dose-dependently prevented cell proliferation through inhibition of the oestrogen activated ERK1/2 signaling pathway but did not show a direct effect on the mediation of ER gene expression [50]. It was later shown that oestrogen responses were also mediated by the GPER/GPER30 receptors, of which HT and oleuropein are agonists [108]. Despite both oestrogen and the polyphenols showing the same mechanism of receptor binding, they have opposite effects. Oestrogen leads to cell proliferation, while polyphenols lead to apoptosis or cell death. Both activate the ERK1/2 pathways but it has been proposed that the length of activation could influence the effect, with prolonged activation leading to apoptosis, and short-term to cell proliferation [108]. Sustained ERK activation has previously been demonstrated to result in inhibition of MCF-7 cell growth [109]. In vivo studies looking at olive leaf polyphenols also appear to support an anti-cancer effect. Oleuropein (125 mg/kg of diet) slowed tumor growth and inhibited cancer metastasis after MCF-7 cell xenograft establishment in mice [110]. OLE dissolved in water (150 and 225 mg/kg/day) reduced tumour volume and weight in mice after breast cancer xenograft [111].

The aromatase (CYP19) enzyme is the catalyst for the rate determining reaction in oestrogen synthesis. Inhibiting CYP19 effectively prevents oestrogen synthesis and because high levels of oestrogen are linked to breast cancer, this holds potential as a treatment [112]. A recent clinical study has shown that amylase inhibitors taken daily for 5 years were successfully able to reduce the incidence of breast cancer in high-risk postmenopausal women [113]. In MCF-7 cells, luteolin suppressed CYP19 transcription potentially via activator protein-1 (AP1) and C/EBP binding to the aromatase promoter [26].

The olive flavones apigenin and luteolin have been shown to act as aryl hydrocarbon receptor (AhR) antagonists in mouse cell lines [114]. Upon ligand binding, AhR is translocated to the nucleus where it activates response elements in the DNA sequence and consequent production of xenobiotic enzymes [115]. Other work has found that AhR in cancer cell lines acts as a tumour suppressor through diminished DNA replication and G0/G1 arrest [116]. Another study has reported that apigenin suppresses the growth of MCF-7 cells, inhibiting the NF-κB signaling pathway, the phosphorylation of IkBα, and nuclear translocation of p65 within the nucleus [27]. Apigenin was not found to inhibit cell survival signaling through mediators such as AKT, ERK, JNK, or p38, but it decreased STAT3 transcriptional activity in the cells, indicating that this compound induces growth-suppressive activity. The transcription factor STAT3 is more specifically involved in inflammatory signaling within cancer tumours and interacts with cytokines [117], thus by inhibiting STAT3, luteolin could also be having an anti-inflammatory effect. In another study oleuropein was cytotoxic to MDA-MB-231 and MCF-7 cells, avoiding damage to normal cells, with apoptosis taking place via induction of the mitochondrial pathway [49]. MCF-7 cell proliferation was inhibited by oleuropein at the S-phase of the cell cycle by an up-regulation of the p21 gene, and inhibition of NF-κB and its target D1 gene expression.

In PC3 and DU145 prostate cancer cell lines, HT has demonstrated the ability to interfere with cell proliferation [51]. HT also activated mitogen-activated protein kinase (MAPK), ERK, p38 MAPK and JNK. However, when inhibited by specific antagonists, HT was still able to inhibit cell growth. The authors concluded that HT was able to induce apoptosis in cancer cells via the generation of superoxide dismutase (SOD) and extracellular ROS.

Work using the prostate cancer cell lines, LNCaP and DU145, found that oleuropein was pro-oxidative, causing loss of viability, but in non-malignant cells (a benign hyperplastic prostatic epithelial cell line) oleuropein acted as an anti-oxidant [48]. The downstream products of EpRE activation were all increased with oleuropein; pAkt, y-glutamylcysteine (y-GCS), heme oxygenase-1 (HO-1) and ROS. Interference with pAkt was proposed as the mechanism enabling cell apoptosis in these prostate cancer cell lines [48].

5.1. *Anti-Inflammatory Properties of Olive Leaf Polyphenols and Their Effects on Cancer*

Inflammation is the natural defense mechanism against foreign threats, and its mechanisms are essential for survival. However, chronic inflammation, even at low levels, has been correlated to many health complications and age-associated diseases, including but not limited to cancer and cardiovascular disease [118]. The NF-κB signaling pathways play a pivotal role in inflammatory response and are an attractive target for preventing inflammation. NF-κB resides inactive within the cytoplasm due to the presence of IκB kinase, an inhibitor enzyme, therefore it can be activated very quickly to initiate cytokine and prostanoid production. There is strong evidence that olive polyphenols are able to interact with these pathways [119–121].

The cyclooxygenase 2 (COX-2) enzyme plays an important role in inflammation as the catalyst for the synthesis for prostanoids and hence an inflammatory response [122]. Cellular studies with OLE polyphenols have found a protective effect in relation to inflammation; a down-regulation of NO and COX-2 [120,123–125]. Inhibition of the Toll-like receptor (TLR) signaling induced by LPS was demonstrated not only by down-regulation of iNOS and COX2, but also by a decrease in ERK1/2, JNK and nuclear factor of kappa light polypeptide gene enhancer in B-cells inhibitor alpha (IκBα) phosphorylation in vitro after oleuropein treatment [120] (Figure 5). In down-regulating this pathway the pro-inflammatory enzymes interleukin 6 (IL-6) and interleukin 1β (IL-1β) and the gene AP-1 were also down-regulated. In human monocytes HT inhibited LPS induced COX-2 and prostanoid production, however, it increased TNF-α. In contrast in human cell models tyrosol down-regulated TNF-α and induced NF-κB, JNK and ERK phosphorylation and COX-2 expression [126] (Figure 5). Lastly the olive flavonoid luteolin regulated IL-1β induced COX-2 expression via ERK, JNK and NF-κB [127].

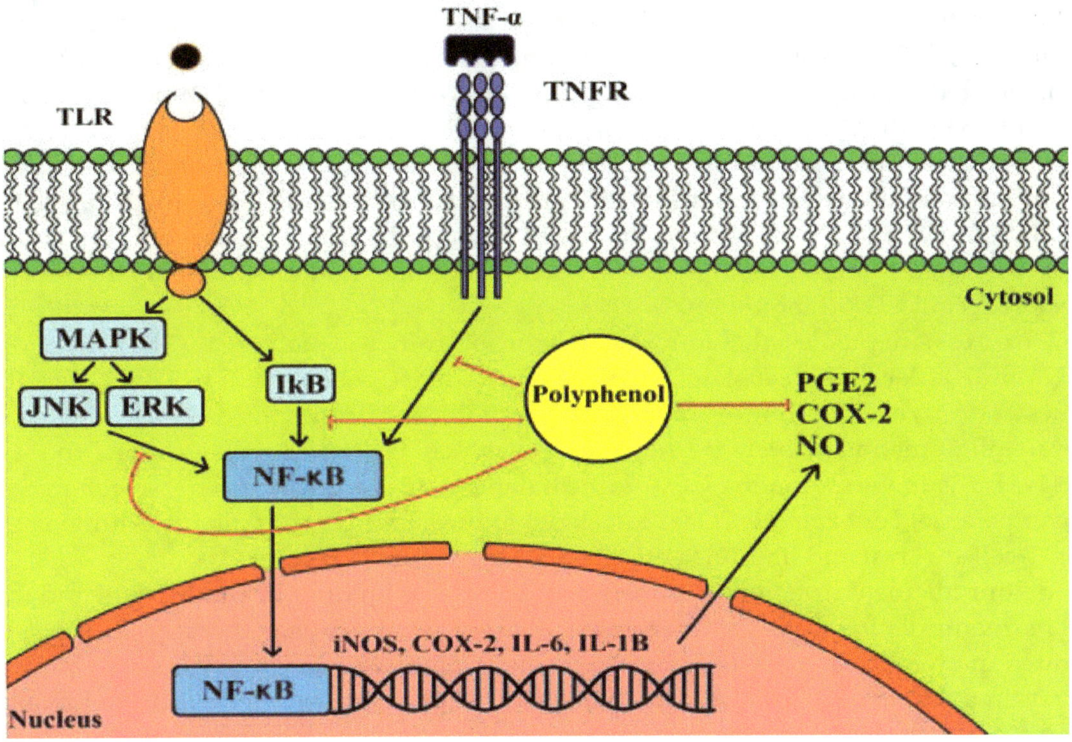

Figure 5. Olive leaf polyphenols may interact with gene and protein expression directly or via an interaction with receptors on the cell membrane. Toll-like receptor (TLR) and tumour necrosis factor receptor (TNFR) activation results in inflammatory gene expression (COX2, IL-6, IL-6 and IL-1β) and prostanoid production. This illustration shows the potential points at which OLE polyphenols could interact if able to enter the cell membrane.

5.2. Cancer, Inflammation and COX2 Expression

An overexpression of COX-2 has been linked to invasiveness of many cancers including human breast cancer [128,129], prostate [130] and colorectal [131]. Drugs that inhibit COX-2 enzymes are able to reduce the risk of breast cancer [132], and have pro-apoptotic effects in the MCF-7 cell line [133] and prostate cancer cell lines [134]. Luteolin, when administered with the COX-2 inhibitor celecoxib, created a synergistic effect in MCF-7 and three other breast cancer cell lines. Interestingly, the ERK1/2 levels were inhibited in the oestrogen receptor positive cell lines, but were increased in the negative cell lines [135]. Down-regulation of the phosphatidylinositide 3-kinase (P13K)/Akt pathway inhibits phosphorylated Akt levels, which in turn stimulates apoptosis. Phosphorylated Akt levels were decreased in all cell lines [135].

A review on breast cancer found all stages of cancer progression corresponded to COX-2 expression [129]. COX-2 is a down-stream product of NF-κB which was down-regulated in MCF-7 treated with oleuropein [49]. In mouse models, COX-2 driven prostaglandin E2 (PGE2) expression in mammary tissue led to an increase of *CYP19* and aromatase-catalysed oestrogen biosynthesis [136]. Samples taken from patients with breast cancer showed a correlation between transcription of *CYP19* and both gene and protein expressions of COX-2 and PGE2 [137]. In a previous study the authors hypothesized that HT and oleuropein were able to inhibit proliferation via competing for oestrogen binding sites [50]. These studies suggest that OLE polyphenols may be acting in MCF-7 to block oestrogen receptor binding and to inhibit COX-2 expression, which appears to down-regulate *CYP19* expression [136].

Another gene that COX-2 can regulate is p53. Work in human mammary tissue has demonstrated that COX-2 represses p53 transcription thereby inhibiting cell apoptosis [138] and it has since been demonstrated that p53 down-regulates aromatase expression in breast adipose stromal cells [139].

Work looking at the effects of oleuropein in MCF-7 has shown that it is able to induce apoptosis via up-regulating p53, and consequently the transcription of Bax/Bcl-2 apoptotic genes [62]. Other studies have also measured a change in p53 and Bax expression with oleuropein inhibition of cervical cancer cells [140] and p53 pathway up-regulation with oleuropein inhibition of colorectal cancer cells [61].

In vivo, luteolin (10 mg/kg/day) reduced both volume and weight of tumors in a prostate xenograft mouse model and in vitro, using the prostate cancer cells PC-3, it down-regulated VEGF phosphorylation of VEGF2 receptor and its downstream inflammatory markers IL-8 and IL-6 [25]. If VEGF is correlated to PGE2, as in the breast cancer models mentioned above, then it could be a downstream effect of COX-2 inhibition.

PGE2 expression pushes the immune response from a T-helper 1 (Th1) (including cells such as Natural killer (NK) cells) to a Th2 (such as mast cells) and Th17 mediated response, which is less effective at fighting off infections or protecting from cancer [141]. This potentiates acute, local inflammation driven by phagocytes, which is less aggressive than the Th1/Th17 response [141]. By down-regulating COX-2, the balance will shift back to Th1, which may improve immune-competence. For example COX-2 knock out in breast cancer cells inhibited tumour growth by enhancing T-cell survival and immune surveillance in tumours [142].

The tumour microenvironment has an important impact on tumour progression and metastasis, therefore its manipulation has been suggested as a target for cancer therapy [143]. It has been demonstrated in breast cancer MCF-7 cells that tumour associated macrophages are able to enhance COX-2 levels in the tumour. Conversely inhibiting COX-2 in macrophages was able to inhibit levels in the tumour [144]. In several human intervention studies with olive polyphenols, COX-2 expression in immune cells was down-regulated [145,146]. In cancer patients this could potentially lead to a down-regulation of COX-2 in tumours and thereby inhibit tumour progression. In other intervention studies the inflammatory markers NF-κB, p65, IKKβ, and IKKα [147] and NF-κB, IL-6 and IL-1β [148] have been down-regulated with olive polyphenols. These studies measured changes after single 40 mL doses of EVOO (containing the olive polyphenols), quantities achievable in an individual's standard diet.

5.3. *Quinone Hypothesis for Anti-Cancer Properties of Olive Leaf*

As quinones, olive leaf polyphenols could bind to the cysteine residues of NF-κB in cancer cells and manipulate gene expression. This would explain the observed gene expression in in vitro models [46,120,126]. A recent study has indicated olive leaf polyphenols in a quinone form could interact with Topoisomerase IIα [149]. The olive leaf polyphenols oleuropein, verbascoside, and HT were categorized by Vann et al. as Topoisomerase IIα poisons. Topoisomerase IIα is an enzyme essential for cell survival, catalysing the breaking and re-joining of the DNA helix to remove tangles and playing an important role in cell replication. Acting as Topoisomerase IIα poisons the polyphenols increased DNA cleavage, this effect was 10–100 times stronger in the presence of an oxidant [149]. This is consistent with the idea that the polyphenols have been transformed into quinone electrophiles, which are then able to bind to cysteine residues. This study also demonstrated that the olive leaf polyphenol tyrosol was unable to act as a poison consistent with its inability to form a quinone and bind to the cysteine residue within Topoisomerase IIα.

Although potentially dangerous in normal cells, Topisomerase IIα is an important target for cancer treatment. Due to the requirement of an oxidant environment, this might explain why no toxicity has been shown in normal cells in comparison to tumour cell models; the quinones were not formed.

6. Conclusions

There is strong evidence from cell models which demonstrates that olive polyphenols, and specifically the combination found in olive leaf, are able to modulate and interact with molecular pathways and in doing so may inhibit the progression and development of cancer. However, it is important to acknowledge that cell models are very different from the complex human body and applying these findings to cancer outcomes in humans is difficult.

Meta-analysis correlating the consumption of a MD and OO in humans to protection from digestive system, prostate and breast cancers [4,12], suggest that the effects may be constrained by bioavailability but also directs to a phytoestrogenic mechanism of action. Not only are the reduced risk of oestrogen related cancers in females correlated to protective effects of phytoestrogens, but a recent meta-analysis has correlated a lower risk of prostate cancer with phytoestrogen consumption [150].

The evidence suggests that olive polyphenols may act differently when in different combinations and at different concentrations. The presence of a glucose molecule, one factor that differentiates olive leaf polyphenols from OO polyphenols, is likely to affect the bioavailability and therefore bioactive properties. Changes to microbiota and microbiota-mediated degradation of polyphenols, demonstrate the glucose molecule has an effect.

Both cell models and human intervention studies demonstrate olive polyphenols are creating an anti-inflammatory change involving NF-κB inhibition. The down-stream products of NF-κB: including COX-2, IL-6, IL-8, IL-1β are expressed at lower levels creating a tumour micro-environment that no longer facilitates progression or development of cancers. This may account for the lower prevalence of cancer in people consuming a MD.

To answer the question "does OLE protect against cancer?" is difficult. Evidence is available in cell and animal models to support the conclusion that OLE does have beneficial effects and there is anecdotal evidence that olive polyphenols have a protective effect against cancer in humans. People consuming the MD have a lower prevalence of cancer, the MD consists of a high content of polyphenols, and olive leaf is an excellent source of many of these polyphenols. However, in order to prove that OLE improves cancer outcomes in humans, clinical trials would be required.

Acknowledgments: Funding was provided to Anna Boss from Comvita, New Zealand Limited, 234 Wilson Road South, Paengaroa, Te Puke 3189.

Author Contributions: All authors contributed to the preparation of this review article.

Abbreviations

The following abbreviations are used in this manuscript:

AhR	Aryl hydrocarbon receptor
AP1	Activator protein-1
EVOO	Extra Virgin Olive oil
HT	Hydroxytyrosol
JNK	c-Jun *N*-terminal kinase
MD	Mediterranean diet
MAPK	Mitogen-activated protein kinase
Nrf2	Nuclear factor (erythroid-derived 2)-like 2
NO	Nitric oxide
OLE	Olive leaf extract
OO	Olive oil
ROS	Reactive oxygen species
TLR	Toll-like receptor

References

1. Hanahan, D.; Weinberg, R.A. Hallmarks of cancer: The next generation. *Cell* **2011**, *144*, 646–674. [CrossRef] [PubMed]

2. Ferlay, J.; Soerjomataram, I.; Dikshit, R.; Eser, S.; Mathers, C.; Rebelo, M.; Parkin, D.M.; Forman, D.D.; Bray, F. Cancer incidence and mortality worldwide: Sources, methods and major patterns in GLOBOCAN 2012. *Int. J. Cancer* **2014**, *136*. [CrossRef] [PubMed]
3. Filomeno, M.; Bosetti, C.; Bidoli, E.; Levi, F.; Serraino, D.; Montella, M.; La Vecchia, C.; Tavani, A. Mediterranean diet and risk of endometrial cancer: A pooled analysis of three Italian case-control studies. *Br. J. Cancer* **2015**, *112*, 1816–1821. [CrossRef] [PubMed]
4. Schwingshackl, L.; Hoffmann, G. Does a Mediterranean-Type Diet Reduce Cancer Risk? *Curr. Nutr. Rep.* **2015**, *5*, 9–17. [CrossRef] [PubMed]
5. Ostan, R.; Lanzarini, C.; Pini, E.; Scurti, M.; Vianello, D.; Bertarelli, C.; Fabbri, C.; Izzi, M.; Palmas, G.; Biondi, F.; et al. Inflammaging and cancer: A challenge for the Mediterranean diet. *Nutrients* **2015**, *7*, 2589–2621. [CrossRef] [PubMed]
6. Marlow, G.; Ellett, S.; Ferguson, I.R.; Zhu, S.; Karunasinghe, N.; Jesuthasan, A.C.; Han, D.; Fraser, A.G.; Ferguson, L.R. Transcriptomics to study the effect of a Mediterranean-inspired diet on inflammation in Crohn's disease patients. *Hum. Genom.* **2013**, *7*, 24. [CrossRef] [PubMed]
7. Panunzio, M.F.; Caporizzi, R.; Antoniciello, A.; Cela, E.P.; Ferguson, L.R.; D'Ambrosio, P. Randomized, controlled nutrition education trial promotes a Mediterranean diet and improves anthropometric, dietary, and metabolic parameters in adults. *Ann. Ig. Med. Prev. Comunità* **2010**, *23*, 13–25.
8. Yubero-Serrano, E.M.; Delgado-Casado, N.; Delgado-Lista, J.; Perez-Martinez, P.; Tasset-Cuevas, I.; Santos-Gonzalez, M.; Caballero, J.; Garcia-Rios, A.; Marin, C.; Gutierrez-Mariscal, F.M.; et al. Postprandial antioxidant effect of the Mediterranean diet supplemented with coenzyme Q10 in elderly men and women. *Age (Dordr)* **2011**, *33*, 579–590. [CrossRef] [PubMed]
9. Camargo, A.; Delgado-Lista, J.; Garcia-Rios, A.; Cruz-Teno, C.; Yubero-Serrano, E.M.; Perez-Martinez, P.; Gutierrez-Mariscal, F.M.; Lora-Aguilar, P.; Rodriguez-Cantalejo, F.; Fuentes-Jimenez, F.; et al. Expression of proinflammatory, proatherogenic genes is reduced by the Mediterranean diet in elderly people. *Br. J. Nutr.* **2012**, *108*, 500–508. [CrossRef] [PubMed]
10. Renna, M.; Rinaldi, V.A.; Gonnella, M. The Mediterranean Diet between traditional foods and human health: The culinary example of Puglia (Southern Italy). *Int. J. Gastron. Food Sci.* **2015**, *2*, 63–71. [CrossRef]
11. Schwingshackl, L.; Hoffmann, G. Monounsaturated fatty acids, olive oil and health status: A systematic review and meta-analysis of cohort studies. *Lipids Health Dis.* **2014**, *13*, 154. [CrossRef] [PubMed]
12. Psaltopoulou, T.; Kosti, R.I.; Haidopoulos, D.; Dimopoulos, M.; Panagiotakos, D.B. Olive oil intake is inversely related to cancer prevalence: A systematic review and a meta-analysis of 13,800 patients and 23,340 controls in 19 observational studies. *Lipids Health Dis.* **2011**, *10*, 127. [CrossRef] [PubMed]
13. Portarena, S.; Baldacchini, C.; Brugnoli, E. Geographical discrimination of extra-virgin olive oils from the Italian coasts by combining stable isotope data and carotenoid content within a multivariate analysis. *Food Chem.* **2017**, *215*, 1–6. [CrossRef]
14. Jabeur, H.; Zribi, A.; Bouaziz, M. Changes in chemical and sensory characteristics of Chemlali extra-virgin olive oil as depending on filtration. *Eur. J. Lipid Sci. Technol.* **2016**. [CrossRef]
15. Aparicio, R.; Harwood, J. Handbook of Olive Oil: Analysis and Properties. Springer Science & Business Media, 2013. Available online: https://books.google.com/books?hl=en&lr=&id=gQrkBwAAQBAJ&pgis=1 (accessed on 8 March 2016).
16. EFSA Panel on Dietetic Products, N. and A. (NDA). Scientific Opinion on the Substantiation of health Claims Related to Polyphenols in Olive and Protection of LDL Particles from Oxidative damage (ID 1333, 1638, 1639, 1696, 2865), Maintenance of Normal Blood HDL Cholesterol Concentrations (ID 1639), Mainte. *EFSA J. 2011* **2011**, *9*. [CrossRef]
17. Farràs, M.; Valls, R.M.; Fernández-Castillejo, S.; Giralt, M.; Solà, R.; Subirana, I.; Motilva, M.-J.; Konstantinidou, V.; Covas, M.-I.; Fitó, M. Olive oil polyphenols enhance the expression of cholesterol efflux related genes in vivo in humans. A randomized controlled trial. *J. Nutr. Biochem.* **2013**, *24*, 1334–1339. [CrossRef] [PubMed]
18. Castañer, O.; Corella, D.; Covas, M.I.; Sorlí, J.V.; Subirana, I.; Flores-Mateo, G.; Nonell, L.; Bulló, M.; de la Torre, R.; Portolés, O.; et al. In vivo transcriptomic profile after a Mediterranean diet in high-cardiovascular risk patients: A randomized controlled trial. *Am. J. Clin. Nutr.* **2013**, *98*, 845–853. [CrossRef] [PubMed]
19. Lockyer, S.; Yaqoob, P.; Spencer, J.P.E.; Rowland, I. Olive leaf phenolics and cardiovascular risk reduction: Physiological effects and mechanisms of action. *Nutr. Aging* **2012**, *1*, 125–140.

20. El, S.N.; Karakaya, S. Olive tree (*Olea europaea*) leaves: Potential beneficial effects on human health. *Nutr. Rev.* **2009**, *67*, 632–638. [CrossRef] [PubMed]
21. Wren, R. Potter's New Cyclopaedia of Botanical Drugs and Preparations. 1994. Available online: https://scholar.google.co.nz/scholar?hl=en&q=R.C.+Wren+%28Ed.%29%2C+Potter%27s+New+Cyclopaedia+of+Botanical+Drugs+and+Preparations%2C+The+C.W.+Daniel%2C+Essex%2C+UK+%281994%29%2C+p.+20&btnG=&as_sdt=1%2C5&as_sdtp=#0 (accessed on 21 October 2015).
22. Ye, J.; Wang, C.; Chen, H.; Zhou, H. Variation Rule of Hydroxytyrosol Content in Olive Leaves. Available online: http://en.cnki.com.cn/Article_en/CJFDTOTAL-LCHX201102015.htm (accessed on 15 May 2015).
23. Mihailova, A.; Abbado, D.; Pedentchouk, N. Differences in *n*-alkane profiles between olives and olive leaves as potential indicators for the assessment of olive leaf presence in virgin olive oils. *Eur. J. Lipid Sci. Technol.* **2015**, *117*, 1480–1485. [CrossRef]
24. Nenadis, N.; Moutafidou, A.; Gerasopoulos, D.; Tsimidou, M.Z. Quality characteristics of olive leaf-olive oil preparations. *Eur. J. Lipid Sci. Technol.* **2010**, *112*, 1337–1344. [CrossRef]
25. Pratheeshkumar, P.; Son, Y.-O.; Budhraja, A.; Wang, X.; Ding, S.; Wang, L.; Hitron, A.; Lee, J.-C.; Kim, D.; Divya, S.P.; et al. Luteolin inhibits human prostate tumor growth by suppressing vascular endothelial growth factor receptor 2-mediated angiogenesis. *PLoS ONE* **2012**, *7*, e52279. [CrossRef] [PubMed]
26. Li, F.; Ye, L.; Lin, S.; Leung, L.K. Dietary flavones and flavonones display differential effects on aromatase (CYP19) transcription in the breast cancer cells MCF-7. *Mol. Cell. Endocrinol.* **2011**, *344*, 51–58. [CrossRef] [PubMed]
27. Seo, H.-S.; Choi, H.-S.; Kim, S.-R.; Choi, Y.K.; Woo, S.-M.; Shin, I.; Woo, J.-K.; Park, S.-Y.; Shin, Y.C.; Ko, S.-G.; et al. Apigenin induces apoptosis via extrinsic pathway, inducing p53 and inhibiting STAT3 and NFκB signaling in HER2-overexpressing breast cancer cells. *Mol. Cell. Biochem.* **2012**, *366*, 319–334. [CrossRef] [PubMed]
28. Barrajón-Catalán, E.; Taamalli, A.; Quirantes-Piné, R.; Roldan-Segura, C.; Arráez-Román, D.; Segura-Carretero, A.; Micol, V.; Zarrouk, M. Differential metabolomic analysis of the potential antiproliferative mechanism of olive leaf extract on the JIMT-1 breast cancer cell line. *J. Pharm. Biomed. Anal.* **2015**, *105*, 156–162. [CrossRef] [PubMed]
29. Gonzalez-Menendez, P.; Hevia, D.; Rodriguez-Garcia, A.; Mayo, J.C.; Sainz, R.M. Regulation of GLUT transporters by flavonoids in androgen-sensitive and -insensitive prostate cancer cells. *Endocrinology* **2014**, *155*, 3238–3250. [CrossRef] [PubMed]
30. Artajo, L.S.; Romero, M.P.; Motilva, M.J. Transfer of phenolic compounds during olive oil extraction in relation to ripening stage of the fruit. *J. Sci. Food Agric.* **2006**, *86*, 518–527. [CrossRef]
31. Luján, R.J.; Capote, F.P.; Marinas, A.; de Castro, M.D.L. Liquid chromatography/triple quadrupole tandem mass spectrometry with multiple reaction monitoring for optimal selection of transitions to evaluate nutraceuticals from olive-tree materials. *Rapid Commun. Mass Spectrom.* **2008**, *22*, 855–864. [CrossRef] [PubMed]
32. Flores, A.; Isabel, M.; Romero-González, R.; Frenich, G.; Vidal, A.; Martínez, L.J. Analysis of phenolic compounds in olive oil by solid-phase extraction and ultra high performance liquid chromatography-tandem mass spectrometry. *Food Chem.* **2012**, *134*, 2465–2472. [CrossRef] [PubMed]
33. Šarolić, M.; Gugić, M.; Friganović, E.; Tuberoso, C.; Jerković, I. Phytochemicals and Other Characteristics of Croatian Monovarietal Extra Virgin Olive Oils from Oblica, Lastovka and Levantinka Varieties. *Molecules* **2015**, *20*, 4395–4409. [CrossRef] [PubMed]
34. Rigane, G.; Ayadi, M.; Boukhris, M.; Sayadi, S.; Bouaziz, M. Characterisation and phenolic profiles of two rare olive oils from southern Tunisia: Dhokar and Gemri-Dhokar cultivars. *J. Sci. Food Agric.* **2013**, *93*, 527–534. [CrossRef] [PubMed]
35. Pereira, A.P.; Ferreira, I.C.; Marcelino, F.; Valentão, P.; Andrade, P.B.; Seabra, R.; Estevinho, L.; Bento, A.; Pereira, J.A. Phenolic Compounds and Antimicrobial Activity of Olive (*Olea europaea L.* Cv. Cobrançosa) Leaves. *Molecules* **2007**, *12*, 1153–1162. [CrossRef] [PubMed]
36. Aouidi, F.; Ayari, S.; Ferhi, H.; Roussos, S.; Hamdi, M. Gamma irradiation of air-dried olive leaves: Effective decontamination and impact on the antioxidative properties and on phenolic compounds. *Food Chem.* **2011**, *127*, 1105–1113. [CrossRef] [PubMed]
37. Japón-Luján, L.; Luque-Rodríguez, J.; Luque de Castro, M. Dynamic ultrasound-assisted extraction of oleuropein and related biophenols from olive leaves. *J. Chromatogr. A* **2006**, *1108*, 76–82. [CrossRef] [PubMed]

38. Japón-Luján, R.; Luque de Castro, M.D. Liquid-liquid extraction for the enrichment of edible oils with phenols from olive leaf extracts. *J. Agric. Food Chem.* **2008**, *56*, 2505–2511. [CrossRef] [PubMed]
39. Oliveras-López, M.-J.; Berná, G.; Jurado-Ruiz, E.; López-García de la Serrana, H.; Martín, F. Consumption of extra-virgin olive oil rich in phenolic compounds has beneficial antioxidant effects in healthy human adults. *J. Funct. Foods* **2014**, *10*, 475–484. [CrossRef]
40. Rosignoli, P.; Fuccelli, R.; Fabiani, R.; Servili, M.; Morozzi, G. Effect of olive oil phenols on the production of inflammatory mediators in freshly isolated human monocytes. *J. Nutr. Biochem.* **2013**, *24*, 1513–1519. [CrossRef] [PubMed]
41. Lockyer, S.; Rowland, I.; Spencer, J.P.E.; Yaqoob, P.; Stonehouse, W. Impact of phenolic-rich olive leaf extract on blood pressure, plasma lipids and inflammatory markers: A randomised controlled trial. *Eur. J. Nutr.* **2016**. [CrossRef] [PubMed]
42. Martín-Peláez, S.; Mosele, J.I.; Pizarro, N.; Farràs, M.; de la Torre, R.; Subirana, I.; Pérez-Cano, F.J.; Castañer, O.; Solà, R.; Fernandez-Castillejo, S.; et al. Effect of virgin olive oil and thyme phenolic compounds on blood lipid profile: implications of human gut microbiota. *Eur. J. Nutr.* **2015**. [CrossRef] [PubMed]
43. Hamdi, H.K.; Castellon, R. Oleuropein, a non-toxic olive iridoid, is an anti-tumor agent and cytoskeleton disruptor. *Biochem. Biophys. Res. Commun.* **2005**, *334*, 769–778. [CrossRef] [PubMed]
44. López de las Hazas, M.-C.; Piñol, C.; Macià, A.; Romero, M.-P.; Pedret, A.; Solà, R.; Rubió, L.; Motilva, M.-J. Differential absorption and metabolism of hydroxytyrosol and its precursors oleuropein and secoiridoids. *J. Funct. Foods* **2016**, *22*, 52–63. [CrossRef]
45. Goldsmith, C.D.; Vuong, Q.V.; Sadeqzadeh, E.; Stathopoulos, C.E.; Roach, P.D.; Scarlett, C.J. Phytochemical Properties and Anti-Proliferative Activity of *Olea europaea L.* Leaf Extracts against Pancreatic Cancer Cells. *Molecules* **2015**, *20*, 12992–3004. [CrossRef] [PubMed]
46. Samet, I.; Han, J.; Jlaiel, L.; Sayadi, S.; Isoda, H. Olive (*Olea europaea*) Leaf Extract Induces Apoptosis and Monocyte/Macrophage Differentiation in Human Chronic Myelogenous Leukemia K562 Cells: Insight into the Underlying Mechanism. *Oxid. Med. Cell. Longev.* **2014**, *2014*, 927619. [CrossRef] [PubMed]
47. Quirantes-Piné, R.; Zurek, G.; Barrajón-Catalán, E.; Bäßmann, C.; Micol, V.; Segura-Carretero, A.; Fernández-Gutiérrez, A. A metabolite-profiling approach to assess the uptake and metabolism of phenolic compounds from olive leaves in SKBR3 cells by HPLC-ESI-QTOF-MS. *J. Pharm. Biomed. Anal.* **2013**, *72*, 121–126. [CrossRef] [PubMed]
48. Acquaviva, R.; Di Giacomo, C.; Sorrenti, V.; Galvano, F.; Santangelo, R.; Cardile, V.; Gangia, S.; D'Orazio, N.; Abraham, N.G.; Vanella, L. Antiproliferative effect of oleuropein in prostate cell lines. *Int. J. Oncol.* **2012**, *41*, 31–38. [PubMed]
49. Elamin, M.H.; Daghestani, M.H.; Omer, S.A.; Elobeid, M.A.; Virk, P.; Al-Olayan, E.M.; Hassan, Z.K.; Mohammed, O.B.; Aboussekhra, A. Olive oil oleuropein has anti-breast cancer properties with higher efficiency on ER-negative cells. *Food Chem. Toxicol.* **2013**, *53*, 310–316. [CrossRef] [PubMed]
50. Sirianni, R.; Chimento, A.; De Luca, A.; Casaburi, I.; Rizza, P.; Onofrio, A.; Iacopetta, D.; Puoci, F.; Andò, S.; Maggiolini, M.; et al. Oleuropein and hydroxytyrosol inhibit MCF-7 breast cancer cell proliferation interfering with ERK1/2 activation. *Mol. Nutr. Food Res.* **2010**, *54*, 833–840. [CrossRef] [PubMed]
51. Luo, C.; Li, Y.; Wang, H.; Cui, Y.; Feng, Z.; Li, H.; Li, Y.; Wang, Y.; Wurtz, K.; Weber, P.; et al. Hydroxytyrosol promotes superoxide production and defects in autophagy leading to anti-proliferation and apoptosis on human prostate cancer cells. *Curr. Cancer Drug Targets* **2013**, *13*, 625–639. [CrossRef] [PubMed]
52. Erbay, Z.; Icier, F. A review of thin layer drying of foods: Theory, modeling, and experimental results. *Crit. Rev. Food Sci. Nutr.* **2010**, *50*, 441–464. [CrossRef] [PubMed]
53. Pandey, K.; Rizvi, S. Plant polyphenols as dietary antioxidants in human health and disease. *Oxid. Med. Cell. Longev.* **2009**, *2*, 270–278. [CrossRef] [PubMed]
54. de Bock, M.; Derraik, J.G.B.; Brennan, C.M.; Biggs, J.B.; Morgan, P.E.; Hodgkinson, S.C.; Hofman, P.L.; Cutfield, W.S. Olive (*Olea europaea L.*) leaf polyphenols improve insulin sensitivity in middle-aged overweight men: A randomized, placebo-controlled, crossover trial. *PLoS ONE* **2013**, *8*, e57622.
55. Jemai, H.; El Feki, A.; Sayadi, S. Antidiabetic and antioxidant effects of hydroxytyrosol and oleuropein from olive leaves in alloxan-diabetic rats. *J. Agric. Food Chem.* **2009**, *57*, 8798–8804. [CrossRef] [PubMed]
56. Kuem, N.; Song, S.J.; Yu, R.; Yun, J.W.; Park, T. Oleuropein attenuates visceral adiposity in high-fat diet-induced obese mice through the modulation of WNT10b- and galanin-mediated signalings. *Mol. Nutr. Food Res.* **2014**, *58*, 2166–2176. [CrossRef] [PubMed]

57. Bendini, A.; Cerretani, L.; Carrasco-Pancorbo, A.; Gómez-Caravaca, A.M.; Segura-Carretero, A.; Fernández-Gutiérrez, A.; Lercker, G. Phenolic Molecules in Virgin Olive Oils: A Survey of Their Sensory Properties, Health Effects, Antioxidant Activity and Analytical Methods. An Overview of the Last Decade Alessandra. *Molecules* **2007**, *12*, 1679–1719. [CrossRef] [PubMed]
58. Nekooeian, A.A.; Khalili, A.; Khosravi, M.B. Oleuropein offers cardioprotection in rats with simultaneous type 2 diabetes and renal hypertension. *Indian J. Pharmacol.* **2015**, *46*, 398–403. [CrossRef] [PubMed]
59. Lee, O.-H.; Lee, B.-Y. Antioxidant and antimicrobial activities of individual and combined phenolics in *Olea europaea* leaf extract. *Bioresour. Technol.* **2010**, *101*, 3751–3754. [CrossRef] [PubMed]
60. Elamin, M.H.; Al-Maliki, S.S. Leishmanicidal and apoptotic activities of oleuropein on Leishmania major. *Int. J. Clin. Pharmacol. Ther.* **2014**, *52*, 880–888. [CrossRef] [PubMed]
61. Cárdeno, A.; Sánchez-Hidalgo, M.; Rosillo, M.A.; Alarcón de la Lastra, C. Oleuropein, a secoiridoid derived from olive tree, inhibits the proliferation of human colorectal cancer cell through downregulation of HIF-1α. *Nutr. Cancer* **2013**, *65*, 147–156. [CrossRef] [PubMed]
62. Hassan, Z.K.; Elamin, M.H.; Omer, S.A.; Daghestani, M.H.; Al-Olayan, E.S.; Elobeid, M.A.; Virk, P. Oleuropein Induces Apoptosis Via the p53 Pathway in Breast Cancer Cells. *Asian Pac. J. Cancer Prev.* **2013**, *14*, 6739–6742. [CrossRef]
63. Han, J.; Talorete, T.P.N.; Yamada, P.; Isoda, H. Anti-proliferative and apoptotic effects of oleuropein and hydroxytyrosol on human breast cancer MCF-7 cells. *Cytotechnology* **2009**, *59*, 45–53. [CrossRef] [PubMed]
64. Granados-Principal, S.; Quiles, J.L.; Ramirez-Tortosa, C.L.; Sanchez-Rovira, P.; Ramirez-Tortosa, M.C. Hydroxytyrosol: from laboratory investigations to future clinical trials. *Nutr. Rev.* **2010**, *68*, 191–206. [CrossRef] [PubMed]
65. Alipieva, K.; Korkina, L.; Orhan, I.E.; Georgiev, M.I. Verbascoside—A review of its occurrence, (bio) synthesis and pharmacological significance. *Biotechnol. Adv.* **2014**, *32*, 1065–1076. [CrossRef] [PubMed]
66. Al-Rimawi, F.; Odeh, I.; Bisher, A.; Abbadi, J.; Qabbajeh, M. Effect of Geographical Region and Harvesting Date on Antioxidant Activity, Phenolic and Flavonoid Content of Olive Leaves. *J. Food Nutr. Res.* **2014**, *2*, 925–930. [CrossRef]
67. Ando, C.; Takahashi, N.; Hirai, S.; Nishimura, K.; Lin, S.; Uemura, T.; Goto, T.; Yu, R.; Nakagami, J.; Murakami, S.; et al. Luteolin, a food-derived flavonoid, suppresses adipocyte-dependent activation of macrophages by inhibiting JNK activation. *FEBS Lett.* **2009**, *583*, 3649–3654. [CrossRef] [PubMed]
68. Shukla, S.; Gupta, S. Apigenin: A promising molecule for cancer prevention. *Pharm. Res.* **2010**, *27*, 962–978. [CrossRef] [PubMed]
69. Guinda, Á.; Pérez-Camino, M.C.; Lanzón, A. Supplementation of oils with oleanolic acid from the olive leaf (*Olea europaea*). *Eur. J. Lipid Sci. Technol.* **2004**, *106*, 22–26. [CrossRef]
70. Tabera, J.; Guinda, A.; Ruiz-Rodríguez, A.; Señoráns, F.J.; Ibáñez, E.; Albi, T.; Reglero, G. Countercurrent supercritical fluid extraction and fractionation of high-added-value compounds from a hexane extract of olive leaves. *J. Agric. Food Chem.* **2004**, *52*, 4774–4779. [CrossRef] [PubMed]
71. Virtamo, J.; Taylor, P.R.; Kontto, J.; Männistö, S.; Utriainen, M.; Weinstein, S.J.; Huttunen, J.; Albanes, D. Effects of α-tocopherol and β-carotene supplementation on cancer incidence and mortality: 18-year postintervention follow-up of the Alpha-tocopherol, Beta-carotene Cancer Prevention Study. *Int. J. Cancer* **2014**, *135*, 178–185. [CrossRef] [PubMed]
72. Menendez, J.A.; Joven, J.; Aragonès, G.; Barrajón-Catalán, E.; Beltrán-Debón, R.; Borrás-Linares, I.; Camps, J.; Corominas-Faja, B.; Cufí, S.; Fernández-Arroyo, S.; et al. Xenohormetic and anti-aging activity of secoiridoid polyphenols present in extra virgin olive oil: A new family of gerosuppressant agents. *Cell Cycle* **2013**, *12*, 555–578. [CrossRef] [PubMed]
73. Joven, J.; Micol, V.; Segura-Carretero, A.; Alonso-Villaverde, C.; Menéndez, J.A. Polyphenols and the modulation of gene expression pathways: Can we eat our way out of the danger of chronic disease? *Crit. Rev. Food Sci. Nutr.* **2014**, *54*, 985–1001. [CrossRef] [PubMed]
74. Fardet, A.; Rock, E. The search for a new paradigm to study micronutrient and phytochemical bioavailability: From reductionism to holism. *Med. Hypotheses.* **2014**, *82*, 181–186. [CrossRef] [PubMed]
75. De Marino, S.; Festa, C.; Zollo, F.; Nini, A.; Antenucci, L.; Raimo, G.; Iorizzi, M. Antioxidant Activity and Chemical Components as Potential Anticancer Agents in the Olive Leaf (*Olea europaea L.* cv Leccino.) Decoction. *Anticancer. Agents Med. Chem.* **2014**, *14*, 1376–1385. [CrossRef] [PubMed]

76. Benavente-garcia, O.; Castillo, J.; Lorente, J.; Ortun, A. Antioxidant activity of phenolics extracted from *Olea europaea L.* leaves. *Food Chem.* **2000**, *68*, 457–462. [CrossRef]
77. Etcheverry, E.P.; Grusak, M.A.; Fleige, L.E. Application of in vitro bioaccessibility and bioavailability methods for calcium, carotenoids, folate, iron, magnesium, polyphenols, zinc, and vitamins B6, B12, D, and E. *Front. Physiol.* **2012**, *3*, 317. [CrossRef] [PubMed]
78. D'Archivio, M.; Filesi, C.; Varì, R.; Scazzocchio, B.; Masella, R. Bioavailability of the polyphenols: Status and controversies. *Int. J. Mol. Sci.* **2010**, *11*, 1321–1342. [CrossRef] [PubMed]
79. De Bock, M.; Thorstensen, E.B.; Derraik, J.G.B.; Henderson, H.V.; Hofman, P.L.; Cutfield, W.S. Human absorption and metabolism of oleuropein and hydroxytyrosol ingested as olive (*Olea europaea L.*) leaf extract. *Mol. Nutr. Food Res.* **2013**, *57*, 2079–2085. [CrossRef] [PubMed]
80. Serra, A.; Rubió, L.; Borràs, X.; Macià, A.; Romero, M.-P.; Motilva, M.-J. Distribution of olive oil phenolic compounds in rat tissues after administration of a phenolic extract from olive cake. *Mol. Nutr. Food Res.* **2012**, *56*, 486–496. [CrossRef] [PubMed]
81. Kendall, M.; Batterham, M.; Callahan, D.L.; Jardine, D.; Prenzler, P.D.; Robards, K.; Ryan, D. Randomized controlled study of the urinary excretion of biophenols following acute and chronic intake of olive leaf supplements. *Food Chem.* **2012**, *130*, 651–659. [CrossRef]
82. Lin, P.; Qian, W.; Wang, X.; Cao, L.; Li, S.; Qian, T. The biotransformation of oleuropein in rats. *Biomed. Chromatogr.* **2013**, *27*, 1162–1167. [CrossRef] [PubMed]
83. Corona, G.; Tzounis, X.; Assunta DessÌ, M.; Deiana, M.; Debnam, E.S.; Visioli, F.; Spencer, J.P.E. The fate of olive oil polyphenols in the gastrointestinal tract: Implications of gastric and colonic microflora-dependent biotransformation. *Free Radic. Res.* **2006**, *40*, 647–658. [CrossRef] [PubMed]
84. Landete, J.M.; Curiel, J.A.; Rodríguez, H.; de las Rivas, B.; Muñoz, R. Study of the inhibitory activity of phenolic compounds found in olive products and their degradation by Lactobacillus plantarum strains. *Food Chem.* **2008**, *107*, 320–326. [CrossRef]
85. Ramírez, E.; Medina, E.; Brenes, M.; Romero, C. Endogenous enzymes involved in the transformation of oleuropein in Spanish table olive varieties. *J. Agric. Food Chem.* **2014**, *62*, 9569–9575. [CrossRef] [PubMed]
86. De Leonardis, A.; Macciola, V.; Cuomo, F.; Lopez, F. Evidence of oleuropein degradation by olive leaf protein extract. *Food Chem.* **2015**, *175*, 568–574. [CrossRef] [PubMed]
87. Yuan, J.-J.; Wang, C.-Z.; Ye, J.-Z.; Tao, R.; Zhang, Y.-S. Enzymatic hydrolysis of oleuropein from Olea europea (olive) leaf extract and antioxidant activities. *Molecules* **2015**, *20*, 2903–2921. [CrossRef] [PubMed]
88. Szablewski, L. Expression of glucose transporters in cancers. *Biochim. Biophys. Acta* **2013**, *1835*, 164–169. [CrossRef] [PubMed]
89. Menendez, J.A.; Vazquez-Martin, A.; Colomer, R.; Brunet, J.; Carrasco-Pancorbo, A.; Garcia-Villalba, R.; Fernandez-Gutierrez, A.; Segura-Carretero, A. Olive oil's bitter principle reverses acquired autoresistance to trastuzumab (Herceptin) in HER2-overexpressing breast cancer cells. *BMC Cancer* **2007**, *7*, 80. [CrossRef] [PubMed]
90. Murphy, M.P.; Holmgren, A.; Larsson, N.-G.; Halliwell, B.; Chang, C.J.; Kalyanaraman, B.; Rhee, S.G.; Thornalley, P.J.; Partridge, L.; Gems, D.; et al. Unraveling the biological roles of reactive oxygen species. *Cell Metab.* **2011**, *13*, 361–366. [CrossRef] [PubMed]
91. de la Puerta, R.; Domínguez, M.E.M.; Rúíz-Gutíerrez, V.; Flavill, J.A.; Hoult, J.R.S. Effects of virgin olive oil phenolics on scavenging of reactive nitrogen species and upon nitrergic neurotransmission. *Life Sci.* **2001**, *69*, 1213–1222. [CrossRef]
92. de la Puerta, R.; Ruiz Gutierrez, V.; Hoult, J.R. Inhibition of leukocyte 5-lipoxygenase by phenolics from virgin olive oil. *Biochem. Pharmacol.* **1999**, *57*, 445–449. [CrossRef]
93. Forman, H.J.; Davies, K.J.A.; Ursini, F. How do nutritional antioxidants really work: Nucleophilic tone and para-hormesis versus free radical scavenging in vivo. *Free Radic. Biol. Med.* **2014**, *66*, 24–35. [CrossRef] [PubMed]
94. Zou, X.; Feng, Z.; Li, Y.; Wang, Y.; Wertz, K.; Weber, P.; Fu, Y.; Liu, J. Stimulation of GSH synthesis to prevent oxidative stress-induced apoptosis by hydroxytyrosol in human retinal pigment epithelial cells: Activation of Nrf2 and JNK-p62/SQSTM1 pathways. *J. Nutr. Biochem.* **2012**, *23*, 994–1006. [CrossRef] [PubMed]
95. Crespo, M.C.; Tomé-Carneiro, J.; Burgos-Ramos, E.; Loria Kohen, V.; Espinosa, M.I.; Herranz, J.; Visioli, F. One-week administration of hydroxytyrosol to humans does not activate Phase II enzymes. *Pharmacol. Res.* **2015**, *95*, 132–137. [CrossRef] [PubMed]

96. Khanal, P.; Oh, W.-K.; Yun, H.J.; Namgoong, G.M.; Ahn, S.-G.; Kwon, S.-M.; Choi, H.-K.; Choi, H.S. p-HPEA-EDA, a phenolic compound of virgin olive oil, activates AMP-activated protein kinase to inhibit carcinogenesis. *Carcinogenesis* **2011**, *32*, 545–553. [CrossRef] [PubMed]
97. Zrelli, H.; Matsuoka, M.; Kitazaki, S.; Zarrouk, M.; Miyazaki, H. Hydroxytyrosol reduces intracellular reactive oxygen species levels in vascular endothelial cells by upregulating catalase expression through the AMPK-FOXO3a pathway. *Eur. J. Pharmacol.* **2011**, *660*, 275–282. [CrossRef] [PubMed]
98. Komatsu, M.; Kurokawa, H.; Waguri, S.; Taguchi, K.; Kobayashi, A.; Ichimura, Y.; Sou, Y.-S.; Ueno, I.; Sakamoto, A.; Tong, K.I.; et al. The selective autophagy substrate p62 activates the stress responsive transcription factor Nrf2 through inactivation of Keap1. *Nat. Cell Biol.* **2010**, *12*, 213–223. [CrossRef] [PubMed]
99. Parzonko, A.; Czerwińska, M.E.; Kiss, A.K.; Naruszewicz, M. Oleuropein and oleacein may restore biological functions of endothelial progenitor cells impaired by angiotensin II via activation of Nrf2/heme oxygenase-1 pathway. *Phytomedicine* **2013**, *20*, 1088–1094. [CrossRef] [PubMed]
100. Ligibel, J.A.; Alfano, C.M.; Courneya, K.S.; Demark-Wahnefried, W.; Burger, R.A.; Chlebowski, R.T.; Fabian, C.J.; Gucalp, A.; Hershman, D.L.; Hudson, M.M.; et al. American Society of Clinical Oncology position statement on obesity and cancer. *J. Clin. Oncol.* **2014**, *32*, 3568–3574. [CrossRef] [PubMed]
101. Anand, P.; Kunnumakkara, A.B.; Kunnumakara, A.B.; Sundaram, C.; Harikumar, K.B.; Tharakan, S.T.; Lai, O.S.; Sung, B.; Aggarwal, B.B. Cancer is a preventable disease that requires major lifestyle changes. *Pharm. Res.* **2008**, *25*, 2097–2116. [CrossRef] [PubMed]
102. Mijatovic, S.A.; Timotijevic, G.S.; Miljkovic, D.M.; Radovic, J.M.; Maksimovic-Ivanic, D.D.; Dekanski, D.P.; Stosic-Grujicic, S.D. Multiple antimelanoma potential of dry olive leaf extract. *Int. J. Cancer* **2011**, *128*, 1955–1965. [CrossRef] [PubMed]
103. Fares, R.; Bazzi, S.; Baydoun, S.E.; Abdel-Massih, R.M. The antioxidant and anti-proliferative activity of the Lebanese *Olea europaea* extract. *Plant Foods Hum. Nutr.* **2011**, *66*, 58–63. [CrossRef] [PubMed]
104. Kaaks, R. Endogenous hormone metabolism as an exposure marker in breast cancer chemoprevention studies. *IARC Sci. Publ.* **2001**, *154*, 149–162. [PubMed]
105. Key, T.; Appleby, P.; Barnes, I.; Reeves, G. Endogenous Hormones and Breast Cancer Collaborative Group. Endogenous sex hormones and breast cancer in postmenopausal women: Reanalysis of nine prospective studies. *J. Natl. Cancer Inst.* **2002**, *94*, 606–616. [PubMed]
106. Bartlett, J.M.S.; Brookes, C.L.; Robson, T.; van de Velde, C.J.H.; Billingham, L.J.; Campbell, F.M.; Grant, M.; Hasenburg, A.; Hille, E.T.M.; Kay, C.; et al. Estrogen receptor and progesterone receptor as predictive biomarkers of response to endocrine therapy: A prospectively powered pathology study in the Tamoxifen and Exemestane Adjuvant Multinational trial. *J. Clin. Oncol.* **2011**, *29*, 1531–1538. [CrossRef] [PubMed]
107. Carrera-González, M.P.; Ramírez-Expósito, M.J.; Mayas, M.D.; Martínez-Martos, J.M. Protective role of oleuropein and its metabolite hydroxytyrosol on cancer. *Trends Food Sci. Technol.* **2013**, *31*, 92–99. [CrossRef]
108. Chimento, A.; Casaburi, I.; Rosano, C.; Avena, P.; De Luca, A.; Campana, C.; Martire, E.; Santolla, M.F.; Maggiolini, M.; Pezzi, V.; et al. Oleuropein and hydroxytyrosol activate GPER/GPR30-dependent pathways leading to apoptosis of ER-negative SKBR3 breast cancer cells. *Mol. Nutr. Food Res.* **2014**, *58*, 478–489. [CrossRef] [PubMed]
109. Kim, B.-W.; Lee, E.-R.; Min, H.-M.; Jeong, H.-S.; Ahn, J.-Y.; Kim, J.-H.; Choi, H.-Y.; Choi, H.; Kim, E.Y.; Park, S.P.; et al. Sustained ERK activation is involved in the kaempferol-induced apoptosis of breast cancer cells and is more evident under 3-D culture condition. *Cancer Biol. Ther.* **2014**, *7*, 1080–1089. [CrossRef]
110. Sepporta, M.V.; Fuccelli, R.; Rosignoli, P.; Ricci, G.; Servili, M.; Morozzi, G.; Fabiani, R. Oleuropein inhibits tumour growth and metastases dissemination in ovariectomised nude mice with MCF-7 human breast tumour xenografts. *J. Funct. Foods.* **2014**, *8*, 269–273. [CrossRef]
111. Milanizadeh, S.; Bigdeli, M.R.; Rasoulian, B.; Amani, D. The Effects of Olive Leaf Extract on Antioxidant Enzymes Activity and Tumor Growth in Breast Cancer. *Thrita* **2014**, *3*. [CrossRef]
112. Osborne, C.; Tripathy, D. Aromatase inhibitors: Rationale and use in breast cancer. *Annu. Rev. Med.* **2005**, *56*, 103–116. [CrossRef] [PubMed]
113. Cuzick, J.; Sestak, I.; Forbes, J.F.; Dowsett, M.; Knox, J.; Cawthorn, S.; Saunders, C.; Roche, N.; Mansel, R.E.; von Minckwitz, G.; et al. Anastrozole for prevention of breast cancer in high-risk postmenopausal women (IBIS-II): An international, double-blind, randomised placebo-controlled trial. *Lancet* **2014**, *383*, 1041–1048. [CrossRef]

114. Amakura, Y.; Tsutsumi, T.; Sasaki, K.; Nakamura, M.; Yoshida, T.; Maitani, T. Influence of food polyphenols on aryl hydrocarbon receptor-signaling pathway estimated by in vitro bioassay. *Phytochemistry* **2008**, *69*, 3117–3130. [CrossRef] [PubMed]
115. Wakabayashi, N.; Slocum, S.L.; Skoko, J.J.; Shin, S.; Kensler, T.W. When NRF2 talks, who's listening? *Antioxid. Redox Signal.* **2010**, *13*, 1649–1663. [CrossRef] [PubMed]
116. Fan, Y.; Boivin, G.P.; Knudsen, E.S.; Nebert, D.W.; Xia, Y.; Puga, A. The aryl hydrocarbon receptor functions as a tumor suppressor of liver carcinogenesis. *Cancer Res.* **2010**, *70*, 212–220. [CrossRef] [PubMed]
117. Yang, L.; Karin, M. Roles of tumor suppressors in regulating tumor-associated inflammation. *Cell Death Differ.* **2014**, *21*, 1677–1686. [CrossRef] [PubMed]
118. Franceschi, C.; Campisi, J. Chronic inflammation (inflammaging) and its potential contribution to age-associated diseases. *J. Gerontol. A Biol. Sci. Med. Sci.* **2014**, *69* (Suppl 1), S4–S9. [CrossRef] [PubMed]
119. Killeen, M.J.; Linder, M.; Pontoniere, P.; Crea, R. NF-κβ signaling and chronic inflammatory diseases: Exploring the potential of natural products to drive new therapeutic opportunities. *Drug Discov. Today* **2014**, *19*, 373–378. [CrossRef] [PubMed]
120. Ryu, S.-J.; Choi, H.-S.; Yoon, K.-Y.; Lee, O.-H.; Kim, K.-J.; Lee, B.-Y. Oleuropein suppresses LPS-induced inflammatory responses in RAW 264.7 cell and zebrafish. *J. Agric. Food Chem.* **2015**, *63*, 2098–2105. [CrossRef] [PubMed]
121. Scoditti, E.; Nestola, A.; Massaro, M.; Calabriso, N.; Storelli, C.; De Caterina, R.; Carluccio, M.A. Hydroxytyrosol suppresses MMP-9 and COX-2 activity and expression in activated human monocytes via PKCα and PKCβ1 inhibition. *Atherosclerosis* **2014**, *232*, 17–24. [CrossRef] [PubMed]
122. Liu, B.; Qu, L.; Yan, S. Cyclooxygenase-2 promotes tumor growth and suppresses tumor immunity. *Cancer Cell Int.* **2015**, *15*, 106. [CrossRef] [PubMed]
123. Scoditti, E.; Calabriso, N.; Massaro, M.; Pellegrino, M.; Storelli, C.; Martines, G.; De Caterina, R.; Carluccio, M.A. Mediterranean diet polyphenols reduce inflammatory angiogenesis through MMP-9 and COX-2 inhibition in human vascular endothelial cells: A potentially protective mechanism in atherosclerotic vascular disease and cancer. *Arch. Biochem. Biophys.* **2012**, *527*, 81–89. [CrossRef] [PubMed]
124. Zhang, X.; Cao, J.; Zhong, L. Hydroxytyrosol inhibits pro-inflammatory cytokines, iNOS, and COX-2 expression in human monocytic cells. *Naunyn Schmied. Arch. Pharmacol.* **2009**, *379*, 581–586. [CrossRef] [PubMed]
125. Fuccelli, R.; Fabiani, R.; Sepporta, M.V.; Rosignoli, P. The hydroxytyrosol-dependent increase of TNF-α in LPS-activated human monocytes is mediated by PGE2 and adenylate cyclase activation. *Toxicol. Vitro* **2015**, *29*, 933–937. [CrossRef] [PubMed]
126. Lamy, S.; Ben Saad, A.; Zgheib, A.; Annabi, B. Olive oil compounds inhibit the paracrine regulation of TNF-α-induced endothelial cell migration through reduced glioblastoma cell cyclooxygenase-2 expression. *J. Nutr. Biochem.* **2015**, *27*, 136–145. [CrossRef] [PubMed]
127. Lamy, S.; Moldovan, P.L.; Ben Saad, A.; Annabi, B. Biphasic effects of luteolin on interleukin-1β-induced cyclooxygenase-2 expression in glioblastoma cells. *Biochim. Biophys. Acta* **2015**, *1853*, 126–135. [CrossRef] [PubMed]
128. Bocca, C.; Ievolella, M.; Autelli, R.; Motta, M.; Mosso, L.; Torchio, B.; Bozzo, F.; Cannito, S.; Paternostro, C.; Colombatto, S.; et al. Expression of COX-2 in human breast cancer cells as a critical determinant of epithelial-to-mesenchymal transition and invasiveness. *Expert Opin. Ther. Targets* **2014**, *18*, 121–135. [CrossRef] [PubMed]
129. Harris, R.E.; Casto, B.C.; Harris, Z.M. Cyclooxygenase-2 and the inflammogenesis of breast cancer. *World J. Clin. Oncol.* **2014**, *5*, 677–692. [CrossRef] [PubMed]
130. Bieniek, J.; Childress, C.; Swatski, M.D.; Yang, W. COX-2 inhibitors arrest prostate cancer cell cycle progression by down-regulation of kinetochore/centromere proteins. *Prostate* **2014**, *74*, 999–1011. [CrossRef] [PubMed]
131. Peng, L.; Zhou, Y.; Wang, Y.; Mou, H.; Zhao, Q. Prognostic significance of COX-2 immunohistochemical expression in colorectal cancer: A meta-analysis of the literature. *PLoS ONE* **2013**, *8*, e58891. [CrossRef] [PubMed]

132. Brasky, T.M.; Bonner, M.R.; Moysich, K.B.; Ambrosone, C.B.; Nie, J.; Tao, M.H.; Edge, S.B.; Kallakury, B.V.S.; Marian, C.; Trevisan, M.; et al. Non-steroidal anti-inflammatory drug (NSAID) use and breast cancer risk in the Western New York Exposures and Breast Cancer (WEB) Study. *Cancer Causes Control* **2010**, *21*, 1503–1512. [CrossRef] [PubMed]
133. Barnes, N.L.P.; Warnberg, F.; Farnie, G.; White, D.; Jiang, W.; Anderson, E.; Bundred, N.J. Cyclooxygenase-2 inhibition: Effects on tumour growth, cell cycling and lymphangiogenesis in a xenograft model of breast cancer. *Br. J. Cancer* **2007**, *96*, 575–582. [CrossRef] [PubMed]
134. Katkoori, V.R.; Manne, K.; Vital-Reyes, V.S.; Rodríguez-Burford, C.; Shanmugam, C.; Sthanam, M.; Manne, U.; Chatla, C.; Abdulkadir, S.A.; Grizzle, W.E. Selective COX-2 inhibitor (celecoxib) decreases cellular growth in prostate cancer cell lines independent of p53. *Biotech. Histochem.* **2013**, *88*, 38–46. [CrossRef] [PubMed]
135. Jeon, Y.W.; Ahn, Y.E.; Chung, W.S.; Choi, H.J.; Suh, Y.J. Synergistic effect between celecoxib and luteolin is dependent on estrogen receptor in human breast cancer cells. *Tumor Biol.* **2015**, *36*, 6349–6359. [CrossRef] [PubMed]
136. Subbaramaiah, K.; Howe, L.R.; Port, E.R.; Brogi, E.; Fishman, J.; Liu, C.H.; Hla, T.; Hudis, C.; Dannenberg, A.J. HER-2/neu status is a determinant of mammary aromatase activity in vivo: Evidence for a cyclooxygenase-2-dependent mechanism. *Cancer Res.* **2006**, *66*, 5504–5511. [CrossRef] [PubMed]
137. Subbaramaiah, K.; Morris, P.G.; Zhou, X.K.; Morrow, M.; Du, B.; Giri, D.; Kopelovich, L.; Hudis, C.A.; Dannenberg, A.J. Increased levels of COX-2 and prostaglandin E2 contribute to elevated aromatase expression in inflamed breast tissue of obese women. *Cancer Discov.* **2012**, *2*, 356–365. [CrossRef] [PubMed]
138. Choi, E.-M.; Heo, J.-I.; Oh, J.-Y.; Kim, Y.-M.; Ha, K.-S.; Kim, J.-I.; Han, J.A. COX-2 regulates p53 activity and inhibits DNA damage-induced apoptosis. *Biochem. Biophys. Res. Commun.* **2005**, *328*, 1107–1112. [CrossRef] [PubMed]
139. Wang, X.; Docanto, M.M.; Sasano, H.; Lo, C.; Simpson, E.R.; Brown, K.A. Prostaglandin E2 inhibits p53 in human breast adipose stromal cells: A novel mechanism for the regulation of aromatase in obesity and breast cancer. *Cancer Res.* **2015**, *75*, 645–655. [CrossRef] [PubMed]
140. Yao, J.; Wu, J.; Yang, X.; Yang, J.; Zhang, Y.; Du, L. Oleuropein Induced Apoptosis in HeLa Cells via a Mitochondrial Apoptotic Cascade Associated With Activation of the c-Jun NH2-Terminal Kinase. *J. Pharmacol. Sci.* **2014**, *125*, 300–311. [CrossRef] [PubMed]
141. Kalinski, P. Regulation of immune responses by prostaglandin E2. *J. Immunol.* **2012**, *188*, 21–28. [CrossRef] [PubMed]
142. Chen, E.P.; Markosyan, N.; Connolly, E.; Lawson, J.A.; Li, X.; Grant, G.R.; Grosser, T.; FitzGerald, G.A.; Smyth, E.M. Myeloid Cell COX-2 deletion reduces mammary tumor growth through enhanced cytotoxic T-lymphocyte function. *Carcinogenesis* **2014**, *35*, 1788–1797. [CrossRef] [PubMed]
143. Quail, D.F.; Joyce, J.A. Microenvironmental regulation of tumor progression and metastasis. *Nat. Med.* **2013**, *19*, 1423–1437. [CrossRef] [PubMed]
144. Li, H.; Yang, B.; Huang, J.; Lin, Y.; Xiang, T.; Wan, J.; Li, H.; Chouaib, S.; Ren, G. Cyclooxygenase-2 in tumor-associated macrophages promotes breast cancer cell survival by triggering a positive-feedback loop between macrophages and cancer cells. *Oncotarget* **2015**, *6*, 29637–29650. [PubMed]
145. Llorente-Cortés, V.; Estruch, R.; Mena, M.P.; Ros, E.; González, M.A.M.; Fitó, M.; Lamuela-Raventós, R.M.; Badimon, L. Effect of Mediterranean diet on the expression of pro-atherogenic genes in a population at high cardiovascular risk. *Atherosclerosis* **2010**, *208*, 442–450. [CrossRef] [PubMed]
146. Camargo, A.; Ruano, J.; Fernandez, J.M.; Parnell, L.D.; Jimenez, A.; Santos-Gonzalez, M.; Marin, C.; Perez-Martinez, P.; Uceda, M.; Lopez-Miranda, J.; et al. Gene expression changes in mononuclear cells in patients with metabolic syndrome after acute intake of phenol-rich virgin olive oil. *BMC Genom.* **2010**, *11*, 253. [CrossRef] [PubMed]
147. Perez-Herrera, P.; Delgado-Lista, J.; Torres-Sanchez, L.; Rangel-Zuñiga, O.; Camargo, A.; Moreno-Navarrete, J.; Garcia-Olid, B.; Quintana-Navarro, G.; Alcala-Diaz, J.; Muñoz-Lopez, C.; et al. The postprandial inflammatory response after ingestion of heated oils in obese persons is reduced by the presence of phenol compounds. *Mol. Nutr. Food Res.* **2012**, *56*, 510–514. [CrossRef] [PubMed]
148. Camargo, A.; Rangel-Zuñiga, O.A.; Haro, C.; Meza-Miranda, E.R.; Peña-Orihuela, P.; Meneses, M.E.; Marin, C.; Yubero-Serrano, E.M.; Perez-Martinez, P.; Delgado-Lista, J.; et al. Olive oil phenolic compounds decrease the postprandial inflammatory response by reducing postprandial plasma lipopolysaccharide levels. *Food Chem.* **2014**, *162*, 161–171. [CrossRef] [PubMed]

149. Vann, K.R.; Sedgeman, C.A.; Gopas, J.; Golan-Goldhirsh, A.; Osheroff, N. Effects of Olive Metabolites on DNA Cleavage Mediated by Human Type II Topoisomerases. *Biochemistry* **2015**, *54*, 4531–4541. [CrossRef] [PubMed]
150. He, J.; Wang, S.; Zhou, M.; Yu, W.; Zhang, Y.; He, X. Phytoestrogens and risk of prostate cancer: A meta-analysis of observational studies. *World J. Surg. Oncol.* **2015**, *13*, 231. [CrossRef] [PubMed]

5

Anticancer Efficacy of Polyphenols and their Combinations

Aleksandra Niedzwiecki *, Mohd Waheed Roomi, Tatiana Kalinovsky and Matthias Rath

Dr. Rath Research Institute, 1260 Memorex Drive, Santa Clara, CA 95050, USA; w.roomi@drrath.com (M.W.R.); t.kalinovksy@drrath.com (T.K.); m.rath@drrath.com (M.R.)

* Correspondence: author@drrath.com

Abstract: Polyphenols, found abundantly in plants, display many anticarcinogenic properties including their inhibitory effects on cancer cell proliferation, tumor growth, angiogenesis, metastasis, and inflammation as well as inducing apoptosis. In addition, they can modulate immune system response and protect normal cells against free radicals damage. Most investigations on anticancer mechanisms of polyphenols were conducted with individual compounds. However, several studies, including ours, have indicated that anti-cancer efficacy and scope of action can be further enhanced by combining them synergistically with chemically similar or different compounds. While most studies investigated the anti-cancer effects of combinations of two or three compounds, we used more comprehensive mixtures of specific polyphenols and mixtures of polyphenols with vitamins, amino acids and other micronutrients. The mixture containing quercetin, curcumin, green tea, cruciferex, and resveratrol (PB) demonstrated significant inhibition of the growth of Fanconi anemia head and neck squamous cell carcinoma and dose-dependent inhibition of cell proliferation, matrix metalloproteinase (MMP)-2 and -9 secretion, cell migration and invasion through Matrigel. PB was found effective in inhibition of fibrosarcoma HT-1080 and melanoma A2058 cell proliferation, MMP-2 and -9 expression, invasion through Matrigel and inducing apoptosis, important parameters for cancer prevention. A combination of polyphenols (quercetin and green tea extract) with vitamin C, amino acids and other micronutrients (EPQ) demonstrated significant suppression of ovarian cancer ES-2 xenograft tumor growth and suppression of ovarian tumor growth and lung metastasis from IP injection of ovarian cancer A-2780 cells. The EPQ mixture without quercetin (NM) also has shown potent anticancer activity in vivo and in vitro in a few dozen cancer cell lines by inhibiting tumor growth and metastasis, MMP-2 and -9 secretion, invasion, angiogenesis, and cell growth as well as induction of apoptosis. The presence of vitamin C, amino acids and other micronutrients could enhance inhibitory effect of epigallocatechin gallate (EGCG) on secretion of MMPs. In addition, enrichment of NM with quercetin (EPQ mix) enhanced anticancer activity of NM in vivo. In conclusion, polyphenols, especially in combination with other polyphenols or micronutrients, have been shown to be effective against multiple targets in cancer development and progression, and should be considered as safe and effective approaches in cancer prevention and therapy.

Keywords: polyphenols; tumor growth; metastasis; Matrigel invasion

---

1. Introduction

Polyphenols comprise a diverse group of secondary metabolites abundant in plants, where they play key roles in regulating growth, metabolism, protecting against UV radiation and various pathogens. More than 8000 polyphenolic compounds have been identified in various plant species. Polyphenols have been subjected to numerous studies, investigating their potential health benefits, including protection against oxidative stress, cardiovascular disease, diabetes, asthma, neurodegenerative disease and even aging [1]. Particular interest in these naturally occurring plant components has been kindled by the search for new chemopreventive agents that are more effective and less toxic than conventional therapies. As such, this group of substances has been studied for anticarcinogenic properties, such as modulating cell proliferation, tumor growth, angiogenesis, metastasis, inflammation and apoptosis [2,3].

Polyphenols are classified based on the number of phenol rings and the structural elements that bind these rings to one another. The groups include: phenolic acids, stilbenes, lignans, and flavonoids. Flavonoids, which have both antioxidant and anti-inflammatory properties, are found in fruits, vegetables, legumes, red wine, and green tea. They are subdivided into six classes: flavonols, flavones, isoflavones, flavanones, anthocyanidins, and flavanols (catechins and proanthocyanidins) [4]. Flavonols, the most ubiquitous flavonoids in foods, are generally present at relatively low concentrations. Quercetin and kaempferol are the main representatives, and their richest sources are onions, curly kale, leeks, broccoli, and blueberries [4].

Flavones, consisting mainly of glycosides of luteolin and apigenin, are less common than flavonols in fruit and vegetables; parsley and celery are the main edible sources of flavones [4]. Flavanones, present in tomatoes and certain aromatic plants such as mint, are present in high concentrations only in citrus fruit. Isoflavones, flavonoids with structural similarities to estrogens, have the ability to bind to estrogen receptors, and thus are classified as phytoestrogens. They are found almost exclusively in leguminous plants. Flavanols occur as catechins (a monomer form) and proanthocyanidins (the polymer form).

Catechins are found in many types of fruit, red wine, green tea and chocolate. Gallocatechin, epigallocatechin, and epigallocatechin gallate (EGCG) are found in teas, seeds of leguminous plants and grapes [5,6]. Green tea, a rich source, contains up to 200 mg catechins in a cup of tea [7]. Flavanols are not glycosylated in foods as are other classes of flavonoids; thus tea epicatechins remain very stable when exposed to heat under acidic pH. Only 15% of these substances are degraded after 7 h in boiling water at pH 5 [8].

Among phenolic acids, hydroxybenzoic acids are found in tea and more common hydroxycinnamic acids are found in cinnamon, coffee, blueberries, kiwis, plums, apples, and cherries [4]. These acids are mostly found as glycosylated derivatives of esters of quinic acid, shikimic acid and tartaric acid [4]. Ferrulic acid is the most abundant phenolic acid found in cereal grains and in wheat; it may represent up to about 90% polyphenols [9].

Stilbenes are found in low quantities in our diet, which may be not sufficient to exercise significant health effects; larger quantities can be provided in concentrated extracts or in the form of purified compounds. Resveratrol is a key stilbene, found especially in red wine and peanuts, which has been extensively studied for its anticarcinogenic and other health effects [10].

Lignans are found in flax seeds, legumes, cereals, grains, fruits, algae, and certain vegetables [4]. Their concentration in linseed is about 1000 times as high as in other food sources [11]. Plant lignin, secoisolariciresinol diglycoside (SDG) and its metabolites have shown promise in reducing carcinogenic tumors, in particular hormone-sensitive ones such as breast, endometrium and prostate tumors [12].

2. Aspects Associated with Bioavailability of Polyphenols

Bioavailability defines the amount of nutrient that is digested, absorbed and metabolized in normal biochemical pathways. Most polyphenols are present in food in the form of esters, glycosides or polymers, and are metabolized by a common pathway. Before absorption, most polyphenols have to be hydrolyzed by intestinal enzymes or microflora present in colon. Only aglycones can be absorbed via the small intestine [13]. Subsequently, during absorption, polyphenols undergo extensive modification by conjugation in the intestinal cells and further processing in the liver through methylation, sulfation and glucuronidation [13]. Therefore, their forms detected in the blood and tissues differ from the ones present in food. In addition, the most biologically active polyphenols are not necessarily the most common ones in the diet.

Metabolic activity of polyphenols is dependent on intrinsic activity, relative absorption from the intestine, rate of metabolism and of elimination. In addition, digestive or hepatic metabolic activity may render the metabolites that reach the blood and target organs to differ in biological activity from their native form. Polyphenol metabolites circulate in the blood bound to proteins, mainly albumin, with binding affinity largely defined by their structural properties [14]. Protein binding can affect the rate of their delivery to cells and tissues.

Polyphenols are able to penetrate tissues, in particular the intestine and liver, where they are metabolized. Their excretion occurs through urine (mainly small conjugates) and more extensively conjugated metabolites are secreted in bile. It appears that the amount of metabolite in urine roughly corresponds to its maximum concentration in plasma. It is quite high for citrus fruit flavanones and decreases from isoflavones to flavonols. Thus, understanding polyphenol bioavailability is essential for determining their health effects.

3. Antitumor Effects of Select Polyphenols

Development of cancer is a multi-stage process that involves initiation, promotion and progression. Dietary polyphenols can affect and modulate multiple diverse biochemical processes and pathways involved in carcinogenesis [15]. In addition, they can act as biological response modifiers supporting immune system function, as well as protecting living cells against damage from free radicals. Although polyphenols in fruits and vegetables are widely implicated in cancer prevention, few protective effects of individual compounds have been firmly confirmed in clinical trials due to differences in dosing, timing and other confounding factors.

Several cancer preventive mechanisms have been identified as affected by polyphenols, including prevention of oxidation, detoxification of xenobiotics, induction of apoptosis, as well as estrogenic/anti-estrogenic activity, stimulating effects on immune system function, anti-inflammatory properties and their effects on the cellular signaling system. Among these are effects on nuclear factors, such as NF-κB or activator protein 1 (AP-1), which play central roles in cellular signaling cascades, regulating DNA transcription, gene expression in response to different stimuli, cell proliferation and survival [16,17]. Most investigations have been conducted with individual polyphenols in order to increase our understanding of biological and cellular mechanisms of their anticancer efficacy. However, final effects of these compounds are largely influenced by their interactions with other natural components, both at the cellular and organ levels. These aspects have been rarely evaluated and studied. Below we will discuss key studies investigating anti-cancer effects of individual polyphenols, as well as their efficacy when used in various combinations, the approach which has been promoted in our research.

3.1. Curcumin

This active ingredient of a rhizome of turmeric has been known for its anti-oxidant properties and many health benefits. It has been demonstrated in different cancer models that curcumin can inhibit cellular proliferation and angiogenesis, block cell cycle progression in tumor cells, and induce apoptosis [18–20]. Aoki et al. demonstrated inhibition of glioma cell xenograft tumor growth by curcumin [21]. Studies by Anand indicate that in addition to modulating cancer cell proliferation, angiogenesis and inducing apoptosis, curcumin can affect cancer invasion, and metastasis [22]. The anti-cancer efficacy of curcumin may involve a variety of mechanisms. Study of pancreatic cancer in nude mice has shown that curcumin can suppress pancreatic cancer cell proliferation and angiogenesis by inhibiting NF-kB-regulated gene products such as cyclin D1, cmyc, Bcl-2, Bcl-xL, and apoptosis protein-1, COX-2, MMP, and vascular endothelial growth factor (VEGF) [18]. Various studies, including the use of lung models, point to curcumin affecting the mechanisms involving inhibition of the signal transducer and activation of transcription Stat3 pathways [23], as well as matrix metalloproteinases and VEGF [18].

Curcumin's anti-tumor effects may also be due to its interactions with arachidonate metabolism and in vivo anti-angiogenic properties [24]. Some studies indicate curcumin interacts with vitamin D receptors, which would explain its preventive properties against colon cancer where vitamin D has strong anti-cancer effects [25]. Curcumin also appears to work in synergy with isoflavones in suppressing prostate specific antigen (PSA) production in prostate cells [26]. Gupta et al. have reviewed clinical trial research on curcumin and have concluded that curcumin, either alone or in combination with other agents, has demonstrated potential against various cancers, including colorectal, pancreatic, breast, prostate, lung, multiple myeloma, and head and neck squamous cell carcinoma [27]. Overall, chemoprevention and anticancer effects of curcumin are multimodal and complex. Molecular pathways and targets modulated by curcumin have been discussed in details in other review articles [28,29].

3.2. *Quercetin*

Cancer preventive effects of quercetin include induction of cell cycle arrest, apoptosis and antioxidant functions [30]. Induction of apoptosis by quercetin in cancer cells during different cell cycle stages without affecting normal cells has been documented in various cancers in vivo and in vitro [30]. Quercetin has been reported to reduce both the risk and progression of cancer through their free radical scavenging activity [31,32]. It protects cells from oxidative stress, inflammation, and DNA damage due to its antioxidant properties and modulates growth of many cancer cell lines by blocking cell cycle progression and tumor cell proliferation and by inducing apoptosis [33–36]. In addition, quercetin provided protection against liver cancer development in rats injected with a cancer inducer [37]. Furthermore, injection of quercetin directly into breast tumors led to a significant reduction of their mass [38]. Epidemiological studies report that intake of quercetin-rich food reduced the risk of gastric cancer by 43% [31] and colon cancer by 32% [39]. Consumption of quercetin was also reported to reduce lung cancer risk by 51% and even in heavy smokers by 65% [32]. Intravenous administration of quercetin in patients with different types of cancer demonstrated decreased activity of the enzyme tyrosine kinase, an enzyme required for tumor growth, in nine of 11 patients [40]. There is a growing interest among scientists in exploring synergistic interactions of quercetin with standard chemotherapeutics. Both in vitro and in vivo studies have shown that quercetin can potentiate the efficacy of concomitant drugs by enhancing their bioavailability and accumulation, and by sensitizing cancer cells to these chemotherapeutics [41]. From a clinical perspective, this would allow dose reduction of toxic drugs, thereby alleviating their severe side effects.

3.3. *Resveratrol*

Resveratrol has demonstrated to be effective in preventing all stages of cancer development and has been found effective in most cancers including prostate, breast, stomach, colon, lung, thyroid and pancreatic cancer cell lines [42]. Bishayee et al. reported that resveratrol can affect carcinogenesis by modulating signal transduction pathways that control cell division and growth, apoptosis, inflammation, angiogenesis and metastasis [43]. In vivo, resveratrol has shown efficacy in preventing and treating skin, esophageal, intestinal, and colon tumors [44]. Various anti-cancer cellular mechanisms of resveratrol have been suggested, including inhibition of angiogenesis, metastasis and induction of apoptosis [38]. Resveratrol has been studied in patients with colon cancer to evaluate the pharmacokinetic and metabolite profiles in these patients [45]. In addition, resveratrol studied in healthy volunteers demonstrated that it is well tolerated and modulates enzyme systems involved in carcinogen activation and detoxification [46]. Resveratrol has promising anti-cancer potential but, because of its poor bioavailability, the best efficacy has been limited to tumors it can come into direct contact with (e.g., skin cancers or gastrointestinal tract cancers).

3.4. *Cruciferous Plant Extracts*

Cruciferous vegetables of the *Brassica* genus, such as broccoli, cabbage, cauliflower and others contain a number of nutrients and phytochemicals with cancer preventive properties, including carotenoids, chlorophyll and fibers. Their unique anti-cancer characteristic relates to being a source of large quantities of sulfur containing natural compounds known as glucosinolates [47]. After hydrolysis they form bioactive isothiocyanates and indole-3-carbinol [48,49]. By 2011 more than 132 glucosinolates with their unique hydrolysis products had been identified in plants [50]. Epidemiological evidence suggests that high intake of cruciferous vegetables can lower risk of some cancers, including colon and lung cancers [48]. Numerous in vitro and in vivo studies suggest that dietary compounds from cruciferous plants may have potent chemopreventive properties by acting through different molecular mechanisms [51–56]. This includes many studies, which have shown that cruciferous vegetables can help prevent the onset and inhibit the progression of colon, breast, prostate, thyroid, cervical, and other cancers [57–66]. It has been shown that cruciferous bioactive components can facilitate detoxification and excretion of carcinogens, protect against oxidative stress, inhibit cancer cell proliferation and increase apoptosis, resulting in inhibition of tumor growth [67].

3.5. *Green Tea*

Green tea extract, rich in catechins, has been subjected to numerous studies and shown to modulate cancer cell growth, metastasis, angiogenesis, and other aspects of cancer progression by affecting different mechanisms [68–73]. The four principal tea catechins are epicatechin (EC), epicatechin-3-gallate (ECG), epigallocatechin (EGC) and epigallocatechin-3-gallate (EGCG) [74]. It has been shown that three of these catechins, EGCG, EGC and ECG, have anticancer preventive activity, and that their combination with an inactive EC has synergistic effect on prostate cancer cells PC-9, by inducing apoptosis and inhibiting proliferation [75].

The most studied of all green tea catechins in relation to cancer is EGCG, which is found at the highest concentration in green tea (10%–15%) [75]. Gupta et al. demonstrated that EGCG potently induced apoptosis and suppressed cell growth in vitro by modulating expression of cell cycle regulatory proteins, activating killer caspases, and suppressing activation of NF-κB [76]. Harakeh et al. demonstrated the anti-proliferative and pro-apoptotic effects of EGCG in HTLV-1-positive and -negative cells. These effects included down-regulation of TGF-alpha, up-regulation of TGF-beta2, increased cell distribution in pre-G(1) phase and upregulation of p53, Bax and p21 proteins expression while down-regulating Bcl-2alpha [73]. EGCG was reported to control and promote IL-23 dependent DNA repair, enhance cytotoxic T-cell activities and block cancer development by inhibiting carcinogenic signal transduction pathways [77]. EGCG was also shown to modulate several biological pathways, including growth factor-mediated pathway, the mitogen activated protein kinase-dependent pathway, and ubiquitin/proteasome degradation pathways [78]. Clinically, in a study of over 8000 individuals, daily consumption of green tea demonstrated delayed cancer onset; furthermore, breast cancer patients experienced a lower recurrence rate and longer remission [75]. Another clinical study found that oral ingestion of EGCG (200 mg per os) for 12 weeks was effective in patients with human papilloma virus-infected cervical lesions [79].

While EGCG is the most studied catechin in cancer, the in vitro study in human pancreatic ductal adenocarcinoma (PDAC) cells showed that two minor green tea catechins, ECG and EG, had much stronger anti proliferative and anti-inflammatory effects, including inhibition of NF-κB, IL8 and uPA, than EGCG [80].

Epigallocatechin gallate (EGCG) has poor bioavailability in rats and humans due to oxidation, metabolism and its efflux. In addition, specific interactions with other polyphenolic compounds can modulate its metabolic efficacy. However, a study by Kale et al. [81] showed that green tea extract consumed together with onion, which is rich in quercetin, can significantly enhance bioavailability of EGCG in humans. Wang et al. confirmed this effect, showing that quercetin affects EGCG by decreasing its methylation [82]. EGCG-quercetin interactions resulted in enhanced anti-proliferative effects of EGCG in androgen-dependent and androgen-independent prostate cancer cells [83]. EGCG bioavailability is affected by numerous compounds as its consumption with cereal and milk resulted in lower EGCG blood levels [84]. This indicates that proper selection of compounds and their combinations are important in achieving the desired biological effect.

4. Benefits of Nutrient Combinations—Pleiotropic Effects

Numerous in vitro and in vivo studies provide support for use of polyphenols in cancer prevention by applying them in combinations with other micronutrients for achieving pleiotropic effects. As mentioned previously, one of major problems with using polyphenols as anticancer agents individually is their poor bioavailability in the human body. In addition, their interactions with other natural compounds in a diet may hinder or complicate consistency of their efficacy [85]. Therefore, specifically designed combinations of several polyphenols or combinations of polyphenols with other natural agents aimed at defined biological targets will expand metabolic effects of constituents of such mixtures in controlled and reproducible ways. In addition, proper combinations of micronutrients enable use of lower doses of individual components without compromising their efficacy, rather than expanding the scope of cellular mechanisms affected. This novel approach opens up a possibility of developing more effective strategies against various human pathologies, including cancer.

Several in vitro and in vivo studies have shown that combinations of two or three polyphenols were more effective in inhibiting cancer growth than treatment with a single compound. Our research has demonstrated that multi-nutrient combinations, through their reciprocal interactions, including synergy, can modulate bioavailability of natural compounds and exercise pleiotropic effects by affecting multiple metabolic pathways involved in carcinogenesis simultaneously. Below we present a few examples of specific and effective anti-cancer nutrient mixtures. They include a combination of different polyphenols and combinations of polyphenols with vitamins and other micronutrients, which were selected to specifically target defined key cellular mechanisms involved in carcinogenesis.

4.1. Anticancer Effects of a Combination of Different Polyphenols

Several studies investigated the efficacy of mixtures containing two or three different polyphenols. These include combinations of EGCG with quercetin in prostate cancer cells [86,87], and EGCG with resveratrol in prostate cancer cell lines [88] and breast cancer MCF-7 cell line [89]. Combinations studied also included curcumin with EGCG and EC in lung cancer cell lines [90,91], curcumin with EGCG in human B-cell chronic leukemia [92] and in xenograft mouse models implanted with MDA-MB-231 breast cancer cells [93] and lung A549 cells [91]. Piao et al. [94] demonstrated anti-cancer effects of a tri-nutrient combination composed of curcumin, resveratrol and epicatechin gallate on cell viability, clonogenic survival, apoptosis and tumor growth in HPV-positive head and neck squamous cell carcinoma.

These findings indicate that more comprehensive mixtures of nutrients with similar or complementary anti-cancer mechanisms would allow for enhanced complementary or synergistic interactions between these compounds, thereby expanding different cancer mechanisms simultaneously and in a controlled fashion. Therefore, we combined the compounds previously investigated in combinations and cruciferous extract in order to enhance and expand their anti-cancer mechanisms through additive and synergistic effects. This mixture of nutrients (PB) included: quercetin, 400 mg; Cruciferex™ (priopprietary extract from cabbage, cauliflower, broccoli and carrots), 400 mg; turmeric root extract containing 95% curcuminoids, 300 mg; resveratrol, 50 mg; and standardized green tea extract (80% polyphenols), 300 mg. See Table 1 for summary of PB studies using in vitro and in vivo approaches. These included human Fanconi anemia head and neck squamous cell carcinoma (HNSCC), which with acute myeloid leukemia, are the major causes of mortality and morbidity in Fanconi anemia patients. We found that nude mice injected with OHSU-974 cells and subsequently fed a diet supplemented with 1% PB demonstrated inhibition of tumor growth by 67.6% ($p < 0.0001$) and tumor burden by 63.6% ($p < 0.0001$) [95]. In vitro study demonstrated dose-dependent inhibition of OSHU-974 cell proliferation, with cell toxicity detected at 27% ($p = 0.0003$) and 48% ($p = 0.0004$) at PB concentrations of 75 and 100 µg/mL, respectively [95]. These cells constitutively secrete matrix metalloproteinase (MMP)-2 and, after stimulation by phorbyl 12-myristate (PMA), also MMP-9. The secretion of MMPs by both stimulated and unstimulated cells was suppressed by PB in a dose-dependent manner, with total block of both at 50 µg/mL, which is below PB's toxicity level [95]. This concentration was also effective in inhibiting cancer cell migration (by scratch test) and invasion through Matrigel, apparently not related to cell toxicity, as no visible morphological changes were detected at this and lower concentrations [95].

Table 1. Anticancer effect of polyphenol mixture containing quercetin, curcumin, green tea, Cruciferex™, and resveratrol (PB) on cancer cell lines.

Cancer Cell Line and in Vivo Design	Tumor Growth Inhibition	In Vitro Inhibition
FA HNSCC Athymic male nude mice injected SQ with 3×10^6 OHSU-974 cells Control group fed regular murine diet and PB group diet supplemented with PB 1% × 4 weeks [95]	Tumor weight by 67.6% ($p < 0.0001$) Tumor burden by 63.6%	Cell proliferation inhibited by 48% at 100 µg/mL PB; MMP-2 and -9 completely blocked at 50 µg/mL PB; cell migration and Matrigel invasion blocked at 50 µg/mL PB
Fibrosarcoma HT-1080 [96]	N/A	HT-1080 cell proliferation inhibited by 80% at 50 µg/mL PB; MMP-2 and -9 completely blocked at 50 µg/mL PB; Matrigel invasion blocked at 25 µg/mL PB; induction of dose-dependent apoptosis
Melanoma A-2058 [97]	N/A	A-2058 cell proliferation inhibited by 80% at 25 µg/mL PB; MMP-2 and -9 completely blocked at 50 µg/mL PB; Matrigel invasion blocked at 50 µg/mL PB; induction of dose-dependent apoptosis

The inhibitory effects of PB were also observed in fibrosarcoma, which is an aggressive and highly metastatic cancer of connective tissue, and in melanoma, which causes the majority of skin cancer-related deaths, secondary to metastasis. The in vitro studies used human fibrosarcoma cell line HT-1080 [96] and melanoma A2058 cells [97]. The study showed that PB inhibited cell proliferation of human fibrosarcoma cells by 60% at 25 µg/mL and 80% at 50 µg/mL, and inhibited both MMP-2 and -9 secretion in a dose-dependent manner, with total inhibition at 50 µg/mL [96]. At PB concentration of 25 µg/mL, invasion of HT-1080 cells through Matrigel was totally blocked [96]. Melanoma cells were more sensitive to PB, as their proliferation was inhibited by 80% at 25 ug/mL and MMP-2 and -9 secretion and Matrigel cell invasion blocked completely at 50 µg/mL, indicating strong anti-invasive properties of this polyphenol mixture [97]. PB also induced cell apoptosis in both cell lines in a dose-dependent fashion.

4.2. *Anticancer Effects of Combinations of Polyphenols, with Vitamins and Other Compounds*

Combinations of polyphenols with mixtures of vitamins, amino acids and other micronutrients are rarely utilized in cancer research. We initiated this multi-targeted approach over a decade ago, demonstrating that a combination of EGCG with specific micronutrients showed anti-proliferative and anti-invasive effects in human breast (MDA-MB-231), colon (HCT 116) and melanoma (A-2058) cancer cells [98]. The investigated combination included EGCG from green tea together with ascorbic acid, lysine, proline, arginine, *N*-acetyl cysteine, selenium, copper and manganese. This mixture, designated as NM, was tested in vitro and in vivo against a few dozen human cancer cell lines. The composition of this specific micronutrient mixture exemplifies the importance of extracellular matrix-mediated processes in developing a general strategy of effective control of cancer. While most of natural compound combinations target intracellular regulatory mechanisms of tumorigenesis, our approach expands it to include connective tissue integrity as a common element involved in tumor growth, invasion and metastasis. The role of this natural anti-cancer barrier is frequently overlooked in therapeutic approaches to cancer. However, all critical metabolic steps in cancer require degradation of basement membrane and extracellular matrix components as the physical barrier restraining growth, migration and invasion of tumor cells. Increased activity of proteinases, such as MMPs and plasmin, accompanied by down-regulation of their natural inhibitors has been correlated with aggressiveness of cancer and angiogenesis, associated with neovascularization of tumors [99,100]. This new approach to curbing cancer growth by strengthening the connective tissue in the body was introduced by Rath in the 1990s [101]. This can be achieved with micronutrients essential for the synthesis and structure of connective tissue (vitamin C, lysine, proline, and copper manganese) and inhibitors of enzymatic breakdown of collagen facilitated by malignant cells (i.e., lysine). In addition to its essential role in collagen production, vitamin C has shown to be an effective anti-cancer agent (pro-oxidant effects) [102,103] and in cancer prevention (antioxidant effects) [104]. The presence of polyphenols in this mixture, in addition to selenium, *N*-acetylcysteine and arginine allows for expanding biological targets and enhancing several cellular mechanisms important in controlling cancer, such as immune system function. The mixture was formulated in two variants in regard to its polyphenol components: including both EGCG and quercetin (EPQ) and containing EGCG (NM) as the sole polyphenol. Both compositions were tested against several human and murine cancer cell lines both in vivo and in vitro.

4.2.1. EGCG in Combination with Vitamin C, Amino Acids and Other Micronutrients

The multiple aspects of anticancer efficacy of the combination of green tea extract rich in EGCG with ascorbic acid, lysine, proline, arginine, *N*-acetylcysteine, selenium, copper and manganese (NM) on several cancer cell lines in vivo and in vitro were presented in a review article [105].

This unique mixture demonstrated potent, significant suppression of hepatic and pulmonary metastasis in a murine model resulting in significant reduction in tumor size and tumor burden in all human cancer cell lines tested. In vitro studies demonstrated that NM was very effective in inhibition of cell proliferation (by MTT assay), MMP secretion (by gelatinase zymography), cell invasion (through Matrigel), cell migration (by scratch test), angiogenesis (VEGF and other angiogenic models), induction of apoptosis (by live green caspase) and induction of pro-apoptotic genes in many diverse cancer cell lines. A more recent study conducted with the NM mixture illustrates its efficacy against multiple parameters of cancer growth and progression in vivo and in vitro. We used an orthotopic breast cancer model to evaluate the development of tumors and metastasis, challenging mice with breast cancer 4T1 cells into the mammary pad, and also studied in vitro activity of NM on cell proliferation, MMP secretion, cell migration and invasion [106]. See Table 2 for summary of results. In contrast to human tumor cell models, murine tumor cell models often metastasize more effectively and display metastatic characteristics more similar to those observed in cancer patients. The 4T1 mammary carcinoma model was chosen since the primary tumor grows in the anatomically correct site and, as in human breast cancer, 4T1 metastatic disease develops spontaneously from the primary tumor. In addition, metastatic spread of 4T1 metastases to other organs and the draining lymph nodes is similar to that of human mammary cancer. The results showed that NM inhibited tumor weight and burden by 50% ($p = 0.02$) and 53.4% ($p < 0.0001$), respectively, and metastasis, by reducing mean number of colonies by 87% ($p < 0.0001$) and mean weight of lungs by 60% ($p = 0.0001$) compared to Control mice [106]. Metastasis to liver, spleen, kidney and heart was significantly reduced with NM supplementation [106].

Table 2. Anticancer effect of the combination of green tea extract with ascorbic acid, lysine, proline, arginine, *N*-acetyl cysteine, selenium, copper and manganese (NM) on breast 4T1 tumor [106].

Tumor Cell Line/In Vivo Design	Tumor Growth and Metastasis	In Vitro Results
Orthotopic injection of 5×10^5 breast cancer 4T1 cells into the mammary pad of Balb C mice Control group fed regular murine diet and NM group diet supplemented with NM 0.5% × 4 weeks	Tumor weight reduced by 50% ($p = 0.02$) and tumor burden by 53.4% ($p < 0.0001$) in NM mice compared to Control mice Lung metastasis inhibited by 87% ($p < 0.0001$) in NM mice compared to Control mice Mean weight of lungs reduced by 60% ($p = 0.0001$) Metastasis to liver, spleen, kidney and heart significantly reduced in NM group compared to Control	Cell proliferation reduced by 50% at 250 μg/mL NM MMP-2 and -9 completely blocked at 1000 μg/mL NM Cell migration and Matrigel invasion blocked at 250 μg/mL NM

4.2.2. Inhibitory Effects of EGCG Applied Individually, and in Combination with Other Micronutrients on MMPs

In a previous study, we compared the anticancer effects of EGCG alone, in green tea and in combinations with micronutrients on the critical aspect of malignancy. Since type IV collagenase matrix metalloproteinases, especially MMP-2 and MMP-9, have been found to promote invasion and metastasis of malignant tumors, we investigated the relative inhibitory effects in MMP-2 and -9 by EGCG, the main polyphenol in green tea extract (GTE) to that of GTE and to that of NM as a whole using four cancer cell lines expressing MMP-2, MMP-9 or both, to determine if there is an additive or synergistic effect from combinations of these agents [107]. The cell lines tested included human fibrosarcoma (HT-1080), hepatocellular carcinoma (SK-Hep-1), glioblastoma (T-98G) and uterine leiomyosarcoma (SK-UT-1). The cells were also treated with PMA 100 ng/mL to study enhanced expression of MMP-9. Secretion of MMPs was assessed by gelatinase zymography. Fibrosarcoma and hepatocellular carcinoma cells expressed both MMP-2 and MMP-9, glioblastoma cells MMP-2 and PMA-induced MMP-9, and uterine leimyosarcoma cells only PMA-induced MMP-9. NM was the most potent dose-dependent inhibitor of MMPs, followed by green tea extract and EGCG. See Table 3 for summary of results. These results suggest the enhanced efficacy of nutrients working in synergy to modulate complex pathways such as MMP expression.

Table 3. Comparative cumulative expression of MMP-2 and -9 in cell lines treated with epigallocatechin gallate (EGCG), green tea extract (GTE) and the nutrient mixture (NM) [107].

	EGCG	GTE	NM	EGCG + PMA	GTE + PMA	NM + PMA
			Fibrosarcoma HT-1080			
MMP-2	7.88	7.47	3.29	0.21	0.20	0
MMP-9	5.74	3.02	1.58	209.06	139.84	93.54
			Hepatocellular carcinoma Sk-Hep-1			
MMP-2	1.21	1.10	0	0.77	0.55	0.29
MMP-9	256.51	187.28	26.59	611.90	593.80	508.28
			Glioblastoma T-98G			
MMP-2	109.97	86.63	65.84	178.16	140.09	53.20
MMP-9	0.37	0.37	0.10	92.69	82.67	52.50
			Uterine leimyosarcoma SK-UT-1			
MMP-2	0	0	0	51.36	49.97	34.30
MMP-9	0	0	0	87.42	87.30	77.95

4.2.3. Quercetin in Enhancing the Micronutrient Mixture Efficacy in Established Breast Cancer Tumors

We observed that including quercetin in the nutrient mixture containing EGCG has beneficial effects when administered to rats at early stages of breast tumor growth. Breast tumors were induced by IP administration of *N*-methyl-*N*-nitrosourea to Wistar rats [108]. After tumors were evident in all rats, the animals were divided into groups and fed one of the following regimens for 60 days: control diet; 30 mg green tea extract alone; 30 mg green tea extract in combination with NM; or a diet containing 30 mg of green tea extract, NM and quercetin. The results showed that tumor size/rat was significantly lower in all supplemented groups than in the Control group. The rats on the diet containing NM and quercetin showed significantly lower values for tumor incidence, mean tumor volume and mean tumor weight compared to the Control, the green tea extract and the NM groups [108]. Rats in the Control group developed 24 carcinomas (mostly of grade III severity), contrasted with six carcinomas (all of which were of grade II severity) in the NM supplemented group containing quercetin. The incidence, mean tumor volume and mean tumor weight of the green tea extract group alone (2.0, 7.27 cc, and 5.33 g, respectively) were higher than those of the NM group (1.4, 3.39 cc, and 1.71 g, respectively), and that was greater than that of the quercetin + NM group (1.0, 2.69 cc, and 1.35 g, respectively); however, the differences did not reach statistical significance. Higher anti-cancer efficacy of the mixture in the presence of quercetin might be related to its effects on EGCG bioavailability, as the results showed that administration of EGCG in the mixture with vitamins, amino acids and trace element (NM) resulted in a modest increase of its plasma concentration to 45.81 ng/mL from 35.84 ng/mL with EGCG administered alone. The enrichment of this mixture with quercetin resulted in increased plasma EGCG level to 65.94 ng/mL.

4.2.4. Anticancer Effects of EGCG plus Quercetin in the Micronutrient Mixture

The studies presented below illustrate the anti-cancer potential of EGCG and quercetin in combination with the micronutrient mixture against ovarian cancer using two different cell lines (ES-2 and A-2780) [109,110]. See Table 4 for summary of results. EPQ contains the following nutrients in the relative amounts indicated: vitamin C (as ascorbic acid and as Mg, Ca ascorbates, and ascorbyl palmitate) 700 mg; L-lysine 1000 mg; L-proline 750 mg; L-arginine 500 mg; *N*-acetyl cysteine 200 mg; standardized green tea extract (80% polyphenol) 1000 mg; quercetin as quercetin dihydrate, from *Saphora japonica* 50 mg; selenium 30 µg; copper 2 mg; manganese 1 mg.

Table 4. Anticancer effect of mixture containing polyphenols quercetin and green tea extract with ascorbic acid, lysine, proline, arginine, *N*-acetyl cysteine, selenium, copper and manganese (EPQ).

Cancer Cell Line and in Vivo Design	Tumor Growth and Metastasis Inhibition	In Vitro Inhibition
Athymic female mice inoculated subcutaneously with 3×10^6 ovarian ES-2 cells Control group fed regular murine diet and EPQ group diet supplemented with EPQ 0.5% × 4 weeks [109]	Tumor weight reduced by 59.2% ($p < 0.0001$) and tumor burden by 59.7% $p < 0.0001$) in EPQ mice	ES-2 cell proliferation inhibited by 35% at 1000 µg/mL EPQ; MMP-2 virtual total block at 1000 µg/mL EPQ; cell migration and Matrigel invasion blocked at 500 µg/mL EPQ
Athymic female mice inoculated intraperitoneally with 2×10^6 ovarian A-2780 cells Control group fed regular murine diet and EPQ group diet supplemented with EPQ 0.5% × 4 weeks [110]	Incidence of ovarian tumors reduced to 1 small tumor in EPQ group contrasted with Control group mice which all developed large ovarian tumors; tumor growth suppressed by 87% ($p < 0.0001$); lung metastasis completely suppressed in EPQ mice, but 100% present in Control mice	A-2780 cell proliferation inhibited by 80% at 1000 µg/mL EPQ; MMP-9 virtual total block at 250 µg/mL EPQ; Matrigel invasion blocked at 250 µg/mL EPQ

Epithelial ovarian carcinoma is the leading cause of death from gynecological malignancy due to metastasis and recurrence. Our previous publication on athymic female mice inoculated with ES-2 ovarian cancer cells showed that dietary intake of EPQ (0.5%, w/w) inhibited weight and burden of tumors by 59.2% ($p < 0.0001$) and 59.7% ($p < 0.0001$), respectively [109] (see Figure 1). A subsequent study on ovarian carcinoma used IP injection of ovarian cancer A-2780 cells into athymic female mice and focused on ovarian tumor growth and lung metastasis [110]. In the A-2780 study, all Control mice developed large ovarian tumors, whereas five out of six mice in the EPQ group developed no tumors, and one, only a small tumor [110]. EPQ suppressed tumor growth by 87% ($p < 0.0001$). In addition, all animals in the Control group had lung metastasis while, in contrast, no metastasis was observed in the EPQ group of mice [110]. In vitro, the effects of EPQ on cell proliferation, MMP secretion, invasion through Matrigel, migration by scratch test and morphology were evaluated in ES-2 [109] and A2780 [110] cells. EPQ exhibited 35% toxicity over the control in ES-2 cells [109] and 80% in A-2780 cells [110] at 1000 µg/mL concentration. ES-2 cells demonstrated only MMP-2, with and without PMA, which was inhibited by EPQ in a dose dependent fashion, with near total inhibition at 1000 µg/mL [109]. A-2780 cells demonstrated only MMP-9 expression, which EPQ inhibited in a dose dependent fashion, with virtual total block at 250 µg/mL concentration [110]. Migration of ES-2 cells by scratch test and invasion through Matrigel were inhibited in a dose dependent manner with total block of invasion and migration at 500 µg/mL [109]. Invasion through Matrigel of A-2780 cells was completely inhibited by EPQ at 250 µg/mL [110]. H&E staining showed no morphological changes below 500 µg/mL EPQ in A-2780 cells [110] and below 1000 µg/mL EPQ in ES-2 cells [109]. See Table 4 for summary of results.

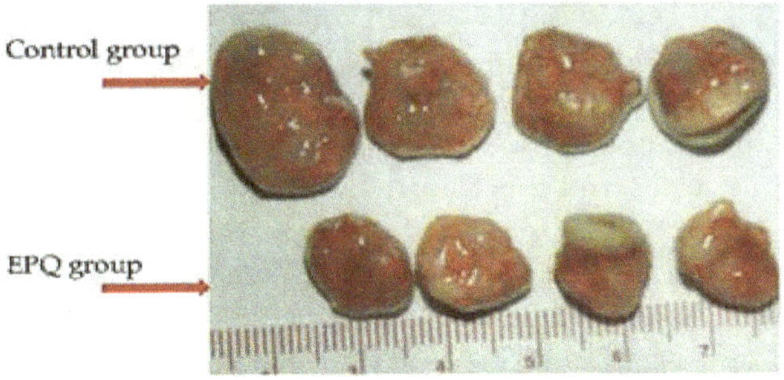

Figure 1. Gross photographs of representative tumors from Control and EPQ groups of mice inoculated with ovarian cancer ES-2 cells. Mean tumor weight and burden of EPQ group tumors were inhibited by 59.2% ($p < 0.0001$) and 59.7% ($p < 0.0001$) compared to Control group, respectively.

An earlier study investigated the efficacy of a combination of polyphenols, quercetin and green tea, on prostate cancer xenograft tumor growth. The results confirmed the synergistic effects of this nutrient combination resulting in tumor growth inhibition by 45%, compared to 15% with quercetin and 21% with green tea only [111]. Although the experimental design and tumor type differed in the Wang studies from our research, both investigations point out to enhance anticancer effects of various nutrient combinations and the importance of connective tissue in confining tumor growth and metastasis.

5. Conclusions

Current cancer therapies based on chemotherapy and radiation are associated with significant side effects. Therefore, there is an urgent need for developing alternate or adjuvant approaches. Polyphenolic compounds, which are abundant from dietary sources, show great promise in cancer treatment, especially considering their safe use. Due to their ability to modulate multiple biological mechanisms involved in cancer initiation and progression, they offer more comprehensive therapeutic effects than single drugs. Bioavailability, as well as curative and preventive properties of these nutrients, can be enhanced and expanded in combination therapies that include natural compounds of the same or different chemical class. Combinations of polyphenols with micronutrients essential for maintaining integrity and stability of extracellular matrix offer expanded anti-cancer benefits. They include targeting complementary metabolic pathways important in curtailing cancer invasion and metastasis. Therefore, future research directions should expand to using natural compounds, especially in combinations, as safe, effective and affordable therapeutic approaches to cancer.

Acknowledgments: The research study was funded by Dr. Rath Health Foundation (Santa Clara, CA, USA), a non-profit organization.

Author Contributions: This review was written by A.N., M.W.R., T.K. and M.R.

References

1. Scalbert, A.; Manach, C.; Morand, C.; Rémésy, C.; Jime'nez, L. Dietary polyphenols and the prevention of diseases. *Crit. Rev. Food Sci. Nutr.* **2005**, *45*, 287–306. [CrossRef] [PubMed]
2. Ramos, S. Cancer chemoprevention and chemotherapy: Dietary polyphenols and signaling pathways. *Mol. Nutr. Food Res.* **2008**, *52*, 507–526. [CrossRef] [PubMed]
3. Fantini, M.; Benvenuto, M.; Masuelli, L.; Frajese, G.V.; Tresoldi, I.; Modesti, A.; Bei, R. In vitro and in vivo antitumoral effects of combinations of polyphenols, or polyphenols and anticancer drugs: Perspectives on cancer treatment. *Int. J. Mol. Sci.* **2015**, *16*, 9236–9282. [CrossRef] [PubMed]
4. Manach, C.; Scalbert, A.; Morand, C.; Rémésy, C.; Jime'nez, L. Polyphenols: Food sources and bioavailability. *Am. J. Clin. Nutr.* **2004**, *79*, 727–747. [PubMed]

5. Arts, I.C.W.; van de Putte, B.; Hollman, P.C.H. Catechin contents of foods commonly consumed in The Netherlands. Fruits, vegetables, staple foods, and processed foods. *J. Agric. Food Chem.* **2000**, *48*, 1746–1751. [CrossRef] [PubMed]
6. Arts, I.C.; van de Putte, B.; Hollman, P.C.H. Catechin contents of foods commonly consumed in The Netherlands. Tea, wine, fruit juices, and chocolate milk. *J. Agric. Food Chem.* **2000**, *48*, 1752–1757. [CrossRef] [PubMed]
7. Lakenbrink, C.; Lapczynski, S.; Maiwald, B.; Engelhardt, U.H. Flavonoids and other polyphenols in consumer brews of tea and other caffeinated beverages. *J. Agric. Food Chem.* **2000**, *48*, 2848–2852. [CrossRef] [PubMed]
8. Zhu, Q.Y.; Zhang, A.Q.; Tsang, D.; Huang, Y.; Chen, Z.Y. Stability of green tea catechins. *J. Agric. Food Chem.* **1997**, *45*, 4624–4628. [CrossRef]
9. Lempereur, I.; Rouau, X.; Abecassis, J. Genetic and agronomic variation in arabinoxylan and ferulic acid contents of durum wheat (Triticum durum L) grain and its milling fractions. *J. Cereal Sci.* **1999**, *25*, 103–110. [CrossRef]
10. Bhat, K.P.; Pezzuto, J.M. Cancer chemopreventive activity of resveratrol. *Ann. N. Y. Acad. Sci.* **2002**, *957*, 210–229. [CrossRef] [PubMed]
11. Adlercreutz, H.; Mazur, W. Phyto-oestrogens and western diseases. *Ann. Med.* **1997**, *29*, 95–120. [CrossRef] [PubMed]
12. Tourė, A.; Xuemin, X. Flax lignans: Source, biosynthesis, metabolism, antioxidant activity, bio-active components, and health benefits. *Compr. Rev. Food Sci. Food Saf.* **2010**, *9*, 261–269. [CrossRef]
13. Scalbert, A.; Williamson, G. Dietary intake and bioavailability of polyphenols. *J. Nutr.* **2000**, *130*, 2073S–2085S. [PubMed]
14. Bogaards, I.J.P.; van Ommen, B.; Falke, H.E.; Willems, M.I.; van Bladeren, P.J. Glutathione S-transferase subunit induction patterns of Brussel sprouts, allyl isothiocyanate and goitrin in rat liver and small intestinal mucosa: A new approach for the identification of inducing xenobiotics. *Food Chem. Toxicol.* **1990**, *28*, 81–88. [CrossRef]
15. Han, X.; Shen, T.; Lou, H. Dietary polyphenols and their biological significance. *Int. J. Mol. Sci.* **2007**, *8*, 950–988. [CrossRef]
16. Shen, S.Q.; Zhang, Y.; Xiang, J.J.; Xiong, C.L. Protective effect of curcumin against liver warm ischemia/reperfusion injury in rat model is associated with regulation of heat shock protein and antioxidant enzymes. *World J. Gastroenterol.* **2007**, *13*, 1953–1961. [CrossRef] [PubMed]
17. Chen, C.; Yu, R.; Owuor, E.D.; Kong, A.N. Activation of antioxidant response element (ARE), mitogen-activated protein kinases (MAPKs) and caspases by major green tea polyphenol components during cell survival and death. *Arch. Pharm. Res.* **2000**, *23*, 605–612. [CrossRef] [PubMed]
18. Kunnumakkara, A.B.; Guha, S.; Krishnan, S.; Diagaradjane, P.; Gelovani, J.; Aggarwal, B.B. Curcumin potentiates antitumor activity of gemcitabine in an orthotopic model of pancreatic cancer through suppression of proliferation, angiogenesis, and inhibition of nuclear factor kappa B-regulated gene products. *Cancer Res.* **2007**, *67*, 3853–3861. [CrossRef] [PubMed]
19. Collett, G.P.; Campbell, F.C. Curcumin induces c-jun *N*-terminal kinase-dependent apoptosis in HCT116 human colon cancer cells. *Carcinogenesis* **2004**, *25*, 2183–2189. [CrossRef] [PubMed]
20. Anto, R.J.; Mukhopadhyay, A.; Denning, K.; Aggarwal, B.B. Curcumin (diferuloylmethane) induces apoptosis through activation of caspase-8, BID cleavage and cytochrome c release: Its suppression by ectopic expression of Bcl-2 and Bcl-xL. *Carcinogenesis* **2002**, *23*, 143–150. [CrossRef] [PubMed]
21. Aoki, H.; Takada, Y.; Kondo, S.; Sawaya, R.; Aggarwal, B.; Kondo, Y. Evidence that curcumin suppresses the growth of malignant gliomas in vitro and in vivo through induction of autophagy: Role of Akt and ERK signaling pathways. *Mol. Pharmacol.* **2007**, *72*, 29–39. [CrossRef] [PubMed]
22. Anand, P.; Sundaram, C.; Jhurani, S.; Kunnumakkara, A.B.; Aggarwal, B.B. Curcumin and cancer: An 'old-age' disease with an 'age-old' solution. *Cancer Lett.* **2008**, *267*, 133–164. [CrossRef] [PubMed]
23. Alexandrov, M.G.; Song, L.J.; Altiok, S.; Gray, J.; Haura, E.B.; Kumar, N.B. Curcumin: A novel Stat3 pathway inhibitor for chemoprevention of lung cancer. *Eur. J. Cancer Prev.* **2012**, *21*, 407–412. [CrossRef] [PubMed]
24. Ng, T.P.; Chiam, P.C.; Lee, T.; Chua, H.C.; Lim, L.; Kua, E.H. Curry consumption and cognitive function in the elderly. *Am. J. Epidemiol.* **2006**, *164*, 898–906. [CrossRef] [PubMed]

25. Bartik, L.; Whitfield, G.K.; Kaczmarska, M.; Lowmiller, C.L.; Moffet, E.W.; Furmick, J.K.; Hernandez, Z.; Haussler, C.A.; Haussler, M.R.; Jurutka, P.W. Curcumin: A novel nutritionally derived ligand of the vitamin D receptor with implications for colon cancer. *J. Nutr. Biochem.* **2010**, *21*, 1153–1161. [CrossRef] [PubMed]
26. Ide, H.; Tokiwa, S.; Sakamaki, K.; Nishio, K.; Isotani, S.; Muto, S.; Hama, T.; Masuda, H.; Horie, S. Combined inhibitory effect of soy flavones and curcumin on the production of prostate specific antigen. *Prostate* **2010**, *70*, 1127–1133. [CrossRef] [PubMed]
27. Gupta, S.C.; Patchva, S.; Aggarwal, B.B. Therapeutic roles of curcumin: Lessons learned from clinical trials. *AAPS J.* **2013**, *15*, 195–218. [CrossRef] [PubMed]
28. Ravindran, J.; Prasad, S.; Aggrawal, B.B. Curcumin and cancer cells: How many ways can curry kill tumor cells selectively? *AAPS J.* **2009**, *11*, 495–510. [CrossRef] [PubMed]
29. Shanmugam, M.K.; Rane, G.; Kanchi, M.M. The multifaceted role of curcumin in cancer prevention and treatment. *Molecules* **2015**, *20*, 2728–2769. [CrossRef] [PubMed]
30. Gibellini, L.; Pinti, M.; Nasi, M.; Montagna, J.P.; De Biasi, S.; Roat, E.; Bertoncelli, L.; Cooper, E.L.; Cossarizza, A. Quercetin and cancer chemoprevention. *Evid. Based Complement. Alternat. Med.* **2011**, *2011*, 591356. [CrossRef] [PubMed]
31. Ekstrom, A.M.; Serafini, M.; Nyren, O.; Wolk, A.; Bosetti, C.; Bellocco, R. Dietary quercetin intake and risk of gastric cancer: Results from a population-based study in Sweden. *Ann. Oncol.* **2011**, *22*, 438–443. [CrossRef] [PubMed]
32. Lam, T.K.; Rotunno, M.; Lubin, J.H.; Wacholder, S.; Consonni, D.; Pesatori, A.C.; Bertazzi, P.A.; Chanock, S.J.; Burdette, L.; Goldstein, A.M.; et al. Dietary quercetin, quercetin-gene interaction, metabolic gene expression in lung tissue and lung cancer risk. *Carcinogenesis* **2010**, *31*, 634–642. [CrossRef] [PubMed]
33. Jeong, J.H.; An, J.Y.; Kwon, Y.T.; Rhee, J.G.; Lee, Y.G. Effects of low dose quercetin: Cancer cell-specific inhibition of cell cycle progression. *J. Cell. Biochem.* **2009**, *106*, 73–82. [CrossRef] [PubMed]
34. Yang, J.H.; Hsia, T.C.; Kuo, H.M.; Chou, P.D.; Chou, C.C.; Wei, Y.H.; Chung, J.G. Inhibition of lung cancer cell growth by quercetin glucuronides via G 2/M arrest and induction of apoptosis. *Drug Metab. Dispos.* **2006**, *34*, 296–304. [CrossRef] [PubMed]
35. Nair, H.K.; Rao, K.V.K.; Aalinkeel, R.; Mahajan, S.; Chawda, R.; Schwartz, S.A. Inhibition of prostate cancer cell colony formation by the flavonoid quercetin correlates with modulation of specific regulatory genes. *Clin. Diagn. Lab. Immunol.* **2004**, *11*, 63–69. [CrossRef] [PubMed]
36. Mu, C.; Jia, P.; Yan, Z.; Liu, X.; Li, X.; Liu, H. Quercetin induces cell cycle G1 arrest through elevating Cdk inhibitors p21 and p27 in human hepatoma cell line (HepG2). *Methods Find. Exp. Clin. Pharmacol.* **2007**, *29*, 179–183. [CrossRef] [PubMed]
37. Seufi, A.M.; Ibrahim, S.S.; Elmagrahby, T.K.; Hafez, E.E. Preventive effect of the flavonoid, quercetin, on hepatic cancer in rats via oxidant/antioxidant activity: Molecular and histological evidences. *J. Exp. Clin. Cancer Res.* **2009**, *28*, 80. [CrossRef] [PubMed]
38. Devipriya, S.; Ganapthy, V.; Shyamaladevi, C.S. Suppression of tumor growth and invasion in 9,10 dimethyl benz (a) anthracene induced mammary carcinoma by the plant bioflavonoid quercetin. *Chem-Biol. Interact.* **2006**, *162*, 106–113. [CrossRef] [PubMed]
39. Theodoratou, E.; Kyle, J.; Cetnarskyj, R.; Farrington, S.M.; Tenesa, A.; Barnetson, R.; Porteous, M.; Dunlop, M.; Campbell, H. Dietary flavonoids and the risk of colorectal cancer. *Cancer Epidemiol. Biomark. Prev.* **2007**, *16*, 684–693. [CrossRef] [PubMed]
40. Ferry, D.R.; Smith, A.; Malkhandi, J.; Fyfe, D.W.; de Takats, P.G.; Anderson, D.; Baker, J.; Kerr, D.J. Phase I clinical trial of the flavonoid quercetin: Pharmacokinetics and evidence for in vivo tyrosine kinase inhibition. *Clin. Cancer Res.* **1996**, *2*, 659–668. [PubMed]
41. Miles, S.L.; McFarland, M.; Niles, R.M. Molecular and physiological actions of quercetin: Need for clinical trials to assess its benefits in human disease. *Nutr. Rev.* **2014**, *72*, 720–734. [CrossRef] [PubMed]
42. Udenigwe, C.C.; Ramprasath, V.R.; Aluko, R.E.; Jones, P.J. Potential of resveratrol in anticancer and anti-inflammatory therapy. *Nutr. Rev.* **2008**, *66*, 445–454. [CrossRef] [PubMed]
43. Bishayee, A. Cancer prevention and treatment with resveratrol: From rodent studies to clinical trials. *Cancer Prev. Res.* **2009**, *2*, 409–418. [CrossRef] [PubMed]
44. Kukreja, A.; Waddhwa, N.; Tiwari, A. Therapeutic role of resveratrol and piceatannol in disease prevention. *J. Blood Disord. Transf.* **2014**, *5*, 1–6. [CrossRef]

45. Patel, K.R.; Brown, V.A.; Jones, D.J.L.; Britton, R.G.; Hemingway, D.; Miller, A.S.; West, K.P.; Booth, T.D.; Perloff, M.; Crowell, J.A.; et al. Clinical pharmacology of resveratrol and its metabolites in colorectal cancer patients. *Cancer Res.* **2010**, *70*, 7392–7399. [CrossRef] [PubMed]
46. Chow, H.H.S.; Garland, L.L.; Hsu, C.H.; Vining, D.R.; Chew, W.M.; Miller, J.A.; Perloff, M.; Crowell, J.A.; Alberts, D.S. Resveratrol modulates drug- and carcinogen-metabolizing enzymes in a healthy volunteer study. *Cancer Prev. Res.* **2010**, *3*, 1168–1175. [CrossRef] [PubMed]
47. Drewnowski, A.; Gomez-Carneros, C. Bitter taste, phytonutrients and the consumer: A review. *Am. J. Clin. Nutr.* **2000**, *72*, 1424–1435. [PubMed]
48. Hidgon, J.V.; Delage, B.; Williams, D.E.; Dashwood, R.H. Cruciferous vegetables and human cancer risk: Epidemiologic evidence and mechanistic basis. *Pharmacol. Res.* **2007**, *55*, 224–236.
49. Holst, B.; Williamson, G. A critical review of the bioavailability of glucosinolates and related compounds. *Nat. Proc. Rep.* **2004**, *21*, 425–447. [CrossRef] [PubMed]
50. Agerbirk, N.; Olsen, C.E. Glucosinolate structures in evolution. *Phytochemistry* **2012**, *77*, 16–45. [CrossRef] [PubMed]
51. Kandala, P.K.; Srivastava, S.K. DIMming ovarian cancer growth. *Curr. Drug Targets* **2012**, *13*, 1869–1875. [CrossRef] [PubMed]
52. Bradlow, H.L. Indole-3-carbinol as a chemopreventive agent in breast and prostate cancer. *In Vivo* **2008**, *22*, 441–446. [PubMed]
53. Beaver, L.M.; Yu, T.W.; Sokolowski, E.I.; Williams, D.E.; Dashwood, R.H.; Ho, E. 3,3′-diindolylmethane, but not indole-3-carbinol, inhibits histone deacetylase activity in prostate cancer cells. *Toxicol. Appl. Pharmacol.* **2012**, *263*, 345–351. [CrossRef] [PubMed]
54. Sepkovic, D.W.; Raucci, L.; Stein, J.; Carlisle, A.D.; Auborn, K.; Ksieski, H.B.; Nyirenda, T.; Bradlow, H.L. 3,3′-Diindolylmethane increases serum interferon-γ levels in the K14-HPV16 transgenic mouse model for cervical cancer. *In Vivo* **2012**, *26*, 207–211. [PubMed]
55. Chinni, S.R.; Li, Y.; Upadhyay, S.; Koppolu, P.K.; Sarkar, F.H. Indole-3-carbinol (I3C) induced cell growth inhibition, G1 cell cycle arrest and apoptosis in prostate cancer cells. *Oncogene* **2001**, *20*, 2927–2937. [CrossRef] [PubMed]
56. Li, Y.; Li, X.; Sarkar, F.H. Gene expression profiles of IC3 and DIM-treated PC3 human prostate cancer dells determined by cDNA microarray analysis. *J. Nutr.* **2003**, *133*, 1011–1019. [PubMed]
57. Aggarwal, B.B.; Ichikawa, H. Molecular targets and anticancer potential of indole-3-carbinol and its derivatives. *Cell Cycle* **2005**, *4*, 1201–1215. [CrossRef] [PubMed]
58. Sarkar, F.H.; Li, Y. Indole-3-carbinol and prostate cancer. *J. Nutr.* **2004**, *134*, 3493S–8349S. [PubMed]
59. Plate, A.Y.; Gallaher, D.D. Effects of indole-3-carbinol and phenethyl isothiocyanate on colon carcinogenesis induced by azoxymethane in rats. *Carcinogenesis* **2006**, *27*, 287–292. [CrossRef] [PubMed]
60. Tadi, K.; Chang, Y.; Ashok, B.T.; Chen, Y.; Moscatello, A.; Schaefer, S.D.; Schantz, S.P.; Policastro, A.J.; Geliebter, J.; Tiwari, R.K. 3,3′-Diindolylmethane, a cruciferous vegetable derived synthetic anti-proliferative compound in thyroid disease. *Biochem. Biophys. Res. Commun.* **2005**, *337*, 1019–1025. [CrossRef] [PubMed]
61. Kim, Y.S.; Milner, J.A. Targets for indole-3-carbinol in cancer prevention. *J. Nutr. Biochem.* **2005**, *16*, 65–73. [CrossRef] [PubMed]
62. Brew, C.T.; Aronchik, I.; Hsu, J.C.; Sheen, J.H.; Dickson, R.B.; Bjeldanes, L.F.; Firestone, G.L. Indole-3-carbinol activates the ATM signaling pathway independent of DNA damage to stabilize p53 and induce G1 arrest of human mammary epithelial cells. *Int. J. Cancer* **2006**, *118*, 857–868. [CrossRef] [PubMed]
63. Chang, X.; Tou, J.C.; Hong, C.; Chen, Y.; Moscatello, A.; Schaefer, S.D.; Schantz, S.P.; Policastro, A.J.; Geliebter, J.; Tiwari, R.K. 3,3′-Diindolylmethane inhibits angiogenesis and the growth of transplantable human breast carcinoma in athymic mice. *Carcinogenesis* **2005**, *26*, 771–778. [CrossRef] [PubMed]
64. Shukla, Y.; Kalra, N.; Katiyar, S.; Siddiqui, I.A.; Arora, A. Chemopreventive effect of indole-3-carbinol on induction of preneoplastic altered hepatic foci. *Nutr. Cancer* **2004**, *50*, 214–220. [CrossRef] [PubMed]
65. Garikapaty, V.P.; Ashok, B.T.; Chen, Y.G.; Mittelman, A.; Iatropoulos, M.; Tiwari, R.K. Anti-carcinogenic and anti-metastatic properties of indole-3-carbinol in prostate cancer. *Oncol. Rep.* **2005**, *13*, 89–93. [CrossRef] [PubMed]
66. Bonnesen, C.; Eggleston, I.M.; Hayes, J.D. Dietary indoles and isothiocyanates that are generated from cruciferous vegetables can both stimulate apoptosis and confer protection against DNA damage in human colon cell lines. *Cancer Res.* **2001**, *61*, 6120–6130. [PubMed]

67. Keck, A.S.; Finley, J.W. Cruciferous vegetables: Cancer protective mechanisms of glucosinolate hydrolysis products and selenium. *Integr. Cancer Ther.* **2004**, *3*, 5–12. [CrossRef] [PubMed]
68. Valcic, S.; Timmermann, B.N.; Alberts, D.S.; Wächter, G.A.; Krutzsch, M.; Wymer, J.; Guillén, J.M. Inhibitory effect of six green tea catechins and caffeine on the growth of four selected human tumor cell lines. *Anticancer Drugs* **1996**, *7*, 461–468. [CrossRef] [PubMed]
69. Mukhtar, H.; Ahmad, N. Tea polyphenols: Prevention of cancer and optimizing health. *Am. J. Clin. Nutr.* **2000**, *71*, S1698–S1702, discussion S1703–S1704.
70. Yang, G.Y.; Liao, J.; Kim, K.; Yurkow, E.J.; Yang, C.S. Inhibition of growth and induction of apoptosis in human cancer cell lines by tea polyphenols. *Carcinogenesis* **1998**, *19*, 611–616. [CrossRef] [PubMed]
71. Taniguchi, S.; Fujiki, H.; Kobayashi, H.; Go, H.; Miyado, K.; Sadano, H.; Shimokawa, R. Effect of (−)-epigallocatechin gallate, the main constituent of green tea, on lung metastasis with mouse B16 melanoma cell lines. *Cancer Lett.* **1992**, *65*, 51–54. [CrossRef]
72. Hara, Y. *Green Tea: Health Benefits and Applications*; Marcel Dekker: New York, NY, USA, 2001.
73. Harakeh, S.; Abu-El-Ardat, K.; Diab-Assaf, M.; Niedzwiecki, A.; El-Sabban, M.; Rath, M. Epigallocatechin-3-gallate induces apoptosis and cell cycle arrest in HTLV-1-positive and -negative leukemia cells. *Med. Oncol.* **2008**, *25*, 30–39. [CrossRef] [PubMed]
74. Cabrera, C.; Gimenez, R.; Lopez, M.C. Determination of tea components with antioxidant activity. *J. Agric. Food Chem.* **2003**, *53*, 4427–4435. [CrossRef] [PubMed]
75. Fujiki, H.; Suganuma, M.; Okabe, S.; Sueoka, E.; Suga, K.; Imai, K.; Nakachi, K.; Kimura, S. Mechanistic findings of green tea as cancer preventive for humans. *Proc. Soc. Exp. Biol. Med.* **1999**, *220*, 225–228. [CrossRef] [PubMed]
76. Gupta, S.; Hastak, K.; Afaq, F.; Ahmad, N.; Mukhtar, H. Essential role of caspases in epigallocatechin-3-gallate-mediated inhibition of nuclear factor kappa B and induction of apoptosis. *Oncogene* **2004**, *23*, 2507–2522. [CrossRef] [PubMed]
77. Ahmed, S.; Wang, N.; Lalonde, M.; Goldberg, V.M.; Haqqi, T.M. Green tea polyphenol epigallocatechin-3-gallate (EGCG) differentially inhibits interleukin-1 beta-induced expression of matrix metalloproteinase-1 and -13 in human chondrocytes. *J. Pharmacol. Exp. Ther.* **2004**, *308*, 767–773. [CrossRef] [PubMed]
78. Khan, N.; Afaq, F.; Saleem, M.; Ahmad, N.; Mukhtar, H. Targeting multiple signaling pathways by green tea polyphenol (−)-epigallocatechin-3-gallate. *Cancer Res.* **2006**, *66*, 2500–2505. [CrossRef] [PubMed]
79. Ahn, W.S.; Yoo, J.; Huh, S.W.; Kim, C.K.; Lee, J.M.; Namkoong, S.E.; Bae, S.M.; Lee, I.P. Protective effects of green tea extracts (polyphenon E and EGCG) on human cervical lesions. *Eur. J. Cancer Prev.* **2003**, *12*, 383–390. [CrossRef] [PubMed]
80. Kurbitz, C.; Heise, D.; Redmer, T.; Goumas, F.; Arlt, A.; Lemke, J.; Rimbach, G.; Kalthoff, H.; Trauzold, A. Epicatechin gallate and catechin gallate are superior to epigallocatechin gallate in growth suppression and anti-inflammatory activities in pancreatic tumor cells. *Cancer Sci.* **2011**, *102*, 728–734. [CrossRef] [PubMed]
81. Kale, A.; Gawande, S.; Kotwal, S.; Netke, S.; Roomi, W.; Ivanov, V.; Niedzwiecki, A.; Rath, M. Studies on the effects of oral administration of nutrient mixture, quercetin and red onions on the bioavailability of epigallocatechin gallate from green tea extract. *Phytother. Res.* **2010**, *24*, S48–S55. [CrossRef] [PubMed]
82. Wang, P.; Herber, D.; Henning, S.M. Quercetin increased bioavailability and decreased methylation of green tea polyphenols in vitro and in vivo. *Food Funct.* **2012**, *3*, 635–642. [CrossRef] [PubMed]
83. Wang, P.; Herber, D.; Henning, S.M. Quercetin increased antiproliferative activity of green tea polyphenol (−)-epigallocatechin gallate in prostate cancer cells. *Nutr. Cancer* **2012**, *64*, 580–587. [CrossRef] [PubMed]
84. Naumovsky, N.; Blades, B.L.; Roach, P.D. Food inhibits the oral bioavailability of the major green tea antioxidant epigallocatechin gallate in humans. *Antioxidants* **2015**, *4*, 373–393. [CrossRef] [PubMed]
85. Williamson, G.; Manach, C. Bioavailability and bioefficacy of polyphenols in humans. II. Review of 93 intervention studies. *Am. J. Clin. Nutr.* **2005**, *81*, 243S–255S. [PubMed]
86. Hsieh, T.C.; Wu, J.M. Targeting CWR22Rv1 prostate cancer cell proliferation and gene expression by combinations of the phytochemicals, EGCG, genistein and quercetin. *Anticancer Res.* **2009**, *29*, 4025–4032. [PubMed]
87. Tang, S.N.; Singh, C.; Nall, D.; Meeker, D.; Shankar, S.; Srivastava, R.K. The dietary bioflavonoid quercetin synergizes with epigallocatechin gallate (EGCG) to inhibit prostate cancer stem cell characterstic, invasion migration and epithelial-mesenchymal transition. *J. Mol. Signal.* **2010**, *5*, 14. [CrossRef] [PubMed]

88. Ahmad, K.A.; Harris, N.H.; Johnson, A.D.; Lindvall, H.C.; Wang, G.; Ahmed, K. Protein kinase CK2 modulates apoptosis induced by resveratrol and epigallocatechin gallate in prostate cancer cells. *Mol. Cancer Ther.* **2007**, *6*, 1006–1012. [CrossRef] [PubMed]
89. Hsieh, T.C.; Wu, J.M. Suppression of cell proliferation and gene expression by combinatorial synergy of EGCG, resveratrol and gamma-tocotrienol in estrogen positive MCF-7 breast cancer cells. *Int. J. Oncol.* **2008**, *33*, 851–859. [PubMed]
90. Saha, A.; Kuzuhara, T.; Echigo, N.; Suganuma, M.; Fujiki, H. New role of (−)epicatechin in enhancing the induction of growth inhibition and apoptosis in human lung cancer cells by curcumin. *Cancer Prev. Res.* **2010**, *3*, 953–962. [CrossRef] [PubMed]
91. Zhou, D.H.; Wang, X.; Yang, M.; Shi, X.; Huang, W.; Feng, Q. Combination of low concentration of (−)epigallocatechin gallate (EGCG) and curcumin strongly suppresses the growth of non small cell lung cancer in vitro and in vivo through causing cell cycle arrest. *Int. J. Mol. Sci.* **2013**, *14*, 12023–12036. [CrossRef] [PubMed]
92. Ghosh, A.K.; Kay, N.E.; Secreto, C.R.; Shanafelt, T.D. Curcumin inhibits prosurvival pathways in chronic lymphocytic leukemia B cells and may overcome their stromal protection in combination with EGCG. *Clin. Cancer Res.* **2009**, *15*, 1250–1258. [CrossRef] [PubMed]
93. Somers-Edgar, T.J.; Scandlyn, M.J.; Stuart, E.C.; Le Nedelec, M.J.; Valentine, S.P.; Rosengren, R.J. The combination of epigallocatechin gallate and curcumin suppresses ER alpha-breast cancer cell growth in vitro and in vivo. *Int. J. Cancer* **2008**, *122*, 1966–1971. [CrossRef] [PubMed]
94. Piao, L.; Mukherjee, S.; Chang, Q.; Xie, X.; Li, H.; Castellanos, M.R.; Banerjee, P.; Iqbal, H.; Ivancic, R.; Wang, X.; et al. TriCurin, a novel formulation of curcumin, epicatechin gallate and resveratrol, inhibits the tumorigenicity of human papillomavirus-positive head and neck squamous cell carcinoma. *Oncotarget* **2016**. [CrossRef] [PubMed]
95. Roomi, M.W.; Kalinovsky, T.; Roomi, N.W.; Niedzwiecki, A.; Rath, M. In vitro and in vivo inhibition of human Fanconi anemia head and neck squamous carcinoma by a phytonutrient combination. *Int. J. Oncol.* **2015**, *46*, 2261–2266. [CrossRef] [PubMed]
96. Roomi, M.W.; Jariwalla, N.; Roomi, N.W.; Rath, M.; Niedzwiecki, A. Abstract 1500: A novel nutrient mixture exhibits antitumor activity in human fibrosarcoma cell line HT-1080. In Proceedings of the 102nd Annual Meeting of the AACR, Orlando, FL, USA, 2–6 April 2011.
97. Roomi, M.W.; Siddiqui, S.; Roomi, N.W.; Niedzwiecki, A.; Rath, M. Abstract 1503: Anti-cancer effects of a nutrient mixture in human melanoma cells A2058: Inhibition of cell proliferation, MMP expression, invasion and apoptosis. In Proceedings of the 102nd Annual Meeting of the AACR, Orlando, FL, USA, 2–6 April 2011.
98. Netke, S.P.; Roomi, M.W.; Ivanov, V.; Niedzwiecki, A.; Rath, M. A specific combination of ascorbic acid, lysine, proline and epigallocatechin gallate inhibits proliferation and extracellular matrix invasion of various human cancer cell lines. *Res. Commun. Pharmacol. Toxicol. Emerg. Drugs* **2003**, *8*, IV37–IV49.
99. Stetler-Stevenson, W.G. The role of matrix metalloproteinases in tumor invasion, metastasis and angiogenesis. *Surg. Oncol. Clin. N. Am.* **2001**, *10*, 383–392. [PubMed]
100. Dano, K.; Andreasen, P.A.; Grondahl-Hansen, J.; Kristensen, P.; Nielsen, L.S.; Skriver, L. Plasminogen activators, tissue degradation and cancer. *Adv. Cancer Res.* **1985**, *44*, 139–266. [PubMed]
101. Rath, M.; Pauling, L. Plasmin-induced proteolysis and the role of apoprotein(a), lysine and synthetic analogs. *Orthomol. Med.* **1992**, *7*, 17–23.
102. Park, S. The effects of high concentrations of vitamin on cancer cells. *Nutrients* **2013**, *5*, 3496–3505. [CrossRef] [PubMed]
103. Chen, Q.; Espey, M.G.; Krishna, M.C.; Mitchell, J.B.; Corpe, C.P.; Buettner, G.R.; Shacter, E.; Levine, M. Pharmacologic ascorbic acid concentrations selectively kill cancer cells: Action as a pro-drug to deliver hydrogen peroxide to tissues. *Proc. Natl. Acad. Sci. USA* **2005**, *102*, 13604–13609. [CrossRef] [PubMed]
104. Lutsenko, E.A.; Carcamo, J.M.; Golde, D.W. Vitamin C prevents DNA mutation induced by oxidative stress. *J. Biol. Chem.* **2001**, *277*, 16895–16899. [CrossRef] [PubMed]
105. Niedzwiecki, A.; Roomi, M.W.; Kalinovsky, T.; Rath, M. Micronutrient synergy—A new tool in effective control of metastasis and other key mechanisms of cancer. *Cancer Metastasis Rev.* **2010**, *29*, 529–543. [CrossRef] [PubMed]
106. Roomi, M.W.; Kalinovsky, T.; Roomi, N.M.; Cha, J.; Rath, M.; Niedzwiecki, A. In vivo and in vitro effects of a nutrient mixture on breast 4T1 cancer progression. *Int. J. Oncol.* **2014**, *44*, 1933–1944. [PubMed]

107. Roomi, M.W.; Monterrey, J.C.; Kalinovsky, T.; Rath, M.; Niedzwiecki, A. Comparative effects of EGCG, green tea, and a nutrient mixture on the patterns of MMP-2 and MMP-9 expression in cancer cell lines. *Oncol. Rep.* **2010**, *24*, 747–757. [PubMed]
108. Kale, A.; Gawande, S.; Kotwal, S.; Netke, S.; Roomi, M.W.; Ivanov, V.; Niedzwiecki, A.; Rath, M. A combination of green tea extract, specific nutrient mixture and quercetin: An effective intervention treatment for the regression of *N*-methyl-*N*-nitrosourea (MNU)-induced mammary tumors in Wistar rats. *Oncol. Lett.* **2010**, *1*, 313–317. [PubMed]
109. Roomi, M.W.; Kalinovsky, T.; Niedzwiecki, A.; Rath, M. A nutrient mixture modulates ovarian ES-2 cancer progression by inhibiting xenograft tumor growth and cellular MMP secretion, migration and invasion. *Int. J. Clin. Exp. Med.* **2016**, *9*, 814–822.
110. Roomi, M.W.; Niedzwiecki, A.; Rath, M. Abstract 4053: A unique nutrient mixture suppresses ovarian cancer growth of A-2780 by inhibiting invasion and MMP-9 secretion. In Proceedings of the 107th Annual Meeting of the AACR, New Orleans, LA, USA, 16–20 April 2016.
111. Wang, P.; Vadgama, J.V.; Said, J.W.; Magyar, C.E.; Doan, N.; Heber, D.; Henning, S.M. Enhanced inhibition of prostate cancer xenograft tumor growth by combining quercetin and green tea. *J. Nutr. Biochem.* **2014**, *25*, 73–80. [CrossRef] [PubMed]

6

Mangiferin and Cancer: Mechanisms of Action

Fuchsia Gold-Smith [1], Alyssa Fernandez [2] and Karen Bishop [1,*]

[1] Auckland Cancer Society Research Center, Faculty of Medical and Health Sciences, University of Auckland, Private Bag 92019, Auckland 1142, New Zealand; fgol315@aucklanduni.ac.nz
[2] Faculty of Medical and Health Sciences, University of Auckland, Private Bag 92019, Auckland 1142, New Zealand; afer098@aucklanduni.ac.nz
[*] Correspondence: k.bishop@auckland.ac.nz

Abstract: Mangiferin, a bioactive compound derived primarily from Anacardiaceae and Gentianaceae families and found in mangoes and honeybush tea, has been extensively studied for its therapeutic properties. Mangiferin has shown promising chemotherapeutic and chemopreventative potential. This review focuses on the effect of mangiferin on: (1) inflammation, with respect to NFκB, PPARγ and the immune system; (2) cell cycle, the MAPK pathway G_2/M checkpoint; (3) proliferation and metastasis, and implications on β-catenin, MMPs, EMT, angiogenesis and tumour volume; (4) apoptosis, with a focus on Bax/Bcl ratios, intrinsic/extrinsic apoptotic pathways and telomerase activity; (5) oxidative stress, through Nrf2/ARE signalling, ROS elimination and catalase activity; and (6) efficacy of chemotherapeutic agents, such as oxaliplatin, etoposide and doxorubicin. In addition, the need to enhance the bioavailability and delivery of mangiferin are briefly addressed, as well as the potential for toxicity.

Keywords: mangiferin; cancer; inflammation; NFκB; oxidative stress; cell cycle; combination therapy; nutraceuticals; bioavailability; hallmarks of cancer

---

1. Introduction

Cancer has been identified as the leading cause of non-communicable disease mortality globally [1], and is responsible for significant morbidity and costs to healthcare systems. Cancer incidence and mortality has been increasing at a greater rate than population growth alone could account for. The International Agency for Research on Cancer (IARC) reported 14.1 million cases and over 8.2 million mortalities due to cancer in 2012 compared to 10 million cases and six million mortalities in 2000 [2] in a baseline population of 7.1 billion and 6.1 billion, respectively [3]. Much of this increase is due to rising cancer burden in less developed countries (LDCs), with 57% of new cases, and 65% of cancer related deaths occurring in LDCs [2]. When standardized by age, the total number of cases per 100,000 population is greater in more developed countries (MDCs) than LDCs (overall age standardized rate: 268 and 148 respectively) [4]. One exception to this pattern is infection-attributable cancers, which are responsible for 26% of the cancer burden in LDCs but only 8% in MDCs [5].

Cancer is less likely to be identified early or treated successfully in LDCs due to reduced access to screening tools and chemotherapeutic drugs. Previously, cancer has been regarded as a MDC disease. However, through the adoption of a more Westernised lifestyle, cancer incidence has been steadily increasing in LDCs. From the data published by Parkin et al., it can be seen that 40%–45% of cancers can be attributable to lifestyle factors such as diet, smoking status, alcohol consumption and lack of physical activity [6]. Some compounds naturally present in the diet, such as mangiferin in mangoes and honeybush tea, are thought to modulate risk of cancer and retard cancer progression.

Mangiferin (1,3,6,7-tetrahydroxyxanthone-C2-β-D glucoside) [7–11] is a polyphenol [8,11–15] found in many plant species, in particular, those from the Anacardiaceae [7,9,16–20] and Gentianaceae families [7,9,13,17,18,20]. For an extensive breakdown of plant sources of mangiferin and mangiferin content, see Matkowski et al. [21].

Mangiferin is not only present in everyday foods, but utilised in a number of natural medicines. In traditional medicine, different cultures have cultivated and processed mangiferin rich plants for the treatment of a range of illnesses including cardiovascular disease, diabetes, infection and cancer [22–24]. In India, Ayurvedic practitioners [22] have used *Salicia chinesis* (saptarangi) [21,25,26] and *Mangifera indica* (mango), which are two species that contain high levels of mangiferin. *Salicia chinesis* has been used for its hypo-lipidaemic, anti-diabetic, hepatoprotective and antioxidant properties. *Salicia chinesis* has now been over-exploited and research is being conducted into how this plant may be grown in a more sustainable way to meet demands [27]. *Mangifera indica* is used not only in Ayurvedic medicine but also used in Cuba [23], China [21,24] and throughout East Asia [21] for its anti-inflammatory, anti-viral, anti-diabetic and anti-cancer properties. *Mangifera indica*, a member of the Gentianaceae family, contains mangiferin [10,20,21,28–30] in its bark (18.33 g/kg dry weight [31]), leaves [15] (old leaves 36.9 g/kg and young leaves 58.12 g/kg dry weight [31]) and root along with the seed, pulp (0 to 2.65 mg/kg dry weight, depending on the variety [32]) and skin of the fruit [7,8,12,20,33–35] (4.94 g/kg dry weight [31]). However, the concentration of mangiferin in the pulp is unlikely to be sufficient to provide significant health benefits, and can vary greatly depending on variety and the maturity of the fruit [32]. Although somewhat lower than levels found in bark and leaves, the mangiferin in the skin [36] and seed/kernel [31], which are usually considered waste products, may provide a promising sustainable option for mangiferin extraction. To date, these mango by-products have been used to enhance the nutritional density of pasta, biscuits, muffins and pancakes [37–40]. Although the phenolic content of these food items increased 2.8–3.9 fold [37,39], the mangiferin content was not reported. However, in the results detailed in the sections hereafter, the concentrations used or administered varied from 12.5 to 100 μg/mL in in vitro studies [12] and approximately 100 mg/kg body weight in in vivo studies [7]. Clearly, the consumption of such quantities is not achievable by consuming fresh mango pulp, but maybe achievable by adding a leaf, bark, and/or seed extract as a supplement to food, or consuming as a liquid (if palatable).

In Cuba, aqueous extracts of *Mangifera indica* bark have become popular [7,12,41,42] for treatment of not only cancer but gastric and dermatological disorders, AIDS and asthma [43]. Stem bark extracts contain polyphenols, terpenoids, steroids, fatty acids and trace elements alongside mangiferin [21,23]. The natural medicine, Vimang® [7,12,42], produced from aqueous extracts of *Mangifera indica*, contains ~20% mangiferin [23] and is available in tablets, creams and syrups. Vimang® is registered as an "anti-inflammatory phytomedicine" by the Cuban Regulatory Health Authorities and is primarily used by those with multiple and different types of cancer. In China, mango leaves [21,24] and *Dobinea delavayi* (Baill.) leaves [44], which both contain mangiferin, are often used in traditional medicines. The greatest dietary source of mangiferin is Honeybush tea, popular in South Africa and obtained from *Cyclopia sp.* [21]. Honeybush tea leaves have been found to consist of up to 4% mangiferin by dry weight [21].

Research into mangiferin has resulted in the identification of a similar compound, namely mangiferin aglycone or norathyriol, which appears to have greater biological activity in some instances. The compound mangiferin aglycone can be artificially synthesized, bypassing any sustainability concerns surrounding mangiferin. The structure of mangiferin and mangiferin aglycone are shown in Figure 1. Mangiferin aglycone has shown greater biological activity in some targets than mangiferin, possibly due to greater water solubility [28], and the former appears to reduce UV-induced skin cancer [8]. Further studies are required to elucidate the degree of similarity in action of mangiferin and mangiferin aglycone.

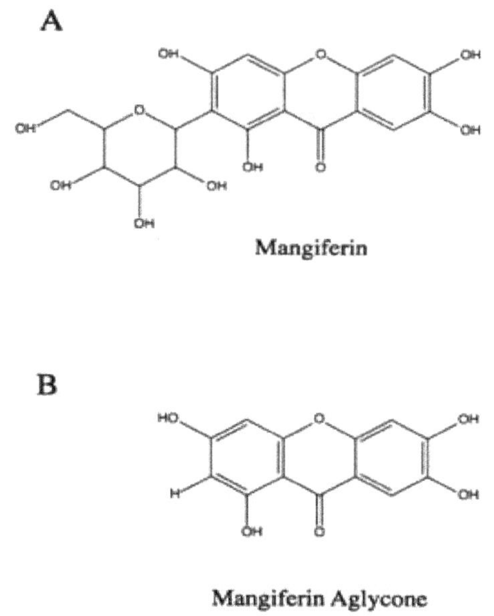

Figure 1. The molecular structure of: (**A**) mangiferin [45]; and (**B**) mangiferin aglycone [46].

Evidence suggests that mangiferin could prove to be a useful, inexpensive compound to not only maintain and improve health in the worried well, but also to significantly improve the outlook for those with certain cancers (e.g., breast cancer [41]) and reduce the likelihood of developing cancer. This is of particular relevance to LDCs, where the more expensive chemotherapeutic drugs may be inaccessible, while mangiferin containing plants are abundant. In MDCs, the potential enhanced synergistic effect seen with major chemotherapeutic drugs may allow for lower dosages of drugs, thus reducing toxicity and providing greater selective toxicity to malignant cells, reducing the extent of side effects [47]. However, it is acknowledged that the quantity of fruit required in order to achieve clinically relevant levels of mangiferin may be unreasonably high. For this reason substitution of flour and sugar with mango processing by product [37,39] may prove an additional and useful method of increasing mangiferin intake.

The anti-cancer properties of mangiferin have been extensively studied over the past few decades. This review article seeks to consolidate the most recent research on the anti-neoplastic properties of mangiferin, with a focus on molecular pathways and uses of mangiferin, in conjunction with known chemotherapeutic agents, to aid further research on this topic.

2. Molecular Mechanisms of the Anti-Cancer Action of Mangiferin

Mangiferin acts through a myriad of mechanisms to exert anti-inflammatory [11,14,20–24,28,29,42,48], immunomodulatory [8,9,14,19,20,23,24,28,29,49], cell cycle arrest, anti-proliferative, anti-apoptotic [48], anti-oxidative [8,11,14,15,19,20,22–24,28–30,36,42,48–51], anti-genotoxic [30] and anti-viral [11,15,20,48] effects which cumulatively result in anti-tumour activity [9,11,15,19–21,23,24,29,41,50]. Mangiferin has demonstrated broad-spectrum efficacy against an array of different cancers in in vitro and in vivo studies [8,11,12,14,21]. To date, evidence suggests that the side effects of mangiferin vary from mild to non-existent [52]; however, there may be some variation according to source of mangiferin.

2.1. Inflammation

The chronic activation of inflammatory processes is widely regarded as an enabling characteristic towards the acquisition of cancer [53]. Approximately 20% of cancers are attributable to chronic inflammation [54], which may be induced by bacterial or viral infections, autoimmune disease, or constant exposure to irritants. Chronic inflammation can drive tumour growth by providing a favourable environment, rich in inflammatory mediators, to enhance cell growth and survival [53,55].

In addition, inflammation involves the production of reactive oxygen species (ROS), which can cause DNA damage, enhancing carcinogenic capabilities [56]. Mangiferin is thought to dampen down the inflammatory response primarily by interference with Nuclear Factor κ-light-chain-enhancer of activated B cells (NFκB) [34].

By reducing inflammation, mangiferin not only provides unfavourable conditions for cancer, but can provide anti-diabetic effects [11,15,19,21,23,24,28,29,50] and reduce risk of cardiovascular disease. Mangiferin also reduces serum glucose levels and lipid levels [8,14,30], further decreasing development and severity of diabetes and cardiovascular disease. Thus, while many medications used to treat these widespread non-communicable diseases may create adverse conditions in the body that may lead to other diseases, mangiferin provides broad spectrum benefits across a range of diseases such as cancers, cardiovascular disease and diabetes [26,33,35,39].

2.1.1. Nuclear Factor κ-Light-Chain-Enhancer of Activated B Cells Activity

The transcription factor NFκB regulates many important processes in inflammation, including the expression of pro-inflammatory cytokines, migration molecules, growth factors and other genes involved in proliferation and survival [34]. NFκB is up-regulated during inflammation. Under inflammatory conditions, ligands bind and activate Toll-like receptors (TLRs) and Interleukin-1 Receptors (IL-1R), triggering the Myeloid Differentiation Primary Response Gene 88 (Myd88) to recruit Interleukin-1 Receptor Activated Kinase 1 (IRAK1) to this receptor-signalling complex for phosphorylation [57,58]. Association of IRAK1 with Myd88 allows phosphorylation by IRAK4 and subsequent autophosphorylation. In its phosphorylated form, IRAK1 interacts with Tumour necrosis factor Receptor-Associated Factor 6 (TRAF6) to form a complex, which signals sequentially through Transforming growth factor beta-activated kinase 1/Transforming growth factor beta-activated kinase 1-binding protein 1 and 2 (TAK1/TAB1/TAB2), NFκB Essential Modulator/Inhibitor of NFκB Kinase subunit-β/Inhibitor of NFκB Kinase subunit-α (NEMO/IKK-β/IKK-α) and Inhibitor of κB (IκB)/p50/p65 complexes to ultimately activate NFκB [57]. Recent findings suggest mangiferin inhibits NFκB activation at various steps in the pathway (Figure 2A,B) [11,47]. NFκB can be activated via the classical or alternative pathways. The classical pathway is regulated by the IκB kinase complex and p50, while the alternative pathway is regulated by IKKα and p52 [59].

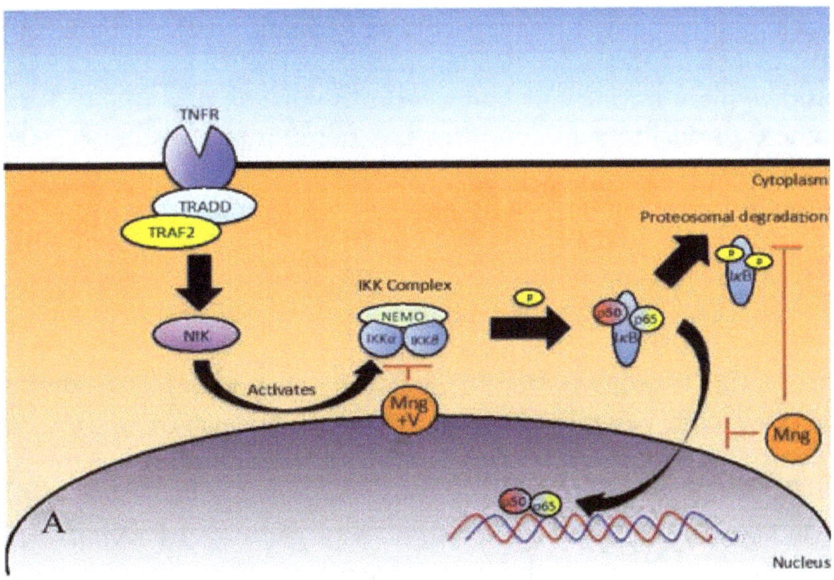

Figure 2. *Cont.*

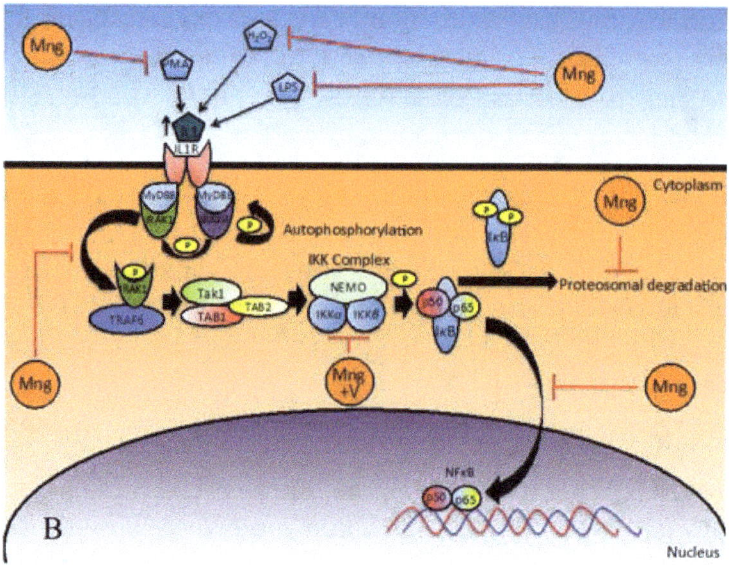

Figure 2. Inhibition of NFκB via the (**A**) classical and (**B**) alternative pathways by mangiferin and Vimang (adapted from [11,45,55]) (abbreviations: Mng, mangiferin; V, Vimang®).

Initial Stimulus for NFκB Activation

When studied, it was found that mangiferin blocks Tumour Necrosis Factor (TNF) [8], lipopolysaccharide (LPS), peptidoglycan (PDG) [60], phorbol-12-myristate-13-acetate (PMA) [11] or hydrogen peroxide (H_2O_2) mediated NFκB activation by inhibiting ROS production [61]. This effect has been demonstrated in U-937 (lymphoma), HeLa (cervical cancer), MCF-7 (breast cancer) and IRB3 AN27 (human foetal neuronal) cell lines [11]. Jeong et al. [60] demonstrated that the inhibitory effect of mangiferin on NFκB expression when induced by LPS and PDG in peritoneal macrophages was elicited in part by inhibition of IRAK1 phosphorylation and consequently activation. In parallel, mangiferin impedes NFκB activation via inflammatory genes [11,48]. Inhibition of IRAK1 by mangiferin may reduce development of resistance to chemotherapeutic drugs. In particular, triple negative breast cancers have been associated with overexpression of IRAK1, and it is reported that inhibition of IRAK1, through the p38-MCL1 pathway, may reverse paclitaxel resistance [62]. Mangiferin, as a component of combination therapy, will be addressed in Section 4.

Subsequent studies have implicated mangiferin in suppressing the TNF signal transduction pathway [11,48], where under normal conditions, canonic interactions of TNF Receptor (TNFR) with Tumour Necrosis Factor Receptor type-1-Associated Death Domain protein (TRADD), TNFR-Associated Factor 2 (TRAF2) and NCK Interacting Kinase (NIK) along with subsequent phosphorylation and degradation of IκBα initiates NFκB activation (Figure 2A) [11]. To identify the site of action, U-937 cells were transfected with TNFR1, TRADD, TRAF2, NIK, IKK and p65 plasmids. Secreted Embryonic Alkaline Phosphatase (SEAP) was used as a reporter gene for NFκB and expression levels were monitored in treated and un-treated cells. Mangiferin inhibited TNFR1, TRADD, TRAF2, NIK and IKK induced SEAP expression but did not have a significant effect on p65 induced SEAP expression. Consequently, mangiferin must act downstream from IKK [11].

Signal Transduction to Activate NFκB

In a study carried out by García-Rivera et al. on estrogen negative MDA-MB231 breast cancer cells, the efficacy of Vimang® (aqueous extract from *Mangifera indica*) was investigated and compared to treatment with either mangiferin only or gallic acid only (another bioactive present in Vimang®) [41]. At baseline, MDA-MB231 cells, which have a mutated p53 gene, demonstrate high NFκB activity [41]. When cells were pre-treated for 4 h with 200 μg/mL Vimang® or 100 μg/mL of mangiferin, there was no change in IKKα expression, but reduced phosphorylation of IKKα and IKKβ was observed [41]. These proteins must be phosphorylated in order to transduce the signal and activate NFκB, thus mangiferin attenuated signal transduction. These authors also report that time taken for IκB phosphorylation and consequently degradation in response to TNF stimulation was doubled and time taken for IκB resynthesis was significantly reduced [41]. The action of mangiferin on IκB degradation has also been reported in a number of other studies [11,41,47,48,63]. Once IκBα is degraded, its inhibitory effect on the NFκB activation pathway is diminished [63] and thus NFκB can freely bind to DNA, allowing transcription and translation of the respective genes and proteins that it regulates [64]. Additionally, mangiferin and Vimang® were found to reduce phosphorylation and translocation of p65 into the nucleus and impeded NFκB/DNA binding in response to TNF [41]. Other studies have also reported that mangiferin affects IκBα and p65 in this way [8,11,48]. García-Rivera et al. revealed that Vimang®, but not mangiferin alone was found to prevent parallel NFκB transactivation [41], emphasising the beneficial effects provided by other bioactive constituents of this aqueous extract.

It is clear that mangiferin is likely to attenuate NFκB expression in a multifaceted way, [34,47] with additional mechanisms yet to be elucidated.

Consequential Effects of NFκB Downregulation

NFκB is implicit in regulating expression of Cyclooxygenase-2 (COX-2), Intercellular Adhesion Molecule-1 (ICAM-1), B Cell Lymphoma-2 (bcl-2), Interleukin-6 (IL-6), Interleukin-8 (IL-8), C-X-C Chemokine Receptor type-4 (CXCR4), X linked Inhibitor of Apoptosis Protein (XIAP) and Vascular Endothelial Growth Factor (VEGF), which are all involved in inflammation, metastasis, cell survival and angiogenesis [11,29,42,48] (more on COX-2 below). As a downregulator of NFκB, mangiferin consequentially reduces expression of the genes listed above [41] and increases apoptosis [8].

IL-6 and IL-8 are both inflammatory cytokines that enhance cell proliferation. In MDA-MB231 cells, proliferation is conditional on autocrine synthesis of inflammatory cytokines and growth factors [41]. Vimang® and mangiferin have each been found to down-regulate IL-6 and IL-8 production when stimulated by TNF [41], thus reducing the inflammatory response.

2.1.2. Peroxisome Proliferator-Activated Receptor γ (PPARγ)

PPARγ is a nuclear receptor that also functions as a transcription factor, regulating expression of genes involved in cell differentiation and tumourigenesis [65]. Under normal circumstances, when the corresponding ligand binds to PPARγ, transcriptional activation of COX-2 is suppressed through a number of mechanisms [66]. COX-2 is one of the key drivers of chronic inflammation through the production of prostaglandins leading to further activation of inflammatory processes [67], and thus COX-2 overexpression favours cancer progression [29]. PPARγ also has a pleiotropic effect on blood glucose levels. PPARγ agonists such as thiazolidinediones are widely used in management of diabetes and have a hypoglycaemic effect [65]. Hyperglycaemia is regarded as an emerging risk factor for cancer development [65]. Mangiferin, like thiazolidinedione may also act to reduce hyperglycaemia, benefiting diabetics and decreasing cancer risk.

Mangiferin increases mRNA expression of the PPARγ gene [68] and thus decreases transcriptional activation of COX-2. This reduces inflammation and creates a less favourable environment for acquisition and proliferation of malignant cells. Mangiferin also impedes expression of COX-2 [41] via upregulation of TGF-β and downregulation of NFκB. Mangiferin may play a beneficial role in modulating PPARγ and COX-2 regulation as evidenced by in vitro studies in MDA-MB231 breast cancer cells [43].

2.1.3. Immune Response

Cancer cells can sometimes escape detection and avoid the immune system, which would otherwise destroy abnormal cells. Cancer cells not only express immune checkpoint proteins that dampen the immune response, but they may also release cytokines and growth factors that promote tumour cell proliferation and minimize apoptosis. By enhancing a patient's immune response a better outcome can be achieved. In in vivo studies, mangiferin has been found to enhance the number and activity of immune cells [9,10].

Rajendran et al. found that in mice treated with benzo(a)pyrene (B(a)P) to induce lung cancer, dosing with mangiferin influenced the types of immune cells present and concentrations of various immunoglobulins [9]. Mangiferin treatment resulted in higher numbers of lymphocytes and neutrophils [9]. Mangiferin treatment of B(a)P mice increased levels of IgG and IgM immunoglobulins and decreased levels of IgA immunoglobulins, relative to animals only receiving B(a)P treatment [9]. In addition, mangiferin inhibited phagocytic capacity and nitric oxide production of macrophages when stimulated with LPS and IFN_{Y} [9]. Thus, with respect to the inflammatory response, less collateral damage is likely to occur. In a later study, it was found that in tumour bearing Swiss mice, mangiferin promoted cytotoxic behaviour of lymphocytes and macrophages against malignant cells, and thus the incidence of fibrosarcoma was reduced [7].

2.2. *Cell Cycle*

Maintenance of a normal cell cycle is essential for homeostasis. It allows cells to be replaced at the same rate as they are lost. Often in cancer, the length of the cell cycle is reduced, allowing aberrant proliferation of malignant cells.

Findings suggest that mangiferin influences the Mitogen Activated Protein Kinase (MAPK) pathway and progression from the G_2/M checkpoint, thus maintaining a more normal cell cycle length, or cell cycle arrest at the appropriate checkpoint [8,13,52].

2.2.1. Mitogen Activated Protein Kinase Pathway

The MAPK pathway is frequently implicated in tumourigenesis as it plays a role in processes such as cell proliferation, growth, differentiation, apoptosis and migration [69]. Mangiferin attenuates MAPK signalling [34] by inhibiting MAPKs p38, Extracellular signal-Regulated Kinase (ERK) and c Jun N-terminal Kinase phosphorylation [60]. Li et al. found that mangiferin aglycone, a metabolite of mangiferin, formed through deglycosylationin vivo, also inhibited ERK1/2 when phosphorylation was induced by UVB [70]. In this study, mangiferin aglycone was found to significantly reduce UV-induced skin cancers in mice, primarily through this interaction with ERK [70]. While further study is required, this suggests a beneficial effect against skin cancer.

2.2.2. G_2/M Checkpoint

Under normal conditions, cells with mutations are not able to undergo mitosis, as there are a number of checkpoints in the cycle that prevent mutated DNA from replicating [71]. Cancer cells must acquire characteristics that allow them to bypass these checkpoints in order to survive and proliferate [71].

The G_2/M checkpoint occurs during the transition from G_2 to mitotic entry. The G_2 phase involves rapid growth of a cell as it prepares for mitosis. Cell progression from the G_2/M checkpoint only occurs in the absence of DNA damage signals [72]. DNA damage can be sensed by Ataxia telangiectasia mutated protein (ATM) and Ataxia Telangiectasia and Rad3-related protein (ATR) which signal via Checkpoint kinase 1 (Chk1) and Checkpoint Kinase 2 (Chk2) to cause degradation of M-phase inducer phosphatase 1 (cdc25a), which results in inhibition of the Cyclin-Dependent Kinase 1 (CDK1)-cyclinB1 complex and thus cell cycle arrest [71,72] (see Figure 3). The cdc2-cyclinB1 complex is often overexpressed in malignant cells, enhancing entry into mitosis in eukaryotic cells. Malignant cells may acquire characteristics, which enable them to escape cell cycle arrest regardless of mutations. Chemotherapeutic agents such as etoposide target malignant cells at the G_2/M checkpoint, thus when cell cycle progression is inhibited, the efficacy of etoposide at inducing apoptosis is increased. Mangiferin is thought to induce G_2/M phase arrest [8], reducing proliferation of malignant cells and increasing efficacy of chemotherapeutic agents that target this phase.

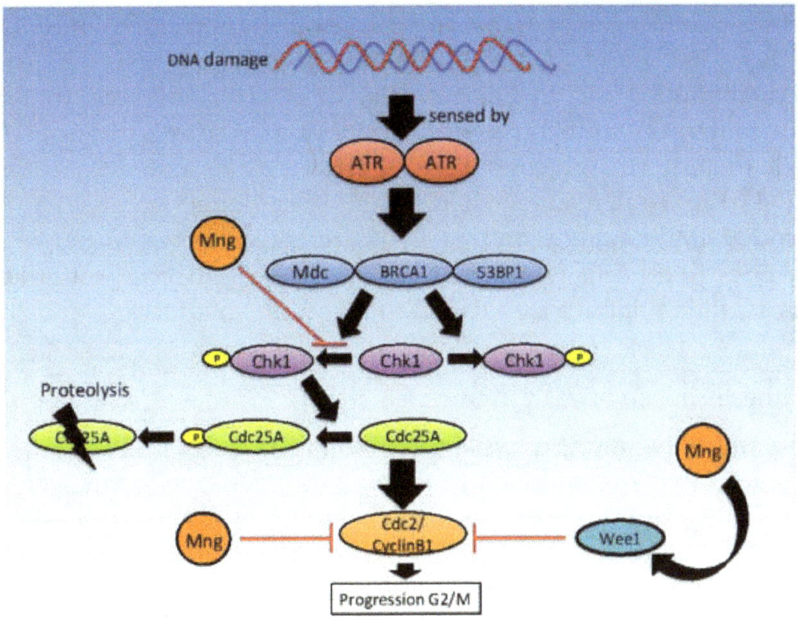

Figure 3. Mangiferin affects the molecular events leading to cell cycle G_2/M phase arrest (Figure adapted from [71]).

Mangiferin has been shown to arrest cell cycle progression in a time dependent manner at the G_2/M phase through suppression of the cdc2-cyclin B1 signalling pathway in MCF-7 cells [8]. This was observed through analysis of cell cycle distribution through flow cytometry, where a greater number of cells were found in the G_2/M phase after incubation with mangiferin [13,52]. These findings are in keeping with results from the Peng et al. study in HL-60 cells [8]. Peng et al. [52] also found that in HL-60 leukaemia cells, gene expression of Chk1, cdc25 and Wee1 was elevated when exposed to low concentrations of mangiferin, but at higher concentrations, Chk1 and cdc25 gene expression was reduced at the mRNA level. Mangiferin has been shown to significantly inhibit phosphorylation of ATR, Chk1 and other proteins with anti-proliferative properties such as Wee1, Akt and Erk1/2, while increasing phosphorylation of cdc2 and cyclinB1 [52]. Lv et al. used a Western blot assay to identify a reduction in cdc2 (cdk1) and cyclinB1 [8] protein levels in response to treatment with mangiferin. Findings suggest that inhibition of the ATR-Chk1 stress response DNA damage pathway by mangiferin is responsible for cell cycle arrest.

While G_2/M phase arrest has been identified in response to mangiferin treatment in a number of cancer cell lines (MCF-7, HL-60, BEL-7404 and CNE2) [16,18,35,52,73], further study is required to determine dosages of mangiferin required to elicit an effect. In addition to G_2/M phase arrest, Lv et al. also suggest that mangiferin may induce G_0/G_1 cell cycle arrest in MCF7 cells [8].

2.3. *Proliferation/Metastasis*

Under normal circumstances, the rate of cell replication and cell death is matched to maintain homeostasis. In cancer cells, the mediators of these processes may be deregulated, allowing cells to proliferate continuously, exceeding rates of cell death. Cancer cells may develop a more motile phenotype, due to deregulation of cell adhesion pathways. Loss of adhesion allows cells to escape their site of origin and spread to other sites, causing secondary malignancies.

Mangiferin is thought to reduce cell proliferation [16] through modulation of β-catenin and consequently metalloproteinase-7 (MMP-7), MMP-9, and EMT (epithelial to mesenchymal transition) [14]. Through NFκB, mangiferin may influence VEGF-A transcription to modulate angiogenesis. Additionally, in in vivo experiments, mangiferin has shown efficacy at reducing tumour volume in mice [14].

In a variety of breast cancer cell lines, mangiferin has been implicated in reduced cell proliferation (MDA-MB-231, BT-549, MCF-7 and T47D) [8,14] and reduced metastasis (MDA-MB-231 and BT-549) in a dose-dependent manner [14]. In HL-60 cells, Li et al. reinforced that mangiferin reduced proliferation [14]. In contrast, Wilkinson et al. found that mangiferin did not suppress proliferation in MCF-7 cells, while mangiferin aglycone did [74]. This may be a result of differential activation of estrogen receptors [74]. Kim et al. also reported no significant effect on proliferation when HeLa cells were treated with 25–200 μM of mangiferin [36] and Garcia-Rivera et al. found no significant inhibition of proliferation in MDA-MB231 cells when treated with mangiferin, but proliferation was inhibited by Vimang® [41]. Thus, further evidence is required to ascertain an effect.

2.3.1. Glycogen Synthase Kinase-3β / β-Catenin

In cancer, aberrant activation of β-catenin is often observed [14]. High levels of expression of β-catenin are associated with proliferation and metastasis. Glycogen synthase kinase -3β (GSK-3β) is capable of phosphorylating and degrading β-catenin [14]. GSK-3β may be inhibited by a number of signals. Mangiferin is hypothesised to suppress the β-catenin pathway [14].

Using a Western blot assay to analyse protein expression in breast cancer cell lines, mangiferin was found to down-regulate β-catenin and decrease levels of inactive GSK-3β, indicating suppression of the β-catenin pathway, which in turn down-regulates MMP-7, MMP-9 and snail expression [14]. Snail can be used as an epithelial/mesenchymal phenotye indicator [14], thus lower levels of snail, which are seen on exposure to mangiferin, favour a more epithelial, less mobile phenotype, while higher expression of snail would indicate a more motile phenotype, allowing malignant cells to metastasise.

2.3.2. Matrix Metalloproteinases

Activation of matrix MMPs is a crucial step towards metastasis as these enzymes facilitate cell escape from the initial site of the malignancy, through degradation of the extracellular matrix. As above, mangiferin has been linked to downregulation of NFκB, which in turn influences downstream expression of MMPs [64,75].

In breast cancer, the matrix metalloproteinases MMP-2, -7 and -9 are often up-regulated [14]. Li et al. have demonstrated through a Western blot assay that of these three enzymes, MMP-2 was not significantly affected while MMP-7 and MMP-9 were down-regulated by mangiferin [14]. MMP-7 and -9 strongly promote cancer progression by allowing malignant cells to metastasise [76]. In LNCaP prostate cancer cells, activation of NFκB by TNF-α increases levels of MMP-9 mRNA and protein present in the cell [75]. Mangiferin is capable of attenuating this effect, ultimately reducing metastasis [75]. In addition to this pathway of MMP-9 activation, Xiao et al. (2015) discovered that mangiferin stimulates miR-15b expression, which in turn down-regulates MMP-9 expression in U87 glioma cells [16], thus reducing the capability of malignant cells to escape the extracellular matrix and metastasise. In the study by Jung et al., mangiferin prevented PMA induced MMP-9 expression without influencing other MMP expression in human astroglioma cell lines: U87MG, U373MG and CRT-MG [19]. MMP-1, -2, -3 and -14 expressions were not influenced by mangiferin [19]. Mangiferin is thought to act by suppressing NFκB and AP-1 binding to the promoter region of MMP-9 and prevents phosphorylation of Akt and MAP kinases (see above section) induced by PMA [19]. Jung et al. also suggest that mangiferin acts on MMP-9 suppressors, *Tissue Inhibitor of Metalloproteinase -1* and -2 (*TIMP-1* and -2). *TIMP-1* and *TIMP-2* mRNA levels were enhanced by the presence of mangiferin, implying another favourable quality of mangiferin [19]. Jung et al. suggest that mangiferin, through these mechanisms, may reduce glioma invasiveness [19]. Overall, published studies indicate that mangiferin may play an important role in reducing expression of MMP-9, limiting cancer invasiveness [16,19].

2.3.3. Epithelial to Mesenchymal Transition

EMT involves the loss of adherence and gain of a motile phenotype and resistance to apoptosis, which may allow motile cancer cells to migrate from their site of origin and survive, causing secondary metastases [53]. β-catenin signalling may also play a role in EMT [14]. Mangiferin appears to enhance epithelial characteristics in breast cancer cell lines and thus help protect against metastasis [14].

Li et al. [14] investigated the effect of mangiferin on EMT through analysis of two mesenchymal-like breast cancer cell lines (MDA-MB-231 and BT-549). Mesenchymal characteristics were reduced upon treatment with mangiferin, whereby cells obtained a more epithelial-like morphology. Associated with these physical observations, increased expression of the epithelial phenotype marker, E-cadherin, and decreased expression of mesenchymal phenotype markers, vimentin, snail and slug were seen [14]. In MDA-MB-231 xenograft mice treated with mangiferin, Western blot analysis revealed the same shift in expression in epithelial and mesenchymal markers with lower expression of active β-catenin, MMP-7, MMP-9 and vimentin (mesenchymal markers) and higher expression of E-cadherin (an epithelial marker) [14], reinforcing the in vitro results. While these results are promising in breast cancer cells, investigation in a more diverse range of cell lines is required to determine if these findings may be applicable to a broader range of breast cancer cell lines as well as other cancer cell lines.

2.3.4. Angiogenesis

Sustained angiogenesis is widely regarded as an enabling characteristic of cancer, as tumours are unable to survive beyond a certain size without their own blood supply [53]. Angiogenic tumours are able to grow and proliferate using nutrients and oxygen from their own blood supply. The VEGF-A protein is known to stimulate angiogenesis [53]. Both mangiferin and Vimang® extracts have demonstrated inhibitory effects on TNF-induced transcription of VEGF-A in MDA-MB231 cells [41]. However, this experiment was carried out over a short time period. Further investigation over longer time periods and evidence from in vivo/ex vivo studies are required to further determine the effect of mangiferin on angiogenesis.

2.3.5. Tumour Volume

Duringin vivo experiments in mice, mangiferin has been found to reduce tumour volume. In C57BL/6J mice inoculated with MCF-7 cells on the neck, a reduction of 89.4% in tumour volume relative to control was seen when mice were medicated with 100 mg/kg of mangiferin. This value was closely comparable to the results obtained from cisplatin treatment (91.5%), an established chemotherapeutic drug [8]. In a similar experiment, the lifespan of these mice was extended at dosages from 10 mg/kg mangiferin and above and 60% of mice survived until the end of the assay period [8], while in the no treatment group, there were no mice surviving after day 40 following MCF-7 inoculation. A high dosage of mangiferin (100 mg/kg) extended lifespan to the same degree as cisplatin, with no significant difference ($p < 0.05$) being observed between these treatments [8]. Dose dependency was observed [8].

These results show that mangiferin can act as a potent chemotherapeutic agent in mice and thus further investigation into mangiferin-based products could benefit treatment of cancer in humans.

2.4. Apoptosis

In order to survive and proliferate, cancer cells must be able to evade apoptosis, despite carrying malignant characteristics [53]. Under normal circumstances, either the intrinsic pathway via the mitochondria, or the extrinsic pathway involving death receptors, can induce apoptosis. The intrinsic pathway generally involves increased permeability of the mitochondrial membrane and the release of cytochrome C to activate initiator procaspase-9, while the extrinsic pathway involves Fas Associated Death Domain (FADD) and procaspase-8 [36] (Figure 4). Apoptosis is the preferred pathway of cell death, as necrotic cell death may induce inflammatory changes due to the release of immune-stimulatory molecules. In order to eradicate cancer, many chemotherapeutic agents seek to induce apoptosis in malignant cells. From the peer reviewed literature, it can be concluded that mangiferin has promising apoptosis inducing properties in a number of cell lines and is involved in regulating apoptosis via multiple targets [8,14,36].

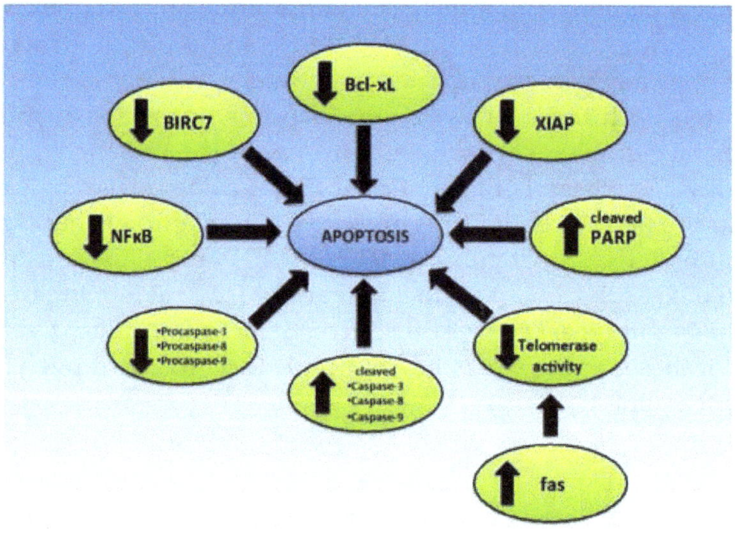

Figure 4. Effect of Mangiferin on proteins implicated in apoptosis.

In 2013, two studies were published that demonstrated a dose dependent increase in apoptosis in response to increasing mangiferin concentration in MDAMB-231, BT-549, MCF7 and T47D breast cancer cell lines [8,14]. Kim et al. reported similar findings in HeLa cells in response to treatment with ethanolic extracts of mango skin or flesh [36]. There are a number of suggested mechanisms by which an increase in apoptosis in these cancer cells may be potentiated. As discussed earlier, mangiferin down-regulates the transcription factor NFκB. It is hypothesized that this dampening of NFκB activity is likely to be responsible for increased apoptosis in HL-60 acute myeloid leukaemia (AML) cells, MCF7 cells and HeLa cells [8,13,35,77].

2.4.1. Mangiferin and Hesperidin in *Cyclopia* Sp. Extracts

Bartoszewski et al. showed in HeLa cells that treatment with *Cyclopia sp.* tea extracts, which are high in mangiferin and hesperidin, caused up-regulation of TRADD and TNFR superfamily member 25 (TRAMP), which are involved in signalling of the extrinsic apoptotic pathway [77]. However, when compared to mangiferin only and hesperidin only, it would appear that hesperidin is a more potent activator of apoptosis in HeLa cells than mangiferin [77]. Regardless, mangiferin did enhance the activity of hesperidin, even when added in low concentrations. Mangiferin itself caused down-regulation of Baculoviral IAP Repeat Containing 7 (BIRC7), which sensitizes cells to death by the extrinsic apoptotic pathway [77].

2.4.2. Bax/Bcl-2

The Bcl-2 protein acts to block programmed cell death while the Bcl-2 associated X protein (Bax) protein favours apoptosis. When the ratio of Bax:Bcl-2 is increased, a cell's sensitivity to apoptosis is increased [78], and consequently malignant cells are less likely to survive. Current literature suggests that the effect of mangiferin on the Bax:Bcl-2 ratio is dependent on cell type, dosage and perhaps the form of mangiferin used [35,79].

Pan et al. found that when CNE2 nasopharyngeal carcinoma cells were treated with mangiferin, the mRNA and protein expression levels of Bcl-2 were consistently down-regulated while Bax was up-regulated [35]. As a consequence, these cells were primed for apoptosis. Bcl-2 was also down-regulated upon treatment with an ethanolic extract of mango skins, which contained mangiferin, mangiferin gallate and isomangiferin gallate [36]. This ultimately resulted in activation of caspase-3, -6, -8 and -9 alongside poly (ADP-ribose) polymerase (PARP) protein [36], favouring cell death. However, Klavitha et al. [22] have found that the reverse applies in the context of excitotoxicity in neurons, whereby mangiferin blocks upregulation of Bax, thus attenuating cell death, making it a promising compound for further research with regard to Parkinson's disease [22]. Furthermore, Bartoszewski et al. demonstrated that on analysis of green fermented *Cyclopia* sp. extracts (in which the primary compounds were mangiferin and hesperidin), there were no significant changes in Bax/Bcl2 mRNA levels or protein levels [77], although Bartoszewski et al. acknowledge that the most likely cause of this disparate finding was low dosage.

In addition to the Bax/Bcl2 ratio, Zhang et al. and Pan et al. reported that apoptosis could be triggered by mangiferin in HL-60 cells due to changes in levels of similar proteins [13,35]. HL-60 cells responded to mangiferin by decreasing levels of Bcl-extra large (Bcl-xL) and XIAP [13,35], resulting in increased apoptosis.

Further experimentation in a wider range of cell lines is required to elucidate what dosage of mangiferin is likely to provide an effect.

2.4.3. Intrinsic/Extrinsic Apoptotic Pathway

To identify whether mangiferin was acting on the intrinsic or extrinsic apoptotic pathway, Kim et al. performed a Western blot experiment to assess expression levels of proteins involved in either the intrinsic pathway, extrinsic pathway or both pathways [36]. Results indicated that there was slightly lower expression levels of BH3 interacting domain (Bid), pro-caspase-3 and pro-caspase-8, but increased expression of cleaved, active forms of PARP, caspase-7 and caspase-9 [36], when HeLa cells were treated with an ethanolic extract of mango peel. Consequently, it is likely that the ethanolic extracts of mango pulp and skin influenced both apoptotic pathways, which is crucial for effective apoptosis. Lv et al. further strengthened the evidence for the role of mangiferin in the intrinsic apoptotic pathway by considering cytochrome C [8]. They found that when MCF-7 cells were treated with mangiferin, cytochrome C concentration in the mitochondria was reduced, while a corresponding increase in cytochrome C concentration was observed in the cytosol. This indicates that cytochrome C was released from the mitochondria in response to mangiferin treatment and thus apoptosis may be induced via the mitochondrial pathway [8]. In addition to these findings, increased expression of caspase-3, -8 and -9, and decreased expression of procaspase-3, -8 and -9 expression was noted, suggesting activation of both intrinsic and extrinsic apoptotic pathways [8]. Based on results from their study, du Plessis-Stoman et al. have suggested that mangiferin may favour apoptotic cell death over necrotic cell death, which has potential to reduce inflammation [48].

2.4.4. Telomerase

Aside from the study of various pathways of apoptosis, in the literature it is reported that mangiferin can inhibit telomerase activity in K562 human leukaemia cells with dose- and time-dependent behaviour [8,35,80], promoting apoptosis. It has been suggested that this may be due to increased *fas* gene expression and protein levels of fas [8]. Enhanced telomerase activity is found in a variety of cancers and is permissive and required for sustained growth of late cancers. Almost all cancers exhibit some form of telomerase reactivation [81]. By reducing telomerase activity, mangiferin can be used to reduce the progression of existing cancers and create an environment in which malignant cells are unlikely to survive.

Mangiferin has demonstrated pro-apoptotic activity in a number of cancer cell lines including K562 leukaemia, MCF-7 breast cancer and CNE2 nasopharyngeal cells [8,35].

2.5. *Oxidative Stress*

Oxidative stress occurs when the burden of ROS is not balanced by antioxidants and detoxification systems. The presence of these excess reactive species can result in cellular damage, particularly to DNA, lipids and proteins. Over time, oxidative stress increases the risk of developing cancer and may exacerbate inflammation. Mangiferin is thought to play a role in: (1) modulating the Nrf2/antioxidant response element (ARE) detoxification pathway (Figure 5); (2) directly detoxifying reactive species; and (3) activating detoxification enzymes such as catalase.

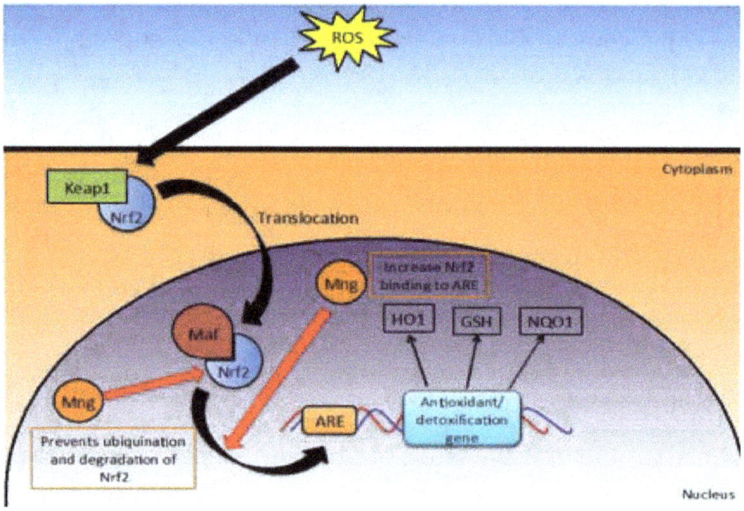

Figure 5. Effect of Mangiferin on the Nrf2/ARE Detoxification Pathway.

2.5.1. Nrf2/ARE Detoxification Pathway

Under normal conditions, Nrf2 gene transcription is inhibited by Kelch-like ECH-associated protein-1 (KEAP-1). However, oxidative stress, dietary components and synthetic chemicals can induce Nrf2 transcription [18]. Consequently, Nrf2 protein can accumulate in the nucleus where it forms heterodimers with musculoaponeurotic fibrosarcoma (maf) protein. This heterodimer signals through the ARE to initiate transcription of a number of phase II detoxification enzymes [17], such as NAD(P)H: quinine reductases (NQO1), glutathione S-transferase (GSH) and heme oxygenase (HO-1) [18]. HO-1, when activated, can translocate into the nucleus to further activate transcription factors relevant to the stimulus [82]. Ultimately, this pathway provides activation of detoxification enzymes when oxidative stresses are presented. Mangiferin manipulates this pathway in such a way that the survival of healthy cells but not malignant cells is enhanced. Mangiferin modulated this Nrf2/ARE signaling pathway at multiple steps [13,17,18].

While mangiferin does not directly influence Nrf2 transcription rates, Zhao et al. have demonstrated that the half-life of Nrf2 is increased due to impaired ubiquitination and thus degradation of the protein [18], which results in higher levels of the protein being present within the cell. Zhang et al. also reported similar findings in human umbilical cord mononuclear blood cells, where mangiferin increased the quantity of Nrf2 accumulating in the nucleus in a time dependent manner [17]. Protein quantity was assessed by microscopy and verified by Western blotting [17]. Additionally, mangiferin increased the binding of Nrf2 to ARE which in turn was shown to increase downstream production of NQO1 (a prominent antioxidant enzyme) when assessed in a Western blot assay [13,17].

Nrf-ARE signaling can provide protection against agents that are chemotherapeutic to normal cells [13] (more on synergistic effects of mangiferin and chemotheraputics later). Similarly, overexpression of Nrf2 in cancer cells can promote resistance to therapy, through up-regulation of antiapoptotic bcl-xL. Mangiferin seems able to differentiate between malignant cells and healthy cells, promoting Nrf2 activation in healthy cells (human umbilical cord mononuclear blood cells) but not cancerous cells (HL-60). Thus, survival is aided in healthy cells by enhanced efficiency of the Nrf2/ARE detoxification pathway while the development of resistance to chemotherapeutics is not permitted in malignant cells [13]. To date, mangiferin is the only known Nrf2 activator that does not confer protection to malignant cells against chemotherapeutic agents [13], making it a promising agent for cancer therapy.

Downstream effects in the Nrf2/ARE detoxification pathway have been further studied upon treatment with Vimang®. Treatment of MDA-MB231 breast cancer cells with 200–400 μL/mL of Vimang® was found to significantly increase HO-1 transcription. However, when treated with mangiferin alone, there was no significant increase in HO-1 transcription [41]. From this result, one may deduce that the Nrf2/ARE detoxification pathway may not have been activated by mangiferin, as was reported earlier in the HL-60 cancer cell line. It is possible that an alternative bioactive, found in Vimang® may be responsible for the up-regulation of HO-1 transcription in the MDA-MB231 breast cancer cells. Overall, results would suggest that mangiferin may provide some benefit through activation of the Nrf-ARE detoxification pathway.

2.5.2. Elimination of Reactive Species

Reactive species must be eliminated promptly to avoid damage to important biological molecules. This may be done directly by antioxidant species, or by inducing and up-regulating detoxification pathways. Mangiferin is an established antioxidant that is able to neutralize a range of reactive species and influence expression and activity of key detoxification enzymes. By performing these actions, oxidative stress and inflammation are reduced.

Mangiferin is able to directly protect against hydroxyl [28], 2,2-diphenyl-1-picrylhydrazyl (DPPH), superoxide, hydrogen peroxide [51], and peroxynitrite free radicals, lipid peroxides [9,21], hypochlorus acid [28] and heavy metal induced reactive oxygen species [15]. Findings from numerous studies can be used to reinforce the notion that mangiferin has greater or comparative antioxidative capacity to other known antioxidants, such as quercetin, baicalein, catechins, phenylpropanoic acids [21], vitamin C, vitamin E and β-carotene [28]. Alongside its antioxidative potential, mangiferin influences ROS production through modulating Fenton-type reactions. Fenton-type reactions usually involve the production of a hydroxyl radical and the oxidation of Fe^{2+} to Fe^{3+}. In the presence of mangiferin, Fenton-type reactions are inhibited by chelating Fe^{2+} ions, reducing production of subsequent ROS [15,29,51]. Additionally, Duang et al. have suggested that mangiferin protects against lipid peroxidation [29]. This protection may in part be responsible for reduced DNA damage and amelioration of cytotoxic action seen in response to ionising radiation in healthy cells [9,83].

Both in vitro and in vivo evidence suggests that mangiferin up-regulates expression of various detoxifying enzymes, resulting in enhanced clearance of ROS. In N2A neuroblastoma cells, Kavintha et al. implicated mangiferin in reducing oxidative stress by providing protection against 1-methyl-4-phenylpyridine (MPP^+) induced cytotoxicity, due to its capability to restore glutathione action and reduce expression of superoxide (SOD) and catalase [22]. In addition to these findings, Matkowski et al. also reported that mangiferin influenced SOD, catalase and glutathione peroxidase in such a way that it halts ROS centred apoptotic pathways through dampening endogenous ROS production [21]. Sarker et al. demonstrated the relationship between mangiferin and glutathione levels by showing that mangiferin increased levels of GSH more than 2× the amount observed on treatment with other anti-oxidants [11]. It has been suggested that mangiferin increases GSH levels by up-regulation of γ-Glutamylcysteine Synthetase (γ-GCS), the enzyme controlling the rate limiting step of GSH synthesis [11]. In vivo studies demonstrate a similar pattern of increased detoxification enzyme activity. In experiments using B(a)P-treated mice, B(a)P attenuated SOD and catalase (see below for more on catalase) activity in lymphocytes, polymorphonuclear cells and macrophages [9]. However, mangiferin co-administration provided a protective effect against these events. Rajendran et al. also found that mangiferin reduced the production of H_2O_2 in B(a)P treated animals [9]. In animals with lung cancer, enhanced activity of glutathione transferase [48], quinine reductase and uridine 5′-diphosphate-glucuronosyl transferase activity has been demonstrated upon treatment with mangiferin [8]. These events each contribute to a reduction in oxidative stress through increased capacity to deal with assault from reactive species. Sarker et al. further suggest that the ability of mangiferin to reduce oxidative stress may also be linked to NFκB down-regulating capabilities, which reduces TNF-induced reactive oxygen intermediate generation [11].

2.5.3. Catalase

Catalase is a detoxification enzyme present in most organisms exposed to oxygen that converts H_2O_2 into water and oxygen. H_2O_2 can cause oxidative damage if not rapidly converted into less toxic species. Mangiferin may directly increase the efficiency of the catalase enzyme by interacting directly with the enzyme, thus reducing oxidative damage that can be done prior to detoxification of H_2O_2 [61]. Increased activity of catalase may modulate downstream signalling pathways that favour an environment that does not promote cancer development and survival. However, not all published findings are consistent with the notion that mangiferin increases catalase activity [11,61].

In silico docking studies using AutoDock and PyMol predict that mangiferin has the capacity to bind to the active site of catalase, but not other oxidase enzymes [61]. The binding of mangiferin to catalase enhanced the activity of catalase by 44% during the in vitro studies conducted by Sahoo et al. [61]. An earlier study by Sarkar et al. reported disparate findings, where mangiferin caused a 0%–23% increase in activity when compared to untreated cells, and did not influence the quantity of enzyme present [11]. In both experiments, U-937 cells were treated alongside other cell lines with 10 μg/mL of mangiferin for 3 h [11].

To further elucidate the effect of mangiferin on catalase activity, Sahoo et al. conducted fluorescent spectrophotometry experiments on catalase in the unbound state (peak at 330 nm, excitation wavelength 280 nm) and subsequently, increasing concentrations of mangiferin were added [61]. As the concentration of mangiferin was increased, the peak at 330 nm decreased in magnitude, suggesting interaction with mangiferin. When the binding constant was calculated (3.1×10^{-7} M^{-1}), this indicated a strong binding affinity between catalase and mangiferin [61]. Mangiferin also proved capable of overriding aminotriazole (ATZ) inhibition of catalase in lipid peroxidation assays [61]. Sahoo et al. further demonstrated that direct quenching of H_2O_2 by mangiferin was not significant, implying that the entire 44% difference found may be attributable to enhanced activity of the catalase enzyme [61].

It has been suggested that increased catalase activity may dampen excessive activation of MAPK/AKT, which is commonly found in malignant cells [61] (See above for MAKP/AKT). Sarker et al. suggested that high expression of catalase would reduce NFκB levels [11]. However, evidence does not support any change in catalase expression, only in the efficiency of this enzyme [11,61]. Increased catalase activity could reduce oxidative stress and inflammation, thus favouring a chemopreventative environment.

2.6. *DNA Damage*

DNA damage facilitates mutations in the genetic material of a cell. Mutation is required to initiate the development of cancer and also expedites the acquisition of characteristics required for a malignant cell to survive. Thus, a higher susceptibility to DNA damage results in a higher incidence of mutation and the development of cancer [84]. The role of mangiferin with regard to DNA damage is controversial.

Studies have reported that mangiferin is capable of protecting not only DNA [42] but also deoxyribose, phospholipids, polyunsaturated fatty acids and proteins [21]. However, Rodeiro et al. [12] found that when aqueous extracts from *Mangifera indica* bark were applied to lymphocytes and lymphoblastic cells, DNA damage was induced. When this effect was further investigated with the compound mangiferin alone, there was a reduction in DNA damage, thus there is likely to be an alternative compound in the extract that is inducing DNA damage [12]. In addition, Rodeiro et al. found that when DNA damage was induced by γ-radiation, the aqueous extract was protective against DNA damage [12].

Radiation Damage

Ionising radiation has been shown to induce DNA damage. In patients undergoing radiotherapy, many healthy cells acquire collateral damage. Mangiferin and mangiferin aglycone have demonstrated protective effects against radiation damage during in vitro studies [28].

Lei et al. demonstrated that pre-treatment of human intestinal epithelial cells with mangiferin aglycone reduced the percentage of cells with double strand breakages in their DNA by 47% when treated with ionizing radiation [28]. This was more effective than the 40% reduction seen following mangiferin pre-treatment. Currently, there are few radioprotective agents, and these agents tend to be associated with high levels of toxicity [28]. Mangiferin may provide some protection to cancer patients undergoing chemotherapy as well as improve efficiency of anti-cancer treatments.

3. Synergistic Effects

The use of many chemotherapeutic agents induces a range of side effects, which can cause serious illness. Mangiferin shows potential to reduce or negate these side effects by selectively targeting malignant cells for cell death and enhancing survival of healthy cells. Mangiferin may potentiate cell death by existing drugs through modulation of NFκB activity [11] and causing cell cycle arrest in malignant cells at the G_2/M checkpoint, leaving cells susceptible to apoptosis induced by chemotherapeutic agents such as etoposide [13]. Through NFκB inhibition, mangiferin is likely to reduce resistance to chemotherapeutic agents in cancer cells [13,48]. Studies using pro-apoptotic agents such as oxaliplatin, etoposide, doxorubicin and paclitaxel have documented additional beneficial effects when co-administered with mangiferin (Table 1).

Table 1. Summary of proposed beneficial effects of co-administration of mangiferin alongside chemotherapeutic agents.

Chemotherapeutic Agent	Cell Line	Reference	Evidence
Oxaliplatin	HeLa, HT29, HL60	[48]	Reduction in oxaliplatin IC50 values; counteracts resistance to oxaliplatin.
Etoposide	HL60, U937	[11,13]	Reduces oxidative stress. Protects normal cells without reducing sensitivity of HL60 to etoposide [13]. Activity of the drug is enhanced by mangiferin [11].
Doxorubicin	MCF7, U937	[13,33]	At high concentrations mangiferin can inhibit P-glycoprotein expression and chemosensitise for doxorubicin therapy [33]. Activity of the drug is enhanced by mangiferin [11].
Paclitaxel	Triple negative breast cancer	[60,62]	IRAK1 overexpression confers a growth advantage [62]. Mangiferin may inhibit *IRAK1* activation [60,62].
Cisplatin	U937	[11]	Inhibits ROS production [8]. Activity of the drug is enhanced by mangiferin; Impedes NFκB activation; Enhanced cell death in the presence of TNF [11].
Vincristine	U937	[11]	Inhibits ROS production [8]. Activity of the drug is enhanced by mangiferin; Impedes NFκB activation; Enhanced cell death in the presence of TNF [11].
Adriamycin	U937	[11]	Inhibits ROS production [8]. Activity of the drug is enhanced by mangiferin; Impedes NFκB activation; Enhanced cell death in the presence of TNF [11].
AraC	U937	[11]	Inhibits ROS production [8]. Activity of the drug is enhanced by mangiferin; Impedes NFκB activation; Enhanced cell death in the presence of TNF [11].

3.1. *Pro-Apoptotic Agents*

While mangiferin (at a concentration of 10 μg/mL) does not trigger apoptotic cell death itself [11], it may enhance action of chemotherapeutic pro-apoptotic agents. Sarker et al. [11] demonstrated that this was due to down-regulation of NFκB by transfecting U-937 cells with an IκBα-double negative construct, blocking NFκB activation and also transfecting with a p65 construct and observing cell death after 36 h by MTT assay, using the Live/Dead cell assay. In IκBα-double negative transfected cells, cell death increased by 12% and increased cell death with TNF from 42% to 53%. Cell death in the presence of mangiferin was increased a further 4%. In p65 overexpressing cells, cell death was not observed in response to treatment with TNF or TNF and mangiferin. By considering SEAP as a reporter gene, IκBα-double negative cells were shown to down-regulate NFκB and p65 overexpressing cells up-regulated NFκB. Thus, it was found that down-regulation of NFκB primes cells for cytotoxic agents [11].

Sarkar et al. reported that the activity of the pro-apoptotic agents cisplatin, vincristine, doxorubicin, etoposide, Adriamycin and AraC was enhanced significantly by co-administration of mangiferin in U-937 cells [11]. Unlike other antioxidants, mangiferin was not found to be toxic to the cells, as it only enhanced cell death when exposed to TNF [11].

Oxidative damage induced by chemotherapeutic drugs correlates with the development of secondary malignancies such as acute myeloid leukaemia (AML). Mangiferin reduces oxidative stress induced by these agents and thus reduces likelihood of developing secondary malignancies [13].

By enhancing apoptotic activity against malignant cells upon treatment with chemotherapeutic agents, lower dosages may be required when co-administered with mangiferin, which may reduce the side effects associated with toxicity.

3.1.1. Oxaliplatin

Oxaliplatin is a platinum-based anti-neoplastic agent used for the treatment of colon or rectal cancer once metastasised. It is often given in conjunction with other chemotherapeutic agents. Common side effects, occurring in >30% of patients, include nausea, vomiting, fatigue, loss of appetite, mouth sores, low blood count, diarrhoea and peripheral neuropathy [85]. Apoptotic efficacy of oxaliplatin is enhanced by the addition of mangiferin, as mangiferin inhibits NFκB (see above) [13,14,48,77] and is thought to increase the sensitivity of malignant cells to apoptotic cell death [48].

Du Plessis-Stoman et al. demonstrated the positive effect of mangiferin on oxaliplatin action in HeLa cells and HT29 cells through use of IC_{50} assays [48]. When stained with tryptan blue, cells treated with oxaliplatin and mangiferin displayed fewer non-viable cells than those treated with oxaliplatin only, indicating that there was less necrosis, suggesting the apoptotic pathway for cell death was preferred [48]. Co-administration of mangiferin with oxaliplatin increased caspase 3 activation in HeLa and HT29 cell lines relative to cells that only received oxaliplatin, further implicating the apoptotic pathway of cell death was favoured, thus reducing inflammation [48].

Du Plessis-Stoman et al. have suggested that mangiferin only exhibits NFκB inhibition when used with platinum containing complexes, as they found that treatment of normal cells with mangiferin alone resulted in increased NFκB activity [48]. When treated with mangiferin and oxaliplatin, the level of NFκB inhibition was similar to cells treated with oxaliplatin alone. However, in the presence of mangiferin, the oxaliplatin IC_{50} was 3.4 times lower in the cells receiving both treatments [48]. In addition, when assessing changes in cell cycle, mangiferin caused a delay in S-phase only when used in conjunction with oxaliplatin [48]. On treatment with oxaliplatin or mangiferin alone, a G_2/M phase cell cycle arrest was noted.

Both oxaliplatin and mangiferin are implicated in the mitochondrial pathway of apoptosis through reduction of mitochondrial membrane potential. However, cells treated with mangiferin and oxaliplatin did not show a significantly different mitochondrial membrane potential to those treated with oxaliplatin alone [48].

Evidence indicates that mangiferin increases the efficacy of oxaliplatin at inducing cell death in malignant cells.

3.1.2. Etoposide

As discussed above (Section 2.5.1 on Nrf2), mangiferin protects against etoposide induced oxidative damage in human umbilical cord blood mononuclear cells by promoting Nrf2 signalling to activate a number of antioxidant enzymes [13]. Side effects such as myelo-suppression are also reduced. As discussed earlier, literature indicated that mangiferin causes G_2/M phase cell cycle arrest. Etoposide targets cells in this phase [86]. In addition, oxidative damage in response to etoposide may result in p53 activation. However, when the effect of mangiferin on etoposide efficacy was studied, HL-60 cells were used, which lack wild type p53, thus further experimentation is required to elucidate this effect [13].

3.1.3. Doxorubicin

Louisa et al. (2014) reported that mangiferin increased the efficacy of doxorubicin in MCF-7 [33]. Cells were initially incubated with a low concentration of doxorubicin for 10 days. The apoptotic rate was measured and found to be reduced, indicating the development of drug resistance. Thereafter, cells were treated with mangiferin and at high concentrations mangiferin significantly reduced cell viability through reduced expression of P-glycoprotein, which acts as a multidrug transporter. The efficacy of mangiferin increased in a concentration dependent manner [33]. In this study it was found that mRNA levels associated with multidrug resistance associated protein-1 and breast cancer resistance protein were unaffected by mangiferin, unlike P-glycoprotein [33].

4. Bioavailability and Delivery of Mangiferin

Extraction, quantification, solubility and bioavailability of polyphenols, including mangiferin, are of relevance to clinical success. Bioavailability is dependent on bioaccessibility (quantity of compound released from the food matrix), solubility in gastrointestinal fluids, cellular uptake, compound metabolism and efficiency of the circulatory system [87,88]. Like many other polyphenols, the optimal health benefits of mangiferin are not fully realised due to poor water solubility and oral bioavailability (1.2% in rats) [89].

Using HPLC-MS, Hou et al. evaluated the pharmacokinetics (PK) of mangiferin following oral administration (0.1 g. 0.3 g and 0.9 g) in healthy male volunteers [90]. The point of maximum plasma concentration (38.64 ng/mL^{-1}) was at approximately 1 h, and was surprisingly low considering the dose of 0.9 g. This outcome supports other published findings such as those reported by [89,91] in rats. Maximal plasma concentrations, both quantity and time, were enhanced when mangiferin was orally administered to rats as a polyherbal formulation, rather than as mangiferin alone [92]. Similarly, Ma et al., in a rat model, found that permeability and plasma concentrations were improved following administration of a phospholipid complex containing mangiferin, relative to administration of mangiferin alone [93]. However, in addition to whole body PK, intratumoral PK, influenced by packing density of solid tumour cells and components of the extracellular matrix, is also important [94], and these challenges could be addressed by co-formulation and innovative delivery modes.

Bioavailability can be influenced by the properties of the food matrix (composition and structure) and hence the oral bioavailability of bioactive compounds, in this case, mangiferin could be improved if the major limiting factors were characterised [88] and modes of delivery designed accordingly. McClements et al. developed a new system for the classification of factors limiting oral bioavailability of nutraceuticals such that the design of food matrices can be optimised for each nutraceutical. The classification system is largely based on bioaccessibility (liberation, solubilisation and interactions), absorption (mucus layer, bilayer permeability and tight-, active- and efflux- transporters), and transformation (chemical degradation and metabolism) [88]. Such a system assists with determining an optimal food matrix design that will maximise oral bioavailability e.g., the encapsulation of a compound with low bilayer permeability or the addition of components that may protect a compound, that is sensitive to metabolism, against enzymes in the gut [88]. Many of these characteristics need to be assessed for mangiferin in order to improve oral bioavailability.

Encapsulation of compounds has improved PK properties in general, and is particularly suitable for compounds such as mangiferin, that are poorly water soluble [50]. Spray-drying formulations can impact on retention of mangiferin in the particle as demonstrated by the comparison of a pectin formulation versus a chitosan polysaccharide, with pectin being found to have a better retention of mangiferin in the particles than a chitosan formulation [50]. Numerous types of nanovehicles have been developed, and many polysaccharide-based nanovehicles have been used for the delivery of anti-cancer drugs, some of which may interact with membrane receptors. (See Caro and Pozo for an overview on the application of polysaccharides as nanovehicles in cancer therapy [95]). Specialised polysaccharide-based nanovehicles may be suitable for the delivery of mangiferin. It is clear that further work is required with respect to improving bioavailability and delivery methods of mangiferin from fruit or supplement to tumour site. The design of a "smart vehicle" for the delivery of mangiferin to the tumour cells, rather than healthy cells, and for avoidance or minimisation of a delivery gradient within the solid tumour, the "smart vehicle" will likely need to be unique to mangiferin and possibly to the cancer type.

5. Toxicity

In addition to bioavailability and delivery of bioactive compound to enhance health, it is critical to consider toxicity of the compound. Being a natural compound, mangiferin exhibits minimal toxicity [34] and is generally regarded as non-toxic [28]. Stem-bark extract from *Mangifera indica* has only shown toxicity in animals when injected intra-peritoneally and after acute exposure [12]. Mangiferin's reported toxic dose in mice is 400 mg/kg [28,50]. In experiments involving blood peripheral lymphocytes and hepatocytes of rats, mangiferin did not induce cytotoxicity, genotoxicity or mutagenicity [12]. However, in a more recent study by Prado et al. [96], oral administration of mangiferin in rodents demonstrated low acute and sub-chronic toxicity. Nonetheless, it is still anticipated that there is a wide safety margin for this compound when taken orally [96]. Due to the polyphenolic structure of mangiferin, it is likely to undergo biotransformation in the liver, and for this reason it is suggested that further investigation into the safety of mangiferin metabolites may be required [23].

6. Conclusions

Evidence strongly supports the link between mangiferin treatment and modulation of many molecular pathways to prevent the development and progression of cancer. Mangiferin is primarily implicated in down-regulating inflammation, causing cell cycle arrest, reducing proliferation/metastasis, promoting apoptosis in malignant cells and protecting against oxidative stress and DNA damage. Perhaps the most promising anti-proliferative effect observed on treatment with mangiferin was that seen during in vivo experiments where mangiferin reduced tumour volume to a similar extent as treatment with cisplatin. Literature consistently shows that mangiferin enhances the efficacy of pro-apoptotic chemotherapeutic agents, with the most evidence supporting synergistic effects with oxaliplatin, etoposide and doxorubicin. This is of particular interest when we consider that mangiferin exhibits low toxicity and has a wide oral safety margin, unlike other compounds with similar activity. However, the bioavailability and delivery of mangiferin requires further research and development.

Ultimately, there is strong evidence, in a number of pathways, for a protective effect of mangiferin. However, in some cases, there may be variation in effect due to dosage, origin of extract or cell line used. Furthermore, low water solubility as well as low oral bioavailability are two factors that limit clinical use at present, and further research efforts targeting appropriate delivery systems are required in order to improve clinical efficacy. In addition, investigations into in vivo effects are required to determine the significance of these results to human health. Clinical trials in humans could substantially improve our understanding of the macroscopic effects of mangiferin. Additionally, further investigation into mangiferin aglycone, may uncover a more sustainable way of achieving greater efficiency than that observed with mangiferin alone.

Acknowledgments: Funding to Fuchsia Gold-Smith from the School of Medicine Foundation. Funding to Karen Bishop from the Auckland Cancer Society Research Center, Auckland, New Zealand.

Author Contributions: All authors conceived of the idea, proofread and edited the manuscript. Fuchsia Gold-Smith and Alyssa Fernandez summarised the literature and Fuchsia Gold-Smith wrote the manuscript. Alyssa Fernandez drew the schematic diagrams and Fuchsia Gold-Smith drew the chemical structures. Karen Bishop guided the development of the manuscript and performed the final manuscript edits.

Abbreviations

The following abbreviations are used in this manuscript:

AML	acute myeloid leukaemia
ARE	antioxidant response element
ATM	Ataxia telangiectasia mutated protein
ATR	Ataxia Telangiectasia and Rad3-related protein
ATZ	aminotriazole
Bax	Bcl-2 associated X protein
bcl-2	B Cell Lymphoma-2
bcl-xL	B Cell Lymphoma-extra large
B(a)P	benzo(a)pyrene
Bid	BH3 interacting domain
BIRC7	Baculoviral IAP Repeat Containing 7
Chk1	Checkpoint kinase 1
CHk2	Checkpoint Kinase 2
CDK1	Cyclin-Dependent Kinase 1
COX	Cyclooxygenase-2
CXCR4	C-X-C Chemokine Receptor type-4
DPPH	2,2-diphenyl-1-picrylhydrazyl
EMT	Epithelial to Mesenchymal Transition
ERK	Extracellular signal-Regulated Kinase
FADD	Fas Associated Death Domain
GSH	glutathione S-transferase
HO-1	heme oxygenase
H_2O_2	hydrogen peroxide
IARC	International Agency for Research on Cancer
ICAM-1	Intercellular Adhesion Molecule-1
IκB	Inhibitor of κB
IKK-α	Inhibitor of NFκB Kinase subunit-α
IKK-β	Inhibitor of NFκB Kinase subunit-β
IL-1R	Interleukin-1 Receptors
IL-6	Interleukin-6
IL-8	Interleukin-8
IRAK1	Interleukin-1 Receptor Activated Kinase 1
IRAK4	Interleukin-1 Receptor Activated Kinase 4
KEAP-1	Kelch-like ECH-associated protein-1
LDC	Less Developed Countries
LPS	lipopolysaccharide
maf	musculoaponeurotic fibrosarcoma
MAPK	Mitogen Activated Protein Kinase
MDCs	More developed countries
MMP	matrix metalloproteinase
MPP^+	1-methyl-4-phenylpyridine
MTT	3-(4,5-dimethyl-2-thiozolyl)-2,5-diphenyl-2H-tetrazolium bromide
Myd88	Myeloid Differentiation Primary Response Gene 88

NEMO	NFκB Essential Modulator
NFκB	Nuclear Factor κ-light-chain-enhancer of activated B cells
NIK	NCK Interacting Kinase
NQO1	NAD(P)H: quinine reductases
Nrf2	Nuclear factor erythroid 2-Related Factor 2
PDG	peptidoglycan
PK	pharmacokinetics
PMA	phorbol-12-myristate-13-acetate
PPAR$_\gamma$	Peroxisome Proliferator-Activated Receptor$_\gamma$
ROS	Reactive oxygen species
SEAP	Secreted Embryonic Alkaline Phosphatase
SOD	superoxide
TAB1	Transforming growth factor beta-activated kinase 1-binding protein 1
TAB2	Transforming growth factor beta-activated kinase 1-binding protein 2
TAK1	Transforming growth factor beta-activated kinase 1
TLRs	Toll-like receptors
TNF	Tumour Necrosis Factor
TNFR	Tumour Necrosis Factor Receptor
TRADD	TNFR with Tumour Necrosis Factor Receptor type-1-Associated Death Domain protein
TRAF2	Tumour Necrosis Factor Receptor-Associated Factor 2
TRAF6	Tumour necrosis factor Receptor-Associated Factor 6
VEGF	Vascular Endothelial Growth Factor
XIAP	X linked Inhibitor of Apoptosis Protein

References

1. WHO. In Health in 2015 from Millenium Development Goals to Sustainable Development Goals 2015. Available online: http://www.who.int/gho/publications/mdgs-sdgs/MDGs-SDGs2015_chapter6.pdf (accessed on 20 April 2016).
2. Torre, L.; Bray, F.; Siegel, R.; Ferlay, J.; Lortet-Tieulent, J.; Jemal, A. Global cancer statistics 2012. *Cancer J. Clin.* **2015**, *65*, 87–108. [CrossRef] [PubMed]
3. United Nations Department of Economic and Social Affairs. *World Population Prospects: The 2012 Revision, Highlights and Advance Tables*; United Nations: New York, NY, USA, 2013.
4. World Cancer Research Fund International. Comparing More and Less Developed Countries. Available online: http://www.wcrf.org/int/cancer-facts-figures/comparing-more-less-developed-countries (accessed on 12 November 2015).
5. Boon, V.; Carr, J.; Klebe, S. The role of viruses in carcinogenesis. *AMSJ* **2013**, *4*, 11–15.
6. Parkin, D.M.; Boyd, L.; Walker, L.C. The fraction of cancer attributable to lifestyle and environmental factors in the UK in 2010. *Br. J. Cancer.* **2011**, *105*, S77–S81. [CrossRef] [PubMed]
7. Rajendran, P.; Rengarajan, T.; Nishigaki, I.; Ekambaram, G.; Sakthisekaran, D. Potent chemopreventive effect of mangiferin on lung carcinogenesis in experimental Swiss albino mice. *J. Cancer Res. Ther.* **2014**, *10*, 1033–1039. [PubMed]
8. Lv, J.; Wang, Z.; Zhang, L.; Wang, H.L.; Liu, Y.; Li, C.; Deng, J.; Yi, W.; Bao, J.K. Mangiferin induces apoptosis and cell cycle arrest in MCF-7 cells both in vitro andin vivo. *J. Anim. Vet. Adv.* **2013**, *12*, 352–359.
9. Rajendran, P.; Jayakumar, T.; Nishigaki, I.; Ekambaram, G.; Nishigaki, Y.; Vetriselvi, J.; Sakthisekaran, D. Immunomodulatory effect of mangiferin in experimental animals with Benzo(a)pyrene-induced lung carcinogenesis. *Int. J. Biomed. Sci.* **2013**, *9*, 68–74. [PubMed]
10. Hu, X.Y.; Deng, J.G.; Wang, L.; Yuan, Y.F. Synthesis and anti-tumor activity evaluation of gallic acid-mangiferin hybrid molecule. *Med. Chem.* **2013**, *9*, 1058–1062. [CrossRef] [PubMed]
11. Sarkar, A.; Sreenivasan, Y.; Ramesh, G.T.; Manna, S.K. β-D-glucoside suppresses tumor necrosis factor-induced activation of nuclear transcription factor κB but potentiates apoptosis. *J. Biol. Chem.* **2004**, *279*, 33768–33781. [CrossRef] [PubMed]
12. Rodeiro, I.; Delgado, R.; Garrido, G. Effects of a Mangifera indica L. stem bark extract and mangiferin on radiation-induced DNA damage in human lymphocytes and lymphoblastoid cells. *Cell Prolif.* **2014**, *47*, 48–55. [CrossRef] [PubMed]

13. Zhang, B.-P.; Zhao, J.; Li, S.-S.; Yang, L.-J.; Zeng, L.-L.; Chen, Y.; Fang, J. Mangiferin activates Nrf2-antioxidant response element signaling without reducing the sensitivity to etoposide of human myeloid leukemia cells in vitro. *APS* **2014**, *35*, 257–266. [PubMed]
14. Li, H.; Huang, J.; Yang, B.; Xiang, T.; Yin, X.; Peng, W.; Cheng, W.; Wan, J.; Luo, F.; Li, H. Mangiferin exerts antitumor activity in breast cancer cells by regulating matrix metalloproteinases, epithelial to mesenchymal transition, and β-catenin signaling pathway. *Toxicol. Appl. Pharmacol.* **2013**, *272*, 180–190. [CrossRef] [PubMed]
15. Das, S.; Nageshwar Rao, B.; Satish Rao, B.S. Mangiferin attenuates methylmercury induced cytotoxicity against IMR-32, human neuroblastoma cells by the inhibition of oxidative stress and free radical scavenging potential. *Chem. Biol. Interact.* **2011**, *193*, 129–140. [CrossRef] [PubMed]
16. Xiao, J.; Liu, L.; Zhong, Z.; Xiao, C.; Zhang, J. Mangiferin regulates proliferation and apoptosis in glioma cells by induction of microRNA-15b and inhibition of MMP-9 expression. *Oncol. Rep.* **2015**, *33*, 2815–2820. [CrossRef] [PubMed]
17. Zhang, B.; Zhao, J.; Li, S.; Zeng, L.; Chen, Y.; Fang, J. Mangiferin activates the Nrf2-ARE pathway and reduces etoposide-induced DNA damage in human umbilical cord mononuclear blood cells. *Pharm. Biol.* **2015**, *53*, 503–511. [CrossRef] [PubMed]
18. Zhao, J.; Zhang, B.; Li, S.; Zeng, L.; Chen, Y.; Fang, J. Mangiferin increases Nrf2 protein stability by inhibiting its ubiquitination and degradation in human HL60 myeloid leukemia cells. *Int. J. Mol. Med.* **2014**, *33*, 1348–1354. [CrossRef] [PubMed]
19. Jung, J.S.; Jung, K.; Kim, D.H.; Kim, H.S. Selective inhibition of MMP-9 gene expression by mangiferin in PMA-stimulated human astroglioma cells: Involvement of PI3K/Akt and MAPK signaling pathways. *Pharmacol. Res.* **2012**, *66*, 95–103. [CrossRef] [PubMed]
20. Das, J.; Ghosh, J.; Roy, A.; Sil, P.C. Mangiferin exerts hepatoprotective activity against D-galactosamine induced acute toxicity and oxidative/nitrosative stress via Nrf2-NFκB pathways. *Toxicol. Appl. Pharmacol.* **2012**, *260*, 35–47. [CrossRef] [PubMed]
21. Matkowski, A.; Kuś, P.; Góralska, E.; Woźniak, D. Mangiferin—A bioactive xanthonoid, not only from mango and not just antioxidant. *Mini Rev. Med. Chem.* **2013**, *13*, 439–455. [CrossRef] [PubMed]
22. Kavitha, M.; Nataraj, J.; Essa, M.M.; Memon, M.A.; Manivasagam, T. Mangiferin attenuates MPTP induced dopaminergic neurodegeneration and improves motor impairment, redox balance and Bcl-2/Bax expression in experimental Parkinson's disease mice. *Chem. Biol. Interact.* **2013**, *206*, 239–247. [CrossRef] [PubMed]
23. Tolosa, L.; Rodeiro, I.; Donato, M.T.; Herrera, J.A.; Delgado, R.; Castell, J.V.; Gómez-Lechón, M.J. Multiparametric evaluation of the cytoprotective effect of the Mangifera indica L. stem bark extract and mangiferin in HepG2 cells. *J. Pharm. Pharmacol.* **2013**, *65*, 1073–1082. [CrossRef] [PubMed]
24. Zou, T.; Wu, H.; Li, H.; Jia, Q.; Song, G. Comparison of microwave-assisted and conventional extraction of mangiferin from mango (Mangifera indica L.) leaves. *J. Sep. Sci.* **2013**, *36*, 3457–3462. [PubMed]
25. Chellan, N.; Joubert, E.; Strijdom, H.; Roux, C.; Louw, J.; Muller, C.J.F. Aqueous extract of unfermented honeybush (Cyclopia maculata) attenuates STZ-induced diabetes and β-cell cytotoxicity. *Planta Med.* **2014**, *80*, 622–629. [CrossRef] [PubMed]
26. Chavan, J.J.; Ghadage, D.M.; Kshirsagar, P.R.; Kudale, S.S. Optimization of extraction techniques and RP-HPLC analysis of antidiabetic and anticancer drug mangiferin from roots of saptarangi (Salacia chinensis L.). *J. Liq. Chromatogr. Relat. Technol.* **2015**, *38*, 963–969. [CrossRef]
27. Chavan, J.J.; Ghadage, D.M.; Bhoite, A.S.; Umdale, S.D. Micropropagation, molecular profiling and RP-HPLC determination of mangiferin across various regeneration stages of Saptarangi (Salacia chinensis L.). *Ind. Crops Prod.* **2015**, *76*, 1123–1132. [CrossRef]
28. Lei, J.; Zhou, C.; Hu, H.; Hu, L.; Zhao, M.; Yang, Y.; Chuai, Y.; Ni, J.; Cai, J. Mangiferin aglycone attenuates radiation-induced damage on human intestinal epithelial cells. *J. Cell. Biochem.* **2012**, *113*, 2633–2642. [CrossRef] [PubMed]
29. Duang, X.Y.; Wang, Q.; Zhou, X.D.; Huang, D.M. Mangiferin: A possible strategy for periodontal disease to therapy. *Med. Hypotheses* **2011**, *76*, 486–488. [CrossRef] [PubMed]
30. Kaivalya, M.; Rao, B.N.; Satish Rao, B.S. Mangiferin: A xanthone attenuates mercury chloride induced cytotoxicity and genotoxicity in HepG2 cells. *J. Biochem. Mol. Toxicol.* **2011**, *25*, 108–116. [CrossRef] [PubMed]

31. Barreto, J.C.; Trevisan, M.T.; Hull, W.E.; Erben, G.; de Brito, E.S.; Pfundstein, B.; Wurtele, G.; Spiegelhalder, B.; Owen, R.W. Characterization and quantitation of polyphenolic compounds in bark, kernel, leaves, and peel of mango (Mangifera indica L.). *J. Agric. Food Chem.* **2008**, *56*, 5599–5610. [CrossRef] [PubMed]
32. Hewavitharana, A.K.; Tan, Z.W.; Shimada, R.; Shaw, P.N.; Flanagan, B.M. Between fruit variability of the bioactive compounds, β-carotene and mangiferin, in mango (Mangifera indica). *Nutr. Diet.* **2013**, *70*, 158–163. [CrossRef]
33. Louisa, M.; Soediro, T.M.; Suyatna, F.D. In vitro modulation of P-glycoprotein, MRP-1 and BCRP expression by mangiferin in doxorubicin-treated MCF-7 cells. *Asian Pac. J. Cancer Prev.* **2014**, *15*, 1639–1642. [CrossRef] [PubMed]
34. Dou, W.; Zhang, J.; Ren, G.; Ding, L.; Sun, A.; Deng, C.; Wu, X.; Wei, X.; Mani, S.; Wang, Z. Mangiferin attenuates the symptoms of dextran sulfate sodium-induced colitis in mice via NF-κB and MAPK signaling inactivation. *Int. Immunopharmacol.* **2014**, *23*, 170–178. [CrossRef] [PubMed]
35. Pan, L.L.; Wang, A.Y.; Huang, Y.Q.; Luo, Y.; Ling, M. Mangiferin induces apoptosis by regulating Bcl-2 and bax expression in the CNE2 nasopharyngeal carcinoma cell line. *Asian Pac. J. Cancer Prev.* **2014**, *15*, 7065–7068. [CrossRef] [PubMed]
36. Kim, H.; Kim, H.; Mosaddik, A.; Gyawali, R.; Ahn, K.S.; Cho, S.K. Induction of apoptosis by ethanolic extract of mango peel and comparative analysis of the chemical constitutes of mango peel and flesh. *Food Chem.* **2012**, *133*, 416–422. [CrossRef] [PubMed]
37. Ramírez-Maganda, J.; Blancas-Benítez, F.J.; Zamora-Gasga, V.M.; García-Magaña, M.d.L.; Bello-Pérez, L.A.; Tovar, J.; Sáyago-Ayerdi, S.G. Nutritional properties and phenolic content of a bakery product substituted with a mango (Mangifera indica)'Ataulfo'processing by-product. *Food Res. Int.* **2015**, *73*, 117–123. [CrossRef]
38. Yatnatti, S.; Vijayalakshmi, D.; Chandru, R. Processing and Nutritive Value of Mango Seed Kernel Flour. *Curr. Res. Nutr. Food Sci. J.* **2014**, *2*, 170–175. [CrossRef]
39. Ajila, C.M.; Aalami, M.; Leelavathi, K.; Prasada Rao, U.J.S. Mango peel powder: A potential source of antioxidant and dietary fiber in macaroni preparations. *Innov. Food Sci. Emerg. Technol.* **2010**, *11*, 219–224. [CrossRef]
40. Bandyopadhyay, K.; Chakraborty, C.; Bhattacharyya, S. Fortification of Mango Peel and Kernel Powder in Cookies Formulation. *J. Acad. Ind. Res.* **2014**, *2*, 661.
41. García-Rivera, D.; Delgado, R.; Bougarne, N.; Haegeman, G.; Vanden Berghe, W. Gallic acid indanone and mangiferin xanthone are strong determinants of immunosuppressive anti-tumour effects of Mangifera indica L. bark in MDA-MB231 breast cancer cells. *Cancer Lett.* **2011**, *305*, 21–31. [CrossRef] [PubMed]
42. Zhang, B.; Fang, J.; Chen, Y. Antioxidant effect of mangiferin and its potential to be a cancer chemoprevention agent. *Lett. Drug Des. Discov.* **2013**, *10*, 239–244. [CrossRef]
43. Telang, M.; Dhulap, S.; Mandhare, A.; Hirwani, R. Therapeutic and cosmetic applications of mangiferin: A patent review. *Expert Opin. Ther. Pat.* **2013**, *23*, 1561–1580. [CrossRef] [PubMed]
44. Cheng, Z.Q.; Yang, D.; Ma, Q.Y.; Yi, X.H.; Zhou, J.; Zhao, Y.X. A new benzophenone from Dobinea delavayi. *Chem. Nat. Compd.* **2013**, *49*, 46–48. [CrossRef]
45. Xu, G.A. Drug Composition for Treating 2 Type Diabetes and its Chronicity Neopathy. Google Patents EP 2070540 A1, 17 June 2009.
46. Zhang, W.; Li, P.; Gong, Y.; Gao, X. Mangiferin Aglycone Crystal form i and Preparation Method Thereof. Google Patents EP 2716637 A1, 9 April 2014.
47. Ahmad, A.; Padhye, S.; Sarkar, F.H. Role of novel nutraceuticals garcinol, plumbagin and mangiferin in the prevention and therapy of human malignancies: Mechanisms of anticancer activity. In *Nutraceuticals and Cancer*; Springer: New York, NY, USA, 2012; Volume 1, pp. 179–199.
48. Du Plessis-Stoman, D.; du Preez, J.G.H.; Van de Venter, M. Combination treatment with oxaliplatin and Mangiferin Causes Increased Apoptosis and downregulation of NFκB in cancer cell lines. *AJOL* **2011**, *8*, 177–184.
49. Hudecová, A.; Kusznierewicz, B.; Rundén-Pran, E.; Magdolenová, Z.; Hašplová, K.; Rinna, A.; Fjellsbo, L.M.; Kruszewski, M.; Lankoff, A.; Sandberg, W.J.; et al. Silver nanoparticles induce premutagenic DNA oxidation that can be prevented by phytochemicals from Gentiana asclepiadea. *Mutagenesis* **2012**, *27*, 759–769. [CrossRef] [PubMed]
50. De Souza, J.R.R.; Feitosa, J.P.A.; Ricardo, N.M.P.S.; Trevisan, M.T.S.; de Paula, H.C.B.; Ulrich, C.M.; Owen, R.W. Spray-drying encapsulation of mangiferin using natural polymers. *Food Hydrocoll.* **2013**, *33*, 10–18. [CrossRef]

51. Kawpoomhae, K.; Sukma, M.; Ngawhirunpat, T.; Opanasopit, P.; Sripattanaporn, A. Antioxidant and neuroprotective effects of standardized extracts of Mangifera indica leaf. *Thai J. Pharm. Sci.* **2010**, *34*, 32–43.
52. Peng, Z.G.; Yao, Y.B.; Yang, J.; Tang, Y.L.; Huang, X. Mangiferin induces cell cycle arrest at G2/M phase through ATR-Chk1 pathway in HL-60 leukemia cells. *Genet. Mol. Res.* **2015**, *14*, 4989–5002. [CrossRef] [PubMed]
53. Hanahan, D.; Weinberg, R.A. Hallmarks of cancer: The next generation. *Cell* **2011**, *144*, 646–674. [CrossRef] [PubMed]
54. Pikarsky, E.; Porat, R.M.; Stein, I.; Abramovitch, R.; Amit, S.; Kasem, S.; Gutkovich-Pyest, E.; Urieli-Shoval, S.; Galun, E.; Ben-Neriah, Y. NF-κB functions as a tumour promoter in inflammation-associated cancer. *Nature* **2004**, *431*, 461–466. [CrossRef] [PubMed]
55. Vendramini-Costa, D.B.; Carvalho, J.E. Molecular link mechanisms between inflammation and cancer. *Curr. Pharm. Des.* **2012**, *18*, 3831–3852. [CrossRef] [PubMed]
56. Yao, J.; Hu, R.; Gou, Q.L. Inflammation and cancer. *Pharm. Biotechnol.* **2011**, *18*, 372–376.
57. Bhoj, V.G.; Chen, Z.J. Ubiquitylation in innate and adaptive immunity. *Nature* **2009**, *458*, 430–437. [CrossRef] [PubMed]
58. Rhyasen, G.W.; Starczynowski, D.T. IRAK signalling in cancer. *Br. J. Cancer* **2015**, *112*, 232–237. [CrossRef] [PubMed]
59. Tully, J.E.; Nolin, J.D.; Guala, A.S.; Hoffman, S.M.; Roberson, E.C.; Lahue, K.G.; van der Velden, J.; Anathy, V.; Blackwell, T.S.; Janssen-Heininger, Y.M.W. Cooperation between classical and alternative NF-κB pathways regulates proinflammatory Responses in Epithelial Cells. *Am. J. Respir. Cell Mol. Biol.* **2012**, *47*, 497–508. [CrossRef] [PubMed]
60. Jeong, J.J.; Jang, S.E.; Hyam, S.R.; Han, M.J.; Kim, D.H. Mangiferin ameliorates colitis by inhibiting IRAK1 phosphorylation in NF-kappaB and MAPK pathways. *Eur. J. Pharmacol.* **2014**, *740*, 652–661. [CrossRef] [PubMed]
61. Sahoo, B.K.; Zaidi, A.H.; Gupta, P.; Mokhamatam, R.B.; Raviprakash, N.; Mahali, S.K.; Manna, S.K. A natural xanthone increases catalase activity but decreases NF-kappa B and lipid peroxidation in U-937 and HepG2 cell lines. *Eur. J. Pharmacol.* **2015**, *764*, 520–528. [CrossRef] [PubMed]
62. Wee, Z.N.; Yatim, S.M.J.M.; Kohlbauer, V.K.; Feng, M.; Goh, J.Y.; Bao, Y.; Lee, P.L.; Zhang, S.; Wang, P.P.; Lim, E. IRAK1 is a therapeutic target that drives breast cancer metastasis and resistance to paclitaxel. *Nat. Commun.* **2015**, *6*, 8746. [CrossRef] [PubMed]
63. DiDonato, J.A.; Mercurio, F.; Karin, M. NF-kappaB and the link between inflammation and cancer. *Immunol. Rev.* **2012**, *246*, 379–400. [CrossRef] [PubMed]
64. Hoesel, B.; Schmid, J.A. The complexity of NF-kappaB signaling in inflammation and cancer. *Mol. Cancer* **2013**, *12*, 86. [CrossRef] [PubMed]
65. Belfiore, A.; Genua, M.; Malaguarnera, R. PPAR-agonists and their effects on IGF-I receptor signaling: Implications for cancer. *PPAR Res.* **2009**, *2009*, 18. [CrossRef] [PubMed]
66. Vandoros, G.P.; Konstantinopoulos, P.A.; Sotiropoulou-Bonikou, G.; Kominea, A.; Papachristou, G.I.; Karamouzis, M.V.; Gkermpesi, M.; Varakis, I.; Papavassiliou, A.G. PPAR-gamma is expressed and NF-kB pathway is activated and correlates positively with COX-2 expression in stromal myofibroblasts surrounding colon adenocarcinomas. *J. Cancer Res. Clin. Oncol.* **2006**, *132*, 76–84. [CrossRef] [PubMed]
67. Hugo, H.J.; Saunders, C.; Ramsay, R.G.; Thompson, E.W. New Insights on COX-2 in Chronic Inflammation Driving Breast Cancer Growth and Metastasis. *J. Mammary Gland Biol.* **2015**, *20*, 109–119. [CrossRef] [PubMed]
68. Mahmoud-Awny, M.; Attia, A.S.; Abd-Ellah, M.F.; El-Abhar, H.S. Mangiferin mitigates gastric ulcer in ischemia/reperfused rats: Involvement of PPAR-γ, NF-κB and Nrf2/HO-1 signaling pathways. *PLoS ONE* **2015**, *10*, e0132497. [CrossRef] [PubMed]
69. Santarpia, L.; Lippman, S.M.; El-Naggar, A.K. Targeting the MAPK-RAS-RAF signaling pathway in cancer therapy. *Expert Opin. Ther. Targets* **2012**, *16*, 103–119. [CrossRef] [PubMed]
70. Li, J.; Malakhova, M.; Mottamal, M.; Reddy, K.; Kurinov, I.; Carper, A.; Langfald, A.; Oi, N.; Kim, M.O.; Zhu, F.; et al. Norathyriol suppresses skin cancers induced by solar ultraviolet radiation by targeting ERK kinases. *Cancer Res.* **2012**, *72*, 260–270. [CrossRef] [PubMed]
71. Shimada, M.; Nakanishi, M. DNA damage checkpoints and cancer. *J. Mol. Histol.* **2006**, *37*, 253–260. [CrossRef] [PubMed]

72. Mitra, J.; Enders, G.H. Cyclin A/Cdk2 complexes regulate activation of Cdk1 and Cdc25 phosphatases in human cells. *Oncogene* **2004**, *23*, 3361–3367. [CrossRef] [PubMed]
73. Huang, H.; Nong, C.; Guo, L.; Meng, G.; Zha, X.L. The proliferation inhibition effect and apoptosis induction of Mangiferin on BEL-7404 human hepatocellular carcinoma cell. *Chin. J. Dig.* **2002**, *6*, 341–343.
74. Wilkinson, A.S.; Taing, M.W.; Pierson, J.T.; Lin, C.N.; Dietzgen, R.G.; Shaw, P.N.; Gidley, M.J.; Monteith, G.R.; Roberts-Thomson, S.J. Estrogen modulation properties of mangiferin and quercetin and the mangiferin metabolite norathyriol. *Food Funct.* **2015**, *6*, 1847–1854. [CrossRef] [PubMed]
75. Dilshara, M.G.; Kang, C.H.; Choi, Y.H.; Kim, G.Y. Mangiferin inhibits tumor necrosis factor-α-induced matrix metalloproteinase-9 expression and cellular invasion by suppressing nuclear factor-κB activity. *BMB Rep.* **2015**, *48*, 559–564. [CrossRef] [PubMed]
76. Roy, R.; Yang, J.; Moses, M.A. Matrix metalloproteinases as novel biomarker s and potential therapeutic targets in human cancer. *J. Clin. Oncol.* **2009**, *27*, 5287–5297. [CrossRef] [PubMed]
77. Bartoszewski, R.; Hering, A.; Marsza, M.; Hajduk, J.S.; Bartoszewska, S.; Kapoor, N.; Kochan, K.; Ochocka, R. Mangiferin has an additive effect on the apoptotic properties of hesperidin in Cyclopia sp. tea extracts. *PLoS ONE* **2014**, *9*, e92128. [CrossRef] [PubMed]
78. Salakou, S.; Kardamakis, D.; Tsamandas, A.C.; Zolota, V.; Apostolakis, E.; Tzelepi, V.; Papathanasopoulos, P.; Bonikos, D.S.; Papapetropoulos, T.; Petsas, T. Increased Bax/Bcl-2 ratio up-regulates caspase-3 and increases apoptosis in the thymus of patients with myasthenia gravis. *In Vivo* **2007**, *21*, 123–132. [PubMed]
79. Kavitha, M.; Manivasagam, T.; Essa, M.M.; Tamilselvam, K.; Selvakumar, G.P.; Karthikeyan, S.; Thenmozhi, J.A.; Subash, S. Mangiferin antagonizes rotenone: Induced apoptosis through attenuating mitochondrial dysfunction and oxidative stress in SK-N-SH neuroblastoma cells. *Neurochem. Res.* **2014**, *39*, 668–676. [CrossRef] [PubMed]
80. Cheng, P.; Peng, Z.; Yang, J.; Song, S. The effect of mangiferin on telomerase activity and apoptosis in Leukemic K562 cells. *Zhong Yao Cai* **2007**, *30*, 306–309. [PubMed]
81. Shay, J.W.; Wright, W.E. Role of telomeres and telomerase in cancer. *Semin. Cancer Biol.* **2012**, *21*, 349–353. [CrossRef] [PubMed]
82. Foresti, R. *Anti-Inflammatory and Antioxidant Activities of Nrf2/HO-1 Activators: In Vitro Studies in Microglia and Retinal Cells*; Univesity of Catania: Paris, France, 2014.
83. Menkovic, N.; Juranic, Z.; Stanojkovic, T.; Raonic-Stevanovic, T.; Šavikin, K.; Zdunić, G.; Borojevic, N. Radioprotective activity of Gentiana lutea extract and mangiferin. *Phytother. Res.* **2010**, *24*, 1693–1696. [CrossRef] [PubMed]
84. Valko, M.; Izakovic, M.; Mazur, M.; Rhodes, C.J.; Telser, J. Role of oxygen radicals in DNA damage and cancer incidence. *Mol. Cell. Biochem.* **2004**, *266*, 37–56. [CrossRef] [PubMed]
85. Chemocare.com. Oxaliplatin. Available online: http://www.chemocare.com/chemotherapy/drug-info/oxaliplatin.aspx (accessed on 2 September 2016).
86. Schonn, I.; Hennesen, J.; Dartsch, D.C. Cellular responses to etoposide: Cell death despite cell cycle arrest and repair of DNA damage. *Apoptosis* **2010**, *15*, 162–172. [CrossRef] [PubMed]
87. Carbonell-Capella, J.M.; Buniowska, M.; Barba, F.J.; Esteve, M.J.; Frígola, A. Analytical methods for determining bioavailability and bioaccessibility of bioactive compounds from fruits and vegetables: A review. *Compr. Rev. Food Sci. Food Saf.* **2014**, *13*, 155–171. [CrossRef]
88. McClements, D.J.; Li, F.; Xiao, H. The Nutraceutical Bioavailability Classification Scheme: Classifying Nutraceuticals According to Factors Limiting their Oral Bioavailability. *Ann. Rev. Food Sci. Technol.* **2015**, *6*, 299–327. [CrossRef] [PubMed]
89. Han, D.; Chen, C.; Zhang, C.; Zhang, Y.; Tang, X. Determination of mangiferin in rat plasma by liquid-liquid extraction with UPLC-MS/MS. *J. Pharm. Biomed. Anal.* **2010**, *51*, 260–263. [CrossRef] [PubMed]
90. Hou, S.; Wang, F.; Li, Y.; Li, Y.; Wang, M.; Sun, D.; Sun, C. Pharmacokinetic study of mangiferin in human plasma after oral administration. *Food Chem.* **2012**, *132*, 289–294. [CrossRef] [PubMed]
91. Liu, Y.; Xu, F.; Zeng, X.; Yang, L.; Deng, Y.; Wu, Z.; Feng, Y.; Li, X. Application of a liquid chromatography/tandem mass spectrometry method to pharmacokinetic study of mangiferin in rats. *J. Chromatogr. B* **2010**, *878*, 3345–3350. [CrossRef] [PubMed]
92. Kammalla, A.K.; Ramasamy, M.K.; Inampudi, J.; Dubey, G.P.; Agrawal, A.; Kaliappan, I. Comparative Pharmacokinetic Study of Mangiferin After Oral Administration of Pure Mangiferin and US Patented Polyherbal Formulation to Rats. *AAPS PharmSciTech* **2015**, *16*, 250–258. [CrossRef] [PubMed]

93. Ma, H.; Chen, H.; Sun, L.; Tong, L.; Zhang, T. Improving permeability and oral absorption of mangiferin by phospholipid complexation. *Fitoterapia* **2014**, *93*, 54–61. [CrossRef] [PubMed]
94. Al-Abd, A.M.; Aljehani, Z.K.; Gazzaz, R.W.; Fakhri, S.H.; Jabbad, A.H.; Alahdal, A.M.; Torchilin, V.P. Pharmacokinetic strategies to improve drug penetration and entrapment within solid tumors. *J. Control Release* **2015**, *219*, 269–277. [CrossRef] [PubMed]
95. Caro, C.; Pozo, D. Polysaccharide Colloids as Smart Vehicles in Cancer Therapy. *Curr. Pharm Des.* **2015**, *21*, 4822–4836. [CrossRef] [PubMed]
96. Prado, Y.; Merino, N.; Acosta, J.; Herrera, J.A.; Luque, Y.; Hernández, I.; Prado, E.; Garrido, G.; Delgado, R.; Rodeiro, I. Acute and 28-day subchronic toxicity studies of mangiferin, a glucosyl xanthone isolated from Mangifera indica L. stem bark. *J. Pharm. Pharm. Res.* **2015**, *3*, 13–23.

7

Quercitrin from *Toona sinensis* (Juss.) M.Roem. Attenuates Acetaminophen-Induced Acute Liver Toxicity in HepG2 Cells and Mice through Induction of Antioxidant Machinery and Inhibition of Inflammation

Van-Long Truong [1,†], Se-Yeon Ko [1,†], Mira Jun [2] and Woo-Sik Jeong [1,*]

1 Department of Smart Food and Drug, College of Biomedical Science & Engineering, Inje University, Gimhae 50834, Korea; truonglongpro@gmail.com (V.-L.T.); kose91@daum.net (S.-Y.K.)
2 Department of Food and Science & Nutrition, Dong-A University, Busan 49315, Korea; mjun@dau.ac.kr
* Correspondence: jeongws@inje.ac.kr
† These authors contributed equally to this work.

Abstract: Quercitrin is found in many kinds of vegetables and fruits, and possesses various bioactive properties. The aim of the present study was to elucidate hepatoprotective mechanisms of quercitrin isolated from *Toona sinensis* (Juss.) M.Roem. (syn. *Cedrela sinensis* Juss.), using acetaminophen (APAP)-treated HepG2 cell and animal models. In an in vitro study, quercitrin suppressed the production of reactive oxygen species and enhanced expression of nuclear factor E2-related factor 2 (Nrf2), activity of antioxidant response element (ARE)-reporter gene, and protein levels of NADPH: quinone oxidoreductase 1 (NQO1), catalase (CAT), glutathione peroxidase (GPx), and superoxide dismutase 2 (SOD-2) in APAP-treated HepG2 cells. In an in vivo study, Balb/c mice were orally administered with 10 or 50 mg/kg of quercitrin for 7 days and followed by the injection with single dose of 300 mg/kg APAP. Quercitrin decreased APAP-caused elevation of alanine aminotransferase and aspartate aminotransferase levels, liver necrosis, the expression of pro-inflammatory factors including inducible nitric oxide synthase, cyclooxygenase 2 and inerleukin-1β, and phosphorylation of kinases including c-Jun N-terminal kinase and p38. Quercitrin restored protein levels of Nrf2, NQO1 and activities and expressions of CAT, GPx, SOD-2. The results suggested that quercitrin attenuates APAP-induced liver damage by the activation of defensive genes and the inhibition of pro-inflammatory genes via the suppressions of JNK and p38 signaling.

Keywords: quercitrin; acetaminophen; hepatoprotection; Nrf2/ARE; antioxidant

---

1. Introduction

Acetaminophen (APAP, marketed as Paracetamol® or Tylenol®), a widely used over-the-counter analgesic and antipyretic drug, is safe and effective at therapeutic dose. However, it can cause acute liver failures such as serve hepatic necrosis, hepatic lesions and cirrhosis, and even death when taken in high doses. APAP-induced hepatotoxicity is initiated by formation of excess reactive intermediate *N*-acetyl-p-benzoquinone imine (NAPQI), which is produced by metabolism of liver cytochrome P450s (CYPs) including CYP2E1, CYP3A4 and CYP1A2 [1]. NAPQI depletes cellular glutathione (GSH) and adenosine triphosphate (ATP), causes mitochrondrial dysfunction and damage, and finally causes DNA fragmentation and apoptosis. Acetaminophen also contributes to overproduction of reactive oxygen species (ROS) [2]. In addition, lipid peroxidation resulting from oxidative stress has been demonstrated to contribute to the initiation and progression of APAP-induced liver damage [3]. Furthermore, accumulating evidence indicates that acetaminophen overdose triggers the transcriptional activation of pro-inflammatory mediators and cytokines such as inducible nitric oxide (iNOS), cyclooxygenase 2 (COX-2), tumor necrosis factor α (TNF-α), and interleukin 1β (IL-1β) [2,4].

N-acetylcysteine (NAC) is used as a clinical antidote for APAP poisoning [5,6]. NAC protects liver from APAP-induced injury by restoring hepatic glutathione and scavenging free radicals [7]. However, NAC therapy has considerable limitations because the therapeutic effect of this drug is quite narrow and it could cause some side-effects such as nausea, anaphylactic reaction, headaches and diarrhea [7,8]. Thus, alternative and effective agents are needed to prevent APAP-induced hepatotoxicity.

Toona sinensis (Juss.) M.Roem. (syn. *Cedrela sinensis* Juss.), a member of the Meliaceae family, is an upland tree that has been used as traditional medicine and nutritious food for a long time in China and Korea. *T. sinensis* leaves contain a variety of bioactive compounds such as gallic acid, methyl gallte, kaemferol, quercetin, rutin, quercitrin, palmitic acid and linoleic acid, etc. [9–12]. Of these compounds, quercitrin (3-rhamnosyl quercetin) (Figure 1), a glycoside of quercetin, has been found as a main bioactive constituent in *T. sinensis* leaves [13,14]. The sugar portion bound to the aglycone in quercitrin has been demonstrated to increase solubility of quercitrin and consequently improve the absorption by interacting with the sodium dependent glucose transport receptor in the small intestine [15,16]. Pharmacological studies have shown that quercitrin has antioxidant [17,18], anti-inflammatory [19,20], and anti-allergic [21] activities. Quercitrin has been demonstrated to exert a protective effect against UV-induced cell death and apoptosis [22,23]. Furthermore, quercitrin has been studied as an anti-cancer agent against non-small cell lung cancer through the modulation of immune response [24]. Our group previously reported that quercitrin from *T. sinensis* leaves potently scavenged free radicals and induced antioxidant enzymes in H_2O_2-treated HepG2 cells [9]. However, the protective mechanisms of quercitrin against APAP-induced hepatotoxicity have not been investigated.

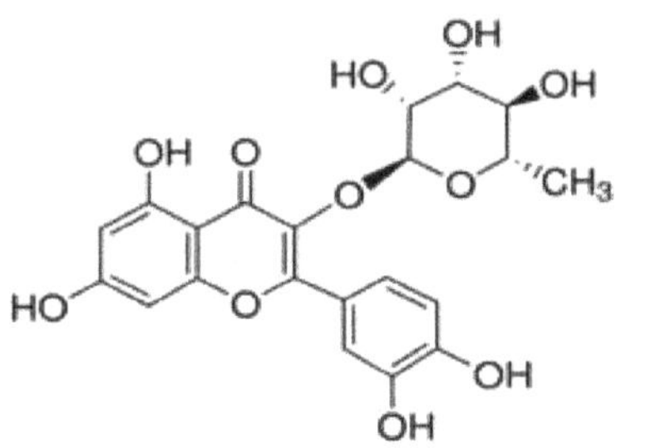

Figure 1. Chemical structure of quercitrin.

In the present study, we examined the hepatoprotective effects of quercitrin in both cell line and animal models of hepatotoxicity challenged by APAP. The stimulating activity of quercitrin on cellular defensive genes including transcription factor nuclear factor E2-related factor 2 (Nrf2), antioxidant response element (ARE)-reporter gene and antioxidant enzymes was determined. The inhibitory effects of quercitrin on liver damage markers of alanine aminotransferase (ALT) and aspartate aminotransferase (AST) as well as inflammatory targets of iNOS, COX-2 and IL-1β were evaluated in APAP-induced hepatotoxic mice. In addition, the modulation of mitogen activated protein kinases (MAPKs) by quercitrin was examined.

2. Materials and Methods

2.1. Chemicals

Acetaminophen, silymarin, MTT [3-(4,5-dimethylthiazol-2-yl)-2,5-diphenyltetrazolium bromide], dimethyl sulphoxide (DMSO), polyethylene glycol (PEG), and triton X-100 were purchased from Sigma-Aldrich (St. Louis, MO, USA). 2′,7′-dichlorodihydrofluorescein diacetate (DCFH-DA) was purchased from Molecular Probe Inc. (Eugene, OR, USA). The colorimetric ALT and AST assay kits were supplied by Young-Dong Co. (Seoul, Korea). Anti-Nrf2 (sc-13032), anti-NQO1 (sc-25591), anti-SOD-2 (sc-18504), anti-GPx (sc-30147), anti-COX-2 (sc-1745), anti-iNOS (sc-651), anti-IL-1β (sc-7884), anti-β-actin (sc-1616), and horseradish peroxidase-conjugated anti-goat immunoglobulin IgG (sc-2350) antibodies were purchased from Santa Cruz Biotechnology Inc. (Santa Cruz, CA, USA). Anti-p-ERK (9101), anti-p-JNK (9251), anti-p-p38 MAPK (9211), anti-CAT (14097), and horseradish peroxidase-conjugated anti-rabbit immunoglobulin IgG (7074) were purchased from Cell Signaling Technology (Beverly, MA, USA). All other reagents used in this study were of the highest grade commercially available.

2.2. Preparation of Quercitrin

Quercitrin from powder of *T. sinensis* (Juss.) M.Roem. leaves, kindly provided by Slow-life Chamjook Farm Corporation (Hamyang, Korea), was isolated according to previous literature [9]. A voucher specimen (Jeong, W.S. 001) of the raw material was deposited at the Herbarium of Kyungpook National University (KNU), Daegu, Korea. Briefly, the powder of *T. sinensis* was extracted three times with 95% ethanol (EtOH) for 24 h in room temperature and concentrated by rotary evaporation at 40 °C. After concentration, the concentrate was suspended in 10% EtOH and then fractionated with a series of organic solvents, including h-hexane, DCM, ethylacetate (EtOAc), n-butanol, and water in sequence. The EtOAc-solution fraction, the most potent antioxidant fraction to both scavenging radicals and antioxidant enzyme activity, was applied onto a silica gel open column. The column was eluted with solvent mixtures of DCM/methanol under gradient conditions to yield 17 fractions. The most potent subfraction (Fr. 10) was purified by recycling preparatory high-performance liquid chromatography (HPLC) and structural analyses were performed using 1H- and 13C-nuclear magnetic resonance (NMR) analysis.

2.3. Cell Culture

Human hepatoma cell line HepG2, obtained from American Type Culture Collection (ATCC, Rockville, MD, USA), was maintained DMEM containing 10% fetal bovine serum (FBS), 100 units/mL penicillin, 100 μg/mL streptomycin, 1% essential amino acids, 1% glutamax in humidified atmosphere of 5% CO_2 at 37 °C. The medium was renewed once every two days.

2.4. Cell Viability Assay

Cell viability was examined using MTT assay. Briefly, HepG2 cells were cultured in a 24-well plate at density of 1×10^5 cells/well. After starvation, cells were treated with a series of various concentrations of quercitrin in the presence of 10 mM APAP for 24 h and then incubated with 5 mg/mL MTT for additional 4 h. The dark blue formazan crystal was solubilized in DMSO and followed by measurement of absorbance at 570 nm with a microplate reader (BioTek Instruments, Winooski, VT, USA).

2.5. ROS Formation Assay

Level of intracellular ROS was measured using DCFH-DA. In viable cells, the DCFH-DA is cleaved by esterase to DCFH and followed oxidizing by ROS to form a highly florescent molecule, DCF. Briefly, HepG2 cells were seeded onto 96-well plates at density of 2×10^4 cells/well and then treated either vehicle (DMSO, 0.1%) or various concentrations of quercitrin in the presence of 10 mM APAP for 24 h. After washing twice with phosphate-buffered saline (PBS), the cells were incubated with 20 μM DCF-DA for 1 h at 37 °C in darkness. The fluorescence that is representative of intracellular reactive oxygen species level was measured at 485/20 nm excitation and 528/20 nm emission using a fluorescence multidetection reader (Synergy HT, BioTek, VT, USA).

2.6. *Assay of Reporter Gene Activity*

HepG2-C8 cell line, kindly donated by Ah-Ng Tony Kong (Rutgers University, New Brunswick, NJ, USA), was established by the table transfection of HepG2 cells with p-ARE-T1-luciferase reporter gene as previously described [25]. After starvation, the HepG2-C8 cells were treated with various concentrations of quercitrin for 24 h and then ARE-luciferase activity was measured using a luciferase kit from Promega (Promega Corp., Madison, WI, USA) according to the manufacturer's instructions. Luciferase activity was normalized against total protein concentration, determined by a BCA protein assay kit (Pierce, Rockford, IL, USA), and expressed as a fold induction over that in vehicle-treated cells.

2.7. *Animals and Experimental Design*

Thirty male Balb/c mice (6 weeks old, 20–25 g) were obtained from Hyochang Science (Daegu, Korea) and allowed free access to standard laboratory diet and distilled water *ad libitum* for at least one week prior to the experiment. The animal room was environmentally controlled at 25 ± 2 °C, 55%–60% humidity, 12 h light/dark cycle. This animal experiment was approved by the Animal Care and Used Committee of Inje University with protocol number 2013-50 (Gimhae, Korea). The mice were randomly divided into six groups with five mice each. Group I (control group) received 50% PEG as a vehicle for 7 days. Group II (quercitrin group) was only administered 50 mg/kg quercitrin for 7 days. Group III (APAP group) received 50% PEG for 7 days. Group IV and V (quercitrin + APAP group) were orally gavaged with 10 or 50 mg/kg of quercitrin, respectively, for 7 consecutive days. Group VI (APAP + silymarin group) was orally administered 50 mg/kg of silymarin (SIL), which is frequently used as a natural hepatoprotectant by its antioxidant and anti-inflammatory properties [26] for 7 days. After 1 h last administration, a single dose of APAP (300 mg/kg) was injected to mice in groups III-VI. After 24 h APAP challenge, all mice were sacrificed to obtain blood and livers for further biochemical analysis.

2.8. *Measurement of Plasma ALT and AST Levels*

Blood samples from mice were centrifuged at 3000× *g*, 4 °C for 10 min to obtain serum supernatant. The ALT and AST activities in serum were measured using commercially available kits (Young-dong Pharm, Seoul, Korea).

2.9. *Assay for Antioxidant Enzymes Activity*

Liver tissues were collected and homogenized in phosphate buffer (pH 7.0) and then tissue homogenates were centrifuged at 10,000× *g*, 4 °C for 10 min to obtain separately supernatant and pellet for further experiments. The protein concentration was determined using a BCA protein assay kit (Pierce, Rockford, IL, USA). CAT activity was determined by the method of Aebi [27]. GPx activity was performed according to the method of Bongdanska et al. [28]. SOD activity was determined by the method of Oyanagui [29]. Enzyme activities were expressed in relation to the vehicle-treated control.

2.10. *Western Blot Analysis*

Cells and liver tissues were homogenized in RIPA buffer and then centrifuged at 10,000× *g*, 4 °C for 10 min to obtain supernatant. Total protein concentration of each sample was determined using a BCA protein assay kit (Pierce, Rockford, IL, USA) according to the manufacturer's instructions. Equal amounts of protein were resolved on SDS-PAGE gels and then transferred onto PVDF membranes (Millipore, Bedford, MA, USA) using a semidry transfer system (Bio-rad, Hercules, CA, USA). After blocking with 5% non-fat milk in PBST (0.1% Tween 20 in PBS) for 2 h at 4 °C, the membranes were incubated overnight with appropriate primary antibodies at 4 °C. Then, the membranes were washed five times with PBST and hybridized with horseradish peroxidase-conjugated anti-rabbit or anti-goat immunoglobulin IgG secondary antibodies for 3 h at 4 °C. After washing five times with

PBST, blots were visualized using enhanced chemiluminescence western blotting reagent (Santa Cruz Biotechnology, Santa Cruz, CA, USA).

2.11. Statistical Analysis

Data were expressed as means ± SD. Statistical comparisons were evaluated using analysis of variance (ANOVA) followed by Tukey's test. $p < 0.05$ was considered as significant.

3. Results

3.1. Protective Effect of Quercitrin against Oxidative Stress in APAP-Induced HepG2 Cells

To investigate the effect of quercitrin on the APAP-induced ROS formation, we measured the intracellular level of ROS using a redox-sensitive fluorescence reagent, DCF-DA. As shown in Figure 2A, exposure of HepG2 cells to APAP remarkably elevated the ROS production by over 2-fold at 24 h when compared to the control. Pre-treatment of quercitrin, however, inhibited the increase of APAP-induced ROS level. The presence of 10, 25, 50 μg/mL quercitrin significantly decreased the ROS formation in HepG2 cells by 0.5-, 0.5-, and 1.3-fold, respectively, compared to APAP-treated cells alone. Enhanced oxidative stress can result in apoptosis and cell death; thus, we tested whether quercitrin rescue APAP-induced cell death using MTT assay. Consequently, 10 mM APAP reduced 30% cell viability, which was restored by quercitrin (Figure 2B).

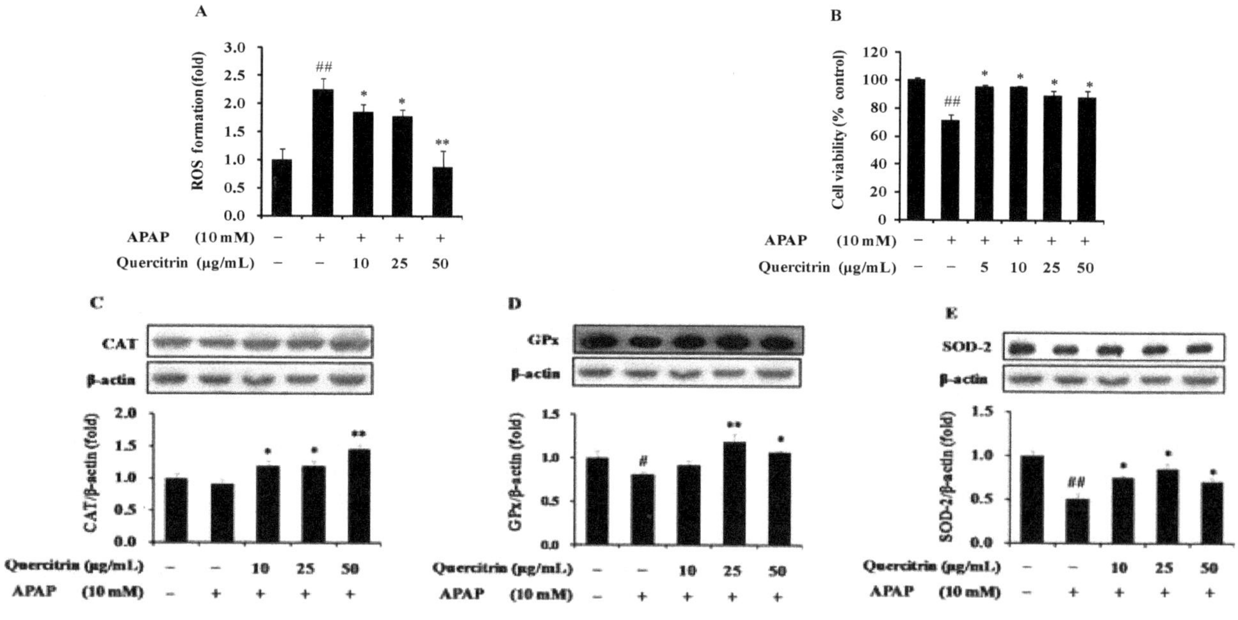

Figure 2. Protective effects of quercitrin on acetaminophen (APAP)-treated HepG2 cells. (**A**) Effect of quercitrin on APAP-mediated reactive oxygen species (ROS) formation; (**B**) Effect of quercitrin on cell viability using MTT assay at 24 h. Effect of quercitrin on protein expressions of (**C**) catalase (CAT); (**D**) glutathione peroxidase (GPx); and (**E**) superoxide dismutase 2 (SOD-2) in APAP-treated HepG2 cells. ROS was presented as the fold induction of vehicle-treated control. Cell viability was normalized as 100% for control (without any treatments). Protein expression levels were normalized with β-actin. All data represent means ± SD of at least three independent experiments. Significant differences were ($^{\#\#}$) $p < 0.01$ or ($^{\#}$) $p < 0.05$ as compared with the control; (**) $p < 0.01$ or (*) $p < 0.05$ as compared with the APAP group.

Antioxidant enzymes including CAT, GPx, and SOD constitute the primary part of enzymatic antioxidant defense system against oxidative stress via directly eliminating ROS. Thus, the effects of quercitrin on expression levels of antioxidant enzymes were examined. The results showed that

APAP significantly reduced protein expressions of GPx and SOD but not CAT compared with control (Figure 2C–E). However, pretreatment with quercitrin for 1 h blocked the effect of APAP on the decreased expression of antioxidant enzymes. Overall, these results obviously suggested that quercitrin prevents APAP-induced ROS formation and cell death through the induction of antioxidant enzymes in HepG2 cells.

3.2. Upregulation of Nrf2/ARE-Mediated Phase II Detoxifying Enzymes by Quercitrin in APAP-Treated HepG2 Cells

To further confirm the role of quercitrin in protection of cells from APAP toxicity, the activation of Nrf2/ARE pathway was evaluated. Nrf2 is considered as a key transcriptional factor responsible for the regulation of phase II detoxifying and/or antioxidant enzymes, which protect cells from cell death-induced APAP toxicity. The basal levels of protein expression of Nrf2 were detected in HepG2 cells. Compared with untreated control, APAP was able to significantly decrease the Nrf2 protein level for up to 24 h (Figure 3A). Further, we investigated the inhibitory effect of quercitrin on APAP-induced the reduction of Nrf2 expression. Results showed that quercitrin has the potential to induce Nrf2 for 24 h. The quercitrin concentration at ⩾25 μg/mL caused a significant increase in protein level of Nrf2. In particular, quercitrin concentration at 50 μg/mL resulted in a strong up-regulation of Nrf2 at 24 h by 1.6-fold compared to control and 2.0-fold compared with APAP alone. In addition, in order to elucidate whether the activation of Nrf2 induces ARE-mediated phase II detoxifying and/or antioxidant enzymes using ARE-reporter gene activity assay, HepG2-C8 cells, stably transfected with a pARE-TI-luciferase reporter gene were exposed to quercitrin for 24 h. As illustrated in Figure 3B, quercitrin enhanced the ARE-luciferase activity. The luciferase activity by quercitrin at the highest concentration of 50 μg/mL reached 2.6-fold compared with that by vehicle-treated control. This result demonstrated the role of Nrf2 in up-regulation of ARE-mediated phase II enzymes. Furthermore, the effect of quercitrin on protein level of a phase II detoxifying enzyme, NQO1, was examined in APAP-treated HepG2 cells. The result showed that treatment with APAP resulted in the decrease of NQO1 protein level; however, pre-treatment of quercitrin restored the APAP-reduced expression level of NQO1, even more than in the control at quercitrin concentration of 25 μg/mL (Figure 3C). These data suggest that quercitrin promotes hepatoprotective system through the activation of Nrf2 and Nrf2/ARE-mediated antioxidant defense mechanism.

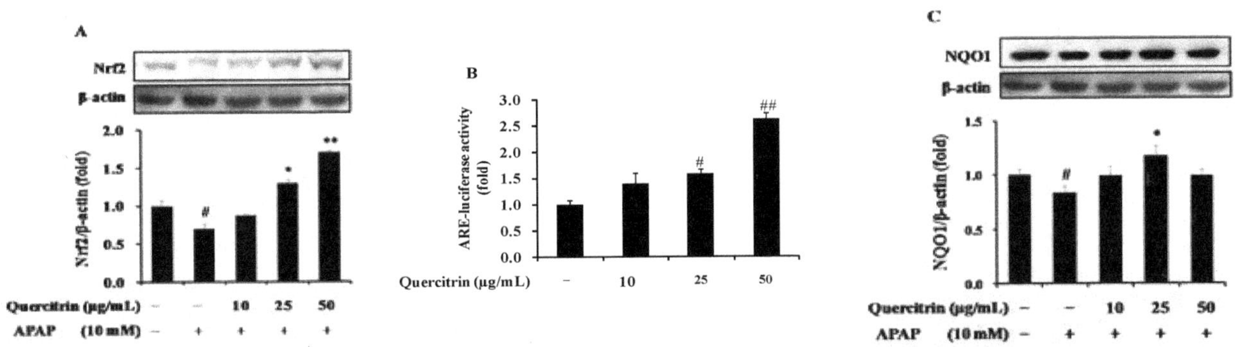

Figure 3. Up-regulation of nuclear factor E2-related factor 2 (Nrf2)/antioxidant response element (ARE)-mediated phase II detoxifying enzyme in APAP-treated HepG2 cells. (**A**) Effect of quercitrin on protein expression of Nrf2; (**B**) Effect of quercitrin on ARE-luciferase activity; (**C**) Effect of quercitrin on protein level of quinone oxidoreductase 1 (NQO1). Luciferase activity was normalized with total protein content and expressed as fold induction of normal control. Protein expression levels were normalized with β-actin. All data represent means ± SD of at least three independent experiments. Significant differences were (##) $p < 0.01$ or (#) $p < 0.05$ as compared with the control; (**) $p < 0.01$ or (*) $p < 0.05$ as compared with APAP group.

3.3. Protective Effect of Quercitrin against APAP-Induced Hepatotoxicity in Vivo

To further investigate the role of quercitrin in protecting liver from APAP-induced toxicity, Balb/c mice were administered quercitrin at a dose of 10 and 50 mg/kg before injection of 300 mg/kg APAP. As shown in Table 1, APAP significantly increased liver weight within 24 h compared with the control and quercitrin alone groups, whereas body weights were comparable among all experimental groups. Oral pre-administration of quercitrin (10 and 50 mg/kg) or SIL (50 mg/kg) reduced the APAP-induced increase of liver weight. In addition, injection of 300 mg/kg APAP highly elevated 14- and 3-fold of serum ALT and AST activities, respectively, compared to the vehicle-treated group, implying that a high dose of APAP caused liver toxicity (Figure 4A,B). Quercitrin treatment significantly prevented the APAP-induced elevation of ALT and AST levels. Similarly, 50 mg/kg of SIL, considered as a positive control in this study, was found to attenuate the ALT and AST activities. Further, the administration of 50 mg/kg quercitrin alone was unlikely to significantly alter the basal activity of these transaminases, suggesting no liver damage caused by quercitrin. Histological (H&E) analysis further revealed that APAP-induced severe hepatic lesions such as hydropic degeneration, inflammation, and hemorrhage were improved by quercitrin pretreatment. Also, a similar result was observed in the positive control group, SIL (Figure 4C). These results prove that quercitrin may be a potential agent in the prevention of APAP-induced liver injury in a mouse model.

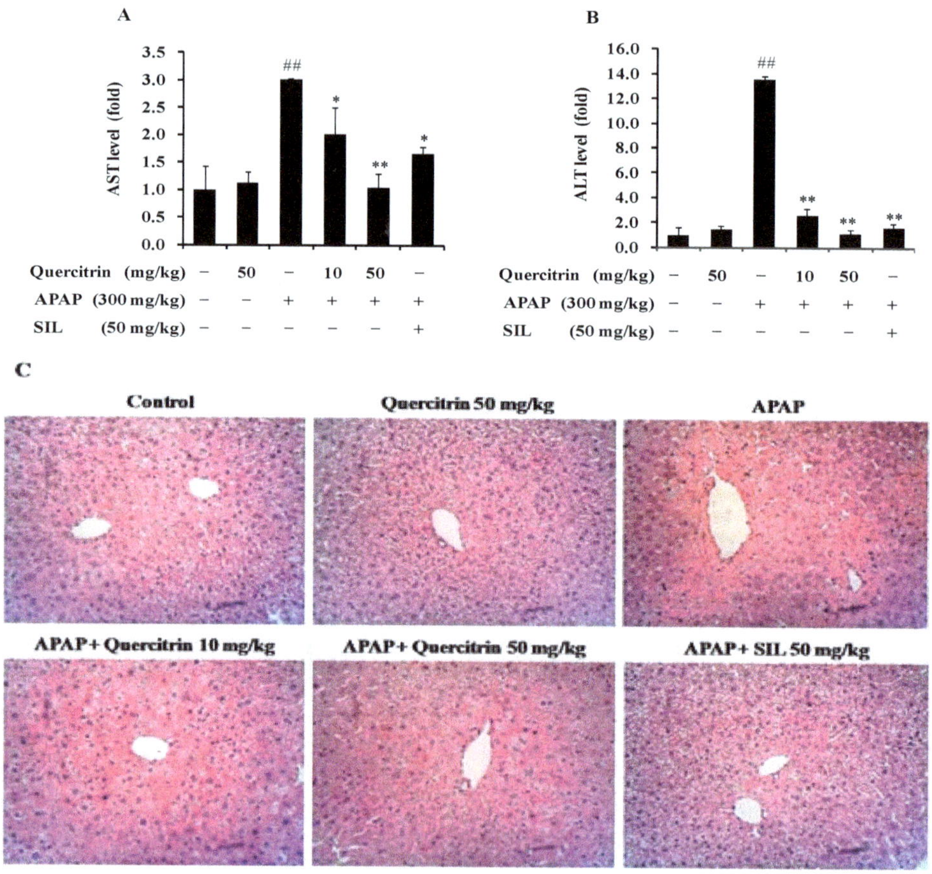

Figure 4. Protective effects of quercitrin on APAP intoxicated mice. Mice were orally administered quercitrin of 10 or 50 mg/kg once a day for seven days. The control group received the same volume of saline. After the seventh gavage of quercitrin or saline, animals received a single injection of APAP (300 mg/kg). All mice were sacrificed at 24 h after APAP injection to obtain blood and liver. Serum ALT (**A**) and AST (**B**) levels; and H&E staining (**C**). All data represent means ± SD of five mice in each group. Significant differences were (##) $p < 0.01$ as compared with the control; (**) $p < 0.01$ or (*) $p < 0.05$ as compared with APAP group.

Table 1. Effect of quercitrin on body weight and liver weight/body weight (%) in APAP intoxicated mice.

Groups	Treatment	Initial Body Weight (g)	Final Body Weight (g)	Liver Weight (g)	Relative Liver Weight (Percentage Ratio)
I	Control	20.12 ± 0.49	23.02 ± 1.36	1.42 ± 0.09	6.19 ± 0.30
II	Quercitrin (50 mg/kg)	19.62 ± 0.59	23.40 ± 0.45	1.53 ± 0.11	6.55 ± 0.53
III	APAP (300 mg/kg)	19.68 ± 0.40	23.37 ± 0.90	1.65 ± 0.11	7.21 ± 0.36 #
IV	Quercitrin (10 mg/kg) + APAP	20.20 ± 0.34	24.1 ± 0.41	1.50 ± 0.10	6.20 ± 0.31 *
V	Quercitrin (50 mg/kg) + APAP	19.92 ± 0.38	23.02 ± 0.97	1.47 ± 0.09	6.40 ± 0.28 *
VI	Silymarin (50 mg/kg) + APAP	19.68 ± 0.85	23.42 ± 0.92	1.50 ± 0.10	6.38 ± 0.19 *

(#) $p < 0.05$ as compared with the control, (*) $p < 0.05$ as compared with APAP group.

3.4. Protective Effect of Quercitrin against APAP-Induced Hepatotoxicity through Enhancement of Activity and Expression of Antioxidant Enzymes

To examine whether quercitrin activates antioxidant defense system in APAP-treated mouse models, we measured activity and protein level of antioxidant enzymes including CAT, GPx, and SOD-2, which importantly contribute to the protection of cells/tissues from oxidative stress through directly neutralizing and eliminating ROS. The results indicated that injection of mice to 300 mg/kg APAP resulted in the reduction in activities of three antioxidant enzymes. Quercitrin pre-administration, however, prevented the APAP-induced decrease of CAT, GPx, and SOD-2 enzyme activities (Figure 5A–C). It is likely that quercitrin, SIL (50 mg/kg), also significantly increased the activities of these enzymes when compared to APAP-treated mice. Interestingly, oral administration of 50 mg/kg quercitrin alone was shown to enhance the CAT and SOD-2 activities but not GPx activity compared to the vehicle-treated control. In order to further confirm the inductive effect as well as the role of quercitrin on liver protection against APAP-induced oxidative stress, protein expression levels of antioxidant enzymes including CAT, GPx, and SOD-2 were determined. The results showed that treatment of 300 mg/kg APAP caused slightly reduced protein expressions of these antioxidant enzymes. However, as expected, quercitrin significantly induced the APAP-abolished CAT, GPx, and SOD-2 proteins, even more than those in the control group (Figure 5D–F). This result is consistent with SIL, which also enhanced the expressions of antioxidant enzymes in APAP-treated mice. Overall, our study supports the use of quercitrin in preventing APAP-mediated liver toxicity.

3.5. Upregulation of NQO1 Expression by Nrf2-Mediated Quercitrin in APAP-Treated Mice

As demonstrated, quercitrin up-regulated Nrf2-mediated phase II detoxifying enzyme in HepG2 cells, thus we confirmed the inductive effect of quercitrin on protein levels of NQO1 in an APAP-treated mouse model. Similar to the in vitro result, exposure of mice to APAP caused a significant attenuate of NQO1 protein level (Figure 6B) but was unlikely to suppress protein expression of Nrf2 after 24 h challenge (Figure 6A) when compared to the untreated control. The presence of quercitrin restored the APAP-reduced protein expression of both Nrf2 and NQO1. Further, the levels of Nrf2 and NQO1 expression induced by quercitrin were even higher than those induced by a positive control, SIL (50 mg/kg) (Figure 6A,B). These results demonstrate the role of quercitrin in the activation of Nrf2/ARE-mediated phase II detoxifying enzyme, implying protection of cells/tissues against APAP-induced toxicity.

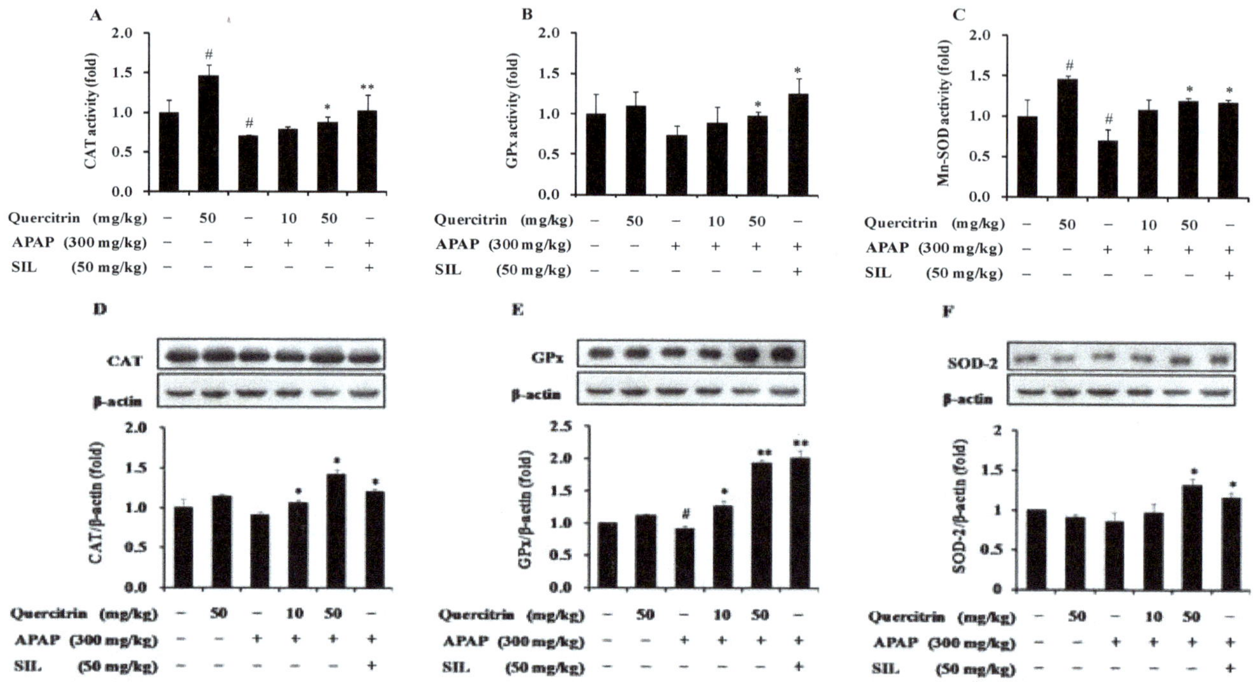

Figure 5. Effects of quercitrin on activities and protein expressions of hepatic antioxidant enzymes in APAP intoxicated mice. The hepatic activities of CAT (**A**); GPx (**B**) and SOD-2 (**C**) were measured as described in Materials and Methods section. The protein levels of CAT (**D**); GPx (**E**) and SOD-2 (**F**) were determined using Western blot analysis. Protein expression levels were normalized with β-actin. All data represent means ± SD of five mice in each group. Significant differences were (#) $p < 0.05$ as compared with the control; (**) $p < 0.01$ or (*) $p < 0.05$ as compared with APAP group.

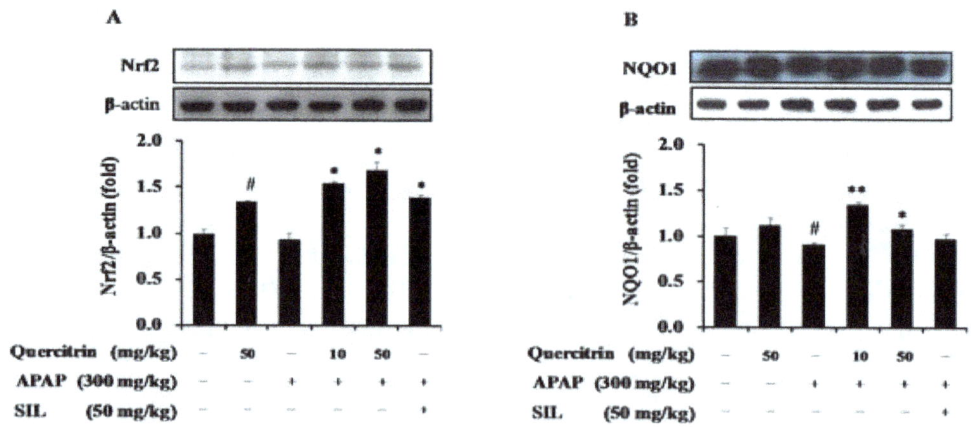

Figure 6. Effects of quercitrin on expressions of Nrf2 and NQO1 in APAP intoxicated mice. The protein levels of Nrf2 (**A**) and NQO1 (**B**) were measured by Western blot analysis as described in Materials and Methods section. Protein expression levels were normalized with β-actin. All data represent means ± SD of five mice in each group. Significant differences were (#) $p < 0.05$ as compared with the control; (**) $p < 0.01$ or (*) $p < 0.05$ as compared with APAP group.

3.6. Quercitrin Attenuates Inflammatory Response in APAP-Treated Mice

In further studies, we evaluated the effects of quercitrin on APAP-induced expression of pro-inflammatory mediators and cytokines implicated in hepatotoxicity. APAP treatment significantly increased protein expression for the pro-inflammatory mediators and cytokine such as iNOS, COX-2 and IL-1β compared to vehicle-treated control, whereas animals receiving quercitrin alone did not show elevated levels of these hepatic inflammatory factors (Figure 7A–C). APAP-enhanced protein expression of iNOS, the enzyme mediating production of nitric oxide, was also inhibited by the presence of quercitrin (Figure 7A). Expression of pro-inflammatory mediator COX-2 that was up-regulated in mice exposing APAP intoxication was reduced in mice pre-treated with quercitrin (Figure 7B). Additionally, quercitrin administration resulted in a decrease in the APAP-induced IL-1β protein level (Figure 7C).

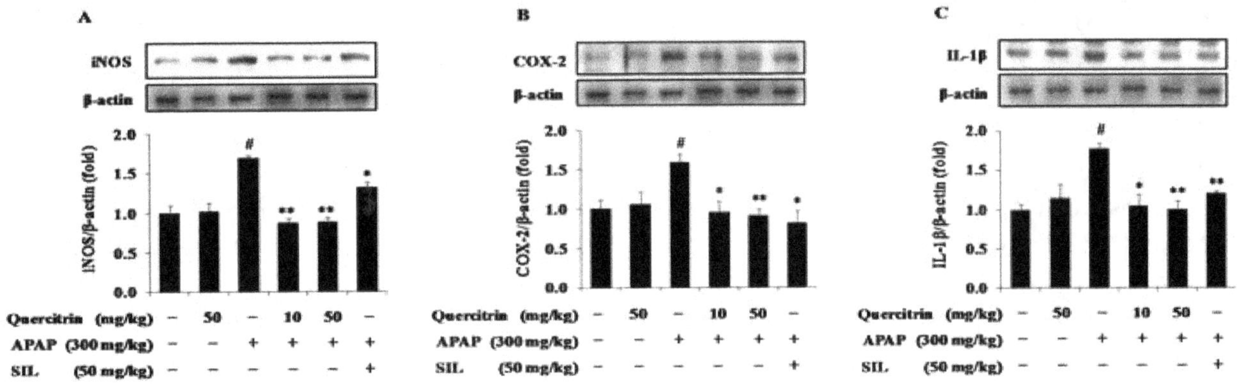

Figure 7. Effects of quercitrin on inflammatory response in APAP intoxicated mice. The hepatic inducible nitric oxide (iNOS) (**A**); cyclooxygenase 2 (COX-2) (**B**) and interleukin 1β (IL-1β) (**C**) levels were evaluated by Western blot analysis. Protein expression levels were normalized with β-actin. All data represent means ± SD of five mice in each group. Significant differences were (#) $p < 0.05$ as compared with the control; (**) $p < 0.01$ or (*) $p < 0.05$ as compared with APAP group.

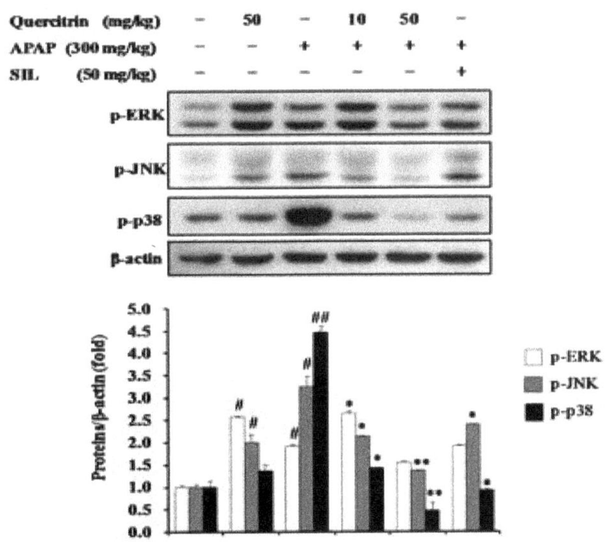

Figure 8. Effects of quercitrin on MAP kinases in APAP intoxicated mice. The phosphorylations of ERK, JNK and p38 MAPK were analyzed by Western blotting. Protein expression levels were normalized with β-actin. All data represent means ± SD of five mice in each group. Significant differences were (##) $p < 0.01$ or (#) $p < 0.05$ as compared with the control; (**) $p < 0.01$ or (*) $p < 0.05$ as compared with APAP group.

3.7. Activation of Cytoprotective Mechanisms by Quercitrin through Regulation of MAPK Pathways in APAP-Treated Mice

To investigate role of quercitrin on the modulation of MAPKs in APAP-treated mice, phosphorylation levels of MAPKs including ERK, JNK, and p38 MAPK were determined using western blotting. As shown in Figure 8, exposure of APAP (300 mg/kg) increased the phosphorylation levels of ERK, JNK, and p38 MAPK in the liver by 2-, 3-, and 4-fold, respectively, when compared to the control group. This suggested that MAPKs involved in APAP-caused hepatotoxicity. On other hand, treatment of quercitrin (50 mg/kg) alone resulted in a significant elevation of phosphorylated ERK and JNK but not phosphorylated p38. Oral administration of quercitrin or SIL, however, strongly inhibited the JNK and p38 MAPK phosphorylations, whereas ERK phosphorylation was slightly decreased at 50 mg/kg quercitrin and there was no change at 50 mg/kg SIL. Overall, our results indicate that the inhibition of APAP-induced phosphorylation levels of JNK and p38 MAPK by quercitrin contributes to protection of liver from toxicity.

4. Discussion

The present study demonstrated the role of quercitrin from *T. sinensis* in the protection of cells/tissues from APAP-induced toxicity. Quercitrin attenuated the ROS formation and cell death induced by APAP overdose through the restoration of antioxidant enzymes as well as enhancement of Nrf2/ARE pathway-mediated cytoprotecive enzymes in HepG2 cells. Moreover, oral administration of quercitrin exhibited protective effects against APAP-caused liver injury in mice, which is consistent with an in vitro test. Indeed, quercitrin pretreatment prevented APAP toxicity, as evidenced by much less liver injury and decreased serum ALT and AST levels. Quercitrin restored the APAP-induced reduction of activities and protein expressions of antioxidant enzymes, including CAT, GPx, and SOD-2 as well as protein level of phase II enzyme NQO1 through the activation of transcription factor Nrf2. In addition, quercitrin exerted the anti-inflammatory property through inhibiting the expression of pro-inflammatory mediators and cytokine such as iNOS, COX-2, IL-1β in APAP-treated liver. Furthermore, inhibition of APAP-mediated phosphorylation levels of JNK and p38 MAPK were considered as a protective mechanism of quercitrin from APAP toxicity in liver. These results, for the first time, demonstrate that antioxidant and anti-inflammatory properties of quercitrin potently contribute to the prevention of APAP-induced liver injury.

Reactive oxygen species (ROS) including free radicals such as superoxide ($O_2 \cdot ^-$), hydroxyl radical ($\cdot OH$), peroxyl radical ($RO_2 \cdot$) and non-radical species such as hydrogen peroxide (H_2O_2) are implicated in the development of various diseases such as aging, cancer, atherosclerosis, fibrosis, and inflammation [30–32]. The accumulation of ROS results in oxidative stress, lipid peroxidation, protein inactivation, DNA damage, loss of cell function, and finally apoptosis and necrosis [33]. Increased oxidative stress and massive impairment of antioxidant defense systems are well-known as the main mechanisms of APAP-caused hepatotoxicity [34]. The major reactive oxygen species generated by APAP toxicity is superoxide ($O_2 \cdot ^-$), which dismutates to molecular oxygen and hydrogen peroxide or reacts with nitric oxide (NO) to produce peroxynitrite ($ONOO^-$), a potent oxidant and nitrating species [35]. A variety of phenomena such as lipid peroxidation, increased ALT and AST, reduced levels of cellular antioxidant enzymes, and DNA damages was observed in APAP toxicity. In this study, we confirmed that ROS levels were dramatically increased, whereas protein expressions and activities of CAT, GPx, and SOD-2 in HepG2 cells and mouse livers significantly decreased after APAP treatment. In addition, HepG2 cell death and liver necrosis were elevated, suggesting that APAP-induced ROS formation results in loss of cell function and ultimately apoptosis. However, quercitrin could inhibit ROS formation and consequently reduce hepatic cell death as well as liver necrosis caused by APAP toxicity. Quercitrin also remarkably abolished plasma ALT and AST levels, which coincided with the decrease of APAP-mediated oxidative damage. Furthermore, the levels of antioxidant enzymes including CAT, GPx, and SOD-2 were restored by pretreatment of quercitrin in APAP-treated HepG2 cells and livers of mice. These results indicate that quercitrin protects cells/livers from APAP-induced oxidative stress through the suppression of ROS production and enhancement of an antioxidant defense system.

Recent studies have demonstrated that transcription factor Nrf2 importantly contributes to cellular defense mechanisms from APAP toxicity [36,37]. Treatment of Nrf2 knockout mice (Nrf2-/-) with APAP results in enhanced hepatotoxicity and mortality compared to wild-type [36]. NAC treatment produced a low efficacy in Nrf2-/- mice, although NAC still exhibited the effective protection against APAP toxicity in wild-type mice [37,38]. Additionally, hepatocyte-specific Kelch-like ECH-associated protein-1 (*keap1*) gene knockout mice that highly express detoxifying enzymes are significantly more resistant to APAP toxicity than wild-type animals [39]. Consequently, up-regulation of phase II antioxidant/detoxifying enzymes by Nrf2/ARE pathway plays a critical role in preventing hepatic damage caused by APAP. To clarify the underlying hepatoprotective mechanism of quercitrin, we investigated the inductive effect of quercitrin on the Nrf2/ARE pathway. The results suggested that protein level of Nrf2 was enhanced by the pre-treatment of quercitrin in both in vitro and in vivo models. Quercitrin also significantly increased the ARE-reporter gene activity in HepG2-C8 cells. Furthermore, quercitrin restored the APAP-induced reduction of phase II enzyme NQO1, which are capable of scavenging oxidative stress and detoxifying/eliminating toxic chemicals. NQO1 has been demonstrated to be capable of lowering NAPQI availability by the conversion of NAPQI back to the parent APAP, prevent adenosine triphosphate (ATP) depletion as well as mitochondrial dysfunction caused by APAP [40,41]. Our findings strongly indicate that quercitrin enhances the hepatic defense system through the activation of Nrf2/ARE-mediated phase II detoxifying/ antioxidant enzymes.

Uncontrolled inflammation initiates the progression of tissue damage and results in the development of many diseases such as Alzheimer's disease, cardiovascular disease, atherosclerosis and cancer [42,43]. During the inflammatory response, pro-inflammatory mediators and cytokines such as iNOS, COX-2, IL-1β, and TNF-α were up-regulated and accumulated in the liver [44]. Numerous evidence has showed that APAP causes early damage, which triggers an inflammatory response with the production of pro-inflammatory factors and innate immune cell infiltration in the liver [45–48]. Thus, inhibition of these mediators and cytokines production is an important mechanism for treatment of inflammation, contributing to preventing APAP-induced hepatotoxicity. In the current study, we confirmed that APAP intoxication resulted in increased expression levels of iNOS, COX-2 as well as IL-1β in the liver. However, mice pre-administered quercitrin exhibited the inhibitory effect on protein expressions of iNOS, COX-2, and IL-1β. These results, for the first time, imply that the hepatoprotective effect of quercitrin may be due to its anti-inflammatory property.

MAP kinases including ERK, JNK, and p38 MAPK play a crucial role in transduction extracellular signals to cellular responses including cellular proliferation, differentiation, development, inflammation and apoptosis in response to various signals produced by growth factors, hormones, cytokines, and xenobiotics as well as oxidative stress [49,50]. A massive study demonstrated that MAP kinases directly implicate in the mechanism of APAP-caused hepatocellular injury. During APAP overdose, JNK is phosphorylated and translocates into mitochondria early in APAP hepatotoxicity in mice, resulting in an initial oxidative stress, induction of mitochorial permeability transition, and inhibition of bioenergetics [35,51]. Additionally, activated JNK can trigger Bax activation, which is responsible for the initial apoptosis-inducing factor (AIF) and endonuclease G release from the mitochondria and early DNA damage, as well as induce iNOS expression, which promotes peroxynitrite formation [52,53]. Furthermore, inhibition of JNK activation or *jnk* gene knockout in mice decreased the liver injury, nuclear DNA fragmentation, and prevented the development of mitochondrial oxidative stress after APAP overdose [51,52,54]. Different from JNK inhibitor, the inhibitors of ERK and p38 MAPK exhibited no protection against APAP toxicity either in vitro or in vivo [52]. Although activations of ERK and p38 MAPK were observed, the roles of ERK and p38 MAPK in APAP-caused heptotoxic mechanism have not been clearly investigated. Overall, the inhibition of JNK phosphorylation contributes to reduction of liver injury induced by APAP challenge. In the present study, we also investigated the inhibition of JNK phosphorylation and concluded it could play a part in the hepatoprotective mechanism of quercitrin against APAP-mediated damage.

5. Conclusions

In conclusion, quercitrin protects against APAP-induced liver injury by enhancing the cellular defense system and lowering inflammatory response. Activation of Nrf2/ARE pathway-mediated cytoprotective proteins by quercitrin may contribute to neutralizing ROS, eliminating toxicants and finally preventing cell death and liver necrosis. Quercitrin also exhibits anti-inflammatory properties through the inhibition of pro-inflammatory mediators including iNOS and COX-2 as well as a cytokine IL-1β in APAP-caused inflammation. Furthermore, the suppression of JNK phosphorylation by quercitrin was identified as a protective mechanism against apoptosis. Our study revealed that quercitrin may have safe therapeutic potential in protecting cell/liver from APAP toxicity.

Acknowledgments: This research was supported by Basic Science Research Program through the National Research Foundation of Korea (NRF) funded by the Ministry of Science, ICT and Future Planning (NRF-2014R1A2A1A11050006).

Author Contributions: Woo-Sik Jeong designed the study and revised the manuscript, Van-Long Truong and Se-Yeon Ko contributed equally to this work, performed experiments and prepared the manuscript, Mira Jun analyzed data.

Abbreviations

The following abbreviations are used in this manuscript:

APAP	Acetaminophen
ALT	Alanine transaminase
ARE	Antioxidant response element
AST	Aspartate aminotransferase
CAT	Catalase
COX-2	Cyclooxygenase-2
CYP	Cytochrome P450
ERK	Extracellular signal regulated kinase
GSH	Glutathione
GPx	Glutathione peroxidase
iNOS	Inducible nitric oxide synthase
JNK	c-Jun N-terminal kinase
Keap 1	Kelch-like ECH-associated protein 1
MAPK	Mitogen activated protein kinase
NAC	*N*-acetylcysteine
NQO1	NADPH:quinone oxidoreductase 1
Nrf2	Nuclear factor erythroid-2-related factor-2
ROS	Reactive oxygen species
SOD	Superoxide dismutase

References

1. Slitt, A.M.L.; Dominick, P.K.; Roberts, J.C.; Cohen, S.D. Effect of ribose cysteine pretreatment on hepatic and renal acetaminophen metabolite formation and glutathione depletion. *Basic Clin. Pharmacol. Toxicol.* **2005**, *96*, 487–494. [CrossRef] [PubMed]
2. Song, E.; Fu, J.; Xia, X.; Su, C.; Song, Y. Bazhen decoction protects against acetaminophen induced acute liver injury by inhibiting oxidative stress, inflammation and apoptosis in mice. *PLoS ONE* **2014**, *9*, e107405. [CrossRef] [PubMed]
3. Noh, J.-R.; Kim, Y.-H.; Hwang, J.H.; Choi, D.-H.; Kim, K.-S.; Oh, W.-K.; Lee, C.-H. Sulforaphane protects against acetaminophen-induced hepatotoxicity. *Food Chem. Toxicol.* **2015**, *80*, 193–200. [CrossRef] [PubMed]
4. Jaeschke, H.; Williams, C.D.; Ramachandran, A.; Bajt, M.L. Acetaminophen hepatotoxicity and repair: The role of sterile inflammation and innate immunity. *Liver Int.* **2012**, *32*, 8–20. [CrossRef] [PubMed]
5. Buckley, N.A.; Whyte, I.M.; O'Connell, D.L.; Dawson, A.H. Oral or intravenous *N*-acetylcysteine: Which is the treatment of choice for acetaminophen (paracetamol) poisoning? *J. Toxicol. Clin. Toxicol.* **1999**, *37*, 759–767. [CrossRef] [PubMed]

6. Flanagan, R.J.; Meredith, T.J. Use of *N*-acetylcysteine in clinical toxicology. *Am. J. Med.* **1991**, *91*, 131S–139S. [CrossRef]
7. Heard, K.J. Acetylcysteine for acetaminophen poisoning. *N. Engl. J. Med.* **2008**, *359*, 285–292. [CrossRef] [PubMed]
8. Sandilands, E.A.; Bateman, D.N. Adverse reactions associated with acetylcysteine. *Clin. Toxicol.* **2009**, *47*, 81–88. [CrossRef] [PubMed]
9. Bak, M.-J.; Jeong, J.-H.; Kang, H.-S.; Jin, K.-S.; Jun, M.; Jeong, W.-S. Stimulation of activity and expression of antioxidant enzymes by solvent fractions and isolated compound from *Cedrela sinensis* leaves in HepG2 cells. *J. Med. Food* **2011**, *14*, 405–412. [CrossRef] [PubMed]
10. Chia, Y.-C.; Rajbanshi, R.; Calhoun, C.; Chiu, R.H. Anti-neoplastic effects of gallic acid, a major component of *Toona sinensis* leaf extract, on oral squamous carcinoma cells. *Molecules* **2010**, *15*, 8377–8389. [CrossRef] [PubMed]
11. Hsiang, C.-Y.; Hseu, Y.-C.; Chang, Y.-C.; Kumar, K.J.S.; Ho, T.-Y.; Yang, H.-L. *Toona sinensis* and its major bioactive compound gallic acid inhibit LPS-induced inflammation in nuclear factor-κB transgenic mice as evaluated byin vivo bioluminescence imaging. *Food Chem.* **2013**, *136*, 426–434. [CrossRef] [PubMed]
12. Su, Y.-F.; Yang, Y.-C.; Hsu, H.-K.; Hwang, S.-L.; Lee, K.-S.; Lieu, A.-S.; Chan, T.-F.; Lin, C.-L. *Toona sinensis* leaf extract has antinociceptive effect comparable with non-steroidal anti-inflammatory agents in mouse writhing test. *BMC Complement. Altern. Med.* **2015**, *15*, 70. [CrossRef] [PubMed]
13. Da Silva, E.R.; Maquiaveli, C.D.C.; Magalhães, P.P. The leishmanicidal flavonols quercetin and quercitrin target *Leishmania* (*Leishmania*) *amazonensis* arginase. *Exp. Parasitol.* **2012**, *130*, 183–188. [CrossRef] [PubMed]
14. Wagner, C.; Fachinetto, R.; Dalla Corte, C.L.; Brito, V.B.; Severo, D.; de Oliveira Costa Dias, G.; Morel, A.F.; Nogueira, C.W.; Rocha, J.B.T. Quercitrin, a glycoside form of quercetin, prevents lipid peroxidation in vitro. *Brain Res.* **2006**, *1107*, 192–198. [CrossRef] [PubMed]
15. Ader, P.; Blöck, M.; Pietzsch, S.; Wolffram, S. Interaction of quercetin glucosides with the intestinal sodium/glucose co-transporter (SGLT-1). *Cancer Lett.* **2001**, *162*, 175–180. [CrossRef]
16. Gee, J.M.; DuPont, M.S.; Rhodes, M.J.C.; Johnson, I.T. Quercetin glucosides interact with the intestinal glucose transport pathway 1. *Free Radic. Biol. Med.* **1998**, *25*, 19–25. [CrossRef]
17. Babujanarthanam, R.; Kavitha, P.; Mahadeva Rao, U.S.; Pandian, M. Quercitrin a bioflavonoid improves the antioxidant status in streptozotocin: Induced diabetic rat tissues. *Mol. Cell. Biochem.* **2011**, *358*, 121–129. [CrossRef] [PubMed]
18. Ham, Y.-M.; Yoon, W.-J.; Park, S.-Y.; Song, G.-P.; Jung, Y.-H.; Jeon, Y.-J.; Kang, S.-M.; Kim, K.-N. Quercitrin protects against oxidative stress-induced injury in lung fibroblast cells via up-regulation of Bcl-xl. *J. Funct. Foods* **2012**, *4*, 253–262. [CrossRef]
19. Camuesco, D.; Comalada, M.; Rodríguez-Cabezas, M.E.; Nieto, A.; Lorente, M.D.; Concha, A.; Zarzuelo, A.; Gálvez, J. The intestinal anti-inflammatory effect of quercitrin is associated with an inhibition in iNOS expression. *Br. J. Pharmacol.* **2004**, *143*, 908–918. [CrossRef] [PubMed]
20. Choi, S.-J.; Tai, B.; Cuong, N.; Kim, Y.-H.; Jang, H.-D. Antioxidative and anti-inflammatory effect of quercetin and its glycosides isolated from mampat (*Cratoxylum formosum*). *Food Sci. Biotechnol.* **2012**, *21*, 587–595. [CrossRef]
21. Cruz, E.A.; Da-Silva, S.A.G.; Muzitano, M.F.; Silva, P.M.R.; Costa, S.S.; Rossi-Bergmann, B. Immunomodulatory pretreatment with *Kalanchoe pinnata* extract and its quercitrin flavonoid effectively protects mice against fatal anaphylactic shock. *Int. Immunopharmacol.* **2008**, *8*, 1616–1621. [CrossRef] [PubMed]
22. Yang, H.-M.; Ham, Y.-M.; Yoon, W.-J.; Roh, S.W.; Jeon, Y.-J.; Oda, T.; Kang, S.-M.; Kang, M.-C.; Kim, E.-A.; Kim, D.; et al. Quercitrin protects against ultraviolet B-induced cell death in vitro and in anin vivo zebrafish model. *J. Photochem. Photobiol. B* **2012**, *114*, 126–131. [CrossRef] [PubMed]
23. Yin, Y.; Li, W.; Son, Y.-O.; Sun, L.; Lu, J.; Kim, D.; Wang, X.; Yao, H.; Wang, L.; Pratheeshkumar, P.; et al. Quercitrin protects skin from UVB-induced oxidative damage. *Toxicol. Appl. Pharmacol.* **2013**, *269*, 89–99. [CrossRef] [PubMed]
24. Cincin, Z.B.; Unlu, M.; Kiran, B.; Bireller, E.S.; Baran, Y.; Cakmakoglu, B. Molecular mechanisms of quercitrin-induced apoptosis in non-small cell lung cancer. *Arch. Med. Res.* **2014**, *45*, 445–454. [CrossRef] [PubMed]

25. Yu, R.; Chen, C.; Mo, Y.-Y.; Hebbar, V.; Owuor, E.D.; Tan, T.-H.; Kong, A.-N.T. Activation of mitogen-activated protein kinase pathways induces antioxidant response element-mediated gene expression via a Nrf2-dependent mechanism. *J. Biol. Chem.* **2000**, *275*, 39907–39913. [CrossRef] [PubMed]
26. Bektur, N.E.; Sahin, E.; Baycu, C.; Unver, G. Protective effects of silymarin against acetaminophen-induced hepatotoxicity and nephrotoxicity in mice. *Toxicol. Ind. Health* **2016**, *32*, 589–600. [CrossRef] [PubMed]
27. Aebi, H. Catalase in vitro. *Methods Enzymol.* **1984**, *105*, 121–126. [PubMed]
28. Bogdanska, J.J.; Korneti, P.; Todorova, B. Erythrocyte superoxide dismutase, glutathione peroxidase and catalase activities in healthy male subjects in republic of macedonia. *Bratisl. Lek. Listy* **2003**, *104*, 108–114. [PubMed]
29. Oyanagui, Y. Reevaluation of assay methods and establishment of kit for superoxide dismutase activity. *Anal. Biochem.* **1984**, *142*, 290–296. [CrossRef]
30. Hybertson, B.M.; Gao, B.; Bose, S.K.; McCord, J.M. Oxidative stress in health and disease: The therapeutic potential of Nrf2 activation. *Mol. Aspects Med.* **2011**, *32*, 234–246. [CrossRef] [PubMed]
31. Lessig, J.; Fuchs, B. Plasmalogens in biological systems: Their role in oxidative processes in biological membranes, their contribution to pathological processes and aging and plasmalogen analysis. *Curr. Med. Chem.* **2009**, *16*, 2021–2041. [CrossRef] [PubMed]
32. Mena, S.; Ortega, A.; Estrela, J.M. Oxidative stress in environmental-induced carcinogenesis. *Mutat. Res.* **2009**, *674*, 36–44. [CrossRef] [PubMed]
33. Valko, M.; Leibfritz, D.; Moncol, J.; Cronin, M.T.D.; Mazur, M.; Telser, J. Free radicals and antioxidants in normal physiological functions and human disease. *Int. J. Biochem. Cell Biol.* **2007**, *39*, 44–84. [CrossRef] [PubMed]
34. Jaeschke, H.; McGill, M.R.; Williams, C.D.; Ramachandran, A. Current issues with acetaminophen hepatotoxicity—A clinically relevant model to test the efficacy of natural products. *Life Sci.* **2011**, *88*, 737–745. [CrossRef] [PubMed]
35. McGill, M.R.; Williams, C.D.; Xie, Y.; Ramachandran, A.; Jaeschke, H. Acetaminophen-induced liver injury in rats and mice: Comparison of protein adducts, mitochondrial dysfunction, and oxidative stress in the mechanism of toxicity. *Toxicol. Appl. Pharmacol.* **2012**, *264*, 387–394. [CrossRef] [PubMed]
36. Enomoto, A.; Itoh, K.; Nagayoshi, E.; Haruta, J.; Kimura, T.; O'Connor, T.; Harada, T.; Yamamoto, M. High sensitivity of Nrf2 knockout mice to acetaminophen hepatotoxicity associated with decreased expression of ARE-regulated drug metabolizing enzymes and antioxidant genes. *Toxicol. Sci.* **2001**, *59*, 169–177. [CrossRef] [PubMed]
37. Chan, K.; Han, X.-D.; Kan, Y.W. An important function of Nrf2 in combating oxidative stress: Detoxification of acetaminophen. *Proc. Natl. Acad. Sci. USA* **2001**, *98*, 4611–4616. [CrossRef] [PubMed]
38. Aleksunes, L.M.; Manautou, J.E. Emerging role of Nrf2 in protecting against hepatic and gastrointestinal disease. *Toxicol. Pathol.* **2007**, *35*, 459–473. [CrossRef] [PubMed]
39. Okawa, H.; Motohashi, H.; Kobayashi, A.; Aburatani, H.; Kensler, T.W.; Yamamoto, M. Hepatocyte-specific deletion of the *keap1* gene activates Nrf2 and confers potent resistance against acute drug toxicity. *Biochem. Biophys. Res. Commun.* **2006**, *339*, 79–88. [CrossRef] [PubMed]
40. Hwang, J.; Kim, Y.-H.; Noh, J.-R.; Gang, G.-T.; Kim, K.-S.; Chung, H.; Tadi, S.; Yim, Y.-H.; Shong, M.; Lee, C.-H. The protective role of NAD(P)H:Quinone oxidoreductase 1 on acetaminophen-induced liver injury is associated with prevention of adenosine triphosphate depletion and improvement of mitochondrial dysfunction. *Arch. Toxicol.* **2015**, *89*, 2159–2166. [CrossRef] [PubMed]
41. Moffit, J.S.; Aleksunes, L.M.; Kardas, M.J.; Slitt, A.L.; Klaassen, C.D.; Manautou, J.E. Role of NAD(P)H:Quinone oxidoreductase 1 in clofibrate-mediated hepatoprotection from acetaminophen. *Toxicology* **2007**, *230*, 197–206. [CrossRef] [PubMed]
42. Lu, H.; Ouyang, W.; Huang, C. Inflammation, a key event in cancer development. *Mol. Cancer Res.* **2006**, *4*, 221–233. [CrossRef] [PubMed]
43. Reddy, S.A.; Shelar, S.B.; Dang, T.-M.; Lee, B.N.-C.; Yang, H.; Ong, S.-M.; Ng, H.-L.; Chui, W.-K.; Wong, S.-C.; Chew, E.-H. Sulforaphane and its methylcarbonyl analogs inhibit the LPS-stimulated inflammatory response in human monocytes through modulating cytokine production, suppressing chemotactic migration and phagocytosis in a NF-κB- and MAPK-dependent manner. *Int. Immunopharmacol.* **2015**, *24*, 440–450. [CrossRef] [PubMed]

44. Chung, H.Y.; Cesari, M.; Anton, S.; Marzetti, E.; Giovannini, S.; Seo, A.Y.; Carter, C.; Yu, B.P.; Leeuwenburgh, C. Molecular inflammation: Underpinnings of aging and age-related diseases. *Ageing Res. Rev.* **2009**, *8*, 18–30. [CrossRef] [PubMed]
45. Dragomir, A.-C.; Sun, R.; Mishin, V.; Hall, L.B.; Laskin, J.D.; Laskin, D.L. Role of galectin-3 in acetaminophen-induced hepatotoxicity and inflammatory mediator production. *Toxicol. Sci.* **2012**, *127*, 609–619. [CrossRef] [PubMed]
46. Hong, S.-W.; Lee, H.-S.; Jung, K.; Lee, H.; Hong, S.-S. Protective effect of fucoidan against acetaminophen-induced liver injury. *Arch. Pharm. Res.* **2012**, *35*, 1099–1105. [CrossRef] [PubMed]
47. Tai, M.; Zhang, J.; Song, S.; Miao, R.; Liu, S.; Pang, Q.; Wu, Q.; Liu, C. Protective effects of luteolin against acetaminophen-induced acute liver failure in mouse. *Int. Immunopharmacol.* **2015**, *27*, 164–170. [CrossRef] [PubMed]
48. Williams, C.D.; Farhood, A.; Jaeschke, H. Role of caspase-1 and interleukin-1β in acetaminophen-induced hepatic inflammation and liver injury. *Toxicol. Appl. Pharmacol.* **2010**, *247*, 169–178. [CrossRef] [PubMed]
49. Chen, C.; Kong, A.-N.T. Dietary cancer-chemopreventive compounds: From signaling and gene expression to pharmacological effects. *Trends Pharmacol. Sci.* **2005**, *26*, 318–326. [CrossRef] [PubMed]
50. Kim, E.K.; Choi, E.-J. Pathological roles of MAPK signaling pathways in human diseases. *Biochim. Biophys. Acta* **2010**, *1802*, 396–405. [CrossRef] [PubMed]
51. Hanawa, N.; Shinohara, M.; Saberi, B.; Gaarde, W.A.; Han, D.; Kaplowitz, N. Role of JNK translocation to mitochondria leading to inhibition of mitochondria bioenergetics in acetaminophen-induced liver injury. *J. Biol. Chem.* **2008**, *283*, 13565–13577. [CrossRef] [PubMed]
52. Gunawan, B.K.; Liu, Z.X.; Han, D.; Hanawa, N.; Gaarde, W.A.; Kaplowitz, N. C-jun n-terminal kinase plays a major role in murine acetaminophen hepatotoxicity. *Gastroenterology* **2006**, *131*, 165–178. [CrossRef] [PubMed]
53. Saito, C.; Lemasters, J.J.; Jaeschke, H. C-jun n-terminal kinase modulates oxidant stress and peroxynitrite formation independent of inducible nitric oxide synthase in acetaminophen hepatotoxicity. *Toxicol. Appl. Pharmacol.* **2010**, *246*, 8–17. [CrossRef] [PubMed]
54. Henderson, N.C.; Pollock, K.J.; Frew, J.; Mackinnon, A.C.; Flavell, R.A.; Davis, R.J.; Sethi, T.; Simpson, K.J. Critical role of c-jun (NH2) terminal kinase in paracetamol-induced acute liver failure. *Gut* **2007**, *56*, 982–990. [CrossRef] [PubMed]

8

Food Matrix Effects of Polyphenol Bioaccessibility from Almond Skin during Simulated Human Digestion

Giuseppina Mandalari [1,2,*], Maria Vardakou [2], Richard Faulks [2], Carlo Bisignano [1], Maria Martorana [1], Antonella Smeriglio [1] and Domenico Trombetta [1]

[1] Dipartimento di Scienze Chimiche, Biologiche, Farmaceutiche ed Ambientali, University of Messina, Sal. Sperone 31, 98166 Messina, Italy; cbisignano@unime.it (C.B.); mmartorana@live.it (M.M.); asmeriglio@unime.it (A.S.); dtrombetta@unime.it (D.T.)

[2] The Model Gut, Institute of Food Research, Norwich Research Park, Colney Lane, Norwich NR4 7UA, UK; M.Vardakou@uea.ac.uk (M.V.); r.faulks147@btinternet.com (R.F.)

* Correspondence: gmandalari@unime.it

Abstract: The goal of the present study was to quantify the rate and extent of polyphenols released in the gastrointestinal tract (GIT) from natural (NS) and blanched (BS) almond skins. A dynamic gastric model of digestion which provides a realistic simulation of the human stomach was used. In order to establish the effect of a food matrix on polyphenols bioaccessibility, NS and BS were either digested in water (WT) or incorporated into home-made biscuits (HB), crisp-bread (CB) and full-fat milk (FM). Phenolic acids were the most bioaccessible class (68.5% release from NS and 64.7% from BS). WT increased the release of flavan-3-ols ($p < 0.05$) and flavonols ($p < 0.05$) from NS after gastric plus duodenal digestion, whereas CB and HB were better vehicles for BS. FM lowered the % recovery of polyphenols, the free total phenols and the antioxidant status in the digestion medium, indicating that phenolic compounds could bind protein present in the food matrix. The release of bioactives from almond skins could explain the beneficial effects associated with almond consumption.

Keywords: almond skin; food matrix; simulated human digestion; polyphenols; bioaccessibility

---

1. Introduction

The presence of polyphenols in almond skin has been related to several health benefits associated with almond (Prunus dulcis Miller D.A. Webb) consumption [1–3]. The antioxidant and free-radical scavenging activity of almond skin polyphenols has been reported [4]. It has been shown that flavonoids and phenolic acids, including flavonols, flavanols, flavanones and simple phenolic acids identified in almond skins may play a role in reducing risk factors against chronic inflammatory diseases and ageing disorders [5,6]. A range of biological effects of flavonoids, including anticancer, antiviral, antimutagenic and anti-inflammatory activities, have been reported [7,8]. Nevertheless, one of the major limiting factors affecting the beneficial effects of polyphenols is their bioaccessibility and subsequent absorption in the gastrointestinal tract (GIT), together with their bio-transformation by the gut microbiota enzymes [9].

This process depends on the physico-chemical properties of the food matrix and its changes during digestion. We refer to bioaccessibility as the proportion of a nutrient or phytochemical compound 'released' from a complex food matrix during digestion and therefore becoming potentially available for absorption in the GIT. A number of studies have reported that food matrix affects polyphenol release in the gut as well as the efficacy by which they are transported across the mucosal epithelium [10,11]. The presence of a food matrix (muffin) decreased the bioaccessibility of certain bioactive compounds, such as protocatechuic acid and luteolin, from raw shelled and roasted salted pistachios during simulated human digestion [12]. Interaction with other food nutrients and the formation of complexes mainly with protein and fat is also known to affect bioaccessibility of phenolic acids [13]. The influence of digestion conditions, such as pH, temperature, bile salts, gastric and pancreatic enzymes on the bioaccessibility of certain polyphenols has been reported [14,15]. Milk has been found to affect bioaccessibility of epicatechin metabolites [16]. We have previously identified a combination of flavonols, flavan-3-ols, hydroxybenzoic acids and flavanones present in almond skin [1]: the major flavonoids were (+)-catechin, (−)-epicatechin, kaempferol and isorhamnetin, both as aglycones or conjugated with rhamnose (Rha) and glucose (Glc). The total phenolic content, expressed as mg gallic acid equivalents (GAE) per 100 g of fresh skin, was higher in natural almond skin (NS, 3474.1 ± 239.8) than blanched almond skin (BS, 278.9 ± 12.0). The blanching process is known to remove most of the water-soluble flavonoids and other polyphenols [1]. BS, obtained by industrial blanching, currently represents a commercially available product. Our previous investigation on the release of almond skin polyphenols during simulated human digestion using a static model demonstrated higher percentages of polyphenols released from NS compared to BS [17].

The aim of the present study was to assess the effect of a range of food matrices on the rate and extent of polyphenol bioaccessibility from NS and BS during simulated human digestion. A dynamic gastric model (DGM) was used to simulate the human stomach [12,18]. Gastric digesta were then subjected to a duodenal phase in order to simulate the full human upper GIT.

2. Materials and Methods

2.1. Production of Test Meals

Natural almonds with intact skin were kindly provided by the Almond Board of California and stored in the dark. NS was removed using liquid-nitrogen as previously reported and milled [17]. BS, provided by ABCO laboratories, was obtained by hot water blanching, dried and powdered. Home-made biscuits (HB) containing NS or BS were prepared using the following ingredients: white flour (200 g), butter at room temperature (100 g), sugar (sucrose, 100 g), eggs (one standard egg) and baked at 180 °C for 12 min. For the digestion experiments, 25 g of HB containing 2 g of either NS or BS were used. Home-made crisp-bread (CB) containing NS or BS was prepared using the following ingredients: baking soda (5 g), hot water (400 mL), salt (1.2 g), fennel seed (1 g), white flour (250 g) and baked at 230 °C for 2–4 min. For the digestion experiments, 34 g of CB containing 2 g of either NS or BS were used.

2.2. Chemicals and Enzymes

Egg *L*-α-phosphatidylcholine (PC, lecithin grade 1, 99% purity) was obtained from Lipid Products (South Nutfield, Surrey, UK). Porcine gastric mucosa pepsin, bovine α-chymotrypsin, pancreatic α-amylase, porcine colipase, porcine pancreatic lipase and bile salts were obtained from Sigma (Poole, Dorset, UK). Lipase for the gastric phase of digestion was a gastric lipase analogue of fungal origin (F-AP15) from Amano Enzyme Inc. (Nagoya, Japan). All flavonoid and other phytochemical standards were obtained from either Sigma-Aldrich (Poole, UK) or Extrasynthese (Genay, France). All solvents were HPLC grade, water was ultra-pure grade, and other chemicals were of AR quality.

2.3. Simulated Human Digestion

Eight meals were prepared as follows and subjected to in vitro gastric and gastric plus duodenal digestion: WT (200 mL) containing either NS (2 g) or BS (2 g), HB (25 g) containing either NS (2 g) or BS (2 g) added to water (240 mL), CB (34 g) containing either NS (2 g) or BS (2 g) added to water (240 mL), FM (200 mL) containing either NS (2 g) or BS (2 g).

2.4. Gastric Digestion

Individual meals were fed onto the DGM in the presence of priming acid (20 mL), as previously reported [18]. In order to replicate the conditions found in the human stomach, samples were processed in two zones: within the fundus/main body of the DGM, where the meals were subjected to inhomogeneous mixing while gastric acid and enzyme secretions were added; in the antrum, where physiological shear and grinding forces were applied in order to mimic the antral shearing and rate of delivery to the duodenum. The composition of the simulated gastric acid solution has also been previously reported [12]. The simulated gastric enzyme solution was prepared by dissolving porcine gastric mucosa pepsin and a gastric lipase analogue from *Rhizopus oryzae* in the above described salt mixture (no acid) at a final concentration of 9000 U/mL and 60 U/mL for pepsin and lipase, respectively. A suspension of single-shelled lecithin liposomes was added to the gastric enzyme solution at a final concentration of 0.127 mM.

A total of six samples (G1–G6) were ejected from the antrum of the DGM at regular intervals during each run (see Table 1 for sampling details) in order to replicate the predicted gastric emptying regimes under physiological conditions. Samples digested in WT were ejected from the antrum of the DGM every 4 min: the amount of gastric acid secretion was 1.5 ± 0.1 mL and 1.6 ± 0.1 mL for NS and BS respectively; the amount of gastric enzyme secretion was 2.8 ± 0.1 mL and 2.7 ± 0.1 mL for NS and BS respectively. Samples digested in HB were ejected from the antrum of the DGM every 4 min: the amount of gastric acid secretion was 6.4 ± 0.1 mL and 6.3 ± 0.1 mL for NS and BS respectively; the amount of gastric enzyme secretion was 11.2 ± 0.2 mL and 11.4 ± 0.1 mL for NS and BS respectively. Samples digested in CB were ejected from the antrum of the DGM every 5 min: the amount of gastric acid secretion was 17.6 ± 0.2 mL and 18.2 ± 0.2 mL for NS and BS respectively; the amount of gastric enzyme secretion was 13.8 ± 0.1 mL and 14.2 ± 0.2 mL for NS and BS respectively. Samples digested in FM were ejected from the antrum of the DGM every 6 min: the amount of gastric acid secretion was 4.4 ± 0.2 mL and 4.6 ± 0.2 mL for NS and BS respectively; the amount of gastric enzyme secretion was 13.1 ± 0.3 mL and 13.8 ± 0.2 mL for NS and BS respectively. A control digestion without addition of gastric enzymes was performed for each meal. Each gastric sample was weighed, its pH recorded and adjusted to 7.0 with NaOH (1 M) in order to inhibit gastric enzyme activity.

Table 1. Simulated human digestion parameters.

Matrix	DGM 1	DGM 2	DGM 3	DGM 4	DGM 5	DGM 6	DD	TDT
	Sampling Time (min)							
Water	4	8	12	16	20	24	120	144
Home-made biscuit	4	8	12	16	20	24	120	144
Crisp bread	5	10	15	20	25	30	120	150
Full-fat milk	6	12	18	24	30	36	120	156

DGM = Gastric sample; DD = Duodenal digestion; TDT = Total digestion time.

2.5. Duodenal Digestion

Individual gastric samples (23 g, G1 to G6) were transferred upon ejection, to a Sterilin plastic tube for duodenal digestion with the addition of simulated bile solution (2.5 mL) and pancreatic enzyme solution (7.0 mL) and incubated at 37 °C under shaking conditions (170 rpm) for 2 h. Simulated bile was prepared fresh daily. It contained lecithin (6.5 mM), cholesterol (4 mM), sodium taurocholate (12.5 mM), and sodium glycodeoxycholate (12.5 mM) in a solution containing NaCl (146.0 mM), CaCl2 (2.6 mM) and KCl (4.8 mM).

Pancreatic enzyme solution contained NaCl (125.0 mM), $CaCl_2$ (0.6 mM), $MgCl_2$ (0.3 mM), and $ZnSO_4 \cdot 7H_2O$ (4.1 μM). Porcine pancreatic lipase (590 U/mL), porcine colipase (3.2 μg/mL), porcine trypsin (11 U/mL), bovine α-chymotrypsin (24 U/mL) and porcine α-amylase (300 U/mL) were added to the pancreatic solution.

2.6. Poliphenols Extraction from Samples before and after Dynamic in Vitro Digestion

All original samples (WT, HB, CB and FM containing NS or BS) and aliquotes obtained from each sample subjected to a dynamic in vitro gastric digestion (NSWT G, NSHB G, NSCB G, NSFM G, BSWT G, BSHB G, BSCB G, BSFM G) and gastric plus duodenal digestion (NSWT G + D, NSHB G + D, NSCB G + D, NSFM G + D, BSWT G + D, BSHB G + D, BSCB G + D, BSFM G + D), were harvested and centrifuged to separate the residual material from the supernatant. The volume of each supernatant was measured; the residues were dried in a forced air heated oven (T °C < 40 °C) and brought to constant weight.

Each residue was extracted with hexane (1:5, w/v) to remove the lipid fraction. The procedure was repeated 3 times. Afterwards it was extracted with a methanol/water mixture (70:30) (1:10, w/v) by shaking for 5 min and sonicating for 10 min. After centrifugation at 12,074 rcf for 10 min, the supernatant was collected. The procedure was repeated 3 times. The supernatants were pooled. In order to precipitate proteins, MeOH (8 mL) and 2M NaOH (600 μL) were added in 10 mL extract. Samples were stirred vigorously and after centrifugation at 5916 rcf for 5 min the supernatant was brought to dryness in a rotavapor. Finally, the residue was resuspended with 10 mL of 1% HCl in MeOH and extracted, using a separatory funnel, with the same volume of ethyl acetate. The extraction was repeated 4 times. The ethyl acetate fractions were combined and evaporated to dryness in a rotavapor. The residue was weighed, solubilised in MeOH, filtered through a Nalgene 0.22 μM nylon filter and subjected to total phenol, radical scavenging activity and HPLC analysis.

For NS and BS digested in water no protein precipitation step was perfermed, given that they were not incorporated into any food matrix.

2.7. Polyphenols Release and Radical Scavenging Activity

Total phenol content was determined colorimetrically by the Folin-Ciocalteu method as modified by Singleton, Orthofer and Lamuela-Raventos [19] using gallic acid as a reference compound. Total phenol content was expressed as mg of gallic acid equivalents (GAE) per 100 g of sample. The anti-radical activity was determined using the stable 2,2-diphenyl-1-picrylhydrazyl radical (DPPH) and the procedure previously described [20]. Results were expressed as mg of extract needed to scavenge 50 μmol of the initial DPPH concentration (SE50). The determination of phenolics and flavonoids was carried out using a Shimadzu high performance liquid chromatography system equipped with an UV–Vis photodiode-array detector (DAD) (SPD-M10AVP, Shimadzu, Kyoto, Japan) and a fluorescence detector (1046A Hewlett Packard, Palo Alto, CA, USA), as previously reported [17].

2.8. Statistical Analysis

All assays were performed in triplicate and expressed as means ± standard deviation (SD). Data analysis was performed using ANOVA tests using SigmaPlot software version 12.0 for Windows (SPSS Inc., Hong Kong, China). To isolate the group or groups that differ from the others, a multiple comparison procedure (*Tukey* Test) was used. Results were considered statistically significant at $p < 0.05$.

3. Results

3.1. Polyphenols Release during Simulated Digestion

The polyphenolic content of the baseline meals (NS WT, NS HB, NS CB and NS FM, BS WT, BS HB, BS CB and BS FM) is reported in Table 2. As expected, the NS meals had a total phenol content nearly ten times higher than the BS meals.

The release of polyphenols as a percentage of the original amount present in each meal (Table 2) after simulated gastric plus duodenal digestion is reported in Figure 1. No polyphenols were detected in blank samples of each meal not containing almond skin. As expected, a high release of bioactive compounds was observed from both NS and BS in WT (Figure 1A).

Table 2. Baseline polyphenols content of natural skins and blanched skins in water (W); home-made biscuits (HB); crisp-bread (CB) and full-fat milk (FM). Values were given as μg/g and represent averages (±SD) of triplicate measurements.

Natural Skin					
Sample	Phenolic acids	Flavonols	Flavan-3-ols	Flavanones	Total phenols
W	2.15 ± 0.11	14.31 ± 1.05	2.37 ± 0.18	3.43 ± 0.22	22.26
HB	17.85 ± 1.02	115.30 ± 8.32	20.82 ± 1.65	30.44 ± 2.21	184.41
CB	12.53 ± 0.89	83.89 ± 4.22	14.72 ± 1.12	21.78 ± 1.44	132.92
FM	2.07 ± 0.12	13.95 ± 1.22	2.15 ± 0.12	3.22 ± 0.17	21.39
Blanched Skin					
Sample	Phenolic acids	Flavonols	Flavan-3-ols	Flavanones	Total phenols
W	0.31 ± 0.02	1.28 ± 0.05	0.62 ± 0.03	0.22 ± 0.02	2.43
HB	2.25 ± 0.14	9.82 ± 0.59	5.18 ± 0.21	1.73 ± 0.102	18.98
CB	1.78 ± 0.12	7.24 ± 0.35	3.65 ± 0.25	1.31 ± 0.09	13.98
FM	0.29 ± 0.01	1.19 ± 0.08	0.60 ± 0.02	0.19 ± 0.01	2. 27

The % release from NS and BS in WT during the gastric phase of digestion was higher for phenolic acids (47.1% from NS and 45.3% from BS) compared with the other classes of polyphenols, with a further increase in the duodenal phase of digestion (68.5% from NS and 64.7% from BS). Lower % release from BS in WT was observed with flavanones after both gastric (29.3%) and gastric plus duodenal incubation (48.2%). Higher release of flavonols (65.6%) and phenolic acids (59.4%) was observed after in vitro gastric plus duodenal digestion from NS (Figure 1A). The % of recovery, calculated from the amount of polyphenols present in the medium at the end of each step of digestion, confirmed the data obtained from the % of release (Figure 2). This data demonstrated a different bioaccessibility across the various classes of polyphenols in the absence of an interfering food matrix. In accordance with our previous investigation [1], high release of polyphenols was detected when NS and BS were incubated in WT. However, the static and dynamic digestion models used affected the rate and extent of bioactives potentially available for absorption in the gut.

The % of release and recovery of polyphenols from NS and BS incorporated into HB are reported in Figures 1B and 2, respectively. Phenolic acids were the class of polyphenols mostly released from NS in the gastric phase, followed by flavonols and flavanones, with an average % release of 40.72 in the gastric compartment. Flavonols had the highest % release from BS in the gastric phase (48.5), followed by flavanones and phenolic acids. For both NS and BS, the gastric + duodenal digestion (G + D) produced only a slight increase in polyphenol release over that observed in the gastric compartment. In addition, higher percentages of phenolic acids and flavonols were released from NSHB G + D.

Higher % of release of phenolic acids, flavonols, flavan-3-ols and flavanones were observed in BSCB G compared with NSCB G, whereas the opposite behaviour was detected in the duodenal phase (Figure 1C). A higher release of phenolic acids was observed in BSCB G (52.7%) compared with BSWT G (45.3%), as well as flavonols both in the gastric (51.4 in BSCB G vs. 33.9 in BSWT G) and in the duodenal phase (63.9 in BSCB G + D vs. 52.3 in BSWT G + D) and flavanones both in the gastric (47.6 in BSCB G vs. 29.3 in BSWT G) and in the duodenal phase (59.8 in BSCB G + D vs. 48.2 in BSWT G + D). The % release data were confirmed by % recovery values (Figure 2).

The % of release and recovery of flavonoids and phenolic acids from NS and BS incorporated into FM are reported in Figures 1D and 2, respectively. The highest % release from NS was detected with flavonols after gastric plus duodenal digestion, followed by flavanones and phenolic acids. About 60% of phenolic acids and flavanones were released from BS in FM after simulated digestion.

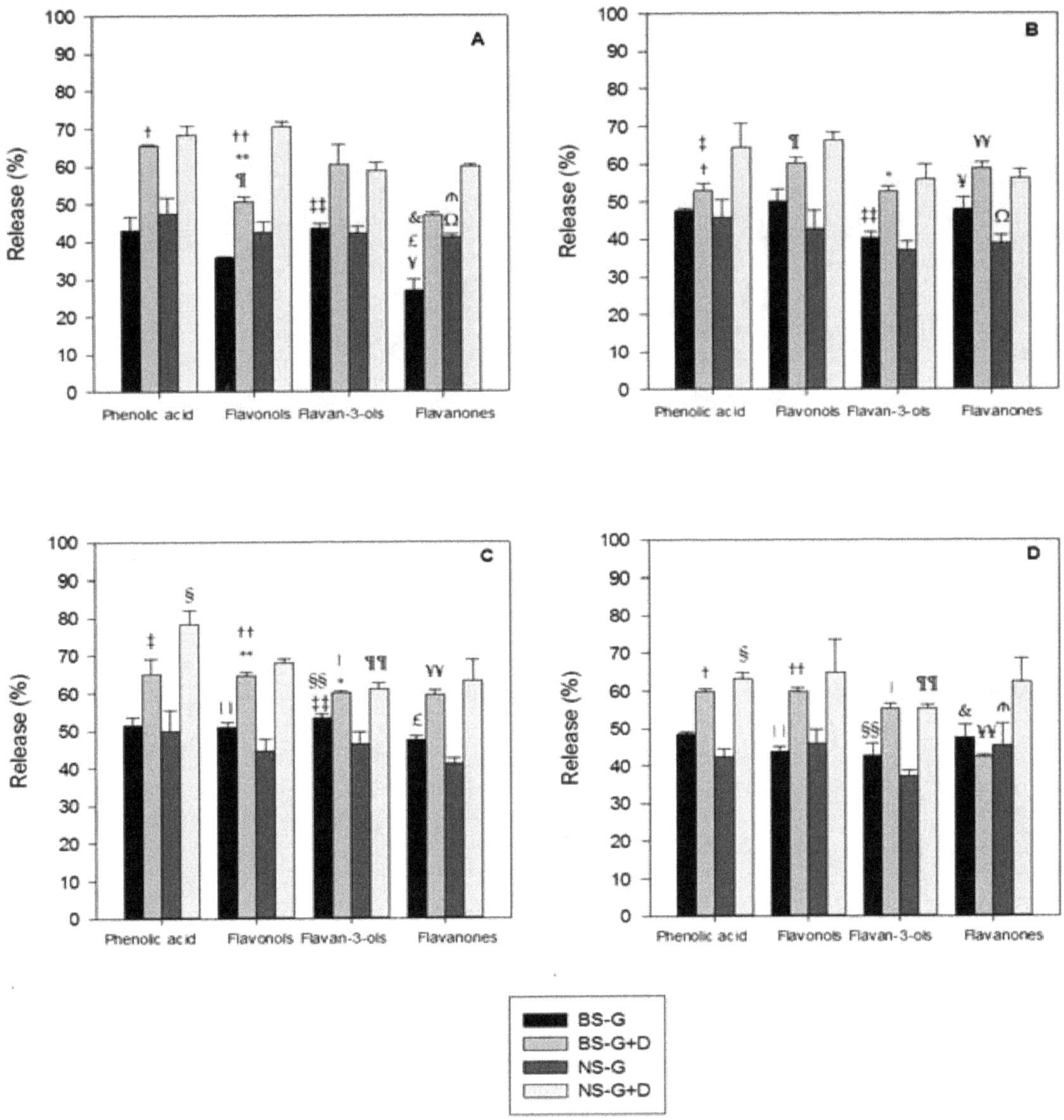

Figure 1. Release of flavonoids and phenolic acids from natural almond skin (NS) and blanched almond skin (BS) in water (**A**); home-made biscuits (**B**); crisp-bread (**C**) and full-fat milk (**D**). Values are given as % phenolic acids, flavanols, flavan-3-ols and flavanones released from the initial amounts presents in the meals (Table 2) during in vitro gastric (G) and gastric + duodenal (G + D) digestion. Values represent averages (±SD) of triplicate measurements. Matching symbols across the four panels indicate significantly different ($p < 0.01$) samples. † Phenolic acid release in BS-G + D significantly different between A, B and D; †† Flavonols release in BS-G + D significantly different between A, C and D; ** Flavonols release in BS-G + D significantly different between A and C; ¶ Flavonols release in BS-G + D significantly different between A and B; ‡‡ Flavan-3-ols release in BS-G significantly different between A, B and C; & Flavanones release in BS-G significantly different between A and D; ¥ Flavanones release in BS-G significantly different between A and B; Ѫ Flavanones release in NS-G significantly different between A and D; Ω Flavanones release in NS-G significantly different between A and B; ‡ Phenolic acid release in BS-G + D significantly different between B and C; * Flavan-3-ols release in BS-G + D significantly different between B and C; ¥¥ Flavanones release in BS-G + D significantly different between B, C and D; § Phenolic acid release in NS-G + D significantly different between C and D; ǀǀ Flavonols release in BS-G significantly different between C and D. §§ Flavan-3-ols release in BS-G significantly different between C and D; ǀ Flavan-3-ols release in BS-G + D significantly different between C and D; ¶¶ Flavan-3-ols release in NS-G+D significantly different between C and D.

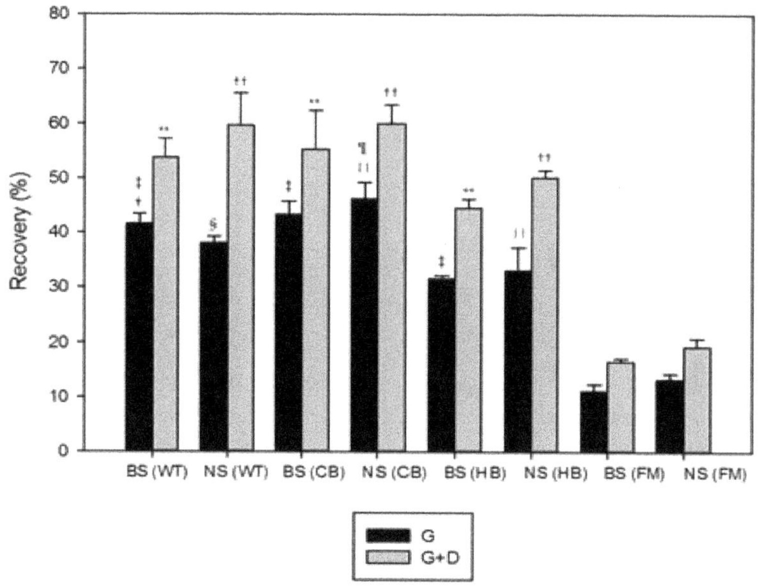

Figure 2. Recovery of total phenolic compounds in the digestion medium from natural almond skin (NS) and blanched almond skin (BS) in water (WT), home-made biscuits (HB), crisp-bread (CB) and full-fat milk (FM). Values are given as % of total phenolic compounds calculated from the amount of polyphenols present in the medium at the end of each step of digestion. Values represent averages (±SD) of triplicate measurements. † $p < 0.01$ vs. BS (CB); ‡ $p < 0.01$ vs. BS (FM); § $p < 0.01$ vs. NS (CB); $^{\|}$ $p < 0.01$ vs. NS (FM); ¶ $p < 0.01$ vs. NS (HB); ** $p < 0.01$ vs. BS (FM); †† $p < 0.01$ vs. NS (FM).

Statistical analysis of Figure 1 showed significant differences in the % of bioactives released from the tested meals: higher release ($p < 0.05$) of phenolic acid was detected from NS in CB vs. FM after G + D, flavan-3-ols from NS in WT vs. FM after G + D and flavonols from NS in WT vs. HB after G + D; higher release ($p < 0.01$) of flavan-3-ols was also observed from NS in CB vs. FM after G + D; higher release ($p < 0.05$) of flavan-3-ols was found from NS in CB vs. FM after G; higher release ($p < 0.01$) of flavanones from BS in HB vs. WT after G and vs. FM after G + D and flavan-3-ols from BS in CB vs. HB after G + D; higher release ($p < 0.01$) of flavanones from BS in FM, CB and HB vs. WT after G + D and of flavonols in CB vs. FM after G; higher release ($p < 0.05$) of phenolic acids from BS in CB vs. WT after G. This data confirmed the presence of a food matrix affected the release of bioactives from almond skin during simulated digestion. Overall WT and CB were good vehicles for the release of polyphenols from NS, whereas HB and CB were optimal for polyphenols bioaccessibility from BS. This could be due to the previous loss of water soluble polyphenols from BS during the industrial blanching process.

Statistical analysis of Figure 2 showed significant differences in the % recovery of polyphenols from the tested meals: higher recovery was observed from both NS and BS in CB vs. HB ($p < 0.05$) and vs. FM ($p < 0.01$) after G + D; higher recovery was also detected from NS in CB vs. WT ($p < 0.01$), FM ($p < 0.01$) and HB ($p < 0.01$) after G, as well as NS in WT vs. HB ($p < 0.05$); lower recovery ($p < 0.01$) was observed with BS in WT vs. CB and FM vs. HB after G. The recovery data also confirmed WT was a good vehicle for bioactives bioaccessibility from NS, whereas CB was optimal for BS.

Significantly ($p < 0.01$) lower % recoveries were obtained with FM from both NS and BS after gastric plus duodenal digestion. We believe the % recovery demonstrated that milk protein were able to bind the free polyphenols present in the digestion medium and the interaction between phenolic compounds and proteins was more pronounced in milk rather than biscuits [21]. Furthermore, complexes made by protein and tannin are less well digested and the amino acid profile may be damaged.

The same trend was also detected when comparing the kinetics (%) of release for flavan-3-ols from NS in WT and FM during the full digestion process (Figure 3). When NS was digested in WT, a steady release of flavan-3-ols over time was observed, corresponding to a significant increase detected for the initial 5 gastric digestion samples. In the presence of FM, the dynamics of release were very similar to WT but at a significantly slower rate.

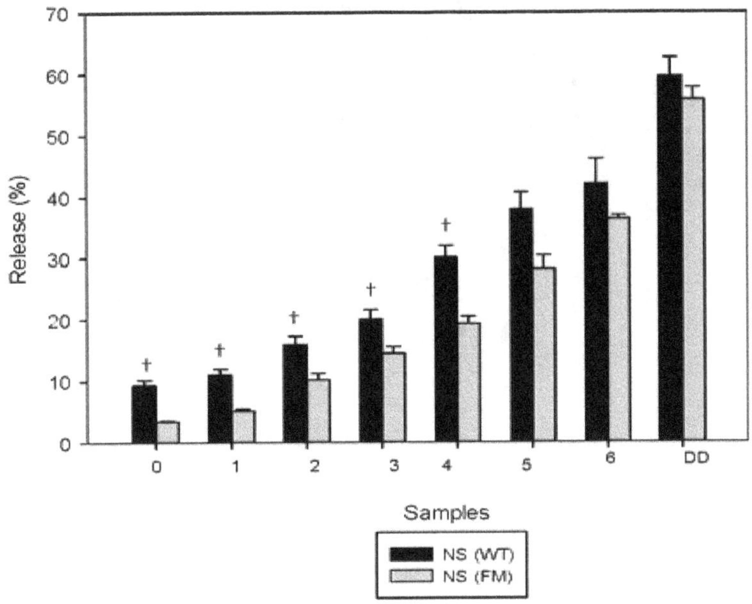

Figure 3. Kinetic of release of flavan-3-ols from natural almond skin (NS) in water and full-fat milk. Values are given as % of flavan-3-ols released from the initial amounts of flavan-3-ols in the meals (Table 2) during in vitro gastric (samples 0 to 6, see Table 1 for sampling time) and gastric + duodenal (DD) digestion. Values represent averages (±SD) of triplicate measurements. SD were always <10%. Water (WT), full-fat milk (FM). $^{+}$ $p < 0.01$ vs. NS (FM).

3.2. Antioxidant Profile during Digestion

The total phenolic content, measured by the Folin-Ciocalteu method, from all the tested meals during digestion is reported in Figure 4A,B. A decrease in the total phenols was observed post in vitro gastric and gastric plus duodenal digestion for both NS and BS in WT, HB, CB and FM. In agreement with the polyphenols release data, significant differences were observed across the four food matrices. A corresponding increase in free total phenols in the digestion medium, expressed as mg GAE/200 mL medium, was observed for WT, HB and CB (Figure 5). However, much lower than expected values of free total phenols were detected in FM, in agreement with the polyphenols recovery data. This data demonstrated that phenolic compounds could bind protein present in the food matrix, thus hindering the antioxidant potential in vitro [21].

In agreement with the total phenolic content, the radical scavenging activity, measured by DPPH, was lower after digestion (Figure 6). As shown in panel A, no statistically significant difference was observed in NS across all matrices; however in panel B, a statistically significant difference in WT vs. CB, HB and FM for sample 6 (last gastric sample) was observed. A corresponding increase of the antioxidant status was detected in the digestion medium, with the exception of FM; a statistically significant difference ($p < 0.01$) was observed in BS digestion media when comparing FM vs. WT, CB and HB and in NS when comparing FM vs. WT and CB (Figure 7).

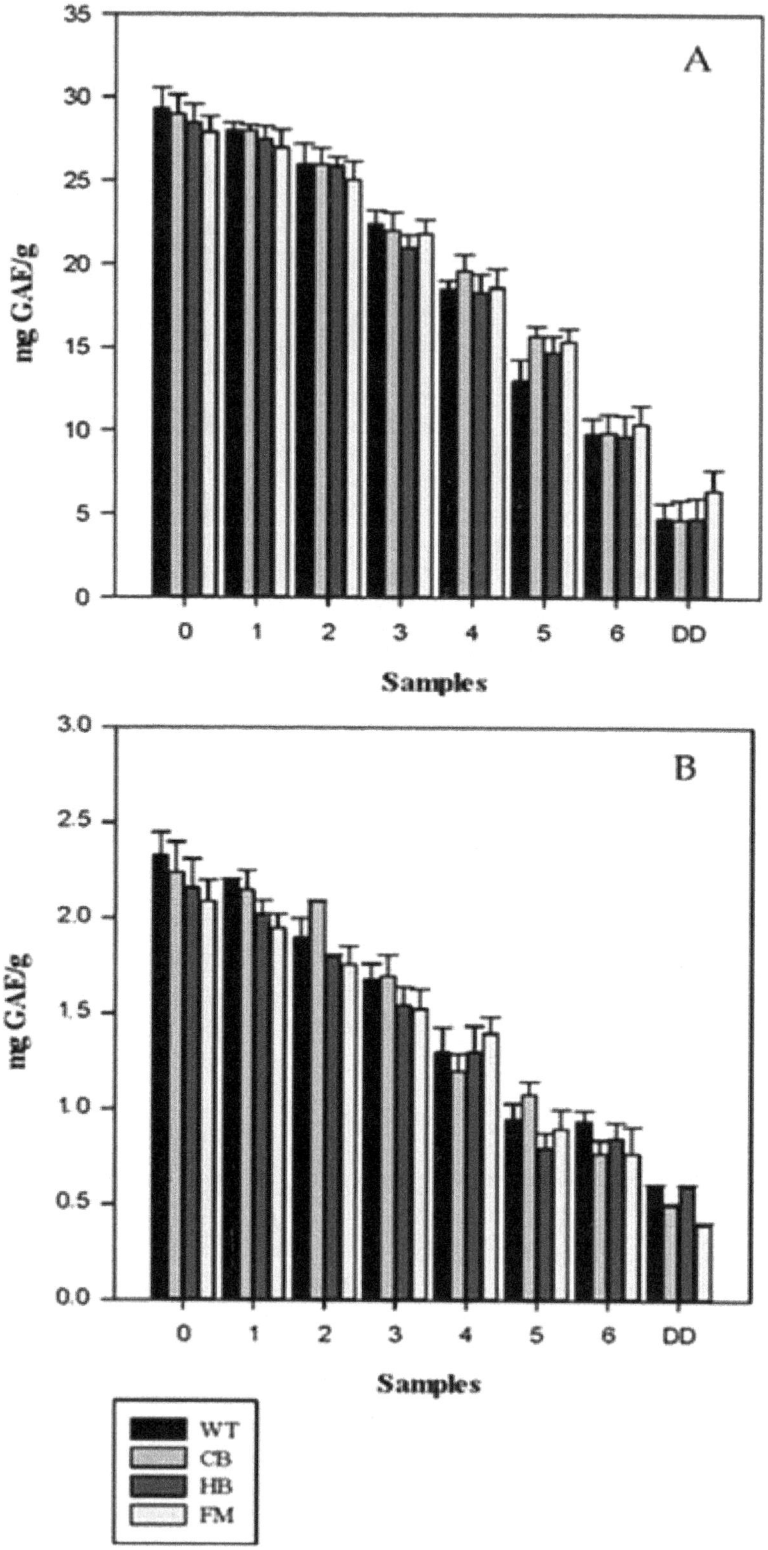

Figure 4. Total phenolic content in natural (NS, panel (**A**)) and blanched (BS, panel (**B**)) almond skin before and after simulated human digestion. Values are expresses in mg GAE/g and they represent mean ± SD of three different experiments. 0 to 6: gastric samples (see Table 1 for sampling time). DD: sample post in vitro gastric + duodenal digestion. Water (WT), home-made biscuits (HB), crisp-bread (CB) and full-fat milk (FM).

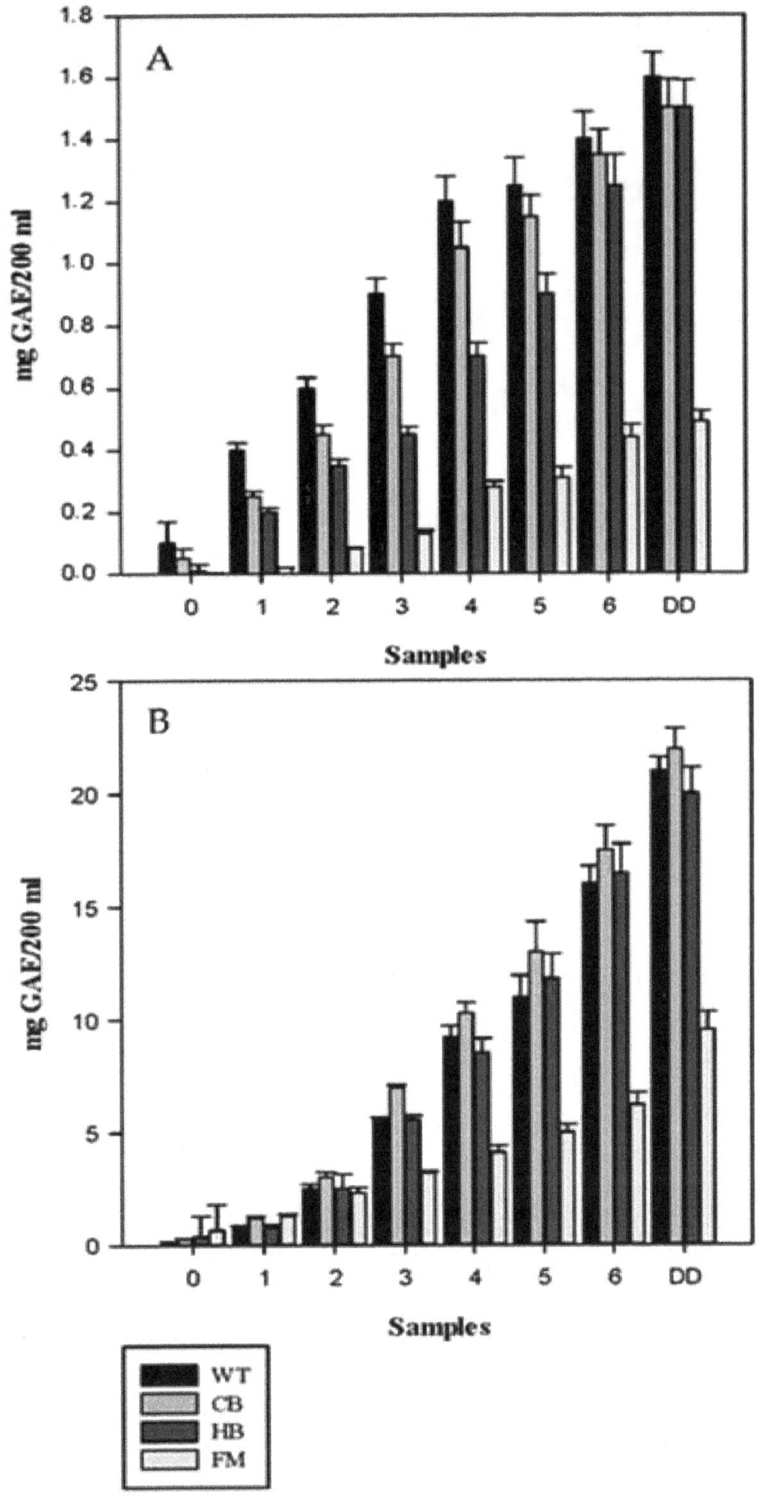

Figure 5. Free total phenols measured in the digestion medium of natural almond skin (**A**) and blanched almond skin (**B**) after in vitro gastric and gastric + duodenal digestion. Values are expressed as mg GAE/200 mL medium. 0 to 6: gastric samples (see Table 1 for sampling time). DD: sample post in vitro gastric + duodenal digestion. Water (WT), home-made biscuits (HB), crisp-bread (CB) and full-fat milk (FM).

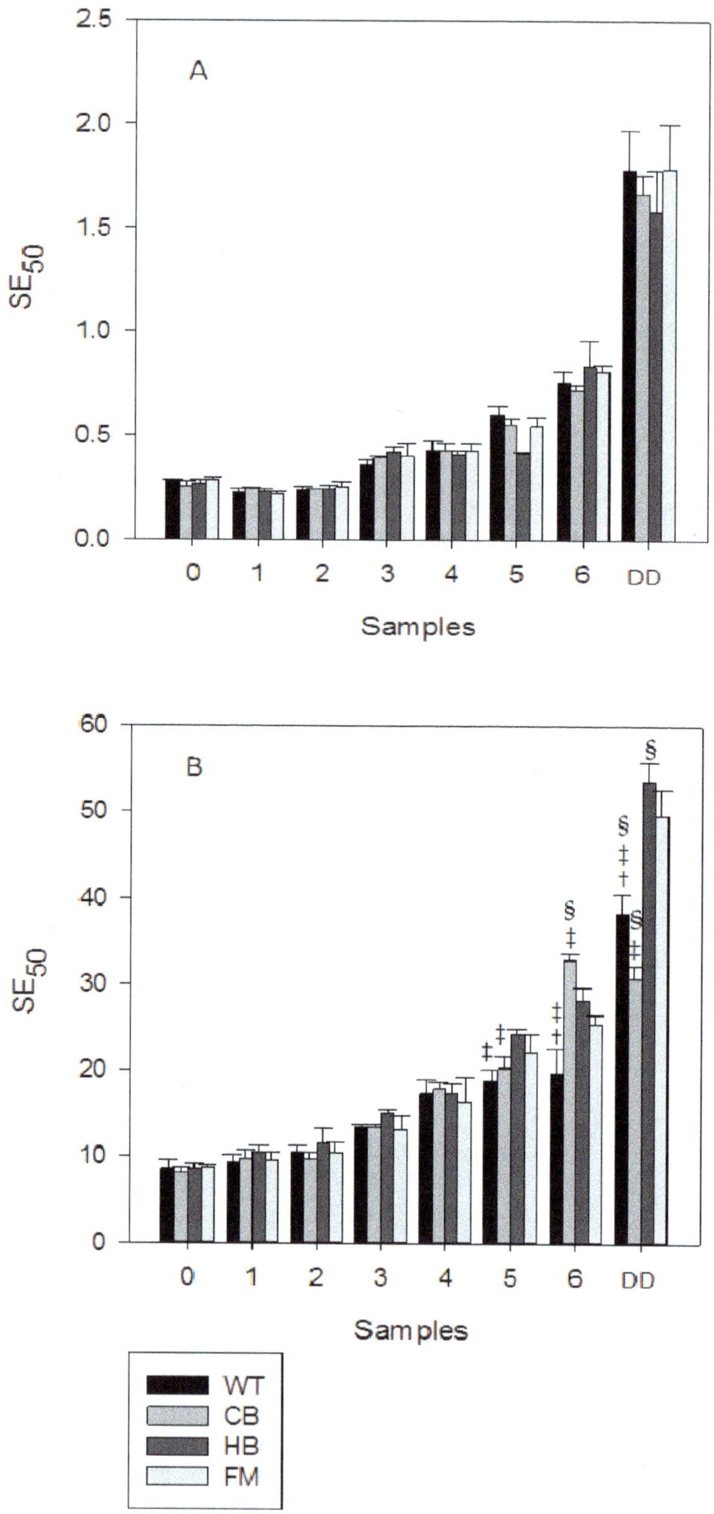

Figure 6. Radical scavenging activity measured in natural (NS, panel (**A**)) and blanched (BS, panel (**B**)) almond skin before and after simulated human digestion. Values are expresses as mg of sample containing the amount needed to scavenge 50 μmol of the initial DPPH solution (SE50) and they represent mean ± SD of three different experiments. 0 to 6: gastric samples (see Table 1 for sampling time). DD: sample post in vitro gastric + duodenal digestion. Water (WT), home-made biscuits (HB), crisp-bread (CB) and full-fat milk (FM). † $p < 0.01$ vs. CB at the same sampling time; ‡ $p < 0.01$ vs. HB at the same sampling time; § $p < 0.01$ vs. FM at the same sampling time.

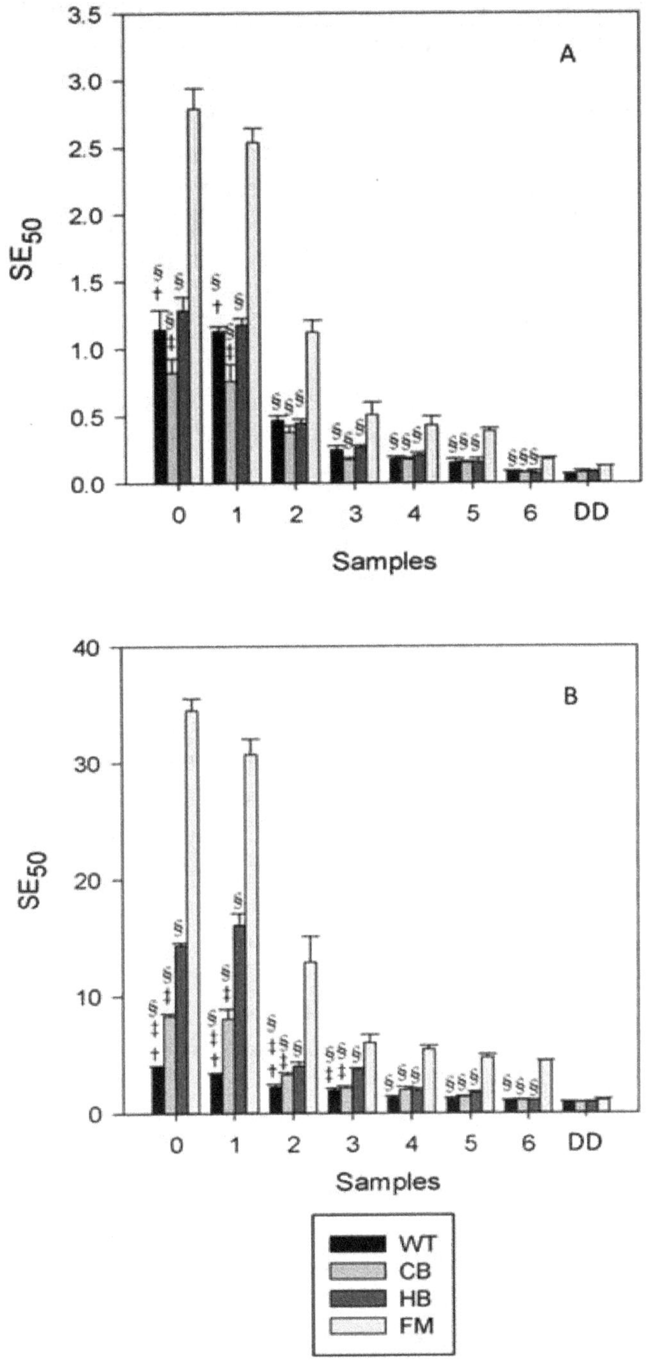

Figure 7. Radical scavenging activity measured in the natural almond skin digestion medium (panel (**A**)) and the blanched almond skin (BS) digestion medium (panel (**B**)) after in vitro gastric and gastric + duodenal digestion. Values are expressed as mg of extract needed to scavenge 50 μmol of the initial DPPH• concentration (SE50). 0 to 6: gastric samples (see Table 1 for sampling time). DD: sample post in vitro gastric + duodenal digestion. Water (WT), home-made biscuits (HB), crisp-bread (CB) and full-fat milk (FM). † $p < 0.01$ vs. CB at the same sampling time; ‡ $p < 0.01$ vs. HB at the same sampling time; § $p < 0.01$ vs. FM at the same sampling time.

4. Discussion

The data presented here has demonstrated that bioaccessibility of polyphenols from almond skin was significantly affected by the type of food matrix used. Given the lack of understanding of the fate of antioxidant compounds in the human body, research focused on the bioaccessibility of polyphenols from solid matrices are extremely important in order to better understand the beneficial effect on the host.

We have previously shown that polyphenols from almond skin were bioaccessible in the upper GIT during simulated human digestion in a static system and most of the release occurred in the gastric phase of digestion [1]. However, in the present study, a considerable further loss of polyphenols was observed during the duodenal phase over that detected in the gastric environment across all the food matrices used (Figure 1). The amount of individual polyphenols released from NS and BS are quite different, although a similar rate was detected across the two skin samples. The use of a dynamic model of digestion (DGM), where the digestion products are removed during the time course of the experiment, has likely affected the rate and release of almond skin polyphenols. A similar trend was observed with lipid bioaccessibility from natural raw and roasted almonds after mastication [22]. A study on polyphenols bioaccessibility from apples indicated the release was mainly achieved during the gastric phase (65% of phenolics and flavonoids), with a slight increase (<10%) during intestinal digestion [23].

In vitro digestion of the cocoa insoluble water fraction, source of polyphenols, lead to a 51% release of the total phenols from the insoluble material, without a reduction of the total antioxidant capacity [24].

In our previous study investigating bioaccessibility of bioactives from pistachios, more of 90% of polyphenols were released in the gastric compartment, with little or no increase in the duodenal phase [12]. The lower % of bioaccessibility in almonds (Figure 1) could be due to the properties of their cell walls, which is known to affect lipid and protein bioaccessibility in the gut [22,25]. Almond skins contain high amount of dietary fiber and several cell wall bound phenolics, including *p*-hydroxybenzoic acid, vanillic acid and *t*-ferulic acid [17]. We have previously shown that complex carbohydrates present in dietary fiber can directly interact with antioxidants and therefore interfere with their bioaccessibility in the gut [26,27]. Furthermore, the polyphenols structure plays a crucial role in relation to their adsorption, which was improved by low degree of hydroxylation and reduced by methylation or methoxylation. An increased degree of polymerization determined enhanced absorption for certain polyphenolic classes, including procyanidins [28]. However, the role of glycosylation still remains controversial [13,28]. Dietary fiber can reduce fat bioaccessibility in the GIT and pectin was found to strongly lower β-carotene bioavailability [29].

The high dietary fiber content in almond skin, as well as the significant amounts of lipids, could have affected the release of phytochemicals, especially in the absence of a food matrix. Dietary fiber could also reduce the rate of antioxidant absorption by physically trapping the bioactive compounds within its matrix in the chyme, thus restricting enzyme diffusion [30]. Therefore, it is hypothesised that certain polyphenols, mainly phenolic acids which are bound to dietary fiber, are not released in the upper GIT but reach the large bowel where they can be metabolised by the gut microbiota. This could also be due to a dietary fiber specific effect on gastrointestinal physiology (e.g., motility and/or secretion) [28]. The polyphenols-carbohydrates interaction could exert positive effects on lipid metabolism and increase the antioxidant activity in the large intestine [13,28].

A number of studies have reported on the effects of a food matrix in a simulated gastrointestinal environment: the findings demonstrated that green tea polyphenols were protected more by the interaction with dairy products, which could help maintain their antioxidant activity during digestion [31] and cheese was identified as an effective matrix for polyphenols protection during gastrointestinal digestion [32]. Stanisavljevic et al. [11] have investigated the changes in polyphenols content and antioxidant activity of chokeberry juice subjected to in vitro gastric digestion in the presence of a food matrix: the results demonstrated a decrease in the total phenolic content, anthocyanin content and DPPH radical scavenging activity immediately after addition of the food matrix. However, the fat content in cocoa samples increased the released of phenolic compounds during duodenal digestion [33]. Lesser et al. [34] have shown that high fat content in meals could either enhance or reduce the absorption of certain flavonoids; polyphenols could also affect the fat adsorption process at the emulsification stage by a direct interaction with phosphatidylcholine or by incorporation within the lipid layer, thus leading to physicochemical property changes of emulsions directly related to lipase activity and fat adsorption decrease, as suggested for tea polyphenols [28]. Moreover, several studies suggested that polyphenols were able to create a positive antioxidant environment at the gastrointestinal level fighting the harmful products of lipid peroxidation [28]. All these interactions could contribute to the well-known beneficial effects of polyphenols.

Another important aspect to discuss is the polyphenols ability to bind proteins, thus affecting the amino acids availability and leading in some cases to protein denaturation (e.g., α-amylase, trypsin, lysozyme) or to their lower digestibility (e.g., β-lactoglobulin) [28,35]. This often affects enzyme activity in a positive way (α-amylase inhibition which could be connected to the prevention of dental injuries) or negative way (when digestive enzymes are involved). It is known, in fact, that protein-polyphenol interactions might influence their adsorption, even though proteins could be carriers of polyphenols through the gastrointestinal tract, thus protecting them from oxidative reactions and increasing their availability at the large intestine [28,35].

In the present study, the fat and protein content in the milk matrix have significantly lowered the release of phenolic acids and flavan-3-ols after simulated human digestion from both NS and BS compared with water, whereas the home-made biscuits decreased bioaccessibility of flavonols (Figure 3). In a recent study [36] the addition of milk decreased the total phenolic, flavonoid and anthocyanin content, although it had no effect on the polyphenols being absorbed in vitro.

It has also been suggested, with respect to what is mentioned above, that the presence of digestible carbohydrates, lipids and other antioxidant compounds may have a beneficial impact on polyphenols bioaccessibility [37]. This could explain the high bioaccessibility detected when almond skins were incorporated in bread.

Even if the bioaccessibility of each antioxidant differs greatly, the potential synergistic effect amongst polyphenols could affect their bioactivity and influence on glycoprotein transporters across the mucosal epithelium. It is well established that a variety of factors, including chemical structure, food matrix, digestion enzymes and interaction with the gut microbiota can directly influence polyphenols bioaccessibility and rate of absorption [38]. A number of studies have indicated some unique technological strategies, including micro-encapsulation, which increase polyphenols bioavailability and therefore increase their beneficial health benefits [39–41].

5. Conclusions

In summary, the results of the present study indicate that the presence of a food matrix had a significant effect on polyphenol bioaccessibility from almond skin in both the gastric and duodenal environments. The dietary fiber present in almond skin may act as barrier to prevent a total release of phytochemicals during digestion. Further studies are warranted in order to investigate absorption of bioactives, which could explain the beneficial health effects associated with almond consumption.

Acknowledgments: We wish to dedicate the present study to our friend and colleague Antonio Tomaino, whose memory will always remain alive in our hearts. This research was funded by the Almond Board of California and the University of Messina (Research & Mobility 2015 Project, project code: RES_AND_MOB_2015_DE_LUCA). We gratefully thank Karen Lapsley from the Almond Board of California for providing the almond samples.

Author Contributions: All authors contributed to the study design. D.T. is the Principal Investigator responsible for study design. G.M. designed the study and wrote the paper. M.V. and R.F. were responsible and performed the experiments of simulated gastric and duodenal digestion. M.M. and A.S. performed instrumental assessment and were responsible for data collection and data analysis; C.B. contributed to interpretation data. All authors approved the final version.

Abbreviations

The following abbreviations are used in this manuscript:

NS	natural almond skin
BS	blanched almond skin
CB	crisp bread water
WT	water
FM	full-fat milk
HB	home-made biscuits
NSWT G	natural almond skin in water post in vitro gastric digestion
NSHB G	natural almond skin in home-made biscuits post in vitro gastric digestion
NSCB G	natural almond skin in crisp-bread post in vitro gastric digestion
NSFM G	natural almond skin in full-fat milk post in vitro gastric digestion
NSWT G + D	natural almond skin in water post in vitro gastric plus duodenal digestion
NSHB G + D	natural almond skin in home-made biscuits post in vitro gastric plus duodenal digestion
NSCB G + D	natural almond skin in crisp-bread post in vitro gastric plus duodenal digestion
NSFM G + D	natural almond skin in full-fat milk post in vitro gastric plus duodenal digestion
BSWT G	blanched almond skin in water post in vitro gastric digestion
BSHB G	blanched almond skin in home-made biscuits post in vitro gastric digestion
BSCB G	blanched almond skin in crisp-bread post in vitro gastric digestion
BSFM G	blanched almond skin in full-fat milk post in vitro gastric digestion
BSWT G + D	blanched almond skin in water post in vitro gastric plus duodenal digestion
BSHB G + D	blanched almond skin in home-made biscuits post in vitro gastric plus duodenal digestion
BSCB G + D	blanched almond skin in crisp-bread post in vitro gastric plus duodenal digestion
BSFM G + D	blanched almond skin in full-fat milk post in vitro gastric plus duodenal digestion

References

1. Mandalari, G.; Tomaino, A.; Rich, G.T.; Lo Curto, R.B.; Arcoraci, T.; Martorana, M.; Martorana, M.; Bisignano, C.; Saija, A.; Parkerd, M.L.; et al. Polyphenol and nutrient release from skin of almonds during simulated human digestion. *Food Chem.* **2010**, *122*, 1083–1088. [CrossRef]
2. Mandalari, G.; Bisignano, C.; Genovese, T.; Mazzon, E.; Wickham, M.S.J.; Paterniti, I.; Cuzzocrea, S. Natural almond skin reduced oxidative stress and inflammation in an experimental model of inflammatory bowel disease. *Int. Immunopharm.* **2011**, *11*, 915–924. [CrossRef] [PubMed]
3. Mandalari, G.; Genovese, T.; Bisignano, C.; Mazzon, E.; Wickham, M.S.J.; di Paola, R.; Bisignano, G.; Cuzzocrea, S. Neuroprotective effects of almond skins in experimental spinal cord injury. *Clin. Nutr.* **2011**, *30*, 221–233. [CrossRef] [PubMed]
4. Chen, C.Y.O.; Blumberg, J.B. In vitro activity of almond skin polyphenols for scavenging free radicals and inducing quinine reductase. *J. Agric. Food Chem.* **2008**, *56*, 4427–4434. [CrossRef] [PubMed]
5. Milbury, P.E.; Chen, C.Y.; Dolnikowski, G.G.; Blumberg, J.B. Determination of flavonoids and phenolics and their distribution in almonds. *J. Agric. Food Chem.* **2006**, *54*, 5027–5033. [CrossRef] [PubMed]
6. Garrido, I.; Monagas, M.; Gómez-Cordovés, C.; Bartolomé, B. Polyphenols and antioxidant properties of almond skins: Influence of industrial processing. *J. Food Sci.* **2008**, *73*, C106–C115. [CrossRef] [PubMed]
7. Benavente-García, O.; Castillo, J. Update on uses and properties of citrus flavonoids: New findings in anticancer, cardiovascular, and anti-inflammatory activity. *J. Agric. Food Chem.* **2008**, *56*, 6185–6205. [CrossRef] [PubMed]
8. Vuorela, S.; Kreander, K.; Karonen, M.; Nieminen, R.; Hämäläinen, M.; Galkin, A.; Laitinen, L.; Salminen, J.P.; Moilanen, E.; Pihlaja, K.; et al. Preclinical evaluation of rapeseed, raspberry, and pine bark phenolics for health related effects. *J. Agric. Food Chem.* **2005**, *53*, 5922–5931. [CrossRef] [PubMed]
9. Stevens, J.F.; Maier, C.S. The chemistry of gut microbial metabolism of polyphenols. *Phytochem. Rev.* **2016**, *15*, 425–444. [CrossRef] [PubMed]
10. Tagliazucchi, D.; Verzelloni, E.; Bertolini, D.; Conte, A. In vitro bioaccessibility and antioxidant activity of grape polyphenols. *Food Chem.* **2010**, *120*, 599–606. [CrossRef]

11. Stanisavljevic, N.; Samardzic, J.; Jankovic, T.; Šavikin, K.; Mojsin, M.; Topalovic, V. Antioxidant and antiproliferative activity of chokeberry juice phenolics during in vitro simulated digestion in the presence of food matrix. *Food Chem.* **2015**, *175*, 516–522. [CrossRef] [PubMed]
12. Mandalari, G.; Bisignano, C.; Filocamo, A.; Chessa, S.; Saro, M.; Torre, G.; Faulks, R.M.; Dugo, P. Bioaccessibility of pistachio polyphenols, xanthophylls, and tocopherols during simulated human digestion. *Nutrition* **2013**, *29*, 338–344. [CrossRef] [PubMed]
13. D'Archivio, M.; Filesi, C.; Varì, R.; Scazzocchio, B.; Masella, R. Bioavailability of the polyphenols: Status and controversies. *J. Mol. Sci.* **2010**, *11*, 1321–1342. [CrossRef] [PubMed]
14. D'Antuono, I.; Garbetta, A.; Linsalata, V.; Minervini, F.; Cardinali, A. Polyphenols from artichoke heads (*Cynara cardunculus* L. subsp. scolymus Hayek): In vitro bio-accessibility, intestinal uptake and bioavailability. *Food Funct.* **2015**, *6*, 1268–1277. [CrossRef] [PubMed]
15. Perez-Vicente, A.; Gil-Izquierdo, A.; Garcia-Viguera, C. In vitro gastrointestinal digestion study of pomegranate juice phenolic compounds, anthocyanins, and vitamin C. *J. Agric. Food Chem.* **2002**, *50*, 2308–2312. [CrossRef] [PubMed]
16. Roura, E.; Andres-Lacueva, C.; Estruch, R.; Mata-Bilbao, M.L.; Izquierdo-Pulido, M.; Waterhouse, A.L.; Lamuela-Raventós, R.M. Milk does not affect the bioavailability of cocoa powder flavonoid in healthy human. *Ann. Nutr. Met.* **2007**, *51*, 493–498. [CrossRef] [PubMed]
17. Mandalari, G.; Tomaino, A.; Arcoraci, T.; Martorana, M.; Lo Turco, V.; Cacciola, F.; Richa, G.T.; Bisignano, C.; Saija, A.; Dugo, P.; et al. Characterization of polyphenols, lipids and dietary fibre from skins of almonds (*Amygdalus communis* L.). *J. Food Comp. Anal.* **2010**, *23*, 166–174. [CrossRef]
18. Pitino, I.; Randazzo, C.L.; Mandalari, G.; Lo Curto, A.; Faulks, R.M.; le Marc, Y.; Bisignano, C.; Caggia, C.; Wickham, M.S. Survival of *Lactobacillus rhamnosus* strains in the upper gastrointestinal tract. *Food Microbiol.* **2010**, *27*, 1121–1127. [CrossRef] [PubMed]
19. Singleton, V.L.; Orthofer, R.; Lamuela-Raventos, R.M. Analysis of total phenols and other oxidation substrates and antioxidants by means of Folin-Ciocalteu reagents. *Methods Enzymol.* **1999**, *299*, 152–178.
20. Bonina, F.; Saija, A.; Tomaino, A.; Lo Cascio, R.; Rapisarda, P.; Dederen, J.C. In vitro antioxidant activity and in vivo photoprotective effect of a red orange extract. *Int. J. Cosmet. Sci.* **1998**, *20*, 331–342.
21. Xu, L.; Diosady, L.L. Removal of phenolic compounds in the production of high-quality canola protein isolates. *Food Res. Int.* **2002**, *35*, 23–30. [CrossRef]
22. Mandalari, G.; Grundy, M.M.; Grassby, T.; Parker, M.L.; Cross, K.L.; Chessa, S.; Bisignano, C.; Barreca, D.; Bellocco, E.; Laganà, G.; et al. The effects of processing and mastication on almond lipid bioaccessibility using novel methods of in vitro digestion modelling and micro-structural analysis. *Br. J. Nutr.* **2014**, *112*, 1521–1529. [CrossRef] [PubMed]
23. Bouayed, J.; Hoffmann, L.; Bohn, T. Total phenolics, flavonoids, anthocyanins and antioxidant activity following simulated gastro-intestinal digestion and dialysis of apple varieties: Bioaccessibility and potential uptake. *Food Chem.* **2011**, *128*, 14–21. [CrossRef] [PubMed]
24. Fogliano, V.; Corollaro, M.L.; Vitaglione, P.; Napolitano, A.; Ferracane, R.; Travaglia, F.; Arlorio, M.; Costabile, A.; Klinder, A.; Gibson, G. In vitro bioaccessibility and gut biotransformation of polyphenols present in the water-insoluble cocoa fraction. *Mol. Nutr. Food Res.* **2011**, *55*, S44–S55. [CrossRef] [PubMed]
25. Grassby, T.; Picout, D.R.; Mandalari, G.; Faulks, R.M.; Kendall, C.W.; Rich, G.T.; Wickham, M.S.; Lapsley, K.; Ellis, P.R. Modelling of nutrient bioaccessibility in almond seeds based on the fracture properties of their cell walls. *Food Funct.* **2014**, *5*, 3096–3106. [CrossRef] [PubMed]
26. Faulks, R.M.; Southon, S. Challenges to understanding and measuring carotenoid bioavailability. *Biochim. Biophys. Acta* **2005**, *1740*, 95–100. [CrossRef] [PubMed]
27. Del Rio, D.; Costa, L.G.; Lean, M.E.; Crozier, A. Polyphenols and health: What compounds are involved? *Nutr. Metab. Cardiovasc. Dis.* **2010**, *20*, 1–6. [CrossRef] [PubMed]
28. Jakobek, L. Interactions of polyphenols with carbohydrates, lipids and proteins. *Food Chem.* **2015**, *175*, 556–567. [CrossRef] [PubMed]
29. Rock, C.L.; Swendseid, M.E. Plasma beta-carotene response in humans after meals supplemented with dietary pectin. *Am. J. Clin. Nutr.* **1992**, *55*, 96–99. [PubMed]
30. Palafox-Carlos, H.; Ayala-Zavala, J.F.; González-Aguilar, G.A. The role of dietary fiber in the bioaccessibility and bioavailability of fruit and vegetable antioxidants. *J. Food Sci.* **2011**, *76*, R6–R15. [CrossRef] [PubMed]

31. Lamothe, S.; Langlois, A.; Bazinet, L.; Couillard, C.; Britten, M. Antioxidant activity and nutrient release from polyphenol-enriched cheese in a simulated gastrointestinal environment. *Food Funct.* **2016**, *7*, 1634–1644. [CrossRef] [PubMed]
32. Lamothe, S.; Azimy, N.; Bazinet, L.; Couillard, C.; Britten, M. Interaction of green tea polyphenols with dairy matrices in a simulated gastrointestinal environment. *Food Funct.* **2014**, *5*, 2621–2631. [CrossRef] [PubMed]
33. Ortega, N.; Reguant, J.; Romero, M.P.; Macià, A.; Motilva, M.J. Effect of fat content on the digestibility and bioaccessibility of cocoa polyphenol by an in vitro digestion model. *J. Agric. Food Chem.* **2009**, *57*, 5743–5749. [CrossRef] [PubMed]
34. Lesser, S.; Cermak, R. Wolffram S. Bioavailability of quercetin in pigs is influenced by the dietary fat content. *J. Nutr.* **2004**, *134*, 1508–1511. [PubMed]
35. Ozdal, T.; Capanoglu, E.; Altay, F. A review on protein–phenolic interactions and associated changes. *Food Res. Int.* **2013**, *51*, 954–970. [CrossRef]
36. Cebeci, F.; Şahin-Yeşilçubuk, N. The matrix effect of blueberry, oat meal and milk on polyphenols, antioxidant activity and potential bioavailability. *Int. J. Food Sci. Nutr.* **2014**, *65*, 69–78. [CrossRef] [PubMed]
37. Bohn, T. Dietary factors affecting polyphenol bioavailability. *Nutr. Rev.* **2014**, *72*, 429–452. [CrossRef] [PubMed]
38. Smeriglio, A.; Barreca, D.; Bellocco, E.; Trombetta, D. Chemistry, pharmacology and health benefits of anthocyanins. *Phytother. Res.* **2016**, *30*, 1265–1286. [CrossRef] [PubMed]
39. Lopez-Rubio, A.; Gavara, R.; Lagaron, J.M. Bioactive packaging: Turning foods into healthier foods through biomaterials. *Trends Food Sci. Technol.* **2006**, *17*, 567–575. [CrossRef]
40. Koga, C.C.; Lee, S.Y.; Lee, Y. Consumer acceptance of bars and gummies with unencapsulated and encapsulated resveratrol. *J. Food Sci.* **2016**, *81*, S1222–S1229. [CrossRef] [PubMed]
41. Neves, A.R.; Martins, S.; Segundo, M.A.; Reis, S. Nanoscale delivery of resveratrol towards enhancement of supplements and nutraceuticals. *Nutrients* **2016**, *8*, 131. [CrossRef] [PubMed]

9

The Anticancer Properties of *Herba Epimedii* and its Main Bioactive Componentsicariin and Icariside II

Meixia Chen [1], Jinfeng Wu [2], Qingli Luo [1], Shuming Mo [1], Yubao Lyu [1], Ying Wei [1] and Jingcheng Dong [1,*]

[1] Department of Integrative Medicine, Huashan Hospital, Fudan University, Shanghai 200040, China; cmx023@126.com (M.C.); qingqingluo2010@163.com (Q.L.); moshuming0703@163.com (S.M.); lvyubao80313@163.com (Y.L.); weiying_acup@126.com (Y.W.)

[2] Department of Dermatology, Huashan Hospital, Fudan University, Shanghai 200040, China; wujinfeng21@163.com

* Correspondence: jcdong2004@126.com

Abstract: Cancer is one of the leading causes of deaths worldwide. Compounds derived from traditional Chinese medicines have been an important source of anticancer drugs and adjuvant agents to potentiate the efficacy of chemotherapeutic drugs and improve the side effects of chemotherapy. *Herba Epimedii* is one of most popular herbs used in China traditionally for the treatment of multiple diseases, including osteoporosis, sexual dysfunction, hypertension and common inflammatory diseases. Studies show *Herba Epimedii* also possesses anticancer activity. Flavonol glycosides icariin and icariside II are the main bioactive components of *Herba Epimedii*. They have been found to possess anticancer activities against various human cancer cell lines in vitro and mouse tumor models in vivo via their effects on multiple biological pathways, including cell cycle regulation, apoptosis, angiogenesis, and metastasis, and a variety of signaling pathways including JAK2-STAT3, MAPK-ERK, and PI3k-Akt-mTOR. The review is aimed to provide an overview of the current research results supporting their therapeutic effects and to highlight the molecular targets and action mechanisms.

Keywords: anticancer properties; *Herba Epimedii*; icariin; icariside II

---

1. Introduction

Cancer is a complex genetic disease involving abnormal cell growth and is continue to be one of the major causes of deaths in both developed and developing countries [1]. According to statistics, there are approximately 14.1 million new cancer cases and 8.2 million deaths in 2012 [2]. It is estimated that new cancer cases will increase to 20 million by 2025. Cancer has been recognized as one of the most crucial health problems all over the world due to its great increased incidence and significant mortality.

Plants have a long history of use in the treatment of cancer and it is reported that more than 3000 plant species have been used [3,4]. The search for anticancer drugs from plant sources started as early as the 1950s, and at present over 60% of anticancer drugs currently used are derived directly or indirectly from natural sources, including plants, marine organisms and micro-organisms [5,6]. One of the successful stories is the discovery and development of the vinca alkaloids, vinblastine and vincristine, isolated from *Catharanthusroseus G. Don* (Apocynaceae) [7], which are the first plant-derived anticancer agents applied to clinical use for the treatment of various cancers [8,9].

Herba Epimedii (Common name: Yin-yang-huo in China, Figure 1) is the dried leaf of *Epimedium brevicornu* Maxim., *Epimedium sagittatum* (Sieb. EtZucc.) Maxim., *Epimedium pubescens* Maxim. or *Epimedium koreanum* Nakaias as recorded in the Chinese Pharmacopoeia (Figure 1) [10]. There are more than 40 kinds of *Epimedium* plants all over the world, mainly distributed in the southwest and central regions of China, although some are found in the temperate and subtropical regions of Asia, Middle East as well as Europe [11]. *Herba Epimedii* has been recorded in the Chinese medical classics *Shen Nong Ben Cao Jing* 400 years ago and has been used in various traditional Chinese formulations. The herb is believed to "nourishing the kidney and reinforcing the Yang" and is proven to have remarkably therapeutic activities. In China and Japan, *Herba Epimedii* alone, or in the formulations, have been widely used for treatment of osteoporosis [12,13], sexual dysfunction [14], hypertension [15] and common inflammatory diseases, such as chronic obstructive pulmonary disease [16]. In addition, *Herba Epimedii* has been shown to exert anticancer effect on cancer cell lines in vitro and also in vivo in mouse tumor model [17].

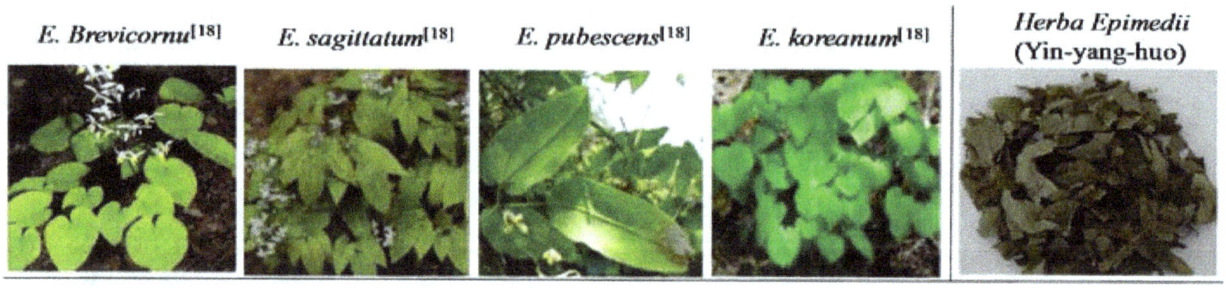

Name	Chemical structure	Molecular formula	MW	Ratio in raw material[19]			
				E. brevicornu	*E. sagittatum*	*E. pubescens*	*E. koreanum*
Icariin	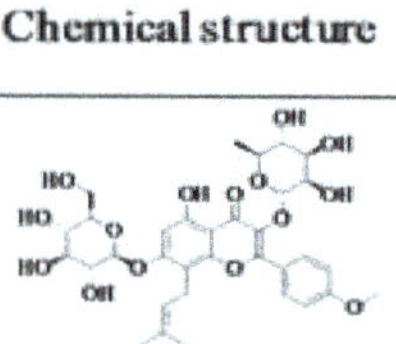	$C_{33}H_{40}O_{15}$	676.66	1.10%	0.806%	0.442%	2.62%
Icarisid II	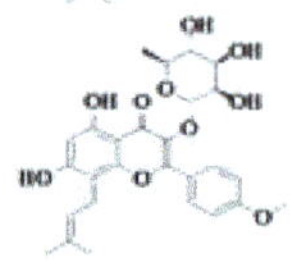	$C_{27}H_{30}O_{10}$	514.52	0.156%	0.365%	0.197%	0.562%

Figure 1. Natural sources and chemical structures of icariin and icariside II [18,19]. Herba Epimedii is made up of the dried leaves of *E. brevicornu*, *E. sagittatum*, *E. pubescens* or *E. koreanum*.

More than 260 constituents have been detected from Herba Epimedii with 141 flavonoids, 31 lignins and multiple other kinds of compounds [11], and the flavonoid glycosides have been confirmed to be the fundamental pharmacologically active constituents [20]. Icariin (Figure 1) is the major active constituent and has been chosen as the chemical marker for quality control of *Herba Epimedii* in Chinese Pharmacopeia. It is specified that the contents of icariin and the total flavonoids are no less than 0.5% and 5.0%, respectively [10]. Icariin has been found to possess a variety of pharmacological activities, including anti-osteoporosis [21], anti-inflammatory [22,23], antioxidant [24], antihepatotoxic [25], antidepressant [26] and neuroprotective effects [27]. It was also demonstrated to improve sexual disorder and to protect against cardiac ischemia/reperfusion injury [28,29] and atherosclerosis [30]. Besides, icariin was reported to exhibit anticancer activity against a series of human cancer cell lines.

Icariside II (Figure 1), another active flavonoid glycoside derived from *Herba Epimedii*, is the major pharmacological metabolite of icariin in vivo and has been reported to be obtained from icariin through enzymatic hydrolysis [31]. Icariside II has been shown to promote osteogenic differentiation of bone marrow derived stromal cells [32]. It shows protective effects on cognitive deficits [33] and cerebral ischemia-reperfusion injury [34] at least in part due to the inhibition of NF-kappaB. Additionally, icariside II has also been demonstrated to possess cytotoxic and cytostatic activities against various cancer cell lines.

The topic of this review will emphasize on the antitumor activities of *Herba Epimudii* and its two main active constituents and the mechanisms of action discovered so far.

2. Anticancer Effects of *Herba Epimedii* in Vitro and in Vivo

Recent studies showed that *Herba Epimedii* could restrain the proliferation of human breast cancer cell lines in vitro as well as inhibit tumor growth in rat model of bone metastasis from breast cancer. The antiproliferative activities of the ethanol extracts from *Herba Epimedii* on two different types of human breast cancer cells were investigated [35]. The 95% ethanol extract significantly inhibited the proliferation of human breast cancer MCF-7 cells in the range of 100–800 μg/mL in a dose dependent manner with an IC_{50} of 528 μg/mL after 72 h treatment. The 70% ethanol extract exhibited a certain activity on the growth of MCF-7 cells, whereas the 20% and 40% ethanol extracts showed no significant antiproliferation activity. The four different ethanol extracts of *Herba Epimedii* showed no obvious antiproliferative activity on human breast cancer MDA-MB-231 cells. In the rat model of bone metastasis from breast cancer, significant increase of 50% Paw withdrawn threshold (50% PWT) and reduction of tumor sizes were observed after oral administration of the decoction of *Herba Epimedii* at a dose of 5 g/kg daily for 20 days. In addition, the bone structural mineral density (BMD) and bone mineral capacity (BMC) were significantly enhanced [36]. In another study, it was found that the *Epimedium sagittatum* extract inhibited the proliferation of various hepatoma and leukemia cell lines, including SK-Hep1, PLC/PRF/5, K562, U937, P3H1 and Raji, with IC_{50} values of 15, 57, 74, 221, 40 and 80 μg/mL, respectively, whereas it showed no inhibition effects to HepG2 and Hep3B cell lines (IC_{50} > 500 μg/mL). The Hep3B was found to be less sensitive to the extract compared with other cell lines, consistent with the reported result that cells with the p53 gene deleted, just like Hep3B cell line, were more resistant to drugs [17].

3. Anticancer Effects of Icariin and Icariside II in Vitro and in Vivo

As for anticancer effects, studies have been performed in various human cancer cell lines. Icariin and icariside are proved to inhibit the growth of human cancer cells in vitro through intervening with multiple signaling pathways which are crucial to tumor growth, progression, invasion and apoptosis. Different concentrations of icariin and icariside II were used in the studies, depending on the types of cancer cell lines. The anticancer activity of icariin and icariside II and the molecular targets on various cancer cell lines were summarized in Table 1.

Table 1. Effects and molecular targets of icariin and icariside II on different cancer cell lines.

Cancer Types	Components	Cell Lines	Concentrations		Effects and Molecular Targets	Reference
			Con. Range	IC_{50}		
Hepatocellular carcinoma	Icariin	HepG2	10 μM	NA	G0/G1↑, S↓, Bcl-2↓	[37]
		SMMC-7721	5–20 μM	around 10 μM	cleaved caspase-3/9↑, mitochondria cytochrome c↓, cytosol cytochrome c↑, cleaved PARP1↑, XIAP↓, MMP↓, Bcl-2↓, Bax↑, p-JNK↑, ROS↑	[38]
Prostate carcinoma	Icariin	PC-3	30 μM	NA	Cyclin D1↓, CDK4↓	[39]
	Icariside II	PC-3	0–40 μM	around 20 μM	MMP↓, cleaved caspase-3/8/9↑, cleaved PARP↑, COX-2↓, iNOS↓, VEGF↓, PGE_2↓	[40]
Esophageal cancer	Icariin	EC109	20–80 μM	106.13 μM (12 h)	cleaved caspase-9↑, ROS↑, NADPH oxidase activity↑, GSH↓, GRP78↑, ATF4↑, CHOP↑, p-PERK↑, p-eIF2α↑, Bcl2↓, PUMA↑	[41]
				73.65 μM (24 h)		
				38.59 μM (36 h)		
		TE1	20–80 μM	115.29 μM (12 h)		
				76.77 μM (24 h)		
				42.21 μM (36 h)		
Ovarian cancer	Icariin	A2780	13–50 μM	NA	caspase-3 activity↑, miR-21↓ PTEN↑ RECK↑ Bcl-2↓	[42]
Lung cancer	Icariin	A549	25–100 μM	118.25 μM (12 h)	ROS↑, caspase 3 activity↑, GSH↓, ERS-related molecules↑(p-PERK, ATF6, GRP78, p-eIF2a, and CHOP), Bcl-2↓, PUMA↑	[43]
				86.21 μM (24 h)		
				56.8 μM (36 h)		
	Icariside II	A549	0–20 μM	NA	vimentin↓, N-cadherin↓, NF-κB↓, p-IκBα↓, p65/IκB↑, p-Akt↓ p-GSK-3β↓	[44]
		H1299	0–20 μM	NA		
Melanoma	Icariin	B16	20–200 μg/mL	84.3μg/mL (72 h)	procaspase-9↓ cleaved caspase-9↑	[45]
	Icariside II	A375	0–100 μM	10.6 μM	G0/G1 phase↑, S↓, G2/M arrest↑, cyclin E↓, CDK2↓, cyclin B1↓, P-CDK1↓, ROS↑, p-p38↑, p-p53↑, p21↑, cleaved caspase-3↑, survivin↓, p-STAT3↓, p-ERK↓, cleaved PARP↑	[46–48]
		SK-MEL-5	0–100 μM	11.1 μM		
Leydig cell tumor	Icariin	MLTC-1	12.5–100 μg/mL	50 μg/mL (48 h)	S↓, Bcl-2↓, Bax↑, cytochrome c↑, cleaved caspase-3/9↑, piwil4↓	[49]
Gastric adenocarcinoma	Icariin	BGC-823	20–200 μg/mL	128 μg/mL	Rac1↓, VASP↓	[50]
Medulloblastoma	Icariin	Daoy	NA	NA	Cyclin A↓, CDK2↓, Cyclin B1↓, cleaved caspase-3↑, cleaved caspase-9↑, PARP↑, Bcl-2↓	[51]
		D341	NA	NA		

Table 1. *Cont.*

Cancer Types	Components	Cell Lines	Concentrations		Effects and Molecular Targets	Reference
			Con. Range	IC_{50}		
Sarcoma	Icariside II	U2OS	0–30 μM	NA	4E-BP1↑, mTORC1↓, p-S6K(Thr389)↓, p-S6(Ser235/236)↓, p-4E-BP1 (Ser65)↓	[52]
		SW1353	0–20 μM	NA		
		S180	0–20 μM	NA		
Hepatoblastoma	Icariside II	HepG2	0–30 μM	NA	$\Delta\psi_m$↓, ROS↑, Bax/Bcl-2↑, cleaved-Bid↑, LAMP1↑, LMP↑, cleaved caspase-8/9/7/3/PARP↑, LC3B-II↑, SQSTM1↑	[53]
Osteosarcoma	Icariside II	MG-63	10–35 μM	NA	p-EGFR↓, p-PI3K↓, p-Akt↓, p-PDK1↓, p-Raf↓, p-mTOR↓, p-PDK1↓, p-PRAS40↓, p-GSK3β↓, p-ERK↓	[54]
		Saos-2	10–35 μM	NA		
		HOS	0–10 μM	NA	HIF-1α↓, VEGF↓, uPAR↓, ADM↓, MMP2↓, Glut4↓, MCT4↓, aldolase A↓, enolase 1↓	[55]
Epidermoid carcinoma	Icariside II	A431 cell line	0–100 μM	NA	cleaved caspase 9↑, cleaved PARP↑, caspase 9↓, PARP↓, p-STAT3↓, p-ERK↓, p-AKT↑, p-EGFR↑↓	[56]
Acute myeloid leukemia	Icariside II	U937	0–50 μM	NA	cleaved PARP↑, procaspase 3↓, Bcl-2↓, Bcl-X_L↓, survivin↓, COX-2↓, p-STAT3↓, p-JAK2↓, p-Src↓	[57]
Breast cancer	Icariside II	MCF-7	0–100 μM	72.73 μM (24 h)	MMP↓, cleaved caspase-3/7/8/9↑, cleaved PARP↑, $\Delta\psi_m$↓, cytosol cyto c↑, cytosol AIF↑, mitochondrial cyto c↓, mitochondrial AIF↓, Fas↑, FADD↑, Bcl-x_L↑, Bax↑, BimL↑	[58]
				57.98 μM (48 h)		
				50.95 μM (72 h)		
				37.75 μM (96 h)		
		MDA-MB-231	0–100 μM	97.14 μM (24 h)		
				62.75 μM (48 h)		
				42.40 μM (72 h)		
				38.65 μM (96 h)		
Multiple myeloma	Icariside II	U266	0-100 μM	NA	p-STAT3↓, p-JAK2↓, p-c-Src↓, SHP-1↑, PTEN↑, cyclin D1↓, Bcl-2↓, Bcl-x_L↓, survivin↓ VEGF↓, COX-2↓, cleaved caspase-3↑, p-PARP↑	[59]

NA, not applicable; ↑, up-regulation; ↓, down-regulation.

Icariin and icariside II have been demonstrated to exhibit in vivo suppressive effects both on tumor weight and tumor volume on a variety of mouse tumor models without obvious side effects (Table 2). Intraperitoneal administration of icariin at the doses of 15–150 mg/kg significantly inhibited tumor growth in xenografted mice models with almost no or very low toxicity to animals. Oral administration of 65 mg/kg icariin was shown to inhibit the growth of melanoma tumor and to inhibit the metastasis of B16 melanoma cells, and the lifespan was apparently pro-longed [45]. At the doses of 10–100 mg/kg, icariside II resulted in significant decrease in tumor weight and volume in cancer cell bearing mice models. All these data suggested that icariin and icariside II indeed have therapeutic potential against cancers.

Table 2. In vivo evaluation of icariin and icariside II in mouse tumor models.

Components	Tumor Models	Transplantation	Treatment	Results	Reference
Icariin	Esophageal cancer EC109	Subcutaneous injection	Given by i.p. 60 and 120 mg/kg every day for 20 days	Significantly inhibit tumor growth	[41]
Icariin	Lung adenocarcinoma A549	Subcutaneous injection	Given by i.p. 100 or 150 mg/kg (5 days/week) for 4 weeks	Significantly inhibit tumor growth	[43]
Icariin	Melanoma B16	Subcutaneous injection into the right flank	Given by p.o. 65 mg/kg every day for 20 days	Apparently inhibit tumor growth	[45]
Icariin	Mammary carcinoma 4 T1-Neu	Subcutaneous inoculation tumor bearing mice	Given by i.p. 100 mg/kg three times a week starting on day 7 until day 28	61% reduction of tumor growth	[60]
Icariin	Hepatoma SMMC-7721	Subcutaneous injectioninto the armpit	Given by i.p. 15, 30, and 60 mg/kg every day for 20 days	38.7%, 54.7%, and 69.9% inhibition in tumor volume, respectively	[38]
Icariin	Hepatoma HepG2	Subcutaneous injection	Given by i.g. 80 mg/kg for 35 days	55.6% inhibition in tumor weight; 47.2% inhibition in tumor volume	[61]
Icariside II	Sarcoma S180	Subcutaneous injection into the right armpit	Given by i.v. 10, 20, 30 mg/kg everyday for 9 days	33.0%, 51.3%, and 62.6% reduction in tumor weight, respectively	[52]
Icariside II	Lung cancer A549	Subcutaneous injection into the flank area	Given by i.v. 30 and 60 mg/kg once every 3 days for 24 consecutive days	Strongly suppress tumor volume	[44]
Icariside II	Liver carcinoma H22	Inoculation	Given by i.v.10, 20, 30 mg/kg everyday for 9 days	Inhibit tumor growth	[53]
Icariside II	Sarcoma S180	Subcutaneous injection into the right flanks	Given by i.p. 10, 20 and 30 mg/kg everyday for 10 days	Inhibit tumor proliferation	[54]
Icariside II	Melanoma B16	Subcutaneous injection into the right flank	Given by i.p. 50 mg/kg and 100 mg/kg 3 times for a week	41% and 49% decrease in tumor volume	[47]

4. Icariin and Icariside II as Adjuvant Therapy

While icariin and icariside II as single agent exhibited antitumor activities towards diverse human cancers, their potentials of potentiating the antitumor activity of a variety of chemotherapeutic drugs as adjuvant agents have shown perspectives in recent years. The combination treatment with the natural bioactive components and the chemotherapeutic drugs could facilitate chemotherapy for patients with cancers and provide a higher efficacy remedy.

Icariin has been shown to potentiate the antitumor activity of arsenic trioxide, temozolomide, doxorubicin, 5-fluorouracil and gemcitabine on a variety of human cancer cell lines, including acute promyelocytic leukemia, glioblastomamultiforme, hepatocellular carcinoma, osteosarcoma, colorectal cancer and gallbladder cancer cell lines, as well as in xenograft murine models (Table 3).

Table 3. Icariin and icariside II used as adjuvant agents in combination with hemotherapeutic drugs.

Component	Chemotherapeutic Drugs	Cancer Types	Cell Lines	Tumor Models	Molecular Targets	Reference
Icariin	Temozolomide	Glioblastomamultiforme	U87MG		NF-κB↓	[62]
Icariin	Arsenic Trioxide	Acute promyelocytic leukemia	HL-60	Xenograft murine model (HepG2)	ROS↑	[63,64]
		Hepatocellular carcinoma	NB4			
			SMMC-7721		ROS↑ NF-κB↓cyclin D1↓ Bcl-2↓Bcl-xL↓ COX-2↓survivin↓ VEGF↓	
			HepG2			
Icariin	Doxorubicin	Osteosarcoma	MG-63/DOX		MDR1↓ PI3K/Akt pathway↓	[65]
Icariin	5-Fluorouracil	Colorectal cancer	HT29	Xenograft murine model (HCT116)	NF-κB↓ cyclin D1↓ caspase-8↑ caspase-9↑ caspase-3↑Bax↑ PARP↑Bcl-xL↑	[66]
			HCT116			
Icariin	Gemcitabine	Gallbladder cancer	GBC-SD	Xenograft murine model (GBC-SD)	NF-κB↓ caspase-3↑ G0/G1 phase arrest↑ Bcl-2↓Bcl-xL↓	[67]
			SGC-996			
Icariside II	Paclitaxel	Melanoma	A375		TLR4–MyD88–ERK↓ caspase-3↑ IL-8 ↓ VEGF↓	[48]
Icariside II	Bortezomib	Multiple myeloma	U266		STAT3↓ JAK2↓ c-Src↓ SHP-1↓ PTEN↓ Bcl-2↓Bcl-xL↓survivin↓cyclin D1↓ COX-2↓ VEGF↓	[59]
	Thalidomide		U266			

The empty cells under tumor model indicates the studies are performed on cells (in vitro) rather than on tumor models (in vivo). ↑, up-regulation; ↓, down-regulation.

Arsenic trioxide (ATO), a traditional Chinese medicine, has been wildly used for the treatment of acute myeloid leukemia (AML) since 1970s in China and has been recommended as the front-line agent. In addition, ATO has exhibited antitumor activity against various solid tumor cell lines. Icariin has demonstrated to potentiate the antitumor activity of ATO in treating AML and hepatocellular carcinoma, at least partially correlated with the increase in the accumulation of intracellular reactive oxygen species (ROS). Of note, the sensitivity of APL cell line NB4 to ATO dues to the reduced glutathione content and the increased ROS production. Adjuvant agent, which promotes the accumulation of ROS, such as icariin, could potentiate the antitumor activity of ATO against APL [63]. Moreover, co-treatment with ATO and icariin resulted in a significant inhibition of tumor growth in xenograft murine model of Hep G2 compared to the treatment with either agent alone by promoting the generation of ROS and suppressing NF-κB without systemic toxicity [64].

Icariin potentiated the anti-tumor activity of temozolimide in glioblastomamultiforme cell line U87MG [62]. The cytotoxicity of doxorubin was enhanced by icariin via the inhibition of ABC1 and down regulation of PI3K/Akt pathway [65]. The combination of icariin and 5-fluorouracil led to the inhibition of tumor growth by suppressing NF-κB activity [66]. Icariin also potentiated the anti-tumor activity of gemcitabine in the treatment of gallbladder cancer by inhibiting NF-κB [67].

Icariside II has been demonstrated an increased inhibitory effect on human melanoma cells and multiple myeloma U266 cells when combined with paclitaxel and bortezomib/thalidomide, respectively (Table 3).

Paclitaxel is a widely used cancer chemotherapeutic drug and exhibits antitumor activity in a variety of human malignancies. It was revealed to induce the activation of the toll-like receptor 4 (TLR4) signaling pathway, which was functionally associated with tumor growth, invasion and chemoresistance [68]. Inhibition of the activation of TLR4-MyD88 has been considered as a novel approach for reversing chemoresistance of paclitaxel. Data from our laboratory demonstrated that Icariside II enhanced paclitaxel-induced apoptosis in human melanoma cells, which might be due to its inhibition on paclitaxel-induced activation of TLR4-MyD88-ERK signaling [48].

Bortezomib (a proteasome inhibitor) and thalidomide (an inhibitor of TNF expression) have been reported to be used for the treatment of multiple myeloma patients. Icariside II has been found to induce the suppression of survival proteins such as Bcl-xL and surviving as well as cleavages of PARP and caspase-3. Co-treatment of icariside II with bortezomib or thalidomide significantly improved the cytotoxic effects of bortezomib and thalidomide from 25% and 20% to 60% and 50% in U266 cells, respectively, accompanied by the further increase of caspase-3 activation and PARP cleavage [59].

Icariin and icariside II have played an excellent adjuvant effects without causing systemic toxicity in the chemotherapeutic treatment of several tumors by interfering with multiple molecular targets in tumor cells. They might be considered as the potential candidates for treating tumors in combination with common chemotherapeutic drugs, thus contributing to the development of the successful therapeutic strategies.

5. Molecular Mechanisms of Anticancer Activity of Icariin and Icariside II

Multiple studies have been performed to investigate the mechanisms by which icariin and icariside II exert their anti-tumor effects. The mechanisms are comprehensive and diverse, involving the regulation of a variety of targets, which play a particularly important role in the process of tumor proliferation, invasion, angiogenesis, metastasis and apoptosis. Besides the effects of icariin and icariside II on numerous signaling proteins and transcription factors, they also regulate the stages of the tumor cells by inhibiting proliferation and inducing apoptosis. In addition, they could play their anti-tumor effect through improving the tumor inflammatory microenvironment (Figure 2). Icariin and icariside II might be considered as potential chemotherapeutic agents for the treatment of various human cancers due to their multiple targets on the cell growth processes.

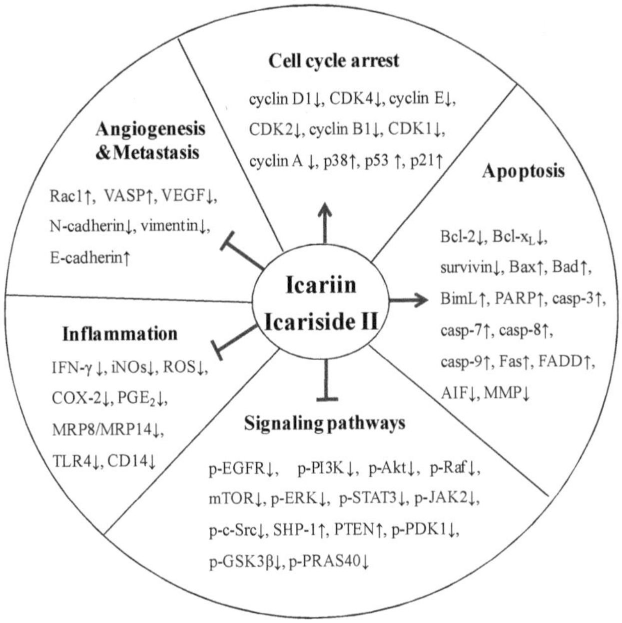

Figure 2. Overview of the anti-cancer effects of icariin and icariside II. Icariin and icariside II stimulate the cell cycle arrest via upregulation of p38, p53, and p21. Icariin and icariside II are involved in the induction of apoptosis and inhibit tumor angiogenesis and metastasis via suppression of multiple signaling pathways. They also have anti-inflammatory effects via downregulation of several factors, such as IFN-γ, iNOs, and COX-2, (← activation; ⊥ inhibition; ↑, up-regulation; ↓, down-regulation).

5.1. Effect on Cell Cycle Regulation

Cell division is divided into two stages: Mitosis (M) and the interlude between two M phases, including G1, S, and G2 phases. In addition, cells in G1 can enter a resting state called G0 just before the DNA replication [69,70]. In normal cells, the cell cycle is a highly regulated event, which is accurately regulated by cyclin dependent kinases (CDKs). The CDKs interact with various corresponding cyclins to form active complexes to ensure that the process at each stage is completely accomplished [71]. Tumor suppressor gene p53 is a vital cell cycle checkpoint regulator at the G1/S and G2/M checkpoints and serves to monitor the accuracy of vital events [72,73]. p38 MARK activation leads to the accumulation of p53 and the p53-induced cell cycle arrest is primarily mediated by the activation of p21 [74].

As shown in Figure 3, there are five active CDKs during the cell cycle, CDK2, CDK4 and CDK6 for G1, CDK2 for S, and CDK1 for both G2 and M. The complexes of cyclin D with CDK4 or CDK6 promote the progression through G1, cyclin E/CDK2 activates G1 into S, cyclin A/CDK2 promotes S progression, cyclin A/CDK1 activates G2 into M, while cyclin B/CDK1 stimulates the mitotic phase [75]. Disorders in the regulatory control of cell cycle could lead to the formation of tumors, characterized by the unlimited cell proliferation and abnormal apoptosis. Overexpression of cyclin D1 has been recognized as one of the distinct features in many types of human tumors [76]. Suppression of deregulated cell cycle progression in cancer cells by inhibiting the activities of CDKs or the cyclins have been considered as an effective strategy to inhibit the proliferation of the tumors [77].

Icariin has been reported to arrest the cell cycle at G0/G1 phase on the HepG2 cells. Icariin treatment for 72 h significantly increased the proportion of cells in G0/G1 phase, while the proportion of cells in S phases was remarkably lower (21.07%, $p < 0.01$) than that of the control group (28.62%) (Figure 3) [37]. Icariin also showed a weak G1 phase arrest accompanied by a mitochondrial transmembrane potential drop by decreasing cyclin D1 and CDK4 in human prostate carcinoma PC-3 cell line [39]. In another report, icariin stimulated S phase arrest in medulloblastoma cells by regulating the cell cycle regulators cyclin A, CDK2 and cyclin B1 [51].

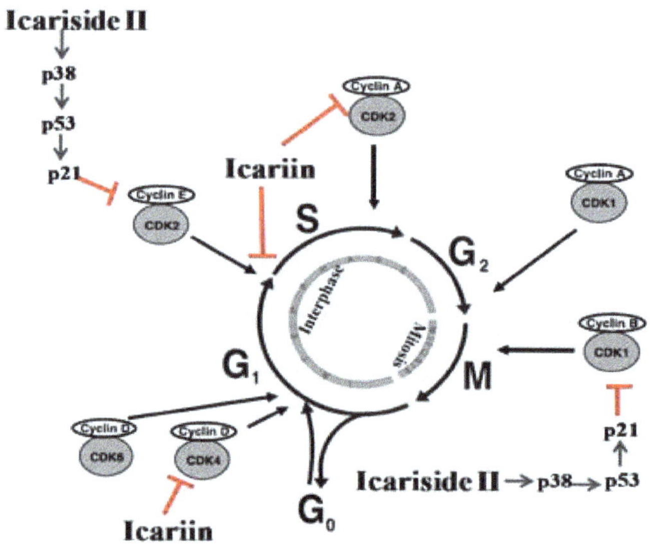

Figure 3. The cell cycle arrest induced by icariin and icariside II. Icariin and icariside II stimulate cell cycle arrest via suppression of the CDKs and cyclins at different stages, (← activation; ⊥ inhibition).

Our study demonstrated that icariside II induced cell cycle arrest at G0/G1 and G2/M phases in A375 human melanoma cell line (Figure 3). After treatment with icariside II at a series of concentrations 0, 25, 50 and 100 μM, the percentage of cells in G0/G1 phase significantly increased with the increase of icariside II concentration and peaked at 100 μM (69.51%), as compared to the control group (44.01%). The cell cycle arrest of A375 cells at G0/G1 phase was found to be correlated with the decreased expression of cyclin E and CDK2, and the arrest at G2/M phase was associated with decreased expression of cyclin B1/CDK1 complex. It was determined that IS inhibits cell proliferation and induces cell cycle arrest through the generation of reactive oxygen species and activation of p38 and p53. These findings were further supported by the evidence that pretreatment with N-acetyl-L-cysteine, SB203580 or pifithrin-α significantly blocked icariside II-induced reduction of cell viability, increase of cell death and cell cycle arrest. Crucially, it was confirmed that these effects were mediated at least in part by activating the ROS-p38-p53 pathway [46].

5.2. Effect on Apoptosis

Apoptosis occurs normally during development to maintain the cell population in normal tissues or occurs as a defense mechanism to selectively eliminate the defective or unwanted cells which are damaged by disease [78]. It has been recognized as a necessary complementary to proliferation and plays a vital role in the development and regulation of the immune system, as well as the removal of damaged cells, and what's more, the disruption of apoptosis is implicated in tumors development [79].

It is well established that there are two main apoptotic pathways: The extrinsic (receptor mediated) and the intrinsic (mitochondrial mediated) signaling pathway (Figure 4). The extrinsic signaling pathway is initiated by the ligation of ligands and corresponding death receptors of the tumor necrosis factor (TNF) receptor subfamily, such as FasL/FasR and TNF-α/TNFR1 [80]. The formation of death-inducing signaling complex (DISC) leads to the autocatalytic activation of procaspase-8 [81]. The intrinsic apoptotic pathway is triggered by cellular stress factors including the negative signals involving the absence of some growth factors, hormones and cytokines and positive signals, including radiation, toxins, hypoxia, viral infections, and free radicals. These stimuli at on the mitochondrial membrane and result in change of themitochondrial permeability transition (MPT), loss of the mitochondrialtransmembrane potential and release of the pro-apopto ticproteins such as cytochrome c and apoptosis inducing factor (AIF) from mitochondria into the cytosol [82]. The released cytochrome c activates Apaf-1 and procaspase-9, resulting in the formation of apopto some [83]. The mitochondrial mediated apoptotic pathway is regulated by the members of the Bcl-2 family proteins [84], which are reported to be implicated with the tumor suppressor protein p53 and comprise two groups of proteins with the opposite function, the anti-apoptotic proteins (e.g., Bcl-2, Bcl-x and Bcl-x_L) and the pro-apoptotic proteins (e.g., Bax, Bid, Bak, Bim and Bik) [85]. The extrinsic pathway can be linked with the intrinsic pathway through caspase-8 by inducing the activation of Bid, in turn, acting on the mitochondrial membrane leading to the release of cytochrome c (Figure 4) [86].

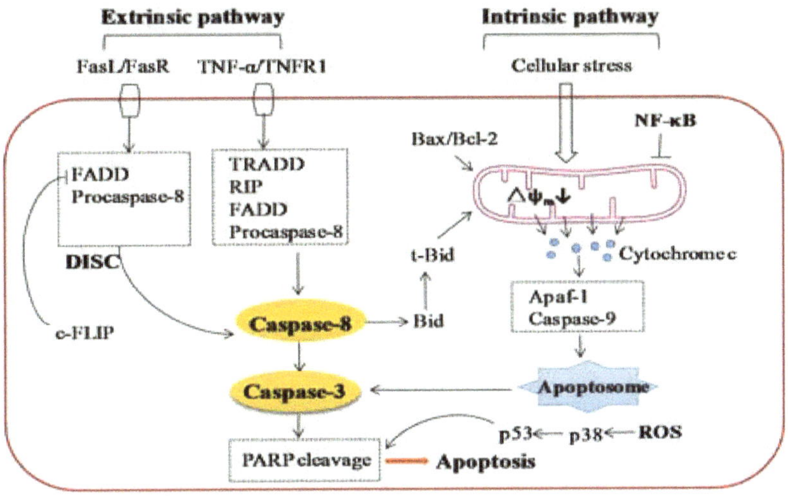

Figure 4. Apoptosis signaling pathways induced by icariin and icariside II. Icariin and icariside II induce apoptosis of tumor cells through two pathways, extrinsic (receptor-mediated) pathway and intrinsic (mitochondria-mediated) pathway. The binding of TNF-α with TNFR1 leads to the formation of TRADD and RIP, then the two factors combine with FADD and procaspase-8, which are resulted from FasL/FasR pathway, leading to the formation of death inducing signaling complex (DISC) and activating caspase-8. Activated caspase-8 stimulates the downstream caspase-3 and PARP, resulting in apoptosis, or cleaves Bid, which is the link between extrinsic pathway and intrinsic pathway, leading to the activation of intrinsic pathway. The cellular stress, activation of t-Bid, or modulation of Bax/Bcl-2 result in the downregulation of mitochondrial membrane potential and subsequent release of cytochrome c. Once released to cytosol, cytochrome c interacts with Apaf-1, resulting in the activation of caspase-9, which then activates caspase-3 resulting in cell death. Activation of NF-κB leads to the activation of several anti-apoptotic factors, which subsequently block the mitochondria-mediated pathway. Tumor cells produce ROS at higher levels, leading to the activation of p38 and p53, and subsequent apoptosis, ($\leftarrow$ activation; $\perp$ inhibition).

Multiple studies have shown that icariin and icariside II can selectively kill cancer cells without apparent toxicity on normal cells by inducing apoptosis in many cancers, including hepatocellular carcinoma, prostate carcinoma, esophageal squamous cell carcinoma, ovarian cancer, lung cancer, melanoma, leydig cell tumor, gastric adenocarcinoma, promyelocytic leukemia, sarcoma, hepatoblastoma, medulloblastoma, osteosarcoma, epidermoid carcinoma, acute myeloid leukemia, breast cancer, and multiple myeloma. It seems that icariin and icariside II induce apoptosis via both extrinsic (caspase induced) and intrinsic (mitochondrial induced) signaling pathways.

Icariside II has been reported to increase the expression of Fas and the Fas-associated death domain (FADD) without changing the level of Daxx, which is also an Fas binding protein inducing apoptosis by activating the JNK pathway, and activate caspase-8 and caspase-3 in MCF-7 breast cancer cells, indicating the involvement of extrinsic apoptosis pathway [58]. It was speculated that the apoptosis induced by icariside II might be occurred by stimulating Fas/FADD signaling independently of FasL and subsequently activating caspase-8. Moreover, the extrinsic signaling pathway might exert its effects on the icariside II-treated MCF-7 cells independent of the intrinsic pathway for the absence truncated Bid (tBid), which is the key molecule linking the two apoptosis pathways.

Several studies have revealed that icariin and icariside II exert their anti-tumor effects by inducing apoptosis via mitochondrial induced signaling pathway, mainly characterized by the loss of mithchondrial membrane potential, release of cytochrome c, activation of caspase-9, caspase-3 and PARP, and elevation of intracellular reactive oxygen species (ROS), which played vital role in cell apoptosis (Table 1). In addition, icariside II has also been shown to induce the release of the apoptosis-inducing factor (AIF) and cytochrome c, and the activation of caspase-9, which are characteristic features of intrinsic apoptosis pathway [58].

Nuclear factor-kappaB (NF-κB), an inducible transcription factor, and its downstream genes were suggested to play an important role in cell proliferation, invasion, apoptosis and chemoresistance [87]. Recent studies have shown that icariin exhibits antitumor activity and potentiates the antitumor effect of several chemotherapeutic drugs via down-regulation of NF-κB in various human cancer cells, generally accompanied by the down-regulation of Bcl-2 and Bcl-x_L [62,64,66,67]. Icariside II has been shown to prohibit invasion of lung cancer A549 and H1299 cells through suppression of Akt/NF-κB pathway [44].

5.3. *Effect on Angiogenesis and Metastasis*

The formation of new blood vessel is one of the key factors responsible for tumor growth and metastasis, not only supply nutrients for the metabolic needs of rapidly proliferating cancer cells but also provide conditions for cancer spread, resulting in malignant tumor growth, invasion and metastasis. Microvascular density in primary tumors is implicated in the numbers of tumor cells entered into the circulation in many tumors. Angiogenesis is regulated by multiple pro-angiogenic genes and signaling molecules including vascular endothelial growth factor (VEGF), basic fibroblast growth factor (bFGF), epidermal growth factor (EGF), platelet-derived growth factors (PDGF), angiopoetin (Ang), hypoxia-inducible factors, and matrix metal oproteinases [88].

Icariin has been shown to significantly prohibit the proliferation of vascular smooth muscle cells (VSMCs) and the activation of ERK1/2. Moreover, icariin also induced G1/S phase cell cycle arrest and decreased the expression of PCNA in VSMCs [89]. Based on these results, it was proposed that the inhibitory effect of icariin on the proliferation of VSMCs might be responsible for the suppression of tumor metastasis.

Effects of icariin and icariside II treatments on the adhesion and metastasis have been investigated in various human tumor cells, including esophageal carcinoma EC109 and TE1 [41], gastric adenocarcinoma BGC-823 [50], and lung cancer A549 and H1299 cell lines [44].

The adhesion and migration of icariin-treated EC109 and TE1 cells were evaluated after incubation in 15 μM ICA for 24 h [41]. The cell adhesion ratio decreased significantly to 47.23% ± 8.97% of that of the control in EC109 cells and 45.98% ± 6.72% of that of the control in TE1 cells, respectively ($p < 0.05$). Similarly, the scratch wound distance significantly increased by 159.23% ± 13.27% in EC109 cells and 179.26% ± 15.14% in TE1 cells, respectively ($p < 0.05$) [41]. Icariin was also reported to significantly inhibit tumor cells migration and invasion of human gastric adenocarcinoma cell line BGC-823 via the down-regulation of Rac1 and VASP [50]. The combination of icariin and the selective siRNA targeting Rac1 and VASP promoted the inhibitory effects. In addition, transfection with Rac1 plasmids pcDNA3-EGFP-Rac1-Q61L resulted in the improvement of expression levels of both Rac1 and VASP. Based on these results, it could be concluded that icariin inhibit the tumor cell invasion and migration through the Rac1-dependent VASP pathway [50]. A study has showed that icariside II prohibited the migration and epithelial-mesenchymal transition (EMT) via the inhibition of N-cadherin and vimentin up-regulation, and E-cadherin down-regulation induced by THP-1-CM in lung cancer A549 and H1299 cells [44].

5.4. *Effect on Multiple Signaling Pathways*

Multiple signaling pathways played vital role in cell survival, apoptosis and metastasis. Targeting various signaling pathways has been considered as a successful option in the treatment of cancer for its potential to avoid drug resistance, which is one of the major drawbacks of most anticancer drugs. Epidermal growth factor receptor (EGFR) is overexpressed in various types of human cancers and its expression is implicated with poor clinical prognosis [90]. Several small molecular kinase inhibitors and antibodies targeting on EGFR have been approved by FDA to treat diverse types of tumors. Activated EGFR recruits a variety of downstream signaling molecules, leading to the activation of major signaling pathways such as JAK2-STAT3, MAPK-ERK, and PI3k-Akt-mTOR, which play vital role in tumor growth, progression, and survival [91].

The inhibitory effects of icariside II on EGFR signaling have been investigated in human epidermoid carcinoma A431 cells [56] and in human osteosarcoma MG-63 and Saos-2 cells [54]. In our study, icariside II was found to inhibit the cell viability of A431 cells, accompanied by the decrease of phosphorylated EGFR. Pretreatment with LY294002 (a phosphatidylinositol 3-kinase (PI3K) inhibitor), EGF (an EGFR agonist) and AG1478 (an EGFR inhibitor) partially reversed the icariside II-induced decrease in cell viability, indicating icariside II effectively inhibited the EGF-induced activation of the EGFR pathway [56]. Icariside II was also found to decrease cell proliferation in MG-63 and Saos-2 cells by inactivating EGFR/mTOR signaling pathway and the decreased cell viability could be reversed partially by the pretreatment of EGF [54].

STAT3 is activated in a broad spectrum of human cancers, such as prostate cancers [92], breast cancer [93], and nasopharyngeal carcinoma [94], and has been implicated as a potential therapeutic target for multiple human cancers. Icariside II exhibited inhibitory effect on STAT3 signaling pathway in human melanoma A375 and SK-MEL-5 cells [47], epidermoid carcinoma A431 cells [56], acute myeloid leukemia U937 cells [57] and multiple myeloma U266 cells [59].

The phosphorylation of STATs is principally mediated via the activation of non-receptor protein tyrosine kinases called as JAK. Data from our laboratory showed that Icariside II dramatically inhibited the proliferation of melanoma A375 and SK-MEL-5 cells in vivo and in vitro by inhibiting the activation of the JAK-STAT3 and MAPK pathways but promoting an unsustained activation peak of the PI3K-AKT pathway [47]. Moreover, we also found icariside II induced apoptosis through inhibition of EGF-induced activation of STAT3 in A431 cells [56]. In U937 and U266 cells, Icariside II decreased the phosphorylation of JAK2 and c-Src, the upstream activators of the STAT pathway, and increased the expression of PTPs such as PTEN and protein tyrosine phosphatase (PTP) SH2 domain-containing phosphatase (SHP)-1 [57,59]. Sodium pervanadate (a PTP inhibitor) prevented Icariside II-induced apoptosis as well as STAT3 inactivation in U937 cells. Furthermore, silencing SHP-1 using specific siRNA significantly blocked STAT3 inactivation and apoptosis induced by Icariside II in U937 cells. All these results support a key role of SHP-1 in the suppression of STAT signaling pathways. In addition, icariside II was proved to reduce the level of STAT3 in MDA-MB-231 (breast adenocarcinoma) and DU145 (prostate carcinoma) cells, in which STAT3 is constitutively active [57].

The mitogen-activated protein kinase (MAPK-ERK, also known as Raf-MEK-ERK) pathway consisted several signal factors and the extracellular signal-regulated kinase-1 and 2 (ERK1/2) are extremely important in human cancers, which then activate ERK [95]. The importance of MAPK-ERK pathways in cancer progression and proliferation has been supported by Shield et al. [96]. Icariside II has been shown to inhibit the activation of ERK in melanoma A375 cells [47,48] and epidermoid carcinoma A431 cells [56]. Our data showed that icariside II treatment could effectively inhibit paclitaxel-induced activation of TLR4-MyD88-ERK signaling pathway in human melanoma A375 cells, which is proposed to be a novel target for reversing chemoresistance to paclitaxel. What's more, icariside II decreased cell proliferation and inactivated Raf-MEK-ERK signaling in osteosarcoma MG-63 and Saos-2 cells [54].

Phosphatidylinostinositol-3-kinase/protein kinase B (PI3K-AKT) signaling was found to play a key role in cell proliferation and is overexpressed in multiple human cancers [97]. As the downstream of PI3K-AKT, the mammalian target of rapamycin (mTOR), is a master growth regulator that senses the presence of growth factors by regulating p70S6K and 4E-binding protein 1 (4E-BP1) [98]. Icariside II, a natural mTOR inhibitor, was found to decrease the phosphorylation of PI3K-PDK1 and dephosphorylated Akt at Thr308 and Ser473 in osteosarcoma MG-63 and Saos-2 cells [54]. Akt activates mTOR by relieving proline-rich Akt substrate 40 (PRAS40)-mediated inhibition of mTOR. In addition, icariside II activated GSK3β, the direct target of Akt, by dephosphorylation atSer9, weakening the stability of transcription factors and cycle-related proteins. The suppression of icariside II on the phosphorylation of PI3K, Akt, PRAS40 was approved by mice bearing osteosarcoma sarcoma-180 cells. In conclusion, icariside II treatment moderated EGF-induced activation of PI3K/Akt/PRAS40 pathway in vitro as well as in vivo [54]. Icariside II was also shown to suppress aberrant energy homeostasis in osteosarcoma U2OS, fibrosarcoma S180 and chondrosarcoma SW1535 cells via suppression of mTORC1 by regulating mTORC1-4E-BP1 axis, suggesting a potential application of icariside II in sarcoma therapy [52]. In addition, icariin was reported to enhance cytotoxicity of doxorubin in the human osteosarcoma doxorubicin (DOX)-resistant MG-63/DOX cell line through down-regulation of PI3K-Akt pathway [65].

5.5. *Anti-Inflammatory Activity*

The hypothesis that chronic inflammation promoted cancer development and progression is strongly supported by the findings that individuals with chronic inflammation of the specific organ are significantly more susceptible to some organ-specific cancers [99]. The induction of myeloid suppressor cells (MDSC), one of the major factors mediating tumor-associated immune suppression, undermines the immune surveillance, thereby providing an environment favorable for tumor growth and allowing proliferation of malignant cells [100]. If inflammation facilitates tumor progression through the induction of more suppressive MDSCby signaling through the toll-like receptor 4 (TLR4) pathway, then it is possible that a decreased pro-inflammatory microenvironment may reduce the potency of MDSC. Data from our laboratory showed that icariin treatment reduced the expression of MRP8/MRP14 and TLR4 on human PBMCs [60]. Administration of icariin inhibited the tumor growth in 4T1-Neu tumor-bearing mice by reducing splenic MDSC accumulation and activation restoration of the functionality of effector CD8+ Tcells [60]. Furthermore, icariin significantly decreased the amounts of nitric oxide and reactive oxygen species in MDSC in vivo. Further, we saw a restoration of IFN-γ production by CD8+T cells and the drops of nitric oxide and reactive oxygen species in tumor bearing mice.

Recent findings demonstrated that cyclooxygenzase-2 (COX-2) is over-expressed in various cancers, including pancreatic cancer [101], gastric carcinoma [102], and prostate cancer [103]. Prostaglandin E_2 (PGE_2), the proflammatory product of elevated COX-2, has been shown to play a crucial role in the progression of malignant tumor. Since COX-2 is increased in inflammatory microenvironment, it is considered as a molecular target for cancer prevention and treatment.

The mechanism of icariside II induced apoptosis in hormone-independent prostate carcinoma PC-3 cells was studied in association with COX-2 [40]. Data showed that Icariside II exerted cytotoxicity with IC_{50} of approximately 20 μM on PC-3 cells. Furthermore, icariside II induced apoptosis via the suppression of COX-2, inducible NO synthase (iNOS), vascular endothelial growth factor (VEGF) and mitochondrial membrane potential, release of cytochrome c, and activation of caspase-8, -9 and, -3 expressions, and cleaved PARP. Moreover, exogeneous PGE2 inhibited PARP cleavage and knockdown of COX-2 enhanced PARP cleavage. These results indicated that icariside II induced mitochondrial dependent apoptosis by initiating the inhibition of COX-2/PGE2 pathway in PC-3 prostate [40]. The apoptosis induced by icariside II in acute myeloid leukemia U937 and multiple myeloma U266 was also found to be associated with the decrease of COX-2 [57,59].

6. Conclusions

A renewed interest emerges in the study of alternative and less toxic remedies for the treatment of many diseases, including cancer. Maximizing efficacy and minimizing side-effects has been recognized as the major goal of the treatment of cancers. *Herba Epimedii* has been traditionally used in clinical due to its multi-purpose activity and low toxicity. Collective data indicate that icariin and icariside II are the main bioactive components of *Herba Epimedii* and are potential anticancer agents towards a broad spectrum of human cancers. They exhibit broad toxicity to various types of human cancer cells by interfering with multiple mechanisms, inhibiting multiple signaling pathways, as well as regulating inflammatory microenvironment. Moreover, icariin and icariside II could be used as chemotherapeutic adjuvant agents in combination with standard drugs to improve the treatment effects and avoid drug resistance. In view of these demonstrated effects, icariin and icariside II could be potential therapeutic intervention agents alone or in combination with current chemotherapeutic drugs for cancers.

Acknowledgments: This work was funded by grant from Development Project of Shanghai Peak Disciplines-Integrative medicine (20150407), The Academy of Integrative Medicine of Fudan University, National Natural Science Foundation of China (81173390), and Shanghai Health and Family Planning Commission (ZYSNXD-CC-HPGC-JD-015).

Author Contributions: Jinfeng Wu and Qingli Luo performed the searching strategy, Meixia Chen analyzed the information and wrote the paper, Shuming Mo and YubaoLv conducted the Figures, Ying Wei revised and proofed the manuscript, Jingcheng Dong revised the manuscript and approved for submission.

References

1. Siegel, R.L.; Miller, K.D.; Jemal, A. Cancer statistics, 2016. *CA Cancer J. Clin.* **2016**, *66*, 7–30. [CrossRef] [PubMed]
2. Ferlay, J.; Soerjomataram, I.; Dikshit, R.; Eser, S.; Mathers, C.; Rebelo, M.; Parkin, D.M.; Forman, D.; Bray, F. Cancer incidence and mortality worldwide: Sources, methods and major patterns in GLOBOCAN 2012. *Int. J. Cancer* **2015**, *136*, E359–E386. [CrossRef] [PubMed]
3. Graham, J.G.; Quinn, M.L.; Fabricant, D.S.; Farnsworth, N.R. Plants used against cancer-an extension of Jonathan Hartwell. *J. Ethnopharmacol.* **2000**, *73*, 347–377. [CrossRef]
4. Amin, A.R.; Kucuk, O.; Khuri, F.R.; Shin, D.M. Perspectives for cancer prevention with natural compounds. *J. Clin. Oncol.* **2009**, *27*, 2712–2725. [CrossRef] [PubMed]
5. Zhang, X.; Chen, L.X.; Ouyang, L.; Cheng, Y.; Liu, B. Plant natural compounds: Targeting pathways of autophagy as anti-cancer therapeutic agents. *Cell Prolif.* **2012**, *45*, 466–476. [CrossRef] [PubMed]
6. Cragg, G.M.; Newman, D.J. Plants as a source of anti-cancer agents. *J. Ethnopharmacol.* **2005**, *100*, 72–79. [CrossRef] [PubMed]
7. Kumar, A.; Patil, D.; Rajamohanan, P.R.; Ahmad, A. Isolation, purification and characterization of vinblastine and vincristine from endophytic fungus Fusarium oxysporum isolated from Catharanthus roseus. *PLoS ONE* **2013**, *8*, e71805. [CrossRef] [PubMed]
8. Nemeth, L.; Somfai, S.; Gal, F.; Kellner, B. Comparative studies concerning the tumour inhibition and the toxicology of vinblastine and vincristine. *Neoplasma* **1970**, *17*, 345–347. [PubMed]
9. Cipriani, D. Clinical experience with vinblastine and vincristine. *Cancro* **1968**, *21*, 185–189. [PubMed]
10. Editorial Committee of China Pharmacopoeia. *The Chinese Pharmacopoeia, Part I*, 2015 ed.; China Chemical Industry Press: Beijing, China, 2015; p. 486.
11. Ma, H.; He, X.; Yang, Y.; Li, M.; Hao, D.; Jia, Z. The genus Epimedium: An ethnopharmacological and phytochemical review. *J. Ethnopharmacol.* **2011**, *134*, 519–541. [CrossRef] [PubMed]
12. Xie, F.; Wu, C.F.; Lai, W.P.; Yang, X.J.; Cheung, P.Y.; Yao, X.S.; Leung, P.C.; Wong, M.S. The osteoprotective effect of Herba epimedii (HEP) extract in vivo and in vitro. *Evid. Based Complement. Altern. Med.* **2005**, *2*, 353–361. [CrossRef] [PubMed]
13. Wang, L.; Li, Y.; Guo, Y.; Ma, R.; Fu, M.; Niu, J.; Gao, S.; Zhang, D. Herba Epimedii: An Ancient Chinese Herbal Medicine in the Prevention and Treatment of Osteoporosis. *Curr. Pharm. Des.* **2016**, *22*, 328–349. [CrossRef] [PubMed]
14. Niu, R. Action of the drug Herba Epimedii on testosterone of the mouse plasma and its accessory sexual organ before and after processing. *China J. Chin. Mater. Med.* **1989**, *14*, 530–574.
15. Yu, L.; Li, H.; Huang, G.; Bai, Y.; Dong, Y. Clinical observations on treatment of 120 cases of coronary heart disease with herba epimedii. *J. Tradit. Chin. Med.* **1992**, *12*, 30–34. [PubMed]
16. Zhao, Y.L.; Song, H.R.; Fei, J.X.; Liang, Y.; Zhang, B.H.; Liu, Q.P.; Wang, J.; Hu, P. The effects of Chinese yam-epimedium mixture on respiratory function and quality of life in patients with chronic obstructive pulmonary disease. *J. Tradit. Chin. Med.* **2012**, *32*, 203–207. [CrossRef]

17. Lin, C.C.; Ng, L.T.; Hsu, F.F.; Shieh, D.E.; Chiang, L.C. Cytotoxic effects of Coptis chinensis and Epimedium sagittatum extracts and their major constituents (berberine, coptisine and icariin) on hepatoma and leukaemia cell growth. *Clin. Exp. Pharmacol. Physiol.* **2004**, *31*, 65–69. [CrossRef] [PubMed]
18. Khan, M.; Maryam, A.; Qazi, J.I.; Ma, T. Targeting Apoptosis and Multiple Signaling Pathways with Icariside II in Cancer Cells. *Int. J. Biol. Sci.* **2015**, *11*, 1100–1112. [CrossRef] [PubMed]
19. Huang, H.; Liang, M.; Zhang, X.; Zhang, C.; Shen, Z.; Zhang, W. Simultaneous determination of nine flavonoids and qualitative evaluation of Herba Epimedii by high performance liquid chromatography with ultraviolet detection. *J. Sep. Sci.* **2007**, *30*, 3207–3213. [CrossRef] [PubMed]
20. Pei, L.K.; Guo, B.L. A review on research of raw material and cut crude drug of Herba epimedii in last ten years. *China J. Chin. Mater. Med.* **2007**, *32*, 466–471.
21. Xie, X.; Pei, F.; Wang, H.; Tan, Z.; Yang, Z.; Kang, P. Icariin: A promising osteoinductive compound for repairing bone defect and osteonecrosis. *J. Biomater. Appl.* **2015**, *30*, 290–299. [CrossRef] [PubMed]
22. Wei, Y.; Liu, B.; Sun, J.; Lv, Y.; Luo, Q.; Liu, F.; Dong, J. Regulation of Th17/Treg function contributes to the attenuation of chronic airway inflammation by icariin in ovalbumin-induced murine asthma model. *Immunobiology* **2015**, *220*, 789–797. [CrossRef] [PubMed]
23. Chen, S.R.; Xu, X.Z.; Wang, Y.H.; Chen, J.W.; Xu, S.W.; Gu, L.Q.; Liu, P.Q. Icariin derivative inhibits inflammation through suppression of p38 mitogen-activated protein kinase and nuclear factor-kappaB pathways. *Biol. Pharm. Bull.* **2010**, *33*, 1307–1313. [CrossRef] [PubMed]
24. Xiong, W.; Chen, Y.; Wang, Y.; Liu, J. Roles of the antioxidant properties of icariin and its phosphorylated derivative in the protection against duck virus hepatitis. *BMC Vet. Res.* **2014**, *10*. [CrossRef] [PubMed]
25. Lee, M.K.; Choi, Y.J.; Sung, S.H.; Shin, D.I.; Kim, J.W.; Kim, Y.C. Antihepatotoxic activity of icariin, a major constituent of Epimedium koreanum. *Planta Med.* **1995**, *61*, 523–526. [CrossRef] [PubMed]
26. Liu, B.; Xu, C.; Wu, X.; Liu, F.; Du, Y.; Sun, J.; Tao, J.; Dong, J. Icariin exerts an antidepressant effect in an unpredictable chronic mild stress model of depression in rats and is associated with the regulation of hippocampal neuroinflammation. *Neuroscience* **2015**, *294*, 193–205. [CrossRef] [PubMed]
27. Liu, B.; Zhang, H.; Xu, C.; Yang, G.; Tao, J.; Huang, J.; Wu, J.; Duan, X.; Cao, Y.; Dong, J. Neuroprotective effects of icariin on corticosterone-induced apoptosis in primary cultured rat hippocampal neurons. *Brain Res.* **2011**, *1375*, 59–67. [CrossRef] [PubMed]
28. Meng, X.; Pei, H.; Lan, C. Icariin Exerts Protective Effect Against Myocardial Ischemia/Reperfusion Injury in Rats. *Cell Biochem. Biophys.* **2015**, *73*, 229–235. [CrossRef] [PubMed]
29. Zhai, M.; He, L.; Ju, X.; Shao, L.; Li, G.; Zhang, Y.; Liu, Y.; Zhao, H. Icariin Acts as a Potential Agent for Preventing Cardiac Ischemia/Reperfusion Injury. *Cell Biochem. Biophys.* **2015**, *72*, 589–597. [CrossRef] [PubMed]
30. Hu, Y.; Liu, K.; Yan, M.; Zhang, Y.; Wang, Y.; Ren, L. Effects and mechanisms of icariin on atherosclerosis. *Int. J. Clin. Exp. Med.* **2015**, *8*, 3585–3589. [PubMed]
31. Xia, Q.; Xu, D.; Huang, Z.; Liu, J.; Wang, X.; Wang, X.; Liu, S. Preparation of icariside II from icariin by enzymatic hydrolysis method. *Fitoterapia* **2010**, *81*, 437–442. [CrossRef] [PubMed]
32. Luo, G.; Gu, F.; Zhang, Y.; Liu, T.; Guo, P.; Huang, Y. Icariside II promotes osteogenic differentiation of bone marrow stromal cells in beagle canine. *Int. J. Clin. Exp. Pathol.* **2015**, *8*, 4367–4377. [PubMed]
33. Yin, C.; Deng, Y.; Gao, J.; Li, X.; Liu, Y.; Gong, Q. Icariside II, a novel phosphodiesterase-5 inhibitor, attenuates streptozotocin-induced cognitive deficits in rats. *Neuroscience* **2016**, *328*, 69–79. [CrossRef] [PubMed]
34. Deng, Y.; Xiong, D.; Yin, C.; Liu, B.; Shi, J.; Gong, Q. Icariside II protects against cerebral ischemia-reperfusion injury in rats via nuclear factor-kappaB inhibition and peroxisome proliferator-activated receptor up-regulation. *Neurochem. Int.* **2016**, *96*, 56–61. [CrossRef] [PubMed]
35. Chen, X.; Tang, L.; Li, Q. Antiproliferative activities of alcohol extracts of Herba Epimedii and Cortex Fraxini on breast cancer cell proliferation: In vitro study. *China Pharm.* **2007**, *18*, 1124–1127.
36. Yao, X.; Jia, L.Q.; Tan, H.Y.; Gao, F.Y.; Cui, J.; Li, H. Effects of Epimedium on rat tumor growth and bone destruction of breast cancer rats with bone metastasis. *Beijing J. Trad. Chin. Med.* **2008**, *27*, 882–884.
37. Wang, Z.M.; Song, N.; Ren, Y.L. Anti-proliferative and cytoskeleton-disruptive effects of icariin on HepG2 cells. *Mol. Med. Rep.* **2015**, *12*, 6815–6820. [CrossRef] [PubMed]
38. Li, S.; Dong, P.; Wang, J.; Zhang, J.; Gu, J.; Wu, X.; Wu, W.; Fei, X.; Zhang, Z.; Wang, Y.; et al. Icariin, a natural flavonol glycoside, induces apoptosis in human hepatoma SMMC-7721 cells via a ROS/JNK-dependent mitochondrial pathway. *Cancer Lett.* **2010**, *298*, 222–230. [CrossRef] [PubMed]

39. Huang, X.; Zhu, D.; Lou, Y. A novel anticancer agent, icaritin, induced cell growth inhibition, G1 arrest and mitochondrial transmembrane potential drop in human prostate carcinoma PC-3 cells. *Eur. J. Pharmacol.* **2007**, *564*, 26–36. [CrossRef] [PubMed]
40. Lee, K.S.; Lee, H.J.; Ahn, K.S.; Kim, S.H.; Nam, D.; Kim, D.K.; Choi, D.Y.; Ahn, K.S.; Lu, J.; Kim, S.H. Cyclooxygenase-2/prostaglandin E2 pathway mediates icariside II induced apoptosis in human PC-3 prostate cancer cells. *Cancer Lett.* **2009**, *280*, 93–100. [CrossRef] [PubMed]
41. Fan, C.; Yang, Y.; Liu, Y.; Jiang, S.; Di, S.; Hu, W.; Ma, Z.; Li, T.; Zhu, Y.; Xin, Z.; et al. Icariin displays anticancer activity against human esophageal cancer cells via regulating endoplasmic reticulum stress-mediated apoptotic signaling. *Sci. Rep.* **2016**, *6*. [CrossRef] [PubMed]
42. Li, J.; Jiang, K.; Zhao, F. Icariin regulates the proliferation and apoptosis of human ovarian cancer cells through microRNA-21 by targeting PTEN, RECK and Bcl-2. *Oncol. Rep.* **2015**, *33*, 2829–2836. [CrossRef] [PubMed]
43. Di, S.; Fan, C.; Yang, Y.; Jiang, S.; Liang, M.; Wu, G.; Wang, B.; Xin, Z.; Hu, W.; Zhu, Y.; et al. Activation of endoplasmic reticulum stress is involved in the activity of icariin against human lung adenocarcinoma cells. *Apoptosis* **2015**, *20*, 1229–1241. [CrossRef] [PubMed]
44. Song, J.; Feng, L.; Zhong, R.; Xia, Z.; Zhang, L.; Cui, L.; Yan, H.; Jia, X.; Zhang, Z. Icariside II inhibits the EMT of NSCLC cells in inflammatory microenvironment via down-regulation of Akt/NF-kappaB signaling pathway. *Mol. Carcinog.* **2016**. [CrossRef] [PubMed]
45. Li, X.; Sun, J.; Hu, S.; Liu, J. Icariin Induced B16 Melanoma Tumor Cells Apoptosis, Suppressed Tumor Growth and Metastasis. *Iran. J. Public Health* **2014**, *43*, 847–848. [PubMed]
46. Wu, J.; Song, T.; Liu, S.; Li, X.; Li, G.; Xu, J. Icariside II inhibits cell proliferation and induces cell cycle arrest through the ROS-p38-p53 signaling pathway in A375 human melanoma cells. *Mol. Med. Rep.* **2015**, *11*, 410–416. [CrossRef] [PubMed]
47. Wu, J.; Xu, J.; Eksioglu, E.A.; Chen, X.; Zhou, J.; Fortenbery, N.; Wei, S.; Dong, J. Icariside II induces apoptosis of melanoma cells through the downregulation of survival pathways. *Nutr. Cancer* **2013**, *65*, 110–117. [CrossRef] [PubMed]
48. Wu, J.; Guan, M.; Wong, P.F.; Yu, H.; Dong, J.; Xu, J. Icariside II potentiates paclitaxel-induced apoptosis in human melanoma A375 cells by inhibiting TLR4 signaling pathway. *Food Chem. Toxicol.* **2012**, *50*, 3019–3024. [CrossRef] [PubMed]
49. Wang, Q.; Hao, J.; Pu, J.; Zhao, L.; Lu, Z.; Hu, J.; Yu, Q.; Wang, Y.; Xie, Y.; Li, G. Icariin induces apoptosis in mouse MLTC-10 Leydig tumor cells through activation of the mitochondrial pathway and down-regulation of the expression of piwil4. *Int. J. Oncol.* **2011**, *39*, 973–980. [PubMed]
50. Wang, Y.; Dong, H.; Zhu, M.; Ou, Y.; Zhang, J.; Luo, H.; Luo, R.; Wu, J.; Mao, M.; Liu, X.; et al. Icariin exterts negative effects on human gastric cancer cell invasion and migration by vasodilator-stimulated phosphoprotein via Rac1 pathway. *Eur. J. Pharmacol.* **2010**, *635*, 40–48. [CrossRef] [PubMed]
51. Sun, Y.; Sun, X.H.; Fan, W.J.; Jiang, X.M.; Li, A.W. Icariin induces S-phase arrest and apoptosis in medulloblastoma cells. *Cell Mol. Biol.* **2016**, *62*, 123–129. [PubMed]
52. Zhang, C.; Yang, L.; Geng, Y.D.; An, F.L.; Xia, Y.Z.; Guo, C.; Luo, J.G.; Zhang, L.Y.; Guo, Q.L.; Kong, L.Y. Icariside II, a natural mTOR inhibitor, disrupts aberrant energy homeostasis via suppressing mTORC1–4E-BP1 axis in sarcoma cells. *Oncotarget* **2016**. [CrossRef] [PubMed]
53. Geng, Y.D.; Zhang, C.; Shi, Y.M.; Xia, Y.Z.; Guo, C.; Yang, L.; Kong, L.Y. Icariside II-induced mitochondrion and lysosome mediated apoptosis is counterbalanced by an autophagic salvage response in hepatoblastoma. *Cancer Lett.* **2015**, *366*, 19–31. [CrossRef] [PubMed]
54. Geng, Y.D.; Yang, L.; Zhang, C.; Kong, L.Y. Blockade of epidermal growth factor receptor/mammalian target of rapamycin pathway by Icariside II results in reduced cell proliferation of osteosarcoma cells. *Food Chem. Toxicol.* **2014**, *73*, 7–16. [CrossRef] [PubMed]
55. Choi, H.J.; Eun, J.S.; Kim, D.K.; Li, R.H.; Shin, T.Y.; Park, H.; Cho, N.P.; Soh, Y. Icariside II from Epimedium koreanum inhibits hypoxia-inducible factor-1alpha in human osteosarcoma cells. *Eur. J. Pharmacol.* **2008**, *579*, 58–65. [CrossRef] [PubMed]
56. Wu, J.; Zuo, F.; Du, J.; Wong, P.F.; Qin, H.; Xu, J. Icariside II induces apoptosis via inhibition of the EGFR pathways in A431 human epidermoid carcinoma cells. *Mol. Med. Rep.* **2013**, *8*, 597–602. [PubMed]
57. Kang, S.H.; Jeong, S.J.; Kim, S.H.; Kim, J.H.; Jung, J.H.; Koh, W.; Kim, J.H.; Kim, D.K.; Chen, C.Y.; Kim, S.H. Icariside II induces apoptosis in U937 acute myeloid leukemia cells: Role of inactivation of STAT3-related signaling. *PLoS ONE* **2012**, *7*, e28706. [CrossRef] [PubMed]

58. Huang, C.; Chen, X.; Guo, B.; Huang, W.; Shen, T.; Sun, X.; Xiao, P.; Zhou, Q. Induction of apoptosis by Icariside II through extrinsic and intrinsic signaling pathways in human breast cancer MCF7 cells. *Biosci. Biotechnol. Biochem.* **2012**, *76*, 1322–1328. [CrossRef] [PubMed]
59. Kim, S.H.; Ahn, K.S.; Jeong, S.J.; Kwon, T.R.; Jung, J.H.; Yun, S.M.; Han, I.; Lee, S.G.; Kim, D.K.; Kang, M.; et al. Janus activated kinase 2/signal transducer and activator of transcription 3 pathway mediates icariside II-induced apoptosis in U266 multiple myeloma cells. *Eur. J. Pharmacol.* **2011**, *654*, 10–16. [CrossRef] [PubMed]
60. Zhou, J.; Wu, J.; Chen, X.; Fortenbery, N.; Eksioglu, E.; Kodumudi, K.N.; Pk, E.B.; Dong, J.; Djeu, J.Y.; Wei, S. Icariin and its derivative, ICT, exert anti-inflammatory, anti-tumor effects, and modulate myeloid derived suppressive cells (MDSCs) functions. *Int. Immunopharmacol.* **2011**, *11*, 890–898. [CrossRef] [PubMed]
61. Yang, J.X.; Fichtner, I.; Becker, M.; Lemm, M.; Wang, X.M. Anti-proliferative efficacy of icariin on HepG2 hepatoma and its possible mechanism of action. *Am. J. Chin. Med.* **2009**, *37*, 1153–1165. [CrossRef] [PubMed]
62. Yang, L.; Wang, Y.; Guo, H.; Guo, M. Synergistic Anti-Cancer Effects of Icariin and Temozolomide in Glioblastoma. *Cell Biochem. Biophys.* **2015**, *71*, 1379–1385. [CrossRef] [PubMed]
63. Wang, Z.; Zhang, H.; Dai, L.; Song, T.; Li, P.; Liu, Y.; Wang, L. Arsenic Trioxide and Icariin Show Synergistic Anti-leukemic Activity. *Cell Biochem. Biophys.* **2015**, *73*, 213–219. [CrossRef] [PubMed]
64. Li, W.; Wang, M.; Wang, L.; Ji, S.; Zhang, J.; Zhang, C. Icariin synergizes with arsenic trioxide to suppress human hepatocellular carcinoma. *Cell Biochem. Biophys.* **2014**, *68*, 427–436. [CrossRef] [PubMed]
65. Wang, Z.; Yang, L.; Xia, Y.; Guo, C.; Kong, L. Icariin enhances cytotoxicity of doxorubicin in human multidrug-resistant osteosarcoma cells by inhibition of ABCB1 and down-regulation of the PI3K/Akt pathway. *Biol. Pharm. Bull.* **2015**, *38*, 277–284. [CrossRef] [PubMed]
66. Shi, D.B.; Li, X.X.; Zheng, H.T.; Li, D.W.; Cai, G.X.; Peng, J.J.; Gu, W.L.; Guan, Z.Q.; Xu, Y.; Cai, S.J. Icariin-mediated inhibition of NF-kappaB activity enhances the in vitro and in vivo antitumour effect of 5-fluorouracil in colorectal cancer. *Cell Biochem. Biophys.* **2014**, *69*, 523–530. [CrossRef] [PubMed]
67. Zhang, D.C.; Liu, J.L.; Ding, Y.B.; Xia, J.G.; Chen, G.Y. Icariin potentiates the antitumor activity of gemcitabine in gallbladder cancer by suppressing NF-kappaB. *Acta Pharmacol. Sin.* **2013**, *34*, 301–308. [CrossRef] [PubMed]
68. Kelly, M.G.; Alvero, A.B.; Chen, R.; Silasi, D.A.; Abrahams, V.M.; Chan, S.; Visintin, I.; Rutherford, T.; Mor, G. TLR-4 signaling promotes tumor growth and paclitaxel chemoresistance in ovarian cancer. *Cancer Res.* **2006**, *66*, 3859–3868. [CrossRef] [PubMed]
69. Nurse, P.; Masui, Y.; Hartwell, L. Understanding the cell cycle. *Nat. Med.* **1998**, *4*, 1103–1106. [CrossRef] [PubMed]
70. Sa, G.; Das, T. Anti cancer effects of curcumin: Cycle of life and death. *Cell Div.* **2008**, *3*, 14. [CrossRef] [PubMed]
71. Elledge, S.J. Cell cycle checkpoints: Preventing an identity crisis. *Science* **1996**, *274*, 1664–1672. [CrossRef] [PubMed]
72. Leonard, C.J.; Canman, C.E.; Kastan, M.B. The role of p53 in cell-cycle control and apoptosis: Implications for cancer. *Important Adv. Oncol.* **1995**, *121*, 33–42.
73. Kastan, M.B.; Canman, C.E.; Leonard, C.J. P53, cell cycle control and apoptosis: Implications for cancer. *Cancer Metastasis Rev.* **1995**, *14*, 3–15. [CrossRef] [PubMed]
74. Bulavin, D.V.; Saito, S.; Hollander, M.C.; Sakaguchi, K.; Anderson, C.W.; Appella, E.; Fornace, A.J., Jr. Phosphorylation of human p53 by p38 kinase coordinates *N*-terminal phosphorylation and apoptosis in response to UV radiation. *EMBO J.* **1999**, *18*, 6845–6854. [CrossRef] [PubMed]
75. Vermeulen, K.; Van Bockstaele, D.R.; Berneman, Z.N. The cell cycle: A review of regulation, deregulation and therapeutic targets in cancer. *Cell Prolif.* **2003**, *36*, 131–149. [CrossRef] [PubMed]
76. Hall, M.; Peters, G. Genetic alterations of cyclins, cyclin-dependent kinases, and Cdk inhibitors in human cancer. *Adv. Cancer Res.* **1996**, *68*, 67–108. [PubMed]
77. Noble, M.; Barrett, P.; Endicott, J.; Johnson, L.; McDonnell, J.; Robertson, G.; Zawaira, A. Exploiting structural principles to design cyclin-dependent kinase inhibitors. *Biochim. Biophys. Acta* **2005**, *1754*, 58–64. [CrossRef] [PubMed]
78. Elmore, S. Apoptosis: A review of programmed cell death. *Toxicol. Pathol.* **2007**, *35*, 495–516. [CrossRef] [PubMed]
79. Cotter, T.G. Apoptosis and cancer: The genesis of a research field. *Nat. Rev. Cancer* **2009**, *9*, 501–507. [CrossRef] [PubMed]
80. Ashkenazi, A.; Dixit, V.M. Death receptors: Signaling and modulation. *Science* **1998**, *281*, 1305–1308. [CrossRef] [PubMed]
81. Kischkel, F.C.; Hellbardt, S.; Behrmann, I.; Germer, M.; Pawlita, M.; Krammer, P.H.; Peter, M.E. Cytotoxicity-Dependent Apo-1 (Fas/Cd95)-Associated Proteins Form a Death-Inducing Signaling Complex (Disc) with the Receptor. *EMBO. J.* **1995**, *14*, 5579–5588. [PubMed]

82. Saelens, X.; Festjens, N.; Vande Walle, L.; van Gurp, M.; van Loo, G.; Vandenabeele, P. Toxic proteins released from mitochondria in cell death. *Oncogene* **2004**, *23*, 2861–2874. [CrossRef] [PubMed]
83. Chinnaiyan, A.M. The apoptosome: Heart and soul of the cell death machine. *Neoplasia.* **1999**, *1*, 5–15. [CrossRef] [PubMed]
84. Cory, S.; Adams, J.M. The Bcl2 family: Regulators of the cellular life-or-death switch. *Nat. Rev. Cancer.* **2002**, *2*, 647–656. [CrossRef] [PubMed]
85. Schuler, M.; Green, D.R. Mechanisms of p53-dependent apoptosis. *Biochem. Soc. Trans.* **2001**, *29*, 684–688. [CrossRef] [PubMed]
86. Igney, F.H.; Krammer, P.H. Death and anti-death: Tumour resistance to apoptosis. *Nat. Rev. Cancer* **2002**, *2*, 277–288. [CrossRef] [PubMed]
87. Aggarwal, B.B. Nuclear factor-kappaB: The enemy within. *Cancer Cell* **2004**, *6*, 203–208. [CrossRef] [PubMed]
88. Cao, Y.; Liu, Q. Therapeutic targets of multiple angiogenic factors for the treatment of cancer and metastasis. *Adv. Cancer Res.* **2007**, *97*, 203–224. [PubMed]
89. Hu, Y.; Liu, K.; Yan, M.; Zhang, Y.; Wang, Y.; Ren, L. Icariin inhibits oxidized low-density lipoprotein-induced proliferation of vascular smooth muscle cells by suppressing activation of extracellular signal-regulated kinase 1/2 and expression of proliferating cell nuclear antigen. *Mol. Med. Rep.* **2016**, *13*, 2899–2903. [PubMed]
90. Ekstrand, A.J.; Sugawa, N.; James, C.D.; Collins, V.P. Amplified and rearranged epidermal growth factor receptor genes in human glioblastomas reveal deletions of sequences encoding portions of the *N*- and/or *C*-terminal tails. *Proc. Natl. Acad. Sci. USA* **1992**, *89*, 4309–4313. [CrossRef] [PubMed]
91. Han, W.; Lo, H.W. Landscape of EGFR signaling network in human cancers: Biology and therapeutic response in relation to receptor subcellular locations. *Cancer Lett.* **2012**, *318*, 124–134. [CrossRef] [PubMed]
92. Mora, L.B.; Buettner, R.; Seigne, J.; Diaz, J.; Ahmad, N.; Garcia, R.; Bowman, T.; Falcone, R.; Fairclough, R.; Cantor, A.; et al. Constitutive activation of Stat3 in human prostate tumors and cell lines: Direct inhibition of Stat3 signaling induces apoptosis of prostate cancer cells. *Cancer Res.* **2002**, *62*, 6659–6666. [PubMed]
93. Dolled-Filhart, M.; Camp, R.L.; Kowalski, D.P.; Smith, B.L.; Rimm, D.L. Tissue microarray analysis of signal transducers and activators of transcription 3 (Stat3) and phospho-Stat3 (Tyr705) in node-negative breast cancer shows nuclear localization is associated with a better prognosis. *Clin. Cancer Res.* **2003**, *9*, 594–600. [PubMed]
94. Hsiao, J.R.; Jin, Y.T.; Tsai, S.T.; Shiau, A.L.; Wu, C.L.; Su, W.C. Constitutive activation of STAT3 and STAT5 is present in the majority of nasopharyngeal carcinoma and correlates with better prognosis. *Brit. J. Cancer* **2003**, *89*, 344–349. [CrossRef] [PubMed]
95. Santarpia, L.; Lippman, S.M.; El-Naggar, A.K. Targeting the MAPK-RAS-RAF signaling pathway in cancer therapy. *Expert. Opin. Ther. Targets* **2012**, *16*, 103–119. [CrossRef] [PubMed]
96. Shields, J.M.; Pruitt, K.; McFall, A.; Shaub, A.; Der, C.J. Understanding Ras: 'It ain't over 'til it's over'. *Trends Cell Biol.* **2000**, *10*, 147–154. [CrossRef]
97. Liu, P.; Cheng, H.; Roberts, T.M.; Zhao, J.J. Targeting the phosphoinositide 3-kinase pathway in cancer. *Nat. Rev. Drug Discov.* **2009**, *8*, 627–644. [CrossRef] [PubMed]
98. Guertin, D.A.; Sabatini, D.M. Defining the role of mTOR in cancer. *Cancer Cell* **2007**, *12*, 9–22. [CrossRef] [PubMed]
99. Shacter, E.; Weitzman, S.A. Chronic inflammation and cancer. *Oncology* **2002**, *16*, 217–229. [PubMed]
100. Bunt, S.K.; Sinha, P.; Clements, V.K.; Leips, J.; Ostrand-Rosenberg, S. Inflammation induces myeloid-derived suppressor cells that facilitate tumor progression. *J. Immunol.* **2006**, *176*, 284–290. [CrossRef] [PubMed]
101. Armstrong, L.; Davydova, J.; Brown, E.; Han, J.; Yamamoto, M.; Vickers, S.M. Delivery of interferon alpha using a novel Cox2-controlled adenovirus for pancreatic cancer therapy. *Surgery* **2012**, *152*, 114–122. [CrossRef] [PubMed]
102. Ristimaki, A.; Honkanen, N.; Jankala, H.; Sipponen, P.; Harkönen, M. Expression of cyclooxygenase-2 in human gastric carcinoma. *Cancer Res.* **1997**, *57*, 1276–1280. [PubMed]
103. Basler, J.W.; Piazza, G.A. Nonsteroidal anti-inflammatory drugs and cyclooxygenase-2 selective inhibitors for prostate cancer chemoprevention. *J. Urol.* **2004**, *171*, S59–S63. [CrossRef] [PubMed]

10

Natural Polyphenols for Prevention and Treatment of Cancer

Yue Zhou [1], Jie Zheng [1], Ya Li [1], Dong-Ping Xu [1], Sha Li [2], Yu-Ming Chen [1] and Hua-Bin Li [1,3,*]

1 Guangdong Provincial Key Laboratory of Food, Nutrition and Health, School of Public Health, Sun Yat-sen University, Guangzhou 510080, China; zhouyue3@mail2.sysu.edu.cn (Y.Z.); zhengj37@mail2.sysu.edu.cn (J.Z.); liya28@mail2.sysu.edu.cn (Y.L.); xudp@mail2.sysu.edu.cn (D.-P.X.); chenyum@mail.sysu.edu.cn (Y.-M.C.)

2 School of Chinese Medicine, The University of Hong Kong, Hong Kong, China; u3003781@connect.hku.hk

3 South China Sea Bioresource Exploitation and Utilization Collaborative Innovation Center, Sun Yat-sen University, Guangzhou 510006, China

* Correspondence: lihuabin@mail.sysu.edu.cn

Abstract: There is much epidemiological evidence that a diet rich in fruits and vegetables could lower the risk of certain cancers. The effect has been attributed, in part, to natural polyphenols. Besides, numerous studies have demonstrated that natural polyphenols could be used for the prevention and treatment of cancer. Potential mechanisms included antioxidant, anti-inflammation as well as the modulation of multiple molecular events involved in carcinogenesis. The current review summarized the anticancer efficacy of major polyphenol classes (flavonoids, phenolic acids, lignans and stilbenes) and discussed the potential mechanisms of action, which were based on epidemiological, in vitro, in vivo and clinical studies within the past five years.

Keywords: polyphenol; flavonoid; anticancer; antioxidant; anti-inflammation

---

1. Introduction

Globally, there were approximately 14.1 million new cancer cases in 2012, and the number was estimated to reach 25 million in 2032. Aside from the high incidence, cancer is also one of the leading causes of death. In 2012 alone, there were about 8.2 million cancer-related deaths, which were mainly attributed to lung, gastric, colorectal, liver, breast, prostate and cervical cancer [1]. The situation urges the research of cancer prevention and treatment. In the last two decades, the anticancer effects of natural polyphenols have become a hot topic in many laboratories. Meanwhile, polyphenols are potential candidates for the discovery of anticancer drugs. Polyphenols are defined as compounds having at least one aromatic ring with one or more hydroxyl functional groups attached. Natural polyphenols refer to a large group of plant secondary metabolites ranging from small molecules to highly polymerized compounds [2]. Polyphenols are widely present in foods and beverages of plant origins (e.g., fruits, vegetables, spices, soy, nuts, tea and wine) [3–5]. Based on chemical structures, natural polyphenols can be divided into five classes, including flavonoids, phenolic acids, lignans, stilbenes and other polyphenols. Flavonoids and phenolic acids are the most common classes, and account for about 60% and 30% of all natural polyphenols, respectively (Table 1) [6]. A plethora of studies have documented the anticancer effects of natural polyphenols [7–11]. Noteworthy examples include anthocyanins from blueberries, epigallocatechin gallate (EGCG) from green tea, resveratrol from red wine and isoflavones from soy. The anticancer efficacy of natural polyphenols has largely been attributed to their potent antioxidant and anti-inflammatory activities as well as their abilities to modulate molecular targets and signaling pathways, which were associated with cell survival, proliferation, differentiation, migration, angiogenesis, hormone activities, detoxification enzymes, immune responses, etc. [12,13].

The present review summarized recent discoveries about the anti-carcinogenic properties of natural polyphenols and discussed the mechanisms of action, which were based on evidence from epidemiological studies, laboratory experiments and clinical trials.

Table 1. The classification of natural polyphenols.

Classification		Representative Members	Major Dietary Sources
flavonoids	anthocyanins	delphinidin, pelargonidin, cyanidin, malvidin	berries, grapes, cherries, plums, pomegranates
	flavanols	epicatechin, epigallocatechin, EGCG, procyanidins	apples, pears, legumes, tea, cocoa, wine
	flavanones	hesperidin, naringenin	citrus fruits
	flavones	apigenin, chrysin, luteolin,	parsley, celery, orange, onions, tea, honey, spices
	flavonols	quercetin, kaempferol, myricetin, isorhamnetin, galangin	berries, apples, broccoli, beans, tea
	isoflavonoids	genistein, daidzein	soy
phenolic acids	hydroxybenoic acid	ellagic acid, gallic acid	pomegranate, grapes, berries, walnuts, chocolate, wine, green tea
	hydroxycinnamic acid	ferulic acid, chlorogenic acid	coffee, cereal grains
lignans		sesamin, secoisolariciresinol diglucoside	flaxseeds, sesame
stilbenes		resveratrol, pterostilbene, piceatannol	grapes, berries, red wine

2. Epidemiological Studies

Evidence from epidemiological studies is inconsistent, especially when considering the results of prospective cohort studies (Table 2). A case-control study in Canada reported favorable effects of a high dietary intake of total flavonoids on lung cancer risks [14]. Apart from this, in a Korean study, for women, the intake of total flavonoids, as well as flavones and anthocyanidins, was inversely associated with the risk of gastric cancer [15]. However, another study in America found no significant association between flavonoids intake and the incidence or survival of gastric cancer [16]. For colorectal cancer, a meta-analysis showed protective roles of high dietary isoflavone intake [17]. Besides, a Spanish case-control study suggested that the dietary intake of total flavonoids (especially certain subclasses) and lignans might decrease colorectal cancer risks [18]. However, large prospective cohorts showed that high habitual consumption of flavonoids could not protect against colorectal cancer [19]. In addition, the Fukuoka study reported no association between total dietary polyphenols and colorectal cancer risks [20]. For hepatocellular carcinoma (HCC), the European Prospective Investigation into Cancer and Nutrition suggested that a high intake of dietary flavanols, but not total flavonoids, might modestly decrease HCC risks [21,22]. In addition, according to a meta-analysis, the risk of breast cancer was reduced in women with a high intake of flavonols and flavones [23]. Studies also suggested that soy isoflavone intake reduced breast cancer risk for Asian women, which was more potent for post-menopausal women (OR 0.46, 95% CI 0.28–0.78) than for premenopausal women (OR 0.63, 95% CI 0.50–0.80). However, for women in Western countries, no significant association could be found, which might due to low levels of isoflavone consumption in the Western population [24,25]. In addition, the estrogen receptor (ER) status might modify the association. For example, a U.S. prospective cohort study showed that a modest inverse trend existed for dietary flavanols intake and the risk of ER-negative breast cancer, but not ER-positive cancer [26]. For prostate cancer, data from a Netherlands cohort study showed that dietary flavonoid intake was correlated with decreased risks of advanced stage prostate cancer but not overall or non-advanced prostate cancer [27]. On the contrary, in a prospective cohort study, the intake of total flavonoids as well as flavan-3-ols, isoflavones, and proanthocyanidins, increased prostate cancer risks [28].

It should be noted that the assessment of polyphenol intakes in many epidemiological studies was based on food questionnaires, which could not provide the exact composition of foods. Therefore, it might be difficult for them to reflect the real impact of natural polyphenols on cancer. In this case, the experimental study in cell culture or animal modes might be a more direct way to assess the anticancer efficacy of natural polyphenols as well as to examine the possible mechanisms involved in this process.

Table 2. Dietary polyphenol intake and cancer risks.

Cancer	Polyphenols	Study Type	Risk Estimates (95% CI)	References
lung cancer	flavonoids	case-control study	0.63 (0.47–0.85)	[14]
gastric cancer	flavonoids	case-control study	no significant association	[16]
	flavonoids	case-control study	0.33 (0.15–0.73)	[15]
colorectal cancer	flavonoids	cohort study	no significant association	[19]
	flavonoids and lignans	case-control study	total flavonoids 0.59 (0.35–0.99); lignans 0.59 (0.34–0.99)	[18]
	polyphenols	case-control study	no significant association	[20]
	isoflavones	meta-analysis	0.76 (0.59–0.98)	[17]
HCC	flavanols	cohort study	0.62 (0.33–0.99)	[22]
breast cancer	flavonoids	meta-analysis	flavonols 0.88 (0.80–0.98); flavones 0.83 (0.76–0.91); no significant association for total flavonoids or other subclasses	[23]
	isoflavones	meta-analysis	0.68 (0.52–0.89)	[25]
	flavanols	cohort study	0.81 (0.67–0.97)	[26]
prostate cancer	flavonoids	cohort study	1.15 (1.04–1.27)	[28]
	flavonoids	cohort study	total catechin 0.73 (0.57–0.95); epicatechin 0.74 (0.57–0.95); kaempferol 0.78 (0.61–1.00); myricetin 0.71 (0.55–0.91)	[27]

3. Experimental Studies

Accumulating evidence from laboratory studies has supported the anticancer properties of natural polyphenols. Given the vast number of studies, a search of PubMed and Web of Science was conducted to identify relevant peer-reviewed articles published in English within 5 years.

3.1. *Anthocyanins*

Anthocyanins (Figure 1), which occur ubiquitously throughout the plant kingdom, are the basis for the bright attractive red, blue and purple colors of fruits and vegetables. In plants, anthocyanins are usually glycosylated with glucose, galactose, arabinose, rutinose, etc. The aglycone forms are known as anthocyanidin, including cyanidin, delphinidin, peonidin, petunidin, pelargonidin, and malvidin [29].

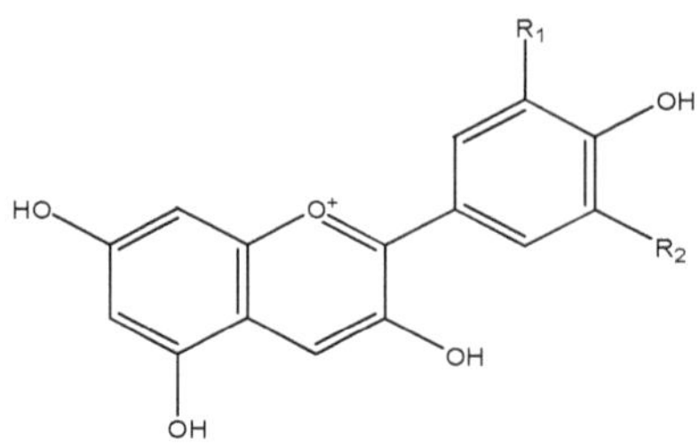

Figure 1. The chemical structures of cyanidin (R_1 = OH, R_2 = H), delphinidin (R_1 = R_2 = OH), peonidin (R_1 = OCH3, R_2 = H), petunidin (R_1 = OCH3, R_2 = OH), pelargonidin (R_1 = R_2 = H) and malvidin (R_1 = R_2 = OCH3).

Among anthocyanins, delphinidin possesses strong anticancer activities. Studies have shown that delphinidin treatment induced apoptosis and cell cycle arrest in several types of cancer. This effect might be due to suppression of the NF-κB pathway [30,31]. The over-expression of human epidermal growth factor receptor 2 (HER2) is usually associated with poor prognosis. A study found that two anthocyanins extracted from black rice, peonidin-3-glucoside and cyaniding-3-glucoside, could induce apoptosis and selectively decrease cell proliferation and tumor growth of HER2 positive breast cancer [32]. In addition, peonidin-3-glucoside treatment significantly suppressed invasion and metastasis of lung cancer cells by down-regulating the matrix metalloproteinase (MMP) [33]. In similar ways, cyanidin-3-*O*-sambubioside from *Acanthopanax sessiliflorus* fruit inhibited angiogenesis and invasion of breast cancer cells [34]. Though anthocyanins are usually considered as antioxidants, a study showed that certain anthocyanins (cyanidin and delphinidin) exhibited oxidative stress-based cytotoxicity to colorectal cancer cells [35]. Another study evaluated the impact of chemical structures on chemopreventive activities of anthocyanins in colon cancer cells. Data indicated that nonacylated monoglycosylated anthocyanins were more potent in inhibiting cancer cell growth, while anthocyanins with pelargonidin aglycone and triglycosylation were weak [36]. On the other hand, it was suggested that a mixture of different anthocyanins might be better than a single one in cancer treatment. For example, a combination of sub-optimal concentration of anthocyanidins synergistically suppressed the growth of lung cancer cells. Meanwhile, in a mice model of lung cancer, a mixture of anthocyanidins from bilberry (0.5 mg/mouse) or delphinidin (1.5 mg/mouse) all inhibited tumor growth, and the effective concentration of delphinidin in the mixture was eight-fold lower than the purified compound [7].

3.2. *Xanthohumol*

Xanthohumol (Figure 2) is a major prenylated chalcone isolated from hops (*Humulus lupulus*). The compound can also be found in beer, but to a much less extent. In some cancers, the xanthohumol-induced cell death was accompanied by apoptosis and S phase cell cycle arrest [37,38]. A study suggested that the apoptosis induced by treatment of xanthohumol (10–40 μM) to HepG2 liver cancer cells was due to modulation of the NF-κB/p53 signaling pathway [39]. Another study reported that xanthohumol treatment (>5 μM) mediated anticancer activity in human liver cancer cells through suppression of the Notch1 signaling pathway [40]. In addition, xanthohumol could block the estrogen signaling pathway. By doing so, it selectively suppressed the growth of ERα-positive breast cancer both in vitro and in vivo [41]. Cysteine X Cysteine chemokine receptor 4 (CXCR4) is over-expressed in many cancers and mediates metastasis of cancer cells to sites expressing its cognate ligand CXCL12. A study demonstrated that xanthohumol treatment dose- and time-dependently decreased expression of CXCR4, thus inhibiting cell invasion induced by CXCL12 in breast and colon cancer cells [42]. In another study, by promoting production of reactive oxygen species (ROS), xanthohumol treatment inhibited the progression of advanced tumor and the growth of poorly differentiated prostate cancer in the transgenic mice [43].

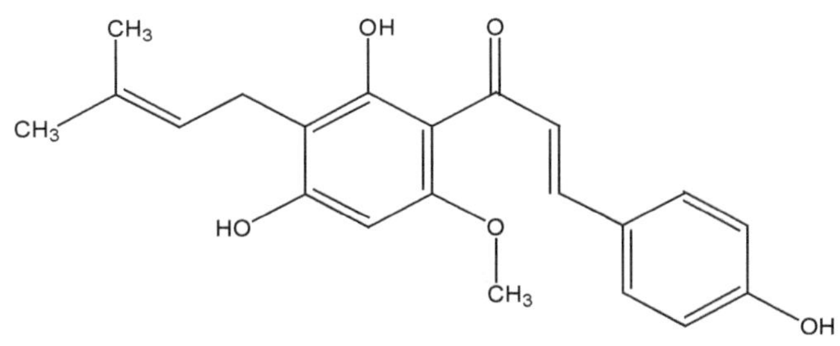

Figure 2. The chemical structure of xanthohumol.

3.3. *Flavanols*

Flavanols, also known as flavan-3-ols, have the most complex structures among subclasses of flavonoid. Flavanols include simple monomers (catechins) as well as oligomers and polymers, the latter two are known as proanthocyanidins or condensed tannins. Flavanols can be commonly found in foodstuffs [29].

3.3.1. EGCG

Smoking is a well-established risk factor of lung cancer. A study showed that EGCG (Figure 3) treatment suppressed nicotine-induced migration and invasion of A549 lung cancer cells in vitro as well as in mice through inhibiting angiogenesis and epithelial-mesenchymal transition (EMT) [9]. The effects of EGCG varied with dose. In CL1-5 lung cancer cells, at concentration of 5–20 μM, EGCG effectively suppressed the invasion and migration through suppressing MMP-2 expression. While at higher concentration (>20 μM), it exhibited anti-proliferation activities through induction of G_2/M cell cycle arrest but not apoptosis [44]. Another study found that several gastric cancer cell lines were sensitive to EGCG (100 μM) induced apoptosis due to inhibition of survivin, a potent anti-apoptotic protein [45]. Many signaling pathways might be affected by EGCG treatment. A study showed that EGCG (20 μM) exerted anti-proliferative effects in gastric cancer cell by preventing the β-catenin oncogenic signaling pathway [46]. Another study on colon cancer suggested that the Akt, extracellular signal-related kinase (ERK) 1/2 and alternative p38MAPK signaling pathways were involved in the chemopreventive effects of EGCG [47]. Besides, there is a growing interest in cancer epigenetics in recent years mainly due to the reversibility of epigenetic alterations. Major epigenetic alterations involve DNA methylation, histone modifications and miRNAs [48]. The combination of EGCG and sodium butyrate inhibited DNA methytransferases and class I histone deacetylases (HDACs) in colorectal cancer cells, thus modulating global DNA methylation and histone modifications [49]. In addition, the cancer stem cell plays a key role in chemoresistance and recurrence. Both in vitro and in vivo studies showed that EGCG could suppress cancer stem cell growth of colorectal cancer as well as breast cancer [50,51]. The anticancer activities of EGCG might involve modulation of hormone activities. It is known that exposure to estrogen is an important risk factor of breast cancer. A study found that EGCG (1 μM) could suppress estrogen (estradiol, E2)-induced breast cancer cell proliferation [52]. In addition, EGCG treatment down-regulated ERα in ER^+/PR^+ breast cancer cells [53]. Treatment of EGCG (20 μM) also inhibited metastasis of breast cancer cells by restoring the balance between MMP and the tissue inhibitor of matrix metalloproteinase (TIMP). Mechanistic studies suggested that the epigenetic induction of TIMP-3 was a key event in this process, which involved modifying the enhancer of zeste homolog 2 and HDAC1 [54]. Androgen deprivation is a main therapy for prostate cancer. It was reported that EGCG could functionally antagonize androgen, leading to suppression of prostate cancer growth both in vitro and in vivo [55].

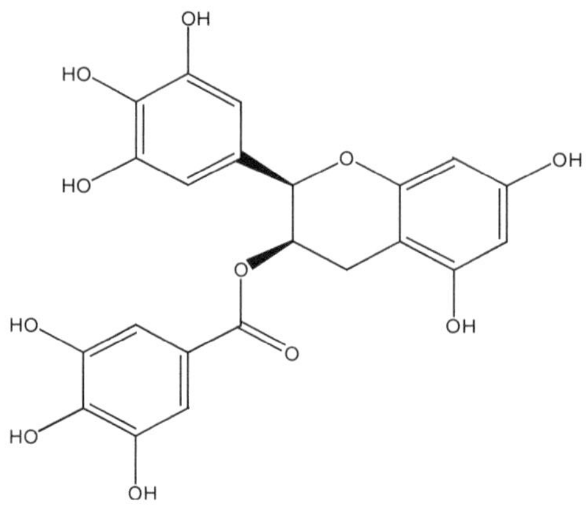

Figure 3. The chemical structure of EGCG.

3.3.2. Procyanidins

A study suggested that procyanidin C1 from Cinnamomi cortex might be able to prevent TGF-β-induced EMT in the A549 lung cancer cells [56]. Another study found that hexmer form of procyanidins from cocoa inhibited the proliferation (50 and 100 μM), induced apoptosis and G_2/M cell cycle arrest in several colorectal cancer cells, which was possibly mediated by the Akt pathway [57]. Procyanidins from Japanese quince also showed pro-apoptotic effects on Caco-2 colon cancer cells, with the oligomer enriched extract showing a more potent pro-apoptotic activity [58]. Besides, data shows that in breast cancer cells, treatment of procyanidins from evening primrose (25–100 μM gallic acid equivalents) decreased cell viability by promoting apoptosis and reduced cell invasion by suppressing angiogenesis propensity [59].

3.4. Flavanones

Flavanones (Figure 4) are abundant in citrus fruits, especially the solid parts of fruit. Major flavanones are naringenin from grapefruit and hesperetin from oranges [2].

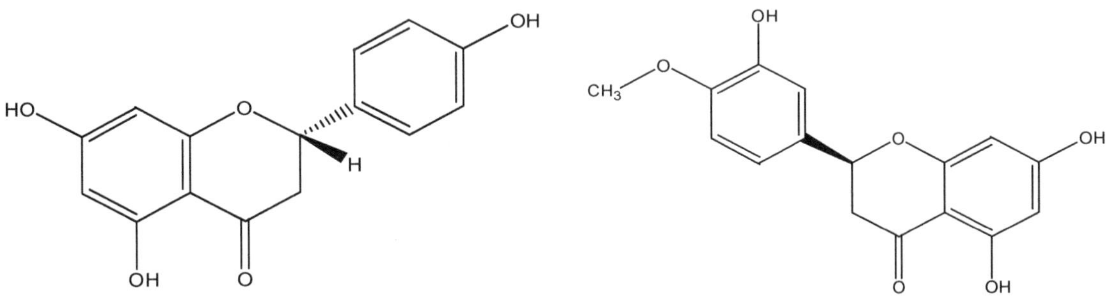

(a) (b)

Figure 4. The chemical structures of naringenin (**a**) and hesperetin (**b**).

3.4.1. Naringenin

In A549 lung cancer cells, naringenin treatment enhanced TRAIL-mediated apoptosis by up-regulating the expression of death receptor 5 [60]. Besides, in SGC-7901 gastric cancer cells, naringenin treatment inhibited cancer cell proliferation, invasion, and migration and induced apoptosis, which might be related to its inhibition of the Akt signaling pathway [61]. Another study in colon cancer cells suggested that the pro-apoptotic activity of naringenin was mediated by the p38-dependent pathway [62]. In HCC cells, naringenin could suppress TPA-induced cancer cell invasion by down-regulating multiple signaling pathways, such as the NF-κB pathway, the ERK and c-Jun N-terminal kinase (JNK) signaling pathway [63]. Besides, naringenin treatment to HepG2 liver cancer cells induced mitochondrial-mediated apoptosis and cell cycle arrest through up-regulation of p53 [64]. In breast cancer cells, naringenin demonstrated anti-estrogenic activity in estrogen-rich status and estrogenic activity in estrogen-deficient status [65]. In addition, oral administration of naringenin suppressed breast cancer metastases after surgery by modulating the host immunity [66].

3.4.2. Hesperetin

In gastric cancer cells, hesperetin treatment (100–400 μM) decreased cell proliferation and induced mitochondria-mediated apoptosis via promoting intracellular ROS accumulation. Meanwhile, the compound (i.p. 20–40 mg/kg thrice a week) significantly suppressed the growth of xenograft tumors in mice model of gastric cancer [67]. Besides, dietary hesperetin showed anti-proliferative activities against chemical-induced colon carcinogenesis. Oral supplements of hesperetin (20 mg/kg/day) reduced the proliferating cell nuclear antigen, the formation of aberrant crypt foci induced by 1,2-dimethylhydrazine in rat [68]. In breast cancer cells, hesperetin (40–200 μM) induced growth inhibition also involved mitochondria-mediated apoptosis, increased ROS and activation of ASK1/JNK pathway [69]. Cancer cells usually have high levels of glucose uptake and metabolism, which plays an important role in tumor growth. A study suggested that the anti-proliferative effects of hesperetin (50–100 μM) on breast cancer were possibly due to the suppression of glucose uptake [70]. Another study found that hesperetin treatment (IC_{50} 40–90 μM) decreased proliferation and induced apoptosis in PC-3 prostate cancer cells, which was likely mediated by inhibition of the NF-κB pathway [71]. In addition, hesperetin (IC_{50} 650 μM) exhibited potential anticancer effects on cervical cancer cells through the induction of both extrinsic and intrinsic apoptosis [72].

3.5. *Flavones*

Flavones (Figure 5) in food are usually the glycosides of apigenin and luteolin. Important dietary sources of flavones are parsley and celery [2].

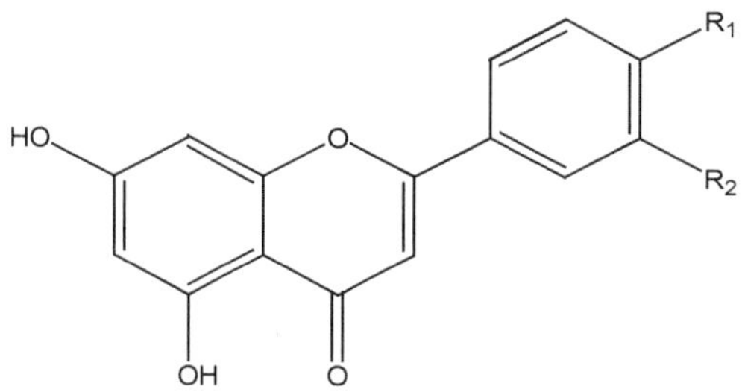

Figure 5. The chemical structures of apigenin (R_1 = OH, R_2 = H), chrysin (R_1 = R_2 = H) and luteolin (R_1 = R_2 = OH).

3.5.1. Apigenin

Apigenin is a common flavonoid widely distributed in plant-based food, such as orange, parsley, onions, tea and wheat sprouts [73]. In H460 lung cancer cells, treatment of apigenin (40–160 μM) induced apoptosis and DNA damage, which was accompanied by increased production of ROS and Ca^{2+} as well as a change of the Bax/Bcl-2 ratio [74]. Apigenin (20 μg/mL) also induced apoptosis in gastric cancer cells, especially in the undifferentiated gastric cancer cells, while showed little cytotoxicity to normal gastric cells [75]. *Helicobacter pylori* infection is known to cause ulcers and is possibly linked to gastric cancer. Atrophic gastritis was suggested to be a critical step in *Helicobacter pylori*-induced carcinogenesis. A study found that apigenin administration (30–60 mg/kg/week) could prevent *Helicobacter pylori*-induced atrophic gastritis as well as gastric cancer development in Mongolian gerbils [76]. Additionally, apigenin treatment (20–120 μM) suppressed proliferation, invasion and migration of several colorectal cancer cell lines. The compound (50 mg/kg) also inhibited tumor growth and metastasis in the orthotopic colorectal cancer model [77].

About 20% of breast cancer cases are HER2-positive, with amplification of human epidermal growth factor receptor (HER2) or over-expression of HER2 protein. These cancers are usually more aggressive and more resistant to hormone treatment than other types of breast cancer. A study found that apigenin treatment (20–100 μM) significantly suppressed growth and caused apoptosis in HER2-positive breast cancer cells, which was possibly mediated by inhibition of the signal transducer and activator of transcription 3 (STAT3) signaling pathway [78]. Another study reported anticancer effects of apigenin on MDA-MB-231 breast cancer cells in vitro (10–40 μM) and in vivo (5 and 25 mg/kg). Possible mechanisms included induction of G_2/M cell cycle arrest and epigenetic alterations. Apigenin inhibited HDACs, which induced acetylation of histone H3 in the $p21^{WAF1/CIP1}$ promoter region, leading to enhanced transcription of $p21^{WAF1/CIP1}$ [79]. Similar epigenetic effects were also found in prostate cancer. Apigenin inhibited HDACs, especially HDAC1 and HDAC3 expression. In this way apigenin treatment (20–40 μM) induced cell cycle arrest and apoptosis in prostate cancer cells and markedly inhibited tumor growth in mice (oral administration: 20 and

50 μg/mouse/day) [80]. In addition, apigenin treatment to mice (20 and 50 μg/mouse/day) markedly decreased tumor volumes of the prostate, inhibited angiogenesis and completely prevented distant organ metastasis, which at least in part, was mediated by the PI3K/Akt/Forkhead box O (FoxO) signaling pathway [81].

3.5.2. Chrysin

Chrysin is a naturally occurring flavone present in honey and propolis as well as the passion flower (*Passiflora caerulea*), and has displayed a variety of bioactivities, such as antioxidant, anti-inflammatory and anticancer activities [82]. AMPK activation is associated with cancer cell apoptosis. A study suggested that AMPK activation might be involved in the growth inhibition and apoptosis induced by chrysin treatment (10 μM) in lung cancer cells, and ROS might be a key regulator in this process [83]. Chrysin (50–100 μM) also exhibited chemopreventive effects in colorectal cancer cells, mainly as a result of TNF-mediated apoptotic cell death, and the aryl hydrocarbon receptor, a transcriptional factor, seemed to modulate this process [84]. Besides, in human triple-negative breast cancer cells, chrysin treatment (5, 10 and 20 μM) dose-dependently inhibited the potential of cancer cells to invasion and migration by down-regulating MMP-10, EMT and the PI3K/Akt signaling pathway [82].

3.5.3. Luteolin

Luteolin is abundant in artichoke as well as several spices, including sage, thyme and oregano. In A549 lung cancer cells, luteolin exhibited significant cytotoxic effects (IC_{50} 40.2 μM) through induction of G_2 cell cycle arrest and apoptosis. The apoptosis was induced in a mitochondria-dependent pathway and was associated with activation of JNK and inhibition of NF-κB (p65) translocation [85]. The micro-environment around cancer cells is highly involved in cancer progression. It was reported that luteolin (1–10 μM) effectively suppressed IL-4 induced polarization of tumor-associated macrophages (major components of cancer cell micro-environment) and consequently inhibited monocyte recruitment and migration of Lewis lung cancer cells [86]. Hypoxia is another important component of cancer micro-environment. In non-small lung cancer cells, high levels of hypoxia are usually related to EMT. Luteolin treatment (5–50 μM) to non-small lung cancer cells could inhibit hypoxia-induced EMT as well as cell viability, proliferation and motility. The effect was at least partly through suppressing the expression of integrin β1 and FAK [87]. More importantly, luteolin administration (i.p. 10 and 30 mg/kg/day) effectively suppressed tumor growth in a lung cancer mice model with EGF receptor mutation and drug resistance [88].

In a human gastric cancer xenograft model, luteolin treatment (i.p. 10 mg/kg/day) significantly suppressed tumor growth, without causing apparent toxicity or weight loss [89]. Luteolin treatment (20–100 μM) also exhibited cytotoxic effect on several colon cancer cell lines through induction of apoptosis and cell cycle arrest. Meantime, the same treatment exerted no evident toxicity on normal differentiated enterocytes [90,91]. These effects of luteolin might be associated with down-regulation of the IGF-1-mediated PI3K/Akt and ERK1/2 pathways, and suppression of synthesis of sphingosine-1-phosphate and ceramide traffic [90,91]. Besides, it was indicated that ERα was a possible target of luteolin. By down-regulating the expression of ERα, luteolin treatment (10–40 μM) suppressed IGF-1-mediated PI3K/Akt pathway, leading to growth inhibition of MCF-7 breast cancer cells accompanied by cell cycle arrest and apoptosis [92]. In the MDA-MB-231 ER-negative breast cancer cells, luteolin treatment also induced cell cycle arrest and apoptosis possibly mediated by EGFR. In addition, luteolin-supplemented diet (0.01% or 0.05%) effectively reduced tumor burden in mice inoculated with MDA-MB-231 cells [93]. Besides, in LNCaP prostate cancer cells, luteolin treatment (30 μM) arrested the cell cycle at G_1/S phase, induced cell apoptosis and inhibited cell invasion. The possible mechanism might be down-regulated expression of prostate-specific antigen by luteolin [94].

3.6. *Flavonols*

Flavonols (Figure 6) are probably the most widely distributed flavonoids in foods, but they are usually present at relatively low concentrations [2]. Representatives of this subclass are quercetin, kaempferol, myricetin, galangin and isorhamnetin.

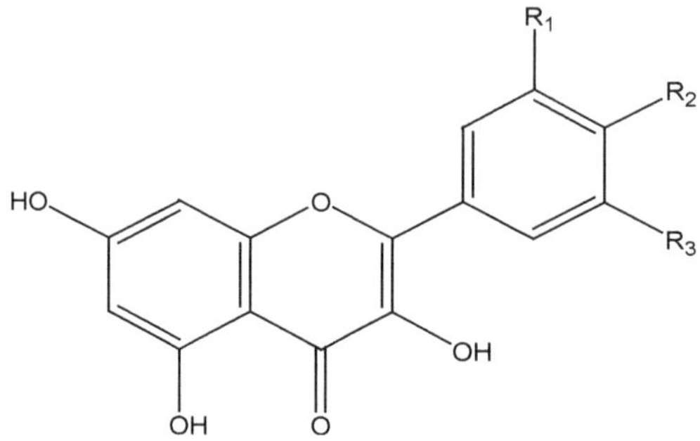

Figure 6. The chemical structures of quercetin (R_1 = H, R_2 = R_3 = OH), kaempferol (R_1 = R_3 = H, R_2 = OH), myricetin (R_1 = R_2 = R_3 = OH), galangin (R_1 = R_2 = R_3 = H) and isorhamnetin (R_1 = H, R_2 = OH, R_3 = OCH3).

3.6.1. Quercetin

Quercetin treatment (IC_{50} 2.30 ± 0.26 μM) to A549 lung cancer cells induced growth inhibition via apoptosis. In similar ways, quercetin (8.4 mg/kg) inhibited the growth of transplanted lung cancer in nude mice [95]. On the other hand, though exposure of gastric cancer cells to quercetin (IC_{50} 40 and 160 μM in two cell lines respectively) led to pronounced apoptosis, the treatment also induced protective autophagy, which impaired the anticancer effects of quercetin [96]. AMPK-mediated signaling pathway, which participates in regulation of energy homeostasis, is important for the adaptive responses of cancer cells and might be critical for the effects of quercetin. A study found that quercetin treatment (i.p. 50 mg/kg/day) significantly decreased tumor volume in the HCT116 colon cancer xenograft model by reducing AMPK activity. Similarly, by inhibiting AMPK, the apoptosis induced by quercetin (100 μM) was more pronounced under hypoxic conditions than normoxic conditions in HCT116 colon cancer cells [97]. Besides, in a mouse model of colorectal cancer, dietary quercetin supplementation (25 mg/kg/day) alleviated several symptoms of cachexia such as body weight, grip strength and muscle mass [98]. Another study found that quercetin treatment (0.05–0.15 mM) to HCC cells effectively inhibited proliferation and induced apoptosis through up-regulation of Bad and Bax, and concomitant down-regulating Bcl-2 and survivin. Importantly, quercetin (i.p. 40 mg/kg/day) also exhibited excellent inhibition effects on tumor growth in mice [99].

The exposure of MCF-7 breast cancer cells to quercetin (50–200 μM) caused a dose- and time-dependent decrease of proliferation through induction of apoptosis, which was accompanied by up-regulation of Bax and down-regulation of Bcl-2 [100]. The inhibition of insulin receptor signaling by quercetin (100 μM) also impairs proliferation of MDA-MB-231 breast cancer cells. Quercetin feeding (50 μg/mouse/day) resulted in a significant decrease of tumor growth in mice model of breast cancer [101]. In another study, quercetin (1–100 μM) inhibited breast cancer cells growth and migration via reversing EMT, which was linked with the modulation of β-catenin as well as its target genes (e.g., cyclin D1 and c-Myc) [102]. VEGFR2-mediated pathway participates in the angiogenesis in cancer development. Quercetin (34 mg/kg/day) inhibited angiogenesis of breast cancer xenograft in mice, which was performed through suppressing this pathway [103]. Besides, dietary quercetin (200 mg/kg body weight thrice a week) protected against prostate carcinogenesis induced by hormone (testosterone) and carcinogen (*N*-methyl-*N*-nitrosourea) in rats [104]. In another preclinical rat model of prostate cancer, oral administration of quercetin (200 mg/kg/day) prevented cancer development by down-regulating the cell survival, proliferative and anti-apoptotic proteins [105]. In HeLa cervical cancer cells, quercetin treatment (110.38 ± 0.66 μM) led to ROS accumulation to induce apoptosis and G_2/M cell cycle arrest [106].

3.6.2. Kaempferol

Kaempferol is a natural flavonol broadly distributed in apples, strawberries, broccoli and beans, and exhibits a wide range of beneficial properties, such as cardioprotective, anti-diabetic, and anti-allergic effects [107]. In A549 lung cancer cells, kaempferol treatment inhibited TGF-β1-induced EMT and migration through suppressing the phosphorylation of smad3 mediated by Akt1 [107]. Another study reported that kaempferol treatment exhibited significant anti-proliferative effects on MKN28 and SGC7901 gastric cancer cells without apparent cytotoxicity to normal gastric epithelial cells. The possible mechanism might be induction of apoptosis and G_2/M cell cycle arrest. More importantly, administration of kaempferol suppressed gastric cancer growth in vivo [108]. In HT-29 colon cancer cells, the treatment of kaempferol (0–60 μM) provoked apoptosis by activating the death receptor pathway and mitochondrial pathway [109]. Another study in SK-HEP-1 human liver cancer cells found G_2/M cell cycle arrest and autophagy following kaempferol treatment, which might be the result of the modulation of CDK1/cyclin B expression and AMPK and AKT signaling pathways [110]. Kaempferol induced apoptosis in MCF-7 breast cancer cells [111]. In the same cell line, treatment of kaempferol (100 μM) also significantly suppressed glucose uptake mediated by GLUT1, which might be another mechanism underlying its anti-proliferative effects [112]. Besides, both in vitro and in vivo study revealed that kaempferol could prevent breast cancer induced by 17β-estradiol or triclosn, an exogenous estrogen [113]. Kaempferol treatment also inhibited breast cell invasion through down-regulating the expression and activity of MMP-9 by blocking the PKCδ/MAPK/AP-1 cascades [114].

3.6.3. Myricetin

Myricetin is rich in berries, walnuts and herbs. Myricetin treatment to gastric cancer cells exhibited anti-proliferative effects by inducing apoptosis and cell cycle arrest [115]. In HCT-15 human colon cancer cells, myricetin treatment induced apoptotic cell death by modulating the Bax/Bcl-2-dependent pathway [116]. Similarly, myricetin also decreased the expression of anti-apoptotic survivin and Bcl-2 and increased the expression of pro-apoptotic Bax in HCC cells and in vivo [117].

3.6.4. Galangin

Galangin is a naturally occurring flavonoid rich in oregano as well as in *Alpinis officinarum*, a common spice in Asia. Galangin treatment (50–200 μM) to SNU-484 human gastric cancer cells dose- and time-dependently inhibited cell proliferation through induction of apoptosis [118]. Besides, in hepG2 liver cancer cells, galangin treatment (10–30 μM) significantly inhibited chemical-induced cell invasion and metastasis by modulating the PKC/ERK pathway [119]. Another study suggested that galangin (79.8–134 μM) could promote ER stress to suppress the proliferation of HCC cells [120].

3.6.5. Isorhamnetin

Isorhamnetin is a natural flavonoid rich in fruits and vegetables as well as tea, and is also an immediate metabolite of quercetin, which has drawn attention for its excellent anti-inflammatory and anticancer activities [121,122].

Treatment of isorhamnetin to A549 lung cancer cells induced apoptotic cell death, which was accompanied by the up-regulation of capase-3, Bax, p53 and the down-regulation of Bcl-2, cyclin D1 and PCNA protein. More importantly, isorhamnetin administration to tumor-bearing mice significantly suppressed tumor growth [123]. Additionally, isorhamnetin suppressed gastric cancer proliferation and invasion, and induced apoptosis by modulating the peroxisome proliferator-activated receptor γ (PPAR γ)-mediated pathway in vitro and in vivo [124]. Another study investigated the anti-proliferative activity of isorhamnetin in several human colorectal cancer cell lines (HT29, HCT116 and SW480), and found that the compound inhibited proliferation of all tested cancer cells by blocking the PI3K/Akt/mTOR pathway [125]. Both in vitro and in vivo experiments suggested that the anticancer property of isorhamnetin in colon cancer involved inhibition of inflammation as well as oncogenic Src activity and consequential loss of nuclear β-catenin [126]. Another study documented the anti-proliferative and pro-apoptotic activities of isorhamnetin in breast cancer cells, which was probably mediated by the Akt and MAPK kinase signaling pathways [121]. Besides, in MDA-MB-231 breast cancer cells, isorhamnetin treatment significantly suppressed cell invasion by down-regulating MMP-2 and MMP-9, which might be associated with the inhibition of p38 MAPK and STAT3 [122].

3.7. *Isoflavones*

Due to structural similarities to estrogen, isoflavones (Figure 7) have been classified as phytoestrogen, another important class of phytochemicals. Genistein and daidzein from soy are representative members of this subclass [2].

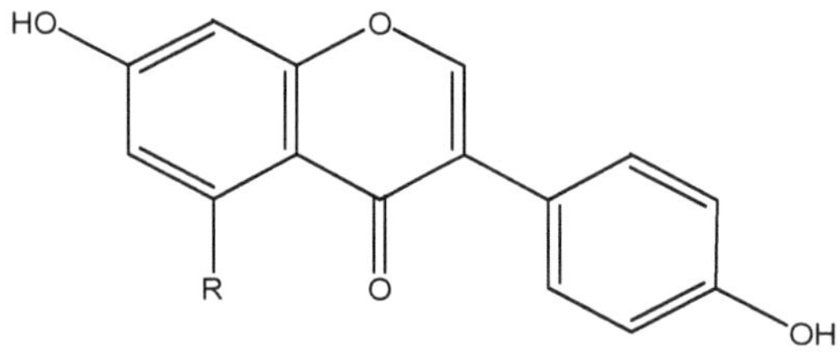

Figure 7. The chemical structures of daidzein (R = H) and genistein (R = OH).

3.7.1. Daidzein

Data indicated that daidzein was an apoptosis inducer in liver cancer cells and treatment of daidzein (200–600 μM) caused mitochondrial-dependent apoptosis mediated by the Bcl-2 family [127]. In an in vitro study, daidzein (50 μM) as well as its metabolites R-equol and S-equol, suppressed the invasion of MDA-MB-231 human breast cancer cells at least partly through the down-regulation of MMP-2 expression [128]. However, another study reported that daidzein treatment (3–10 μM) up-regulated proto-oncogene BRF2 in ER-positive breast cancer cells but not ER-negative cells. Female mice treated with a high-isoflavone commercial diet showed significantly increased BRF2 expression [129].

3.7.2. Genistein

Genistein is the most abundant isoflavonoid contained in soy as well as soy products and is also a major active component of hormonal supplements for menopausal women [10]. In H446 lung cancer cells, genistein treatment (25–75 μM) effectively suppressed the cell proliferation and migration, which was accompanied by induction of apoptosis and G_2/M cell cycle arrest. Importantly, the treatment also suppressed the expression of Forehead box protein M1 and its target genes regulating cell cycle or apoptosis, such as survivin, cyclin B1 and Cdc25. Therefore, the effects of genistein were at least partly mediated by Forkhead box protein M1 [130]. In addition, genistein treatment (15 μM) to gastric cancer cells suppressed the cancer cell stem-like abilities, includingself-renewal, drug resistance and carcinogenicity, which might be due to down-regulation of stemness related genes as well as drug resistance gene ABCG2. Meantime, genistein (i.p. 1.5 mg/kg/day) significantly decreased the weight and size of gastric cancer inoculated in nude mice [131]. Besides, genistein (25–100 μM) exhibited anti-proliferative and pro-apoptotic effects on colon cancer cells. The study indicated that inhibition of oncogenic miR-95, Akt and SGK as well as phosphorylation of Akt could be involved in these anticancer effects. Moreover, genistein treatment (i.p. 20, 50, 80 mg/kg/day) to mice significantly decreased the weight and size of transplanted colorectal cancer [132]. Oral administration of genistein also inhibited angiogenesis and suppressed metastasis of colorectal cancer to distant organs in mice [133].

According to in vitro studies, the anticancer effects of genistein on colorectal cancer might involve the suppression of Wnt, NF-κB signaling pathways [134,135]. Additionally, in nude mice inoculated with liver cancer cells, oral administration of genistein (50 mg/kg/day) significantly suppressed the intrahepatic metastasis [136].

Genistein treatment (5, 10 or 20 μM) elicited growth inhibition of MDA-MB-231 breast cancer cells, which was accompanied by apoptosis and G_2/M cell cycle arrest. This effect might be mediated by down-regulation of the NF-κB activity via the Notch-1 pathway [137]. In MCf-7 breast cancer cells, genistein treatment (15 and 30 μM) also inhibited cell growth, induced apoptosis and decreased the $CD44^{+}CD24^{-}$ cancer stem cells. Importantly, genistein (i.p. 20 and 50 mg/kg/day) could also target breast cancer stem cells to reduce the volume and weight of xenograft tumors in nude mice. The effects might be correlated with down-regulation of Hedgehog-Gli1 signaling pathway [138]. However, some studies found that genistein has adverse effects on breast cancer treatment. A study suggested that the ERα/ERβ ratio could be a determinant of genistein functions in breast cancer. In breast cancer with a low ERα/ERβ ratio (e.g., T4D7 cells), genistein treatment might be harmless or even beneficial, while in breast cancer with a high ratio (e.g., MCF-7 cells), the treatment might be counterproductive [139]. Genistein (10 μM) could also affect the expression and function of ATP-binding cassette drug transporters in breast cancer cells. The effect resulted in an increase of efflux and resistance of chemotherapeutic drugs (doxorubicin and mitoxantrone) in MCF-7 cells [10]. Moreover, in athymic mice model of breast cancer, a low dose long-term treatment of genistein ($\leq$500 ppm) led to tumor growth as well as more aggressive and advanced phenotypes [140]. Genistein was also reported to have different effects on prostate cancer cells. In LAPC-4 cells with wild androgen receptor, genistein treatment (0.5–50 μM) dose dependently suppressed cell proliferation and androgen receptor. However, in LNCaP cells with T877A mutant androgen receptor, genistein promoted cancer cell growth and androgen receptor at physiological concentration (0.5–5 μM), but showed inhibitory activities at higher concentration. Similar biphasic activities of genistein were also observed in PC-3 cells transfected with androgen receptor mutants [141]. In addition, the exposure of HeLa cervical cancer cells to genistein (IC_{50} 100 μM) led to growth inhibition mediated by apoptosis and G_2/M cell cycle arrest and suppressed cell migration by modulating MMP-9 and TIMP-1 [142].

3.8. Phenolic Acids

Phenolic acids (Figure 8) can be mainly classified into two groups, hydroxybenzoic acid and hydroxycinnamic acid. Hydroxybenzoic acids present in few edible plants and are not considered to be of high nutritional interest. The other group is more common in food, but its consumption is highly variable, depending on intake of coffee [2].

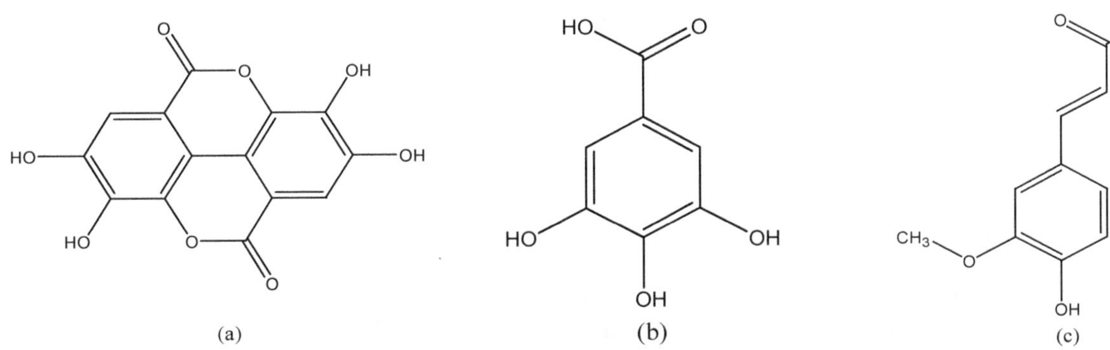

(a) (b) (c)

Figure 8. The chemical structures of (**a**) ellagic acid; (**b**) gallic acid and (**c**) ferulic acid.

3.8.1. Ellagic Acid

Ellagic acid is a dietary flavonoid abundantly in pomegranate, grapes, strawberries and walnuts [143]. Ellagic acid (50–200 μM) exerted anti-proliferative and pro-apoptotic effects in colon cancer cell lines in a concentration dependent manner [144]. Besides, in a chemical-induced liver cancer rat model, oral administration of ellagic acid (30 mg/kg/day) normalized the permeability of mitochondrial outer membrane and alleviated inflammation-mediated cancer cell proliferation [145]. Ellagic acid (10–40 μg/mL) also showed growth inhibitory effects on MCF-7 breast cancer cells, which was accompanied by G_0/G_1 cell cycle arrest. The modulation of the TGF-β/Smads signaling pathway was suggested to be the potential mechanism [143]. Furthermore, exposure to ellagic acid (i.p. 50 and 100 mg/kg/day) suppressed tumor growth and angiogenesis in mice implanted with breast cancer cells [146]. In another study, non-cytotoxic dose of ellagic acid (25 and 50 μM) to androgen independent prostate cancer cells markedly suppressed the cell invasion and motility. The effect might be the result of down-regulation of MMPs [147]. Besides, at higher dose (10–100 μM), ellagic acid treatment was found to induce growth inhibition and caspase-dependent apoptosis in PC3 prostate cancer cells in a dose responsive manner [148].

3.8.2. Gallic Acid

Gallic acid is widely distributed in plant-based food in free forms as well as part of hydrolyzable tannins. Blackberry, raspberry, walnuts, chocolate, wine, green tea and vinegar are rich sources of the compound. Gallic acid possesses various pharmacological activities, such as anti-microbial, anti-inflammatory and anticancer activities [149,150]. Exposure to gallic acid (3.5 μM) inhibited migration of AGS gastric cancer cells, which was possibly mediated by up-regulation of RhoB as well as down-regulation of AKT/small GTPase signals and NF-κB activity. In addition to this, compared with the control, feeding with gallic acid solution (0.25% and 0.5%) significantly decreased tumor size and weight in mice models of gastric cancer [151]. The ROS-dependent pro-apoptotic effects of gallic acid led to decreased viability of different cancer cells, such as HCT-15 colon cancer cells (200 μM) and LNCaP prostate cancer cells (80 μg/mL) [149,152]. Besides, gallic acid treatment selectively inhibited growth of liver cancer cells through the mitochondria-mediated apoptotic pathways (IC_{50} for cancer cells 28.5 ± 1.6 μg/mL and 22.1 ± 1.4 μg/mL, for normal human hepatocytes 80.9 ± 4.6 μg/mL) [153]. Studies on MCF-7 breast cancer cells also showed that gallic acid treatment inhibited cell proliferation (IC_{50} 80.5 μM) and induced apoptosis via both the extrinsic and intrinsic pathways [150]. Additionally, exposure to gallic acid (25 and 50 μM) suppressed the invasion and migration of PC-3 prostate cancer cells through down-regulation of MMP-2 and MMP-9 [154]. In another study, gallic acid (50, 100, and 200 μM) in PC-3 prostate cancer cells provoked DNA damage and inhibited expression of DNA repair genes, which contributed to gallic-induced growth inhibition [155]. Treatment with gallic acid (10–40 μg/mL) decreased cell viability, proliferation, invasion and angiogenesis HeLa and HTB-35 cervical cancer cells, but showed less cytotoxicity on normal cells (HUVEC), indicating a potential role of the compound in cervical cancer treatment [156].

3.8.3. Ferulic Acid

The main dietary sources of ferulic acid are cereal grains, particularly the outer parts of grain. The compound has attracted great attention due to its therapeutic activities against various diseases, such as cancer, cardiovascular and neurodegenerative diseases [157,158].

It was reported that ferulic acid was a pro-oxidant at high concentration or in the presence of metal ions such as copper. Since the increased level of copper was observed in many cancers, and cancer cells are usually under greater oxidative stress than normal cells, the pro-oxidant ability of ferulic acid might lead to selective cytotoxicity to cancer cells [157]. Ferulic acid (10 μg/mL) also decreased cell viability and enhanced efficacy of radiotherapy in two cervical cancer cell lines (HeLa and ME-180), possibly through promotion of ROS [159]. Another study on prostate cancer found that the effects of ferulic acid varied with cell types. Ferulic acid treatment caused cell cycle arrest in PC-3 cells (IC_{50} 300 μM), and led to apoptosis in LNCaP cells (IC_{50} 500 μM) [158].

3.9. Lignans

Lignans (Figure 9) are widely present in plants, such as flaxseed, sesame, and seeds of *Arctium lappa*. Secoisolariciresinol diglucoside (SDG) is a natural lignan rich in flaxseed, and can be converted into more biologically active lignans (enterodiol and enterolactone) by human colon bacteria. These lignans are structurally similar to estradiol; thus, they may have anticancer effects for hormone-related cancers, such as breast, prostate and colon cancer. For example, SDG was reported to possess selective estrogen receptor modulating effects and display anti-estrogenic activity in a high estrogen environment. Treatment with SDG (100 ppm in diet) normalized some biomarkers changed by carcinogen in mammary gland tissue of mice [160]. In another study, enterolactone modulated expression of genes involved in cell proliferation and cell cycle of MDA-MB-231 breast cancer cells (IC_{50} 261.9 ± 10.5 μM) [161].

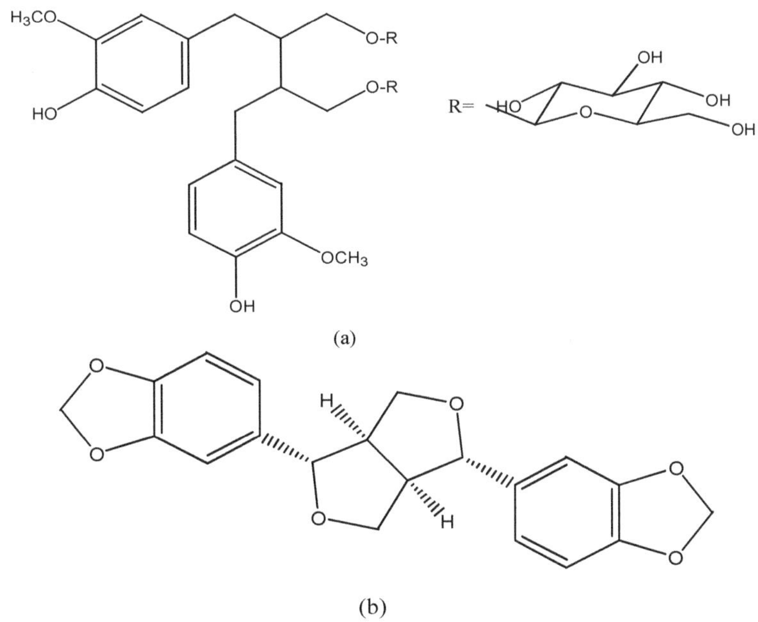

Figure 9. The chemical structures of (**a**) Secoisolariciresinol diglucoside and (**b**) sesamin.

Sesamin is a major lipid soluble lignan from sesame oil. Sesamin treatment (1, 10 and 50 μM) dose-dependently decreased cell viability and increased apoptosis in MCF-7 breast cancer cells. The lignan (10–100 μM) also inhibited the pro-angiogenic activity of macrophages in MCF-7 cells by down-regulating VEGF and MMP-9 [162]. Besides, it was suggested that STAT3 played an important role in sesamin (25–125 μM) induced G_2/M cell cycle arrest and apoptosis in HepG2 cells [163]. Sesamin (10–100 μg/mL) could suppress lipopolysaccharide-induced proliferation and invasion of PC3 prostate cancer cells by modulating the p38-MAPK and NF-κB signaling pathways. Likewise, sesamin pretreatment (10 mg/kg every three days, injection) suppressed PC3 cells-derived tumor growth triggered by lipopolysaccharide in mice [164].

3.10. Stilbenes

Natural stilbenes (Figure 10) are another important group of polyphenols. Though they only exist in a limited group of plant families, the prominent health benefits of resveratrol, an important member of this class, have attracted a lot of studies into natural stilbenes.

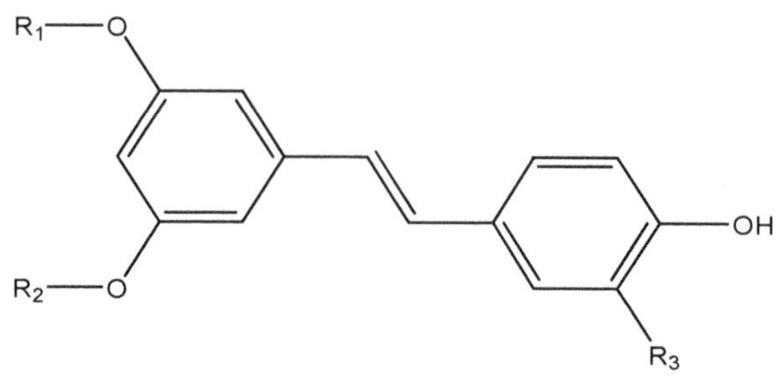

Figure 10. The chemical structures of resveratrol ($R_1 = R_2 = R_3 = H$), pterostilbene ($R_1 = R_2 = CH3$, $R_3 = OH$), piceatannol ($R_1 = R_2 = H$, $R_3 = OH$).

3.10.1. Resveratrol

Resveratrol is predominantly found in red wine, grapes and berries. X-ray repair cross complement group 1 (XRCC1) participates in base excision repair. It was reported that resveratrol treatment (5–50 μM) could suppress XRCC1 expression, thus leading to enhanced chemosensitivity to etoposide (a topoisomerase II inhibitor) of human non-small-cell lung cancer cell lines [165]. Besides, it was reported that 20 μM resveratrol treatment significantly suppressed invasion and metastasis of A549 lung cancer cells by inhibiting EMT [11].

In gastric cancer cells, resveratrol treatment (25 and 50 μM) arrested cancer cells in the G_1 phase, resulting in senescence instead of apoptosis. In similar ways, resveratrol (40 mg/kg/day) inhibited gastric cancer development in nude mice [166]. However, at higher concentrations (50–200 μM), resveratrol induced DNA damage and apoptosis in human gastric adenocarcinoma cells via promoting generation of ROS [167]. Resveratrol induced apoptosis in different colon cancer cell lines via modulating diverse targets. For example, resveratrol induced caspase-8 and -3 dependent apoptosis via ROS-triggered autophagy in HT-29 (IC_{50} 150 μM) and COLO 201 (IC_{50} 75 μM) human colon cancer cells [168]. A study reported that the indirect DNA-damaging effects of resveratrol (30 μM) in colon cancer cells were mainly caused by overproduction of ROS [169]. Another study suggested that the DNA damage induced by resveratrol (25 μM) was due to topoisomerase II poisoning rather than promoting ROS production [170]. Besides, resveratrol (50 μM) suppressed expression of multi-drug resistance protein 1 (MDR1) and drug efflux in drug-resistant colorectal cancer cells [171]. Activating mutations in Kras contribute to sporadic colorectal cancer. An in vivo study found that dietary supplements of resveratrol (equivalent to 105 and 210 mg daily for humans) protected against formation and growth of colorectal cancer by suppressing expression of Kras [172]. In addition, in colorectal cancer patients, following oral administration of resveratrol, high concentrations of resveratrol conjugates (mainly RSV-3-*O*-sulfate, RSV-3-*O*-glucuronide and RSV-4′-*O*-glucuronide) were found in the colorectum. Mixture of these conjugates exhibited synergistic anticancer effects by inducing DNA damage and apoptosis in human colorectal cancer cells. Therefore, despite the low bioavailability of resveratrol, the anti-carcinogenic properties could also be achieved by its main metabolites [173]. Cancer stem cells possess the ability to self-renew and are important for tumor generation. Three signaling pathways regulated the self-renewal of breast cancer stem cells are Wnt, Notch and Hedgehog. It was reported that resveratrol could inhibit the Wnt/β-catenin signaling pathway in breast cancer stem cells. Accordingly, resveratrol treatment (i.v. 100 mg/kg/day) to mice significantly suppressed tumor growth as well as the breast cancer stem cells in primary xenografts [174]. Resveratrol is also a powerful chemopreventive agent against liver cancer. At low concentration, resveratrol treatment (25–100 μM) inhibited metastasis of HCC cells and decreased expression of urokinase-type plasminogen activator (u-PA), which involved down-regulation of the SP-1 signaling pathway [175]. Besides, in *N*-nitrosodiethylamine treated rat, the oral administration of resveratrol (20 mg/kg/day) either at early or advanced stages of liver carcinogenesis was equally effective, possibly mediated by apoptosis [176]. In androgen independent prostate cancer cells, resveratrol treatment (25–100 μM) induced autophagy-mediated cell death [177]. In addition, oral administration of resveratrol (30 mg/kg thrice a week) to mice inhibited proliferation, induced apoptosis, and suppressed angiogenesis and metastasis of prostate cancer [178]. In several cervical cancer cells, resveratrol treatment (150–250 μM) caused cell cycle arrest and apoptosis [179].

3.10.2. Pterostilbene

Pterostilbene is a natural dimethoxylated analog of resveratrol mainly found in blueberries. The hydroxyl group substitution with methoxyl groups gives pterostilbene greater lipophilicity, oral bioavailability and biological half-life than resveratrol.

Pinostilbene is a major metabolite of pterostilbene in the colon of mice. At physiologically relevant concentrations (20 and 40 μM), it significantly inhibited cell growth, and induced apoptosis and S phase arrest of human colon cancer cells. Therefore, pinostilbene might be important for the anticancer effects of orally administered pterostilbene [180]. In addition, pterostilbene treatment (25–75 μM) was able to induce apoptosis in breast cancer cells via Bax activation and over-expression [181]. MicroRNAs (miRNAs) are small non-coding RNAs, which control post-transcriptional expression of genes. It was suggested that miRNAs are highly involved in the development of cancer [48]. A study reported that pterostilbene treatment inhibited EMT and metastasis of breast cancer cells (2.5–10 μM). Mechanistic investigations also showed an up-regulation of miR-205 following pterostilbene treatment, which inhibited the Src/Fak signaling and suppressed tumor growth and metastasis in MDA-MB-231-bearing NOD/SCID mice (i.p. 10 mg/kg thrice a week) [182]. Another study found that pterostilbene treatment selectively killed breast cancer stem cells (IC_{50} 25 μM) and sensitized these cells to chemotherapeutic drug paclitaxel [183]. Besides, pterostilbene treatment (80 μM) activated AMPK in both p53 positive and negative human prostate cancer cells, but the cell fate following AMPK activation was affected by p53 status. In p53 positive LNCaP cells, pterostilbene caused G_1 cell cycle arrest by increasing p53 expression, while in p53 negative PC3 cells, pterostilbene treatment induced apoptosis [184]. In another study, pterostilbene (i.p. 50 mg/kg/day) inhibited tumor growth in mice models of prostate cancer [185].

3.10.3. Piceatannol

Piceatannol is a hydroxylated analog of resveratrol present in a variety of foods, for example, grapes, berries, passion fruit, and white tea. In colorectal cancer cells, piceatannol treatment (30 μM) induced apoptosis by up-regulating miR-129, and thus down-regulating Bcl-2, which is a known target of miR-129 [186]. Besides, in prostate cancer cells, treatment with piceatannol (25 and 50 μM) inhibited proliferation, and induced cell cycle arrest and apoptosis, which might be associated with down-regulated mTOR [187]. Piceatannol was also a potential anti-invasive and anti-metastasis agent on prostate cancer cells. The oral administration of piceatannol (20 mg/kg/day) significantly suppressed the metastasis of prostate cancer to lung in mice [188].

The anticancer activities and potential mechanisms of the polyphenols reviewed in this section were summarized in Table 3 and Figure 11. Due to the critical role of cancer stem cells in cancer development and treatment, the anti-cancer stem cell effects of polyphenols were summarized in Table 4. It should be noted that curcumin is not discussed in this section because it has been extensively reviewed [189–191]. Besides, the bioavailability of many polyphenols is low, which might hamper their application in cancer treatment (Table 5) [6].

Table 3. The in vitro and in vivo anticancer activities of natural polyphenols.

Polyphenol	Study Type	Dose	Main Effects	References
Lung Cancer				
peonidin-3-glucoside	in vitro	10–40 μM	inhibiting cancer cell invasion, motility, secretion of MMPs and u-PA	[33]
anthocyanidins	in vivo	0.5 mg/mouse	inhibiting tumor growth	[7]
xanthohumol	in vitro	14–42 μM	inducing apoptosis and cell cycle arrest	[38]
EGCG	in vitro	5–20 μM	suppressing cancer cell invasion, migration, MMP-2	[44]
EGCG	in vivo	NA [1]	suppressing nicotine-induced angiogenesis	[9]
procyanidin C1	in vitro	1.25–40 μg/mL	inhibiting TGF-β-induced EMT	[56]
naringenin	in vitro	100 μM	enhancing TRAIL-mediated apoptosis	[60]
apigenin	in vitro	40–160 μM	inducing apoptosis and DNA damage	[74]
chrysin	in vitro	10 μM	inducing apoptosis, AMPK activation, ROS	[83]
luteolin	in vitro	5–50 μM	inducing apoptosis, cell cycle arrest, inhibiting monocyte recruitment, migration, EMT	[85–87]
luteolin	in vivo	10–30 mg/kg	suppressing tumor growth	[88]
quercetin	in vivo	8.4 mg/kg	suppressing tumor growth	[95]
kaempferol	in vitro	10–50 μM	inhibiting TGF-β1-induced EMT and migration	[107]
isorhamnetin	in vivo	NA	suppressing tumor growth	[123]
genistein	in vitro	25–75 μM	suppressing cancer cell proliferation and migration, accompanied by apoptosis and cell cycle arrest	[130]
resveratrol	in vitro	5–50 μM	decreasing XRCC1 expression, enhancing chemosensitivity, suppressing invasion, metastasis	[13,165]
Gastric Cancer				
EGCG	in vitro	20–100 μM	inducing apoptosis, down-regulating survivin, the β-catenin signaling pathway	[45,46]
naringenin	in vitro	20–80 μM	inducing apoptosis, inhibiting cancer cell proliferation, invasion, migration and the AKT pathway	[61]
hesperetin	in vivo	20–40 mg/kg	suppressing tumor growth	[67]
apigenin	in vitro	20 μg/mL	inducing apoptosis	[75]
apigenin	in vivo	30–60 mg/kg	preventing *Helicobacter pylori*-induced atrophic gastritis and carcinogenesis	[76]
luteolin	in vivo	10 mg/kg	suppressing tumor growth	[89]
quercetin	in vitro	40–160 μM	inducing apoptosis and protective autophagy	[96]
kaempferol	in vivo	20 mg/kg	suppressing tumor growth	[108]
myricetin	in vitro	20–40 μM	inducing apoptosis and cell cycle arrest	[115]
galangin	in vitro	50–200 μM	inducing apoptosis	[118]
isorhamnetin	in vivo	1 mg/kg	increasing PPAR-γ, decreasing Bcl-2 and CD31	[124]
gallic acid	in vivo	0.25% and 0.5% in water	decreasing tumor size and weight	[151]
resveratrol	in vitro	50–200 μM	inducing apoptosis, DNA damage, ROS production	[167]
resveratrol	in vivo	40 mg/kg	suppressing tumor growth	[166]

Table 3. *Cont.*

Polyphenol	Study Type	Dose	Main Effects	References
Colorectal Cancer				
delphinidin	in vitro	30–240 μM	inducing apoptosis, cell cycle arrest, oxidative stress	[30]
cyanidin	in vitro	100 μM	inducing oxidative stress	[35]
EGCG	in vitro	1–50 μM	inducing epigenetic alteration, apoptosis, MAPK and Akt pathways activation	[47,49]
procyanidins	in vitro	50 and 100 μM	inducing apoptosis and cell cycle arrest	[57]
naringenin	in vitro	50–200 μM	inducing apoptosis	[62]
hesperetin	in vivo	20 mg/kg	suppressing chemical-induced carcinogenesis	[68]
apigenin	in vivo	50 mg/kg	inhibiting tumor growth and metastasis	[77]
chrysin	in vitro	50–100 μM	inducing TNF-mediated apoptotic cell death	[84]
luteolin	in vitro	20-100 μM	inducing apoptosis and cell cycle arrest	[90]
quercetin	in vivo	25–50 mg/kg	suppressing tumor growth by reducing AMPK activity and alleviating cachexia symptoms	[97,98]
kaempferol	in vitro	0–60 μM	inducing apoptosis	[109]
myricetin	in vitro	NA	inducing apoptosis	[116]
isorhamnetin	in vivo	200 g/kg in diet	suppressing mortality, tumor number, tumor burden and chemical-induced inflammatory responses	[126]
genistein	in vivo	20–80 mg/kg	decreasing the weight and size of transplanted tumor, inhibiting angiogenesis and metastasis	[132,133]
ellagic acid	in vitro	50–200 μM	inducing apoptosis	[144]
gallic acid	in vitro	200 μM	inducing apoptosis	[149]
resveratrol	in vitro	25–150 μM	inducing apoptosis, DNA damage and suppressing drug resistance	[168–171]
resveratrol	in vivo	equal to 105 and 210 mg for human	suppressing tumor development by modulation of Kras	[172]
piceatannol	in vitro	30 μM	inducing apoptosis mediated by miR-129	[186]
Liver Cancer				
xanthohumol	in vitro	5–40 μM	inducing apoptosis, modulating the NF-κB/p53 and the Notch1 signaling pathways	[39,40]
naringenin	in vitro	25–200 μM	suppressing TPA-induced cancer cell invasion, inducing apoptosis and cell cycle arrest	[63,64]
quercetin	in vivo	40 mg/kg	suppressing tumor growth	[99]
kaempferol	in vitro	25–100 μM	inducing cell cycle arrest and autophagy	[110]
myricetin	in vivo	100 mg/kg	suppressing chemical-induced carcinogenesis	[117]
galangin	in vitro	10–134 μM	inhibiting chemical-induced cell invasion, metastasis, promoting ER stress	[119,120]
daidzein	in vitro	200–600 μM	inducing apoptosis	[127]
genistein	in vivo	50 mg/kg	suppressing the intrahepatic metastasis	[136]
ellagic acid	in vivo	30 mg/kg	suppressing chemical-induced carcinogenesis	[145]
gallic acid	in vitro	22.1–28.5 μg/mL	inducing apoptosis	[153]
sesamin	in vitro	25–125 μM	inducing apoptosis and cell cycle arrest mediated by STAT3	[163]

Table 3. *Cont.*

Polyphenol	Study Type	Dose	Main Effects	References
Liver Cancer				
resveratrol	in vitro	25–100 μM	inhibiting metastasis, decreasing expression of u-PA, down-regulating the SP-1 signaling pathway	[175]
resveratrol	in vivo	20 mg/kg	suppressing chemical-induced carcinogenesis	[176]
Breast Cancer				
anthocyanins	in vivo	6 mg/kg	suppressing the growth of HER2-positive tumor	[32]
cyanidin-3-*O*-sambubioside	in vitro	1–30 μM	inhibiting angiogenesis and invasion	[34]
xanthohumol	in vitro	NA	decreasing expression of CXCR4, inhibiting cell invasion induced by CXCL12	[42]
xanthohumol	in vivo	0.3 and 1.0 mg/kg	blocking the estrogen singling pathway, selectively suppressing the growth of ERα-positive breast cancer	[41]
EGCG	in vitro	1–40 μM	suppressing estrogen-induced cancer cell proliferation, down-regulating ERα , inhibiting metastasis by restoring the balance between MMP and TIMP	[52–54]
procyanidins	in vitro	25–100 μM	inducing apoptosis, reducing invasion, angiogenesis	[59]
naringenin	in vivo	100 mg/kg	suppressing lung metastases by the host immunity	[66]
hesperetin	in vitro	40–200 μM	inducing apoptosis, ROS production and activation of ASK1/JNK pathway, suppressing glucose uptake	[69,70]
apigenin	in vitro	20–100 μM	suppressing growth and causing apoptosis possibly mediated by the STAT3 signaling pathway	[78]
apigenin	in vivo	5–25 mg/kg	inducing cell cycle arrest through epigenetic change	[79]
chrysin	in vitro	5–20 μM	inhibiting cancer cell invasion and migration	[84]
luteolin	in vitro	10–40 μM	down-regulating ERα expression, inducing apoptosis and cell cycle arrest	[92]
luteolin	in vivo	0.01%–0.05% in diet	reducing tumor burden	[93]
quercetin	in vitro	1–200 μM	inducing apoptosis, suppressing the insulin receptor signaling and EMT	[100–102]
quercetin	in vivo	34 mg/kg	inhibiting angiogenesis	[103]
kaempferol	in vitro	100 μM	inducing apoptosis and suppressing glucose uptake	[111,112]
kaempferol	in vivo	100 mg/kg	preventing cancer development induced by estrogen	[113]
isorhamnetin	in vitro	10–40 μM	inhibiting cancer cell adhesion, migration, invasion	[122]
daidzein	in vitro	3–50 μM	decreasing invasion, MMP-2 expression, up-regulating proto-oncogene BRF2 in ER-positive cancer cells	[128,129]
genistein	in vitro	5–20 μM	inducing apoptosis, cell cycle arrest, increasing drug resistance	[10,137]
genistein	in vivo	≤500 ppm	enhancing tumor growth	[140]
ellagic acid	in vitro	10–40 μg/mL	inducing cell cycle arrest	[143]

Table 3. *Cont.*

Polyphenol	Study Type	Dose	Main Effects	References
Breast Cancer				
ellagic acid	in vivo	50–100 mg/kg	suppressing tumor growth and angiogenesis	[146]
gallic acid	in vitro	80.5 μM	inducing apoptosis	[150]
SDG	in vivo	100 ppm in diet	normalizing some biomarkers changed by carcinogen	[160]
enterolactone	in vitro	261.9 ± 10.5 μM	modulating expression of genes involved in cell proliferation and cell cycle	[161]
sesamin	in vitro	1–100 μM	inducing apoptosis and inhibiting the pro-angiogenic activity of macrophages	[162]
pterostilbene	in vitro	25–75 μM	inducing apoptosis	[181]
pterostilbene	in vivo	10 mg/kg	suppressing tumor growth and metastasis	[182]
Prostate Cancer				
delphinidin	in vitro	3–90 μM	inducing apoptosis and cell cycle arrest	[31]
xanthohumol	in vivo	50 μg/mouse	suppressing tumor growth and progression	[43]
EGCG	in vivo	1 mg 3×/week	antagonizing androgen, suppressing tumor growth	[55]
hesperetin	in vitro	40–90 μM	inducing apoptosis, inhibiting the NF-κB pathway	[71]
apigenin	in vivo	20 and 50 μg/mouse	suppressing tumor growth, angiogenesis, metastasis	[81]
luteolin	in vitro	30 μM	inducing apoptosis, cell cycle arrest, inhibiting invasion	[94]
quercetin	in vivo	200 mg/kg	inhibiting carcinogenesis induced by hormone and carcinogen	[104]
genistein	in vitro	0.5–50 μM	different effects dependent on androgen receptor	[141]
ellagic acid	in vitro	10–100 μM	inducing apoptosis, inhibiting cell invasion, motility	[147,148]
gallic acid	in vitro	25–200 μM	provoking DNA damage, down-regulating DNA repair genes, invasion and migration	[154,155]
ferulic acid	in vitro	300–500 μM	inducing apoptosis and cell cycle arrest	[158]
sesamin	in vivo	10 mg/kg	suppressed tumor growth induced by LPS	[164]
resveratrol	in vitro	25–100 μM	inducing autophagy-mediated cell death	[177]
resveratrol	in vivo	30 mg/kg	inducing apoptosis, suppressing angiogenesis and metastasis	[178]
pterostilbene	in vitro	80 μM	inducing apoptosis and cell cycle arrest	[184]
pterostilbene	in vivo	50 mg/kg	suppressing tumor growth	[185]
piceatannol	in vitro	25 and 50 μM	inducing apoptosis and cell cycle arrest	[187]
piceatannol	in vivo	20 mg/kg	suppressing lung metastasis	[188]
Cervical Cancer				
hesperetin	in vitro	650 μM	inducing apoptosis	[72]
quercetin	in vitro	110.38 μM	inducing apoptosis and cell cycle arrest	[106]
genistein	in vitro	100 μM	inducing apoptosis, cell cycle arrest, suppressing cell migration	[142]
gallic acid	in vitro	10–40 μg/mL	decreasing cell proliferation, invasion, angiogenesis	[156]
ferulic acid	in vitro	10 μg/mL	enhancing efficacy of radiotherapy	[159]
resveratrol	in vitro	150–250 μM	inducing apoptosis and cell cycle arrest	[179]

[1] NA, stands for not available.

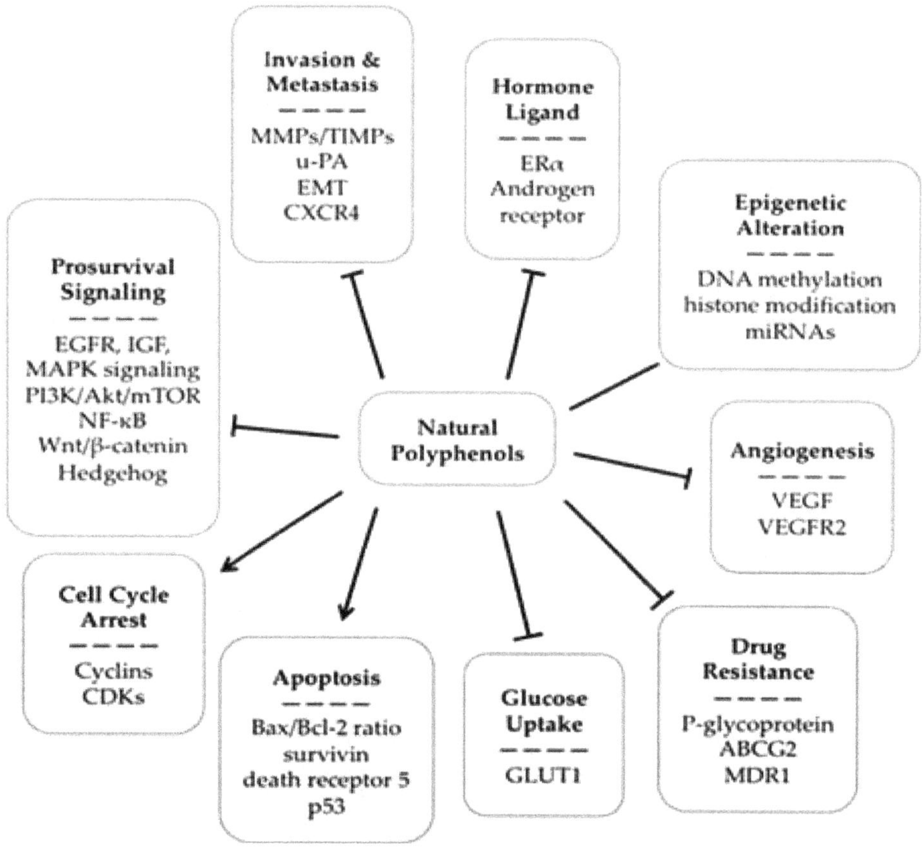

Figure 11. Mechanisms of the anticancer activities of natural polyphenols → stands for activation, – for regulation, ⊥ for inhibition.

Table 4. The anti-cancer stem cell effects of polyphenols.

Compound	Cancer	Study Type	Dose	Effect	References
EGCG	colorectal cancer	in vivo	100 μM	Inhibiting tumor growth of spheroid-derived cancer stem cell xenografts	[50]
	breast cancer	in vivo	16.5 mg/kg	decreasing tumor growth, the expression of VEGF-D and peritumoral lymphatic vessel density	[51]
genistein	gastric cancer	in vivo	1.5 mg/kg	decreasing tumor weight and size	[131]
	breast cancer	in vivo	20–50 mg/kg	targeting breast cancer stem cells to reduce the growth of xenograft tumors and inhibiting the Hedgehog-Gli1 signaling pathway	[138]
resveratrol	breast cancer	in vivo	100 mg/kg	inhibited the Wnt/β-catenin signaling pathway, tumor growth and cancer stem cells	[174]
pterostilbene	breast cancer	in vitro	25 μM	decreasing cancer stem cells and drug resistance	[183]

Table 5. The bioavailability of some natural polyphenols.

Compound	Subject	Treatment	Urine Concentration	Plasm Concentration
anthocyanins	human	black berries 200 g (960 μmol) *	total urinary excretion of anthocyanin metabolites 0.160%	NA
EGCG	human	2 mg/kg	NA	mean Cmax 0.09 μmol/L, Tmax 2 h
naringenin	human	fresh orange segments 150 g (11.8 mg/150 g fresh weight) *	mean urinary excretion 12.5%	mean Cmax 0.08 μmol/L, Tmax 5.88 h
hesperetin	human	fresh orange segments 150 g (79.7 mg/150 g fresh weight) *	mean urinary excretion 4.53%	mean Cmax 0.09 μmol/L, Tmax 7 h
quercetin	human	dry shallot skin 1.4 mg/kg (4.93 μmol/g fresh weight) *	NA	mean Cmax 3.95 μmol/L, Tmax 2.78 h
isorhamnetin	rat	0.25 mg/kg	NA	mean Cmax 0.18 μmol/L, Tmax 8 h
daidzein	human	soy milk 750 mL/day (5.4 mg/250 mL) *	148.35 μmol/24 h after 5 days	196.1 nmol/L after 5 days
genistein	human	soy milk 750 mL/day (16.98 mg/250 mL) *	2077.7 μmol/24 h after 5 days	797.04 nmol/L after 5 days
ellagic acid	human	freeze-dried black raspberry 45 g/day (0.3 mg/g dry weight) *	NA	mean Cmax 0.01 μmol/L, Tmax 1.98 h
gallic acid	human	grape skin extract 18 g (0.7 mg/g dry weight) *	5.9 μmol after 24 h	NA
ferulic acid	rat	5.15 mg/kg	mean urinary excretion 43.4%	mean Cmax 1.68 μmol/L, Tmax 1 h
resveratrol	human	1 mg/kg trans-resveratrol	mean urinary excretion 26%	0.75 μg/mL after 1.5 h

* Indicates content of the compound in food; NA, stands for not available.

4. Clinical Trials

Though numerous studies have demonstrated that natural polyphenol could be potential candidates for anticancer therapy, clinical studies in this area are relatively few and the therapeutic efficacy is sometimes non-significant. A review of early clinical investigations on polyphenolic phytochemicals suggested tea polyphenols could be used for the prevention of premalignancy, but evidence was less convincing for curcumin and soy isoflavones [192]. Table 6 summarized some clinical evidence about the use of natural polyphenol in cancer treatment. The clinical trials in this section were identified from the PubMed database using the MeSH term "neoplasms" combined with "polyphenols".

Table 6. Summary of clinical trials with polyphenols in various cancers.

Subject	Treatment	Outcome	References
54 patients with localized prostate cancer	synthetic genistein (30 mg) daily for 3–6 weeks	decreasing level of serum prostate specific antigen (PSA)	[193]
158 men aged 50–75 with rising prostate specific antigen	isoflavone (60 mg) daily for 12 months	reducing prostate cancer incidence for patients aged 65 or more	[194]
86 patients with localized prostate cancer	soy isoflavone (80 mg total isoflavones, 51 mg aglucon units) daily for 6 weeks	no significant change in serum hormone levels, total cholesterol, or PSA	[195]
10 breast cancer patients undergoing radiotherapy	EGCG (400 mg) thrice daily for 2–8 weeks	enhancing efficacy of radiotherapy	[196]

Table 6. *Cont.*

Subject	Treatment	Outcome	References
147 patients with prostate cancer	flaxseed (30 mg) daily for 30 days	significant inverse association between total urinary enterolignans and enterolactone and Ki67 in the tumor tissue	[197]
87 patients with resected colorectal cancer or polypectomy	flavonoid mixture (20 mg apigenin and 20 mg EGCG) for 3–4 years	reducing recurrence rate of colon neoplasia in patients with resected colon cancer	[198]
5 familial adenomatous polyposis patients with colectomy	curcumin (480 mg) and quercetin (20 mg) thrice daily for 6 months	reducing polyp number and size from baseline without appreciable toxicity	[199]
85 patients with prostate cancer	isoflavones (40 mg) and curcumin (100 mg) daily for 6 months	decreasing level of serum PSA	[200]
44 smokers with 8 or more aberrant crypt foci	curcumin (2 or 4 g) daily for 30 days	decreasing number of aberrant crypt foci	[201]
126 patients with colorectal cancer	curcumin (360 mg) thrice daily for 10–30 days	increasing body weight and expression of p53, suppressing serum level of TNF-α	[202]

5. Conclusions

The epidemiological studies about the relationship between dietary polyphenol consumption and cancer risks yielded different results. The difficult in assessing intake of dietary polyphenols and the diversity of polyphenols might contribute to the inconsistent results. On the other hand, the vast majority of laboratory studies supported anticancer activities of natural polyphenols, such as anthocyanins, EGCG, resveratrol and curcumin. The mechanisms of action mainly included modulation of molecular events and signaling pathways associated with cell survival, proliferation, differentiation, migration, angiogenesis, hormone activities, detoxification enzymes, immune responses, etc. Besides, the anticancer effects of polyphenol varied with cancer types, cell lines and doses. It is of note that some polyphenols, such as genistein and daidzein, have been suggested to have adverse effects on hormone-related cancer. Therefore, the use of these polyphenols in cancer treatment should be cautious. In addition, clinical trials about the anticancer actions of polyphenol are limited. In the future, more epidemiological studies employing biomarkers of polyphenols are needed to assess the impact of dietary polyphenols on cancer risks. Besides, the anticancer activities of more polyphenols need to be assessed and compared, and the mechanisms of action require further study. Larger, randomized clinical trials need to be carried out to provide more reliable evidence. Additionally, the bioavailability of polyphenols should be evaluated and improved. Special attention should be paid to the safety of polyphenols.

Acknowledgments: This work was supported by the National Natural Science Foundation of China (No. 81372976), Key Project of Guangdong Provincial Science and Technology Program (No. 2014B020205002), and the Hundred-Talents Scheme of Sun Yat-sen University.

Author Contributions: Yue Zhou, Sha Li and Hua-Bin Li conceived this paper; Yue Zhou, Jie Zheng, Ya Li and Dong-Ping Xu wrote this paper; and Sha Li, Yu-Ming Chen and Hua-Bin Li revised the paper.

References

1. WHO | Cancer. Available online: http://www.who.int/mediacentre/factsheets/fs297/en/ (accessed on 17 May 2016).

2. Manach, C.; Scalbert, A.; Morand, C.; Remesy, C.; Jimenez, L. Polyphenols: Food sources and bioavailability. *Am. J. Clin. Nutr.* **2004**, *79*, 727–747. [PubMed]
3. Zhou, Y.; Li, Y.; Zhou, T.; Zheng, J.; Li, S.; Li, H.B. Dietary natural products for prevention and treatment of liver cancer. *Nutrients* **2016**, *8*, 156. [CrossRef] [PubMed]
4. Fu, L.; Xu, B.T.; Xu, X.R.; Qin, X.S.; Gan, R.Y.; Li, H.B. Antioxidant capacities and total phenolic contents of 56 wild fruits from South China. *Molecules* **2010**, *15*, 8602–8617. [CrossRef] [PubMed]
5. Deng, G.F.; Lin, X.; Xu, X.R.; Gao, L.; Xie, J.; Li, H.B. Antioxidant capacities and total phenolic contents of 56 vegetables. *J. Funct. Foods* **2013**, *5*, 260–266. [CrossRef]
6. Neveu, V.; Perez-Jimenez, J.; Vos, F.; Crespy, V.; du Chaffaut, L.; Mennen, L.; Knox, C.; Eisner, R.; Cruz, J.; Wishart, D.; et al. Phenol-Explorer: An online comprehensive database on polyphenol contents in foods. *Database* **2010**, *2010*, 24. [CrossRef] [PubMed]
7. Kausar, H.; Jeyabalan, J.; Aqil, F.; Chabba, D.; Sidana, J.; Singh, I.P.; Gupta, R.C. Berry anthocyanidins synergistically suppress growth and invasive potential of human non-small-cell lung cancer cells. *Cancer Lett.* **2012**, *325*, 54–62. [CrossRef] [PubMed]
8. Li, A.N.; Li, S.; Zhang, Y.; Xu, X.R.; Chen, Y.; Li, H.B. Resources and biological activities of Natural Polyphenols. *Nutrients* **2014**, *6*, 6020–6047. [CrossRef] [PubMed]
9. Shi, J.; Liu, F.; Zhang, W.; Liu, X.; Lin, B.; Tang, X. Epigallocatechin-3-gallate inhibits nicotine-induced migration and invasion by the suppression of angiogenesis and epithelial-mesenchymal transition in non-small cell lung cancer cells. *Oncol. Rep.* **2015**, *33*, 2972–2980. [CrossRef] [PubMed]
10. Rigalli, J.P.; Tocchetti, G.N.; Arana, M.R.; Villanueva, S.S.; Catania, V.A.; Theile, D.; Ruiz, M.L.; Weiss, J. The phytoestrogen genistein enhances multidrug resistance in breast cancer cell lines by translational regulation of ABC transporters. *Cancer Lett.* **2016**, *376*, 165–172. [CrossRef] [PubMed]
11. Wang, H.; Zhang, H.; Tang, L.; Chen, H.; Wu, C.; Zhao, M.; Yang, Y.; Chen, X.; Liu, G. Resveratrol inhibits TGF-beta1-induced epithelial-to-mesenchymal transition and suppresses lung cancer invasion and metastasis. *Toxicology* **2013**, *303*, 139–146. [CrossRef] [PubMed]
12. Li, F.; Li, S.; Li, H.B.; Deng, G.F.; Ling, W.H.; Xu, X.R. Antiproliferative activities of tea and herbal infusions. *Food Funct.* **2013**, *4*, 530–538. [CrossRef] [PubMed]
13. Li, F.; Li, S.; Li, H.; Deng, G.; Ling, W.; Wu, S.; Xu, X.; Chen, F. Antiproliferative activity of peels, pulps and seeds of 61 fruits. *J. Funct. Foods* **2013**, *5*, 1298–1309. [CrossRef]
14. Christensen, K.Y.; Naidu, A.; Parent, M.E.; Pintos, J.; Abrahamowicz, M.; Siemiatycki, J.; Koushik, A. The risk of lung cancer related to dietary intake of flavonoids. *Nutr. Cancer* **2012**, *64*, 964–974. [CrossRef] [PubMed]
15. Woo, H.D.; Lee, J.; Choi, I.J.; Kim, C.G.; Lee, J.Y.; Kwon, O.; Kim, J. Dietary flavonoids and gastric cancer risk in a Korean population. *Nutrients* **2014**, *6*, 4961–4973. [CrossRef] [PubMed]
16. Petrick, J.L.; Steck, S.E.; Bradshaw, P.T.; Trivers, K.F.; Abrahamson, P.E.; Engel, L.S.; He, K.; Chow, W.H.; Mayne, S.T.; Risch, H.A.; et al. Dietary intake of flavonoids and oesophageal and gastric cancer: Incidence and survival in the United States of America (USA). *Br. J. Cancer* **2015**, *112*, 1291–1300. [CrossRef] [PubMed]
17. Tse, G.; Eslick, G.D. Soy and isoflavone consumption and risk of gastrointestinal cancer: A systematic review and meta-analysis. *Eur. J. Nutr.* **2016**, *55*, 63–73. [CrossRef] [PubMed]
18. Zamora-Ros, R.; Not, C.; Guino, E.; Lujan-Barroso, L.; Garcia, R.M.; Biondo, S.; Salazar, R.; Moreno, V. Association between habitual dietary flavonoid and lignan intake and colorectal cancer in a Spanish case-control study (the Bellvitge Colorectal Cancer Study). *Cancer Causes Control* **2013**, *24*, 549–557. [CrossRef] [PubMed]
19. Nimptsch, K.; Zhang, X.; Cassidy, A.; Song, M.; O'Reilly, E.J.; Lin, J.H.; Pischon, T.; Rimm, E.B.; Willett, W.C.; Fuchs, C.S.; et al. Habitual intake of flavonoid subclasses and risk of colorectal cancer in 2 large prospective cohorts. *Am. J. Clin. Nutr.* **2016**, *103*, 184–191. [CrossRef] [PubMed]
20. Wang, Z.J.; Ohnaka, K.; Morita, M.; Toyomura, K.; Kono, S.; Ueki, T.; Tanaka, M.; Kakeji, Y.; Maehara, Y.; Okamura, T.; et al. Dietary polyphenols and colorectal cancer risk: The Fukuoka colorectal cancer study. *World J. Gastroenterol.* **2013**, *19*, 2683–2690. [CrossRef] [PubMed]
21. Zamora-Ros, R.; Agudo, A.; Lujan-Barroso, L.; Romieu, I.; Ferrari, P.; Knaze, V.; Bueno-de-Mesquita, H.B.; Leenders, M.; Travis, R.C.; Navarro, C.; et al. Dietary flavonoid and lignan intake and gastric adenocarcinoma risk in the European Prospective Investigation into Cancer and Nutrition (EPIC) study. *Am. J. Clin. Nutr.* **2012**, *96*, 1398–1408. [CrossRef] [PubMed]

22. Zamora-Ros, R.; Fedirko, V.; Trichopoulou, A.; Gonzalez, C.A.; Bamia, C.; Trepo, E.; Nothlings, U.; Duarte-Salles, T.; Serafini, M.; Bredsdorff, L.; et al. Dietary flavonoid, lignan and antioxidant capacity and risk of hepatocellular carcinoma in the European prospective investigation into cancer and nutrition study. *Int. J. Cancer* **2013**, *133*, 2429–2443. [CrossRef] [PubMed]
23. Hui, C.; Qi, X.; Qianyong, Z.; Xiaoli, P.; Jundong, Z.; Mantian, M. Flavonoids, flavonoid subclasses and breast cancer risk: A meta-analysis of epidemiologic studies. *PLoS ONE* **2013**, *8*, e54318. [CrossRef] [PubMed]
24. Chen, M.; Rao, Y.; Zheng, Y.; Wei, S.; Li, Y.; Guo, T.; Yin, P. Association between soy isoflavone intake and breast cancer risk for pre- and post-menopausal women: A meta-analysis of epidemiological studies. *PLoS ONE* **2014**, *9*, e89288. [CrossRef] [PubMed]
25. Xie, Q.; Chen, M.L.; Qin, Y.; Zhang, Q.Y.; Xu, H.X.; Zhou, Y.; Mi, M.T.; Zhu, J.D. Isoflavone consumption and risk of breast cancer: A dose-response meta-analysis of observational studies. *Asia Pac. J. Clin. Nutr.* **2013**, *22*, 118–127. [PubMed]
26. Wang, Y.; Gapstur, S.M.; Gaudet, M.M.; Peterson, J.J.; Dwyer, J.T.; McCullough, M.L. Evidence for an association of dietary flavonoid intake with breast cancer risk by estrogen receptor status is limited. *J. Nutr.* **2014**, *144*, 1603–1611. [CrossRef] [PubMed]
27. Geybels, M.S.; Verhage, B.A.; Arts, I.C.; van Schooten, F.J.; Goldbohm, R.A.; van den Brandt, P.A. Dietary flavonoid intake, black tea consumption, and risk of overall and advanced stage prostate cancer. *Am. J. Epidemiol.* **2013**, *177*, 1388–1398. [CrossRef] [PubMed]
28. Wang, Y.; Stevens, V.L.; Shah, R.; Peterson, J.J.; Dwyer, J.T.; Gapstur, S.M.; McCullough, M.L. Dietary flavonoid and proanthocyanidin intakes and prostate cancer risk in a prospective cohort of US men. *Am. J. Epidemiol.* **2014**, *179*, 974–986. [CrossRef] [PubMed]
29. Crozier, A.; Jaganath, I.B.; Clifford, M.N. Dietary phenolics: Chemistry, bioavailability and effects on health. *Nat. Prod. Rep.* **2009**, *26*, 1001–1043. [CrossRef] [PubMed]
30. Yun, J.M.; Afaq, F.; Khan, N.; Mukhtar, H. Delphinidin, an anthocyanidin in pigmented fruits and vegetables, induces apoptosis and cell cycle arrest in human colon cancer HCT116 cells. *Mol. Carcinog.* **2009**, *48*, 260–270. [CrossRef] [PubMed]
31. Bin, H.B.; Asim, M.; Siddiqui, I.A.; Adhami, V.M.; Murtaza, I.; Mukhtar, H. Delphinidin, a dietary anthocyanidin in pigmented fruits and vegetables: A new weapon to blunt prostate cancer growth. *Cell Cycle* **2008**, *7*, 3320–3326.
32. Liu, W.; Xu, J.; Wu, S.; Liu, Y.; Yu, X.; Chen, J.; Tang, X.; Wang, Z.; Zhu, X.; Li, X. Selective anti-proliferation of HER2-positive breast cancer cells by anthocyanins identified by high-throughput screening. *PLoS ONE* **2013**, *8*, e81586. [CrossRef] [PubMed]
33. Ho, M.L.; Chen, P.N.; Chu, S.C.; Kuo, D.Y.; Kuo, W.H.; Chen, J.Y.; Hsieh, Y.S. Peonidin 3-glucoside inhibits lung cancer metastasis by downregulation of proteinases activities and MAPK pathway. *Nutr. Cancer* **2010**, *62*, 505–516. [CrossRef] [PubMed]
34. Lee, S.J.; Hong, S.; Yoo, S.H.; Kim, G.W. Cyanidin-3-*O*-sambubioside from *Acanthopanax sessiliflorus* fruit inhibits metastasis by downregulating MMP-9 in breast cancer cells MDA-MB-231. *Planta Med.* **2013**, *79*, 1636–1640. [CrossRef] [PubMed]
35. Cvorovic, J.; Tramer, F.; Granzotto, M.; Candussio, L.; Decorti, G.; Passamonti, S. Oxidative stress-based cytotoxicity of delphinidin and cyanidin in colon cancer cells. *Arch. Biochem. Biophys.* **2010**, *501*, 151–157. [CrossRef] [PubMed]
36. Jing, P.; Bomser, J.A.; Schwartz, S.J.; He, J.; Magnuson, B.A.; Giusti, M.M. Structure-function relationships of anthocyanins from various anthocyanin-rich extracts on the inhibition of colon cancer cell growth. *J. Agric. Food Chem.* **2008**, *56*, 9391–9398. [CrossRef] [PubMed]
37. Yong, W.K.; Abd, M.S. Xanthohumol induces growth inhibition and apoptosis in ca ski human cervical cancer cells. *Evid.-Based Complement. Altern. Med.* **2015**, *2015*, 921306. [CrossRef] [PubMed]
38. Yong, W.K.; Ho, Y.F.; Malek, S.N. Xanthohumol induces apoptosis and S phase cell cycle arrest in A549 non-small cell lung cancer cells. *Pharmacogn. Mag.* **2015**, *11*, S275–S283. [PubMed]
39. Zhao, X.; Jiang, K.; Liang, B.; Huang, X. Anticancer effect of xanthohumol induces growth inhibition and apoptosis of human liver cancer through NF-kappaB/p53-apoptosis signaling pathway. *Oncol. Rep.* **2016**, *35*, 669–675. [PubMed]

40. Kunnimalaiyaan, S.; Sokolowski, K.M.; Balamurugan, M.; Gamblin, T.C.; Kunnimalaiyaan, M. Xanthohumol inhibits Notch signaling and induces apoptosis in hepatocellular carcinoma. *PLoS ONE* **2015**, *10*, e127464. [CrossRef] [PubMed]
41. Yoshimaru, T.; Komatsu, M.; Tashiro, E.; Imoto, M.; Osada, H.; Miyoshi, Y.; Honda, J.; Sasa, M.; Katagiri, T. Xanthohumol suppresses oestrogen-signalling in breast cancer through the inhibition of BIG3-PHB2 interactions. *Sci. Rep.* **2014**, *4*, 7355. [CrossRef] [PubMed]
42. Wang, Y.; Chen, Y.; Wang, J.; Chen, J.; Aggarwal, B.B.; Pang, X.; Liu, M. Xanthohumol, a prenylated chalcone derived from hops, suppresses cancer cell invasion through inhibiting the expression of CXCR4 chemokine receptor. *Curr. Mol. Med.* **2012**, *12*, 153–162. [CrossRef] [PubMed]
43. Vene, R.; Benelli, R.; Minghelli, S.; Astigiano, S.; Tosetti, F.; Ferrari, N. Xanthohumol impairs human prostate cancer cell growth and invasion and diminishes the incidence and progression of advanced tumors in TRAMP mice. *Mol. Med.* **2012**, *18*, 1292–1302. [CrossRef] [PubMed]
44. Deng, Y.T.; Lin, J.K. EGCG inhibits the invasion of highly invasive CL1-5 lung cancer cells through suppressing MMP-2 expression via JNK signaling and induces G2/M arrest. *J. Agric. Food Chem.* **2011**, *59*, 13318–13327. [CrossRef] [PubMed]
45. Onoda, C.; Kuribayashi, K.; Nirasawa, S.; Tsuji, N.; Tanaka, M.; Kobayashi, D.; Watanabe, N. (−)-Epigallocatechin-3-gallate induces apoptosis in gastric cancer cell lines by down-regulating survivin expression. *Int. J. Oncol.* **2011**, *38*, 1403–1408. [PubMed]
46. Tanaka, T.; Ishii, T.; Mizuno, D.; Mori, T.; Yamaji, R.; Nakamura, Y.; Kumazawa, S.; Nakayama, T.; Akagawa, M. (−)-Epigallocatechin-3-gallate suppresses growth of AZ521 human gastric cancer cells by targeting the DEAD-box RNA helicase p68. *Free Radic. Biol. Med.* **2011**, *50*, 1324–1335. [CrossRef] [PubMed]
47. Cerezo-Guisado, M.I.; Zur, R.; Lorenzo, M.J.; Risco, A.; Martin-Serrano, M.A.; Alvarez-Barrientos, A.; Cuenda, A.; Centeno, F. Implication of Akt, ERK1/2 and alternative p38MAPK signalling pathways in human colon cancer cell apoptosis induced by green tea EGCG. *Food Chem. Toxicol.* **2015**, *84*, 125–132. [CrossRef] [PubMed]
48. Thakur, V.S.; Deb, G.; Babcook, M.A.; Gupta, S. Plant phytochemicals as epigenetic modulators: Role in cancer chemoprevention. *AAPS J.* **2014**, *16*, 151–163. [CrossRef] [PubMed]
49. Saldanha, S.N.; Kala, R.; Tollefsbol, T.O. Molecular mechanisms for inhibition of colon cancer cells by combined epigenetic-modulating epigallocatechin gallate and sodium butyrate. *Exp. Cell Res.* **2014**, *324*, 40–53. [CrossRef] [PubMed]
50. Toden, S.; Tran, H.M.; Tovar-Camargo, O.A.; Okugawa, Y.; Goel, A. Epigallocatechin-3-gallate targets cancer stem-like cells and enhances 5-fluorouracil chemosensitivity in colorectal cancer. *Oncotarget* **2016**, *7*, 16158–16171. [CrossRef] [PubMed]
51. Mineva, N.D.; Paulson, K.E.; Naber, S.P.; Yee, A.S.; Sonenshein, G.E. Epigallocatechin-3-gallate inhibits stem-like inflammatory breast cancer cells. *PLoS ONE* **2013**, *8*, e73464.
52. Tu, S.H.; Ku, C.Y.; Ho, C.T.; Chen, C.S.; Huang, C.S.; Lee, C.H.; Chen, L.C.; Pan, M.H.; Chang, H.W.; Chang, C.H.; et al. Tea polyphenol (−)-epigallocatechin-3-gallate inhibits nicotine- and estrogen-induced alpha9-nicotinic acetylcholine receptor upregulation in human breast cancer cells. *Mol. Nutr. Food Res.* **2011**, *55*, 455–466. [CrossRef] [PubMed]
53. De Amicis, F.; Russo, A.; Avena, P.; Santoro, M.; Vivacqua, A.; Bonofiglio, D.; Mauro, L.; Aquila, S.; Tramontano, D.; Fuqua, S.A.; et al. In vitro mechanism for downregulation of ER-alpha expression by epigallocatechin gallate in ER+/PR+ human breast cancer cells. *Mol. Nutr. Food Res.* **2013**, *57*, 840–853. [CrossRef] [PubMed]
54. Deb, G.; Thakur, V.S.; Limaye, A.M.; Gupta, S. Epigenetic induction of tissue inhibitor of matrix metalloproteinase-3 by green tea polyphenols in breast cancer cells. *Mol. Carcinog.* **2015**, *54*, 485–499. [CrossRef] [PubMed]
55. Siddiqui, I.A.; Asim, M.; Hafeez, B.B.; Adhami, V.M.; Tarapore, R.S.; Mukhtar, H. Green tea polyphenol EGCG blunts androgen receptor function in prostate cancer. *FASEB J.* **2011**, *25*, 1198–1207. [CrossRef] [PubMed]
56. Kin, R.; Kato, S.; Kaneto, N.; Sakurai, H.; Hayakawa, Y.; Li, F.; Tanaka, K.; Saiki, I.; Yokoyama, S. Procyanidin C1 from Cinnamomi Cortex inhibits TGF-beta-induced epithelial-to-mesenchymal transition in the A549 lung cancer cell line. *Int. J. Oncol.* **2013**, *43*, 1901–1906. [PubMed]

57. Choy, Y.Y.; Fraga, M.; Mackenzie, G.G.; Waterhouse, A.L.; Cremonini, E.; Oteiza, P.I. The PI3K/Akt pathway is involved in procyanidin-mediated suppression of human colorectal cancer cell growth. *Mol. Carcinog.* **2016**. [CrossRef] [PubMed]
58. Gorlach, S.; Wagner, W.; Podsedek, A.; Szewczyk, K.; Koziolkiewicz, M.; Dastych, J. Procyanidins from Japanese quince (*Chaenomeles japonica*) fruit induce apoptosis in human colon cancer Caco-2 cells in a degree of polymerization-dependent manner. *Nutr. Cancer* **2011**, *63*, 1348–1360. [CrossRef] [PubMed]
59. Lewandowska, U.; Szewczyk, K.; Owczarek, K.; Hrabec, Z.; Podsedek, A.; Sosnowska, D.; Hrabec, E. Procyanidins from evening primrose (*Oenothera paradoxa*) defatted seeds inhibit invasiveness of breast cancer cells and modulate the expression of selected genes involved in angiogenesis, metastasis, and apoptosis. *Nutr. Cancer* **2013**, *65*, 1219–1231. [CrossRef] [PubMed]
60. Jin, C.Y.; Park, C.; Hwang, H.J.; Kim, G.Y.; Choi, B.T.; Kim, W.J.; Choi, Y.H. Naringenin up-regulates the expression of death receptor 5 and enhances TRAIL-induced apoptosis in human lung cancer A549 cells. *Mol. Nutr. Food Res.* **2011**, *55*, 300–309. [CrossRef] [PubMed]
61. Bao, L.; Liu, F.; Guo, H.B.; Li, Y.; Tan, B.B.; Zhang, W.X.; Peng, Y.H. Naringenin inhibits proliferation, migration, and invasion as well as induces apoptosis of gastric cancer SGC7901 cell line by downregulation of AKT pathway. *Tumour Biol.* **2016**. [CrossRef] [PubMed]
62. Song, H.M.; Park, G.H.; Eo, H.J.; Jeong, J.B. Naringenin-Mediated ATF3 Expression Contributes to Apoptosis in Human Colon Cancer. *Biomol. Ther. (Seoul)* **2016**, *24*, 140–146. [CrossRef] [PubMed]
63. Yen, H.R.; Liu, C.J.; Yeh, C.C. Naringenin suppresses TPA-induced tumor invasion by suppressing multiple signal transduction pathways in human hepatocellular carcinoma cells. *Chem. Biol. Interact.* **2015**, *235*, 1–9. [CrossRef] [PubMed]
64. Arul, D.; Subramanian, P. Naringenin (citrus flavonone) induces growth inhibition, cell cycle arrest and apoptosis in human hepatocellular carcinoma cells. *Pathol. Oncol. Res.* **2013**, *19*, 763–770. [CrossRef] [PubMed]
65. Kim, S.; Park, T.I. Naringenin: A partial agonist on estrogen receptor in T47D-KBluc breast cancer cells. *Int. J. Clin. Exp. Med.* **2013**, *6*, 890–899. [PubMed]
66. Qin, L.; Jin, L.; Lu, L.; Lu, X.; Zhang, C.; Zhang, F.; Liang, W. Naringenin reduces lung metastasis in a breast cancer resection model. *Protein Cell* **2011**, *2*, 507–516. [CrossRef] [PubMed]
67. Zhang, J.; Wu, D.; Vikash; Song, J.; Wang, J.; Yi, J.; Dong, W. Hesperetin induces the apoptosis of gastric cancer cells via activating mitochondrial pathway by increasing reactive oxygen species. *Dig. Dis. Sci.* **2015**, *60*, 2985–2995. [CrossRef] [PubMed]
68. Aranganathan, S.; Nalini, N. Antiproliferative efficacy of hesperetin (citrus flavanoid) in 1,2-dimethylhydrazine-induced colon cancer. *Phytother. Res.* **2013**, *27*, 999–1005. [CrossRef] [PubMed]
69. Palit, S.; Kar, S.; Sharma, G.; Das, P.K. Hesperetin induces apoptosis in breast carcinoma by triggering accumulation of ROS and activation of ASK1/JNK pathway. *J. Cell. Physiol.* **2015**, *230*, 1729–1739. [CrossRef] [PubMed]
70. Yang, Y.; Wolfram, J.; Boom, K.; Fang, X.; Shen, H.; Ferrari, M. Hesperetin impairs glucose uptake and inhibits proliferation of breast cancer cells. *Cell Biochem. Funct.* **2013**, *31*, 374–379. [CrossRef] [PubMed]
71. Sambantham, S.; Radha, M.; Paramasivam, A.; Anandan, B.; Malathi, R.; Chandra, S.R.; Jayaraman, G. Molecular mechanism underlying hesperetin-induced apoptosis by in silico analysis and in prostate cancer PC-3 cells. *Asian Pac. J. Cancer Prev.* **2013**, *14*, 4347–4352. [CrossRef] [PubMed]
72. Alshatwi, A.A.; Ramesh, E.; Periasamy, V.S.; Subash-Babu, P. The apoptotic effect of hesperetin on human cervical cancer cells is mediated through cell cycle arrest, death receptor, and mitochondrial pathways. *Fundam. Clin. Pharmacol.* **2013**, *27*, 581–592. [CrossRef] [PubMed]
73. Zhu, Y.; Wu, J.; Li, S.; Wang, X.; Liang, Z.; Xu, X.; Xu, X.; Hu, Z.; Lin, Y.; Chen, H.; et al. Apigenin inhibits migration and invasion via modulation of epithelial mesenchymal transition in prostate cancer. *Mol. Med. Rep.* **2015**, *11*, 1004–1008. [CrossRef] [PubMed]
74. Lu, H.F.; Chie, Y.J.; Yang, M.S.; Lu, K.W.; Fu, J.J.; Yang, J.S.; Chen, H.Y.; Hsia, T.C.; Ma, C.Y.; Ip, S.W.; et al. Apigenin induces apoptosis in human lung cancer H460 cells through caspase- and mitochondria-dependent pathways. *Hum. Exp. Toxicol.* **2011**, *30*, 1053–1061. [CrossRef] [PubMed]
75. Chen, J.; Chen, J.; Li, Z.; Liu, C.; Yin, L. The apoptotic effect of apigenin on human gastric carcinoma cells through mitochondrial signal pathway. *Tumor Biol.* **2014**, *35*, 7719–7726. [CrossRef] [PubMed]

76. Kuo, C.H.; Weng, B.C.; Wu, C.C.; Yang, S.F.; Wu, D.C.; Wang, Y.C. Apigenin has anti-atrophic gastritis and anti-gastric cancer progression effects in Helicobacter pylori-infected Mongolian gerbils. *J. Ethnopharmacol.* **2014**, *151*, 1031–1039. [CrossRef] [PubMed]
77. Chunhua, L.; Donglan, L.; Xiuqiong, F.; Lihua, Z.; Qin, F.; Yawei, L.; Liang, Z.; Ge, W.; Linlin, J.; Ping, Z.; et al. Apigenin up-regulates transgelin and inhibits invasion and migration of colorectal cancer through decreased phosphorylation of AKT. *J. Nutr. Biochem.* **2013**, *24*, 1766–1775. [CrossRef] [PubMed]
78. Seo, H.S.; Jo, J.K.; Ku, J.M.; Choi, H.S.; Choi, Y.K.; Woo, J.K.; Kim, H.I.; Kang, S.Y.; Lee, K.M.; Nam, K.W.; et al. Induction of caspase-dependent extrinsic apoptosis by apigenin through inhibition of signal transducer and activator of transcription 3 (STAT3) signalling in HER2-overexpressing BT-474 breast cancer cells. *Biosci. Rep.* **2015**, *35*, e00276. [CrossRef] [PubMed]
79. Tseng, T.H.; Chien, M.H.; Lin, W.L.; Wen, Y.C.; Chow, J.M.; Chen, C.K.; Kuo, T.C.; Lee, W.J. Inhibition of MDA-MB-231 breast cancer cell proliferation and tumor growth by apigenin through induction of G2/M arrest and histone H3 acetylation-mediated p21 expression. *Environ. Toxicol.* **2016**. [CrossRef] [PubMed]
80. Pandey, M.; Kaur, P.; Shukla, S.; Abbas, A.; Fu, P.; Gupta, S. Plant flavone apigenin inhibits HDAC and remodels chromatin to induce growth arrest and apoptosis in human prostate cancer cells: In vitro and in vivo study. *Mol. Carcinog.* **2012**, *51*, 952–962. [CrossRef] [PubMed]
81. Shukla, S.; Bhaskaran, N.; Babcook, M.A.; Fu, P.; Maclennan, G.T.; Gupta, S. Apigenin inhibits prostate cancer progression in TRAMP mice via targeting PI3K/Akt/FoxO pathway. *Carcinogenesis* **2014**, *35*, 452–460. [CrossRef] [PubMed]
82. Yang, B.; Huang, J.; Xiang, T.; Yin, X.; Luo, X.; Huang, J.; Luo, F.; Li, H.; Li, H.; Ren, G. Chrysin inhibits metastatic potential of human triple-negative breast cancer cells by modulating matrix metalloproteinase-10, epithelial to mesenchymal transition, and PI3K/Akt signaling pathway. *J. Appl. Toxicol.* **2014**, *34*, 105–112. [CrossRef] [PubMed]
83. Shao, J.J.; Zhang, A.P.; Qin, W.; Zheng, L.; Zhu, Y.F.; Chen, X. AMP-activated protein kinase (AMPK) activation is involved in chrysin-induced growth inhibition and apoptosis in cultured A549 lung cancer cells. *Biochem. Biophys. Res. Commun.* **2012**, *423*, 448–453. [CrossRef] [PubMed]
84. Ronnekleiv-Kelly, S.M.; Nukaya, M.; Diaz-Diaz, C.J.; Megna, B.W.; Carney, P.R.; Geiger, P.G.; Kennedy, G.D. Aryl hydrocarbon receptor-dependent apoptotic cell death induced by the flavonoid chrysin in human colorectal cancer cells. *Cancer Lett.* **2016**, *370*, 91–99. [CrossRef] [PubMed]
85. Cai, X.; Ye, T.; Liu, C.; Lu, W.; Lu, M.; Zhang, J.; Wang, M.; Cao, P. Luteolin induced G2 phase cell cycle arrest and apoptosis on non-small cell lung cancer cells. *Toxicol. Vitro* **2011**, *25*, 1385–1391. [CrossRef] [PubMed]
86. Choi, H.J.; Choi, H.J.; Chung, T.W.; Ha, K.T. Luteolin inhibits recruitment of monocytes and migration of Lewis lung carcinoma cells by suppressing chemokine (C-C motif) ligand 2 expression in tumor-associated macrophage. *Biochem. Biophys. Res. Commun.* **2016**, *470*, 101–106. [CrossRef] [PubMed]
87. Ruan, J.; Zhang, L.; Yan, L.; Liu, Y.; Yue, Z.; Chen, L.; Wang, A.Y.; Chen, W.; Zheng, S.; Wang, S.; et al. Inhibition of hypoxia-induced epithelial mesenchymal transition by luteolin in non-small cell lung cancer cells. *Mol. Med. Rep.* **2012**, *6*, 232–238. [PubMed]
88. Hong, Z.; Cao, X.; Li, N.; Zhang, Y.; Lan, L.; Zhou, Y.; Pan, X.; Shen, L.; Yin, Z.; Luo, L. Luteolin is effective in the non-small cell lung cancer model with L858R/T790M EGF receptor mutation and erlotinib resistance. *Br. J. Pharmacol.* **2014**, *171*, 2842–2853. [CrossRef] [PubMed]
89. Lu, J.; Li, G.; He, K.; Jiang, W.; Xu, C.; Li, Z.; Wang, H.; Wang, W.; Wang, H.; Teng, X.; et al. Luteolin exerts a marked antitumor effect in cMet-overexpressing patient-derived tumor xenograft models of gastric cancer. *J. Transl. Med.* **2015**, *13*, 42. [CrossRef] [PubMed]
90. Lim, D.Y.; Cho, H.J.; Kim, J.; Nho, C.W.; Lee, K.W.; Park, J.H. Luteolin decreases IGF-II production and downregulates insulin-like growth factor-I receptor signaling in HT-29 human colon cancer cells. *BMC Gastroenterol.* **2012**, *12*, 9. [CrossRef] [PubMed]
91. Abdel, H.L.; Di Vito, C.; Marfia, G.; Ferraretto, A.; Tringali, C.; Viani, P.; Riboni, L. Sphingosine Kinase 2 and Ceramide Transport as Key Targets of the Natural Flavonoid Luteolin to Induce Apoptosis in Colon Cancer Cells. *PLoS ONE* **2015**, *10*, e143384. [CrossRef] [PubMed]
92. Wang, L.M.; Xie, K.P.; Huo, H.N.; Shang, F.; Zou, W.; Xie, M.J. Luteolin inhibits proliferation induced by IGF-1 pathway dependent ERalpha in human breast cancer MCF-7 cells. *Asian Pac. J. Cancer Prev.* **2012**, *13*, 1431–1437. [CrossRef] [PubMed]

93. Lee, E.J.; Oh, S.Y.; Sung, M.K. Luteolin exerts anti-tumor activity through the suppression of epidermal growth factor receptor-mediated pathway in MDA-MB-231 ER-negative breast cancer cells. *Food Chem. Toxicol.* **2012**, *50*, 4136–4143. [CrossRef] [PubMed]
94. Tsui, K.H.; Chung, L.C.; Feng, T.H.; Chang, P.L.; Juang, H.H. Upregulation of prostate-derived Ets factor by luteolin causes inhibition of cell proliferation and cell invasion in prostate carcinoma cells. *Int. J. Cancer* **2012**, *130*, 2812–2823. [CrossRef] [PubMed]
95. Zheng, S.Y.; Li, Y.; Jiang, D.; Zhao, J.; Ge, J.F. Anticancer effect and apoptosis induction by quercetin in the human lung cancer cell line A-549. *Mol. Med. Rep.* **2012**, *5*, 822–826. [CrossRef] [PubMed]
96. Wang, K.; Liu, R.; Li, J.; Mao, J.; Lei, Y.; Wu, J.; Zeng, J.; Zhang, T.; Wu, H.; Chen, L.; et al. Quercetin induces protective autophagy in gastric cancer cells: Involvement of Akt-mTOR- and hypoxia-induced factor 1alpha-mediated signaling. *Autophagy* **2011**, *7*, 966–978. [CrossRef] [PubMed]
97. Kim, H.S.; Wannatung, T.; Lee, S.; Yang, W.K.; Chung, S.H.; Lim, J.S.; Choe, W.; Kang, I.; Kim, S.S.; Ha, J. Quercetin enhances hypoxia-mediated apoptosis via direct inhibition of AMPK activity in HCT116 colon cancer. *Apoptosis* **2012**, *17*, 938–949. [CrossRef] [PubMed]
98. Velazquez, K.T.; Enos, R.T.; Narsale, A.A.; Puppa, M.J.; Davis, J.M.; Murphy, E.A.; Carson, J.A. Quercetin supplementation attenuates the progression of cancer cachexia in ApcMin/+ mice. *J. Nutr.* **2014**, *144*, 868–875. [CrossRef] [PubMed]
99. Dai, W.; Gao, Q.; Qiu, J.; Yuan, J.; Wu, G.; Shen, G. Quercetin induces apoptosis and enhances 5-FU therapeutic efficacy in hepatocellular carcinoma. *Tumor Biol.* **2015**, *5*, 6307–6313. [CrossRef] [PubMed]
100. Duo, J.; Ying, G.G.; Wang, G.W.; Zhang, L. Quercetin inhibits human breast cancer cell proliferation and induces apoptosis via Bcl-2 and Bax regulation. *Mol. Med. Rep.* **2012**, *5*, 1453–1456. [PubMed]
101. Wang, F.; Yang, Y. Quercetin suppresses insulin receptor signaling through inhibition of the insulin ligand-receptor binding and therefore impairs cancer cell proliferation. *Biochem. Biophys. Res. Commun.* **2014**, *452*, 1028–1033. [CrossRef] [PubMed]
102. Srinivasan, A.; Thangavel, C.; Liu, Y.; Shoyele, S.; Den, R.B.; Selvakumar, P.; Lakshmikuttyamma, A. Quercetin regulates beta-catenin signaling and reduces the migration of triple negative breast cancer. *Mol. Carcinog.* **2016**, *55*, 743–756. [CrossRef] [PubMed]
103. Zhao, X.; Wang, Q.; Yang, S.; Chen, C.; Li, X.; Liu, J.; Zou, Z.; Cai, D. Quercetin inhibits angiogenesis by targeting calcineurin in the xenograft model of human breast cancer. *Eur. J. Pharmacol.* **2016**, *781*, 60–68. [CrossRef] [PubMed]
104. Sharmila, G.; Athirai, T.; Kiruthiga, B.; Senthilkumar, K.; Elumalai, P.; Arunkumar, R.; Arunakaran, J. Chemopreventive effect of quercetin in MNU and testosterone induced prostate cancer of Sprague-Dawley rats. *Nutr. Cancer* **2014**, *66*, 38–46. [CrossRef] [PubMed]
105. Sharmila, G.; Bhat, F.A.; Arunkumar, R.; Elumalai, P.; Raja, S.P.; Senthilkumar, K.; Arunakaran, J. Chemopreventive effect of quercetin, a natural dietary flavonoid on prostate cancer in in vivo model. *Clin. Nutr.* **2014**, *33*, 718–726. [CrossRef] [PubMed]
106. Bishayee, K.; Ghosh, S.; Mukherjee, A.; Sadhukhan, R.; Mondal, J.; Khuda-Bukhsh, A.R. Quercetin induces cytochrome-c release and ROS accumulation to promote apoptosis and arrest the cell cycle in G_2/M, in cervical carcinoma: Signal cascade and drug-DNA interaction. *Cell Prolif.* **2013**, *46*, 153–163. [CrossRef] [PubMed]
107. Jo, E.; Park, S.J.; Choi, Y.S.; Jeon, W.K.; Kim, B.C. Kaempferol suppresses transforming growth factor-beta1-induced epithelial-to-mesenchymal transition and migration of A549 lung cancer cells by inhibiting Akt1-mediated phosphorylation of smad3 at threonine-179. *Neoplasia* **2015**, *17*, 525–537. [CrossRef] [PubMed]
108. Song, H.; Bao, J.; Wei, Y.; Chen, Y.; Mao, X.; Li, J.; Yang, Z.; Xue, Y. Kaempferol inhibits gastric cancer tumor growth: An in vitro and in vivo study. *Oncol. Rep.* **2015**, *33*, 868–874. [CrossRef] [PubMed]
109. Lee, H.S.; Cho, H.J.; Yu, R.; Lee, K.W.; Chun, H.S.; Park, J.H. Mechanisms underlying apoptosis-inducing effects of Kaempferol in HT-29 human colon cancer cells. *Int. J. Mol. Sci.* **2014**, *15*, 2722–2737. [CrossRef] [PubMed]
110. Huang, W.W.; Tsai, S.C.; Peng, S.F.; Lin, M.W.; Chiang, J.H.; Chiu, Y.J.; Fushiya, S.; Tseng, M.T.; Yang, J.S. Kaempferol induces autophagy through AMPK and AKT signaling molecules and causes G2/M arrest via downregulation of CDK1/cyclin B in SK-HEP-1 human hepatic cancer cells. *Int. J. Oncol.* **2013**, *42*, 2069–2077. [PubMed]

111. Liao, W.; Chen, L.; Ma, X.; Jiao, R.; Li, X.; Wang, Y. Protective effects of kaempferol against reactive oxygen species-induced hemolysis and its antiproliferative activity on human cancer cells. *Eur. J. Med. Chem.* **2016**, *114*, 24–32. [CrossRef] [PubMed]
112. Azevedo, C.; Correia-Branco, A.; Araujo, J.R.; Guimaraes, J.T.; Keating, E.; Martel, F. The chemopreventive effect of the dietary compound kaempferol on the MCF-7 human breast cancer cell line is dependent on inhibition of glucose cellular uptake. *Nutr. Cancer* **2015**, *67*, 504–513. [CrossRef] [PubMed]
113. Kim, S.H.; Hwang, K.A.; Choi, K.C. Treatment with kaempferol suppresses breast cancer cell growth caused by estrogen and triclosan in cellular and xenograft breast cancer models. *J. Nutr. Biochem.* **2016**, *28*, 70–82. [CrossRef] [PubMed]
114. Li, C.; Zhao, Y.; Yang, D.; Yu, Y.; Guo, H.; Zhao, Z.; Zhang, B.; Yin, X. Inhibitory effects of kaempferol on the invasion of human breast carcinoma cells by downregulating the expression and activity of matrix metalloproteinase-9. *Biochem. Cell. Biol.* **2015**, *93*, 16–27. [CrossRef] [PubMed]
115. Feng, J.; Chen, X.; Wang, Y.; Du, Y.; Sun, Q.; Zang, W.; Zhao, G. Myricetin inhibits proliferation and induces apoptosis and cell cycle arrest in gastric cancer cells. *Mol. Cell. Biochem.* **2015**, *408*, 163–170. [CrossRef] [PubMed]
116. Kim, M.E.; Ha, T.K.; Yoon, J.H.; Lee, J.S. Myricetin induces cell death of human colon cancer cells via BAX/BCL2-dependent pathway. *Anticancer Res.* **2014**, *34*, 701–706. [PubMed]
117. Iyer, S.C.; Gopal, A.; Halagowder, D. Myricetin induces apoptosis by inhibiting P21 activated kinase 1 (PAK1) signaling cascade in hepatocellular carcinoma. *Mol. Cell. Biochem.* **2015**, *407*, 223–237. [CrossRef]
118. Kim, D.A.; Jeon, Y.K.; Nam, M.J. Galangin induces apoptosis in gastric cancer cells via regulation of ubiquitin carboxy-terminal hydrolase isozyme L1 and glutathione S-transferase P. *Food Chem. Toxicol.* **2012**, *50*, 684–688. [CrossRef] [PubMed]
119. Chien, S.T.; Shi, M.D.; Lee, Y.C.; Te, C.C.; Shih, Y.W. Galangin, a novel dietary flavonoid, attenuates metastatic feature via PKC/ERK signaling pathway in TPA-treated liver cancer HepG2 cells. *Cancer Cell Int.* **2015**, *15*, 15. [CrossRef] [PubMed]
120. Su, L.; Chen, X.; Wu, J.; Lin, B.; Zhang, H.; Lan, L.; Luo, H. Galangin inhibits proliferation of hepatocellular carcinoma cells by inducing endoplasmic reticulum stress. *Food Chem. Toxicol.* **2013**, *62*, 810–816. [CrossRef] [PubMed]
121. Hu, S.; Huang, L.; Meng, L.; Sun, H.; Zhang, W.; Xu, Y. Isorhamnetin inhibits cell proliferation and induces apoptosis in breast cancer via Akt and mitogenactivated protein kinase kinase signaling pathways. *Mol. Med. Rep.* **2015**, *12*, 6745–6751. [PubMed]
122. Li, C.; Yang, D.; Zhao, Y.; Qiu, Y.; Cao, X.; Yu, Y.; Guo, H.; Gu, X.; Yin, X. Inhibitory effects of isorhamnetin on the invasion of human breast carcinoma cells by downregulating the expression and activity of matrix metalloproteinase-2/9. *Nutr. Cancer* **2015**, *67*, 1191–1200. [CrossRef] [PubMed]
123. Li, Q.; Ren, F.Q.; Yang, C.L.; Zhou, L.M.; Liu, Y.Y.; Xiao, J.; Zhu, L.; Wang, Z.G. Anti-proliferation effects of isorhamnetin on lung cancer cells in vitro and in vivo. *Asian Pac. J. Cancer Prev.* **2015**, *16*, 3035–3042. [CrossRef] [PubMed]
124. Ramachandran, L.; Manu, K.A.; Shanmugam, M.K.; Li, F.; Siveen, K.S.; Vali, S.; Kapoor, S.; Abbasi, T.; Surana, R.; Smoot, D.T.; et al. Isorhamnetin inhibits proliferation and invasion and induces apoptosis through the modulation of peroxisome proliferator-activated receptor gamma activation pathway in gastric cancer. *J. Biol. Chem.* **2012**, *287*, 38028–38040. [CrossRef] [PubMed]
125. Li, C.; Yang, X.; Chen, C.; Cai, S.; Hu, J. Isorhamnetin suppresses colon cancer cell growth through the PI3KAktmTOR pathway. *Mol. Med. Rep.* **2014**, *9*, 935–940. [PubMed]
126. Saud, S.M.; Young, M.R.; Jones-Hall, Y.L.; Ileva, L.; Evbuomwan, M.O.; Wise, J.; Colburn, N.H.; Kim, Y.S.; Bobe, G. Chemopreventive activity of plant flavonoid isorhamnetin in colorectal cancer is mediated by oncogenic Src and beta-catenin. *Cancer Res.* **2013**, *73*, 5473–5484. [CrossRef] [PubMed]
127. Park, H.J.; Jeon, Y.K.; You, D.H.; Nam, M.J. Daidzein causes cytochrome c-mediated apoptosis via the Bcl-2 family in human hepatic cancer cells. *Food Chem. Toxicol.* **2013**, *60*, 542–549. [CrossRef] [PubMed]
128. Magee, P.J.; Allsopp, P.; Samaletdin, A.; Rowland, I.R. Daidzein, R-(+)equol and S-(−)equol inhibit the invasion of MDA-MB-231 breast cancer cells potentially via the down-regulation of matrix metalloproteinase-2. *Eur. J. Nutr.* **2014**, *53*, 345–350. [CrossRef] [PubMed]

129. Koo, J.; Cabarcas-Petroski, S.; Petrie, J.L.; Diette, N.; White, R.J.; Schramm, L. Induction of proto-oncogene BRF2 in breast cancer cells by the dietary soybean isoflavone daidzein. *BMC Cancer* **2015**, *15*, 905. [CrossRef] [PubMed]
130. Tian, T.; Li, J.; Li, B.; Wang, Y.; Li, M.; Ma, D.; Wang, X. Genistein exhibits anti-cancer effects via down-regulating FoxM1 in H446 small-cell lung cancer cells. *Tumor Biol.* **2014**, *35*, 4137–4145. [CrossRef] [PubMed]
131. Huang, W.; Wan, C.; Luo, Q.; Huang, Z.; Luo, Q. Genistein-inhibited cancer stem cell-like properties and reduced chemoresistance of gastric cancer. *Int. J. Mol. Sci.* **2014**, *15*, 3432–3443. [CrossRef] [PubMed]
132. Qin, J.; Teng, J.; Zhu, Z.; Chen, J.; Huang, W.J. Genistein induces activation of the mitochondrial apoptosis pathway by inhibiting phosphorylation of Akt in colorectal cancer cells. *Pharm. Biol.* **2016**, *54*, 74–79. [CrossRef] [PubMed]
133. Xiao, X.; Liu, Z.; Wang, R.; Wang, J.; Zhang, S.; Cai, X.; Wu, K.; Bergan, R.C.; Xu, L.; Fan, D. Genistein suppresses FLT4 and inhibits human colorectal cancer metastasis. *Oncotarget* **2015**, *6*, 3225–3239. [CrossRef] [PubMed]
134. Luo, Y.; Wang, S.X.; Zhou, Z.Q.; Wang, Z.; Zhang, Y.G.; Zhang, Y.; Zhao, P. Apoptotic effect of genistein on human colon cancer cells via inhibiting the nuclear factor-kappa B (NF-kappaB) pathway. *Tumor Biol.* **2014**, *35*, 11483–11488. [CrossRef] [PubMed]
135. Lepri, S.R.; Zanelatto, L.C.; Da, S.P.; Sartori, D.; Ribeiro, L.R.; Mantovani, M.S. Effects of genistein and daidzein on cell proliferation kinetics in HT29 colon cancer cells: The expression of CTNNBIP1 (beta-catenin), APC (adenomatous polyposis coli) and BIRC5 (survivin). *Hum. Cell* **2014**, *27*, 78–84. [CrossRef] [PubMed]
136. Dai, W.; Wang, F.; He, L.; Lin, C.; Wu, S.; Chen, P.; Zhang, Y.; Shen, M.; Wu, D.; Wang, C.; et al. Genistein inhibits hepatocellular carcinoma cell migration by reversing the epithelial-mesenchymal transition: Partial mediation by the transcription factor NFAT1. *Mol. Carcinog.* **2015**, *54*, 301–311. [CrossRef] [PubMed]
137. Pan, H.; Zhou, W.; He, W.; Liu, X.; Ding, Q.; Ling, L.; Zha, X.; Wang, S. Genistein inhibits MDA-MB-231 triple-negative breast cancer cell growth by inhibiting NF-kappaB activity via the Notch-1 pathway. *Int. J. Mol. Med.* **2012**, *30*, 337–343. [PubMed]
138. Fan, P.; Fan, S.; Wang, H.; Mao, J.; Shi, Y.; Ibrahim, M.M.; Ma, W.; Yu, X.; Hou, Z.; Wang, B.; et al. Genistein decreases the breast cancer stem-like cell population through Hedgehog pathway. *Stem Cell Res. Ther.* **2013**, *4*, 146. [CrossRef] [PubMed]
139. Pons, D.G.; Nadal-Serrano, M.; Torrens-Mas, M.; Oliver, J.; Roca, P. The phytoestrogen genistein affects breast cancer cells treatment depending on the ERalpha/ERbeta ratio. *J. Cell. Biochem.* **2016**, *117*, 218–229. [CrossRef] [PubMed]
140. Andrade, J.E.; Ju, Y.H.; Baker, C.; Doerge, D.R.; Helferich, W.G. Long-term exposure to dietary sources of genistein induces estrogen-independence in the human breast cancer (MCF-7) xenograft model. *Mol. Nutr. Food Res.* **2015**, *59*, 413–423. [CrossRef] [PubMed]
141. Mahmoud, A.M.; Zhu, T.; Parray, A.; Siddique, H.R.; Yang, W.; Saleem, M.; Bosland, M.C. Differential effects of genistein on prostate cancer cells depend on mutational status of the androgen receptor. *PLoS ONE* **2013**, *8*, e78479. [CrossRef] [PubMed]
142. Hussain, A.; Harish, G.; Prabhu, S.A.; Mohsin, J.; Khan, M.A.; Rizvi, T.A.; Sharma, C. Inhibitory effect of genistein on the invasive potential of human cervical cancer cells via modulation of matrix metalloproteinase-9 and tissue inhibitors of matrix metalloproteinase-1 expression. *Cancer Epidemiol.* **2012**, *36*, e387–e393. [CrossRef] [PubMed]
143. Chen, H.S.; Bai, M.H.; Zhang, T.; Li, G.D.; Liu, M. Ellagic acid induces cell cycle arrest and apoptosis through TGF-beta/Smad3 signaling pathway in human breast cancer MCF-7 cells. *Int. J. Oncol.* **2015**, *46*, 1730–1738. [PubMed]
144. Yousef, A.I.; El-Masry, O.S.; Abdel, M.M. Impact of cellular genetic make-up on colorectal cancer cell lines response to ellagic acid: Implications of small interfering RNA. *Asian Pac. J. Cancer Prev.* **2016**, *17*, 743–748. [CrossRef] [PubMed]
145. Srigopalram, S.; Jayraaj, I.A.; Kaleeswaran, B.; Balamurugan, K.; Ranjithkumar, M.; Kumar, T.S.; Park, J.I.; Nou, I.S. Ellagic acid normalizes mitochondrial outer membrane permeabilization and attenuates inflammation-mediated cell proliferation in experimental liver cancer. *Appl. Biochem. Biotechnol.* **2014**, *173*, 2254–2266. [CrossRef] [PubMed]

146. Wang, N.; Wang, Z.Y.; Mo, S.L.; Loo, T.Y.; Wang, D.M.; Luo, H.B.; Yang, D.P.; Chen, Y.L.; Shen, J.G.; Chen, J.P. Ellagic acid, a phenolic compound, exerts anti-angiogenesis effects via VEGFR-2 signaling pathway in breast cancer. *Breast Cancer Res. Treat.* **2012**, *134*, 943–955. [CrossRef] [PubMed]
147. Pitchakarn, P.; Chewonarin, T.; Ogawa, K.; Suzuki, S.; Asamoto, M.; Takahashi, S.; Shirai, T.; Limtrakul, P. Ellagic acid inhibits migration and invasion by prostate cancer cell lines. *Asian Pac. J. Cancer Prev.* **2013**, *14*, 2859–2863. [CrossRef] [PubMed]
148. Malik, A.; Afaq, S.; Shahid, M.; Akhtar, K.; Assiri, A. Influence of ellagic acid on prostate cancer cell proliferation: A caspase-dependent pathway. *Asian Pac. J. Trop. Med.* **2011**, *4*, 550–555. [CrossRef]
149. Subramanian, A.P.; Jaganathan, S.K.; Mandal, M.; Supriyanto, E.; Muhamad, I.I. Gallic acid induced apoptotic events in HCT-15 colon cancer cells. *World J. Gastroenterol.* **2016**, *22*, 3952–3961. [CrossRef] [PubMed]
150. Wang, K.; Zhu, X.; Zhang, K.; Zhu, L.; Zhou, F. Investigation of gallic acid induced anticancer effect in human breast carcinoma MCF-7 cells. *J. Biochem. Mol. Toxicol.* **2014**, *28*, 387–393. [CrossRef] [PubMed]
151. Ho, H.H.; Chang, C.S.; Ho, W.C.; Liao, S.Y.; Lin, W.L.; Wang, C.J. Gallic acid inhibits gastric cancer cells metastasis and invasive growth via increased expression of RhoB, downregulation of AKT/small GTPase signals and inhibition of NF-kappaB activity. *Toxicol. Appl. Pharmacol.* **2013**, *266*, 76–85. [CrossRef] [PubMed]
152. Russell, L.J.; Mazzio, E.; Badisa, R.B.; Zhu, Z.P.; Agharahimi, M.; Oriaku, E.T.; Goodman, C.B. Autoxidation of gallic acid induces ROS-dependent death in human prostate cancer LNCaP cells. *Anticancer Res.* **2012**, *32*, 1595–1602. [PubMed]
153. Sun, G.; Zhang, S.; Xie, Y.; Zhang, Z.; Zhao, W. Gallic acid as a selective anticancer agent that induces apoptosis in SMMC-7721 human hepatocellular carcinoma cells. *Oncol. Lett.* **2016**, *11*, 150–158. [CrossRef] [PubMed]
154. Liu, K.C.; Huang, A.C.; Wu, P.P.; Lin, H.Y.; Chueh, F.S.; Yang, J.S.; Lu, C.C.; Chiang, J.H.; Meng, M.; Chung, J.G. Gallic acid suppresses the migration and invasion of PC-3 human prostate cancer cells via inhibition of matrix metalloproteinase-2 and -9 signaling pathways. *Oncol. Rep.* **2011**, *26*, 177–184. [PubMed]
155. Liu, K.C.; Ho, H.C.; Huang, A.C.; Ji, B.C.; Lin, H.Y.; Chueh, F.S.; Yang, J.S.; Lu, C.C.; Chiang, J.H.; Meng, M.; et al. Gallic acid provokes DNA damage and suppresses DNA repair gene expression in human prostate cancer PC-3 cells. *Environ. Toxicol.* **2013**, *28*, 579–587. [CrossRef] [PubMed]
156. Zhao, B.; Hu, M. Gallic acid reduces cell viability, proliferation, invasion and angiogenesis in human cervical cancer cells. *Oncol. Lett.* **2013**, *6*, 1749–1755. [PubMed]
157. Sarwar, T.; Zafaryab, M.; Husain, M.A.; Ishqi, H.M.; Rehman, S.U.; Rizvi, M.M.; Tabish, M. Redox cycling of endogenous copper by ferulic acid leads to cellular DNA breakage and consequent cell death: A putative cancer chemotherapy mechanism. *Toxicol. Appl. Pharmacol.* **2015**, *289*, 251–261. [CrossRef] [PubMed]
158. Eroglu, C.; Secme, M.; Bagci, G.; Dodurga, Y. Assessment of the anticancer mechanism of ferulic acid via cell cycle and apoptotic pathways in human prostate cancer cell lines. *Tumor Biol.* **2015**, *36*, 9437–9446. [CrossRef] [PubMed]
159. Karthikeyan, S.; Kanimozhi, G.; Prasad, N.R.; Mahalakshmi, R. Radiosensitizing effect of ferulic acid on human cervical carcinoma cells in vitro. *Toxicol. Vitro* **2011**, *25*, 1366–1375. [CrossRef] [PubMed]
160. Delman, D.M.; Fabian, C.J.; Kimler, B.F.; Yeh, H.; Petroff, B.K. Effects of flaxseed lignan secoisolariciresinol diglucosideon preneoplastic biomarkers of cancer progression in a model of simultaneous breast and ovarian cancer development. *Nutr. Cancer* **2015**, *67*, 857–864. [CrossRef] [PubMed]
161. Xiong, X.Y.; Hu, X.J.; Li, Y.; Liu, C.M. Inhibitory effects of enterolactone on growth and metastasis in human breast cancer. *Nutr. Cancer* **2015**, *67*, 1324–1332. [CrossRef] [PubMed]
162. Lee, C.C.; Liu, K.J.; Wu, Y.C.; Lin, S.J.; Chang, C.C.; Huang, T.S. Sesamin inhibits macrophage-induced vascular endothelial growth factor and matrix metalloproteinase-9 expression and proangiogenic activity in breast cancer cells. *Inflammation* **2011**, *34*, 209–221. [CrossRef] [PubMed]
163. Deng, P.; Wang, C.; Chen, L.; Wang, C.; Du, Y.; Yan, X.; Chen, M.; Yang, G.; He, G. Sesamin induces cell cycle arrest and apoptosis through the inhibition of signal transducer and activator of transcription 3 signalling in human hepatocellular carcinoma cell line HepG2. *Biol. Pharm. Bull.* **2013**, *36*, 1540–1548. [CrossRef] [PubMed]
164. Xu, P.; Cai, F.; Liu, X.; Guo, L. Sesamin inhibits lipopolysaccharide-induced proliferation and invasion through the p38-MAPK and NF-kappaB signaling pathways in prostate cancer cells. *Oncol. Rep.* **2015**, *33*, 3117–3123. [PubMed]

165. Ko, J.C.; Syu, J.J.; Chen, J.C.; Wang, T.J.; Chang, P.Y.; Chen, C.Y.; Jian, Y.T.; Jian, Y.J.; Lin, Y.W. Resveratrol enhances etoposide-induced cytotoxicity through down-regulating ERK1/2 and AKT-Mediated X-ray repair cross-complement group 1 (XRCC1) protein expression in human non-small-cell lung cancer cells. *Basic Clin. Pharmacol. Toxicol.* **2015**, *117*, 383–391. [CrossRef] [PubMed]
166. Yang, Q.; Wang, B.; Zang, W.; Wang, X.; Liu, Z.; Li, W.; Jia, J. Resveratrol inhibits the growth of gastric cancer by inducing G1 phase arrest and senescence in a Sirt1-dependent manner. *PLoS ONE* **2013**, *8*, e70627. [CrossRef] [PubMed]
167. Wang, Z.; Li, W.; Meng, X.; Jia, B. Resveratrol induces gastric cancer cell apoptosis via reactive oxygen species, but independent of sirtuin1. *Clin. Exp. Pharmacol. Physiol.* **2012**, *39*, 227–232. [CrossRef]
168. Miki, H.; Uehara, N.; Kimura, A.; Sasaki, T.; Yuri, T.; Yoshizawa, K.; Tsubura, A. Resveratrol induces apoptosis via ROS-triggered autophagy in human colon cancer cells. *Int. J. Oncol.* **2012**, *40*, 1020–1028. [PubMed]
169. Colin, D.J.; Limagne, E.; Ragot, K.; Lizard, G.; Ghiringhelli, F.; Solary, E.; Chauffert, B.; Latruffe, N.; Delmas, D. The role of reactive oxygen species and subsequent DNA-damage response in the emergence of resistance towards resveratrol in colon cancer models. *Cell Death Dis.* **2014**, *5*, e1533. [CrossRef] [PubMed]
170. Demoulin, B.; Hermant, M.; Castrogiovanni, C.; Staudt, C.; Dumont, P. Resveratrol induces DNA damage in colon cancer cells by poisoning topoisomerase II and activates the ATM kinase to trigger p53-dependent apoptosis. *Toxicol. Vitro* **2015**, *29*, 1156–1165. [CrossRef] [PubMed]
171. Wang, Z.; Zhang, L.; Ni, Z.; Sun, J.; Gao, H.; Cheng, Z.; Xu, J.; Yin, P. Resveratrol induces AMPK-dependent MDR1 inhibition in colorectal cancer HCT116/L-OHP cells by preventing activation of NF-kappaB signaling and suppressing cAMP-responsive element transcriptional activity. *Tumor Biol.* **2015**, *36*, 9499–9510. [CrossRef] [PubMed]
172. Saud, S.M.; Li, W.; Morris, N.L.; Matter, M.S.; Colburn, N.H.; Kim, Y.S.; Young, M.R. Resveratrol prevents tumorigenesis in mouse model of Kras activated sporadic colorectal cancer by suppressing oncogenic Kras expression. *Carcinogenesis* **2014**, *35*, 2778–2786. [CrossRef] [PubMed]
173. Aires, V.; Limagne, E.; Cotte, A.K.; Latruffe, N.; Ghiringhelli, F.; Delmas, D. Resveratrol metabolites inhibit human metastatic colon cancer cells progression and synergize with chemotherapeutic drugs to induce cell death. *Mol. Nutr. Food Res.* **2013**, *57*, 1170–1181. [CrossRef] [PubMed]
174. Fu, Y.; Chang, H.; Peng, X.; Bai, Q.; Yi, L.; Zhou, Y.; Zhu, J.; Mi, M. Resveratrol inhibits breast cancer stem-like cells and induces autophagy via suppressing Wnt/beta-catenin signaling pathway. *PLoS ONE* **2014**, *9*, e102535.
175. Yeh, C.B.; Hsieh, M.J.; Lin, C.W.; Chiou, H.L.; Lin, P.Y.; Chen, T.Y.; Yang, S.F. The antimetastatic effects of resveratrol on hepatocellular carcinoma through the downregulation of a metastasis-associated protease by SP-1 modulation. *PLoS ONE* **2013**, *8*, e56661. [CrossRef] [PubMed]
176. Rajasekaran, D.; Elavarasan, J.; Sivalingam, M.; Ganapathy, E.; Kumar, A.; Kalpana, K.; Sakthisekaran, D. Resveratrol interferes with *N*-nitrosodiethylamine-induced hepatocellular carcinoma at early and advanced stages in male Wistar rats. *Mol. Med. Rep.* **2011**, *4*, 1211–1217. [PubMed]
177. Selvaraj, S.; Sun, Y.; Sukumaran, P.; Singh, B.B. Resveratrol activates autophagic cell death in prostate cancer cells via downregulation of STIM1 and the mTOR pathway. *Mol. Carcinog.* **2015**, *5*, 818–831. [CrossRef] [PubMed]
178. Ganapathy, S.; Chen, Q.; Singh, K.P.; Shankar, S.; Srivastava, R.K. Resveratrol enhances antitumor activity of TRAIL in prostate cancer xenografts through activation of FOXO transcription factor. *PLoS ONE* **2010**, *5*, e15627. [CrossRef] [PubMed]
179. Garcia-Zepeda, S.P.; Garcia-Villa, E.; Diaz-Chavez, J.; Hernandez-Pando, R.; Gariglio, P. Resveratrol induces cell death in cervical cancer cells through apoptosis and autophagy. *Eur. J. Cancer Prev.* **2013**, *22*, 577–584. [CrossRef] [PubMed]
180. Sun, Y.; Wu, X.; Cai, X.; Song, M.; Zheng, J.; Pan, C.; Qiu, P.; Zhang, L.; Zhou, S.; Tang, Z.; et al. Identification of pinostilbene as a major colonic metabolite of pterostilbene and its inhibitory effects on colon cancer cells. *Mol. Nutr. Food Res.* **2016**. [CrossRef] [PubMed]
181. Moon, D.; McCormack, D.; McDonald, D.; McFadden, D. Pterostilbene induces mitochondrially derived apoptosis in breast cancer cells in vitro. *J. Surg. Res.* **2013**, *180*, 208–215. [CrossRef] [PubMed]

182. Su, C.M.; Lee, W.H.; Wu, A.T.; Lin, Y.K.; Wang, L.S.; Wu, C.H.; Yeh, C.T. Pterostilbene inhibits triple-negative breast cancer metastasis via inducing microRNA-205 expression and negatively modulates epithelial-to-mesenchymal transition. *J. Nutr. Biochem.* **2015**, *26*, 675–685. [CrossRef] [PubMed]
183. Wu, C.H.; Hong, B.H.; Ho, C.T.; Yen, G.C. Targeting cancer stem cells in breast cancer: Potential anticancer properties of 6-shogaol and pterostilbene. *J. Agric. Food Chem.* **2015**, *63*, 2432–2441. [CrossRef] [PubMed]
184. Lin, V.C.; Tsai, Y.C.; Lin, J.N.; Fan, L.L.; Pan, M.H.; Ho, C.T.; Wu, J.Y.; Way, T.D. Activation of AMPK by pterostilbene suppresses lipogenesis and cell-cycle progression in p53 positive and negative human prostate cancer cells. *J. Agric. Food Chem.* **2012**, *60*, 6399–6407. [CrossRef] [PubMed]
185. Dhar, S.; Kumar, A.; Rimando, A.M.; Zhang, X.; Levenson, A.S. Resveratrol and pterostilbene epigenetically restore PTEN expression by targeting oncomiRs of the miR-17 family in prostate cancer. *Oncotarget* **2015**, *6*, 27214–27226. [CrossRef] [PubMed]
186. Zhang, H.; Jia, R.; Wang, C.; Hu, T.; Wang, F. Piceatannol promotes apoptosis via up-regulation of microRNA-129 expression in colorectal cancer cell lines. *Biochem. Biophys. Res. Commun.* **2014**, *452*, 775–781. [CrossRef] [PubMed]
187. Hsieh, T.C.; Lin, C.Y.; Lin, H.Y.; Wu, J.M. AKT/mTOR as novel targets of polyphenol piceatannol possibly contributing to inhibition of proliferation of cultured prostate cancer cells. *ISRN Urol.* **2012**, *2012*, 272697. [CrossRef] [PubMed]
188. Kwon, G.T.; Jung, J.I.; Song, H.R.; Woo, E.Y.; Jun, J.G.; Kim, J.K.; Her, S.; Park, J.H. Piceatannol inhibits migration and invasion of prostate cancer cells: Possible mediation by decreased interleukin-6 signaling. *J. Nutr. Biochem.* **2012**, *23*, 228–238. [CrossRef] [PubMed]
189. Devassy, J.G.; Nwachukwu, I.D.; Jones, P.J. Curcumin and cancer: Barriers to obtaining a health claim. *Nutr. Rev.* **2015**, *73*, 155–165. [CrossRef] [PubMed]
190. Vallianou, N.G.; Evangelopoulos, A.; Schizas, N.; Kazazis, C. Potential anticancer properties and mechanisms of action of curcumin. *Anticancer Res.* **2015**, *35*, 645–651. [PubMed]
191. Shanmugam, M.; Rane, G.; Kanchi, M.; Arfuso, F.; Chinnathambi, A.; Zayed, M.; Alharbi, S.; Tan, B.; Kumar, A.; Sethi, G. The Multifaceted Role of Curcumin in Cancer Prevention and Treatment. *Molecules* **2015**, *20*, 2728–2769. [CrossRef] [PubMed]
192. Thomasset, S.C.; Berry, D.P.; Garcea, G.; Marczylo, T.; Steward, W.P.; Gescher, A.J. Dietary polyphenolic phytochemicals—Promising cancer chemopreventive agents in humans? A review of their clinical properties. *Int. J. Cancer* **2007**, *120*, 451–458. [CrossRef] [PubMed]
193. Lazarevic, B.; Boezelijn, G.; Diep, L.M.; Kvernrod, K.; Ogren, O.; Ramberg, H.; Moen, A.; Wessel, N.; Berg, R.E.; Egge-Jacobsen, W.; et al. Efficacy and safety of short-term genistein intervention in patients with localized prostate cancer prior to radical prostatectomy: A randomized, placebo-controlled, double-blind Phase 2 clinical trial. *Nutr. Cancer* **2011**, *63*, 889–898. [CrossRef] [PubMed]
194. Miyanaga, N.; Akaza, H.; Hinotsu, S.; Fujioka, T.; Naito, S.; Namiki, M.; Takahashi, S.; Hirao, Y.; Horie, S.; Tsukamoto, T.; et al. Prostate cancer chemoprevention study: An investigative randomized control study using purified isoflavones in men with rising prostate-specific antigen. *Cancer Sci.* **2012**, *103*, 125–130. [CrossRef] [PubMed]
195. Hamilton-Reeves, J.M.; Banerjee, S.; Banerjee, S.K.; Holzbeierlein, J.M.; Thrasher, J.B.; Kambhampati, S.; Keighley, J.; Van Veldhuizen, P. Short-term soy isoflavone intervention in patients with localized prostate cancer: A randomized, double-blind, placebo-controlled trial. *PLoS ONE* **2013**, *8*, e68331.
196. Zhang, G.; Wang, Y.; Zhang, Y.; Wan, X.; Li, J.; Liu, K.; Wang, F.; Liu, K.; Liu, Q.; Yang, C.; et al. Anti-cancer activities of tea epigallocatechin-3-gallate in breast cancer patients under radiotherapy. *Curr. Mol. Med.* **2012**, *12*, 163–176. [CrossRef] [PubMed]
197. Azrad, M.; Vollmer, R.T.; Madden, J.; Dewhirst, M.; Polascik, T.J.; Snyder, D.C.; Ruffin, M.T.; Moul, J.W.; Brenner, D.E.; Demark-Wahnefried, W. Flaxseed-derived enterolactone is inversely associated with tumor cell proliferation in men with localized prostate cancer. *J. Med. Food* **2013**, *16*, 357–360. [CrossRef] [PubMed]
198. Hoensch, H.; Groh, B.; Edler, L.; Kirch, W. Prospective cohort comparison of flavonoid treatment in patients with resected colorectal cancer to prevent recurrence. *World J. Gastroenterol.* **2008**, *14*, 2187–2193. [CrossRef] [PubMed]
199. Cruz-Correa, M.; Shoskes, D.A.; Sanchez, P.; Zhao, R.; Hylind, L.M.; Wexner, S.D.; Giardiello, F.M. Combination treatment with curcumin and quercetin of adenomas in familial adenomatous polyposis. *Clin. Gastroenterol. Hepatol.* **2006**, *4*, 1035–1038. [CrossRef] [PubMed]

200. Ide, H.; Tokiwa, S.; Sakamaki, K.; Nishio, K.; Isotani, S.; Muto, S.; Hama, T.; Masuda, H.; Horie, S. Combined inhibitory effects of soy isoflavones and curcumin on the production of prostate-specific antigen. *Prostate* **2010**, *70*, 1127–1133. [CrossRef] [PubMed]
201. Carroll, R.E.; Benya, R.V.; Turgeon, D.K.; Vareed, S.; Neuman, M.; Rodriguez, L.; Kakarala, M.; Carpenter, P.M.; McLaren, C.; Meyskens, F.J.; et al. Phase IIa clinical trial of curcumin for the prevention of colorectal neoplasia. *Cancer Prev. Res.* **2011**, *4*, 354–364. [CrossRef] [PubMed]
202. He, Z.Y.; Shi, C.B.; Wen, H.; Li, F.L.; Wang, B.L.; Wang, J. Upregulation of p53 expression in patients with colorectal cancer by administration of curcumin. *Cancer Investig.* **2011**, *29*, 208–213. [CrossRef] [PubMed]

11

YAP Inhibition by Resveratrol via Activation of AMPK Enhances the Sensitivity of Pancreatic Cancer Cells to Gemcitabine

Zhengdong Jiang [1], Xin Chen [1], Ke Chen [1], Liankang Sun [1], Luping Gao [1], Cancan Zhou [1], Meng Lei [1], Wanxing Duan [1], Zheng Wang [1], Qingyong Ma [1,*] and Jiguang Ma [2,*]

1 Department of Hepatobiliary Surgery, First Affiliated Hospital of Xi'an Jiaotong University, Xi'an 710061, China; jiang.19900708@stu.xjtu.edu.cn (Z.J.); chenxin.77@stu.xjtu.edu.cn (X.C.); ck532128@stu.xjtu.edu.cn (K.C.); sunliankang@stu.xjtu.edu.cn (L.S.); gaoluping@stu.xjtu.edu.cn (L.G.); trytofly@stu.xjtu.edu.cn (C.Z.); leimeng7@stu.xjtu.edu.cn (M.L.); 0556029@fudan.edu.cn (W.D.); zheng.wang11@mail.xjtu.edu.cn (Z.W.)

2 Department of Anesthesiology, First Affiliated Hospital of Xi'an Jiaotong University, Xi'an 710061, China

* Correspondence: qyma56@xjtu.edu.cn (Q.M.); jgma86@xjtu.edu.cn (J.M.)

Abstract: Resveratrol, a natural polyphenol present in most plants, inhibits the growth of numerous cancers both in vitro and in vivo. Aberrant expression of YAP has been reported to activate multiple growth-regulatory pathways and confer anti-apoptotic abilities to many cancer cells. However, the role of resveratrol in YES-activated protein (YAP) expression and that of YAP in pancreatic cancer cells' response to gemcitabine resistance remain elusive. In this study, we found that resveratrol suppressed the proliferation and cloning ability and induced the apoptosis of pancreatic cancer cells. These multiple biological effects might result from the activation of AMP-activation protein kinase (AMPK) (Thr172) and, thus, the induction of YAP cytoplasmic retention, Ser127 phosphorylation, and the inhibition of YAP transcriptional activity by resveratrol. YAP silencing by siRNA or resveratrol enhanced the sensitivity of gemcitabine in pancreatic cancer cells. Taken together, these findings demonstrate that resveratrol could increase the sensitivity of pancreatic cancer cells to gemcitabine by inhibiting YAP expression. More importantly, our work reveals that resveratrol is a potential anticancer agent for the treatment of pancreatic cancer, and YAP may serve as a promising target for sensitizing pancreatic cancer cells to chemotherapy.

Keywords: pancreatic cancer; resveratrol; AMPK; YAP; gemcitabine

---

1. Introduction

Pancreatic ductal adenocarcinoma (PDAC) is one of the most malignant and lethal tumors, with an overall five-year survival rate less than 7% [1]. Over recent decades, the prognosis of patients with this malignancy has not improved due to aggressive local invasion, metastases, and resistance to chemotherapy [2]. Currently, surgical resection is the only opportunity for curing pancreatic cancer at an early stage. Unfortunately, only approximately 20% of patients are eligible for surgical resection at the time of diagnosis, with most patents losing the opportunity for radical surgery. At present, gemcitabine is the first-line chemotherapeutic agent for pancreatic cancer patients. However, a low response rate to gemcitabine is common in the clinic, and less than 20% of patients experience the ideal effects of gemcitabine [3]. In recent years, FOLFIRINOX (oxaliplatin, irinotecan, fluorouracil, and leucovorin) has become the recommended frontline chemotherapeutic regimen for metastatic pancreatic cancer patients [4]. However, the seriously adverse reaction and acquired drug resistance associated with FOLFIRINOX limits its cytotoxic efficacy. Therefore, a novel target for enhancing current chemotherapy is clearly needed to improve the outcomes of patients with pancreatic cancer.

The Hippo pathway was first discovered by genetic mosaic screens in *Drosophila melanogaster* [5,6], and increasing evidence has demonstrated that the Hippo pathway also limits organ size in mammalian systems [7,8]. The YES-associated protein (YAP), a main component of the Hippo pathway, has been proved to be overexpressed and to participate in the tumorigenesis of a variety of cancers, including breast cancer [9], lung cancer [10], ovarian cancer [11], liver cancer [12], and pancreatic cancer [13,14]. YAP functions as an oncogene and promotes the survival of cancer cells by regulating cancer cell proliferation and apoptosis. The abnormal overexpression of YAP has also been reported to be linked to disease progression and poor prognosis in breast cancer patients [15]. However, whether aberrant YAP expression causes resistance of pancreatic cancer cells to chemotherapy is currently unclear. We hypothesized that overexpression of YAP might be closely correlated to the sensitivity of gemcitabine treatment in pancreatic cancer cells.

Resveratrol (*trans-3,4′,5-trihydroxystilbene*, Res) is a natural polyphenolic phytoalexin that was first isolated by Takaoka from the roots of white hellebore in 1939. Since then, resveratrol has been widely found in plants (such as grape skin, red wine, berries, and peanuts) and in traditional Chinese medicines (such as Rheum officinale Baill and Polygonum cuspidatum) [16,17]. Numerous studies have shown that resveratrol exhibits antioxidant activity, anti-inflammatory activity, and protective activity against cardiac diseases and metabolic disorders [18]. Over the past several years, many reports have demonstrated that resveratrol acts as a cancer chemo-preventive agent to induce growth inhibition, cell cycle arrest, apoptosis, and changes in biomarker expression in several human cancer cell lines [19–21]. Our previous study showed that resveratrol plays an important role in suppressing the proliferation of pancreatic cancer cells via the PI-3K/Akt/NF-κB signaling pathway [22] and the hedgehog signaling pathway [23,24]. However, whether resveratrol can inhibit YAP expression and its molecular mechanism have not been elucidated.

In the present study, we tested the hypothesis that resveratrol is able to inhibit YAP expression via activation of the AMP-activated protein kinase (AMPK) pathway and inhibit the proliferation ability of pancreatic cancer cells. YAP is associated with resistance to gemcitabine chemotherapy and targeting YAP via resveratrol can enhance the sensitivity of pancreatic cancer cells to gemcitabine. Our findings indicate that YAP is a novel molecular target for improving the efficacy of current chemotherapeutic regimens for patients with pancreatic cancer and improving their long-term outcomes.

2. Materials and Methods

All experimental protocols were approved by the Ethical Committee of the First Affiliated Hospital of Medical College, Xi'an Jiaotong University, Xi'an, China.

2.1. Reagents

Resveratrol (>99% pure) and MTT (3-(4,5-dimethyl-2-thiazolyl)-2,5-diphenyl-2-H-tetrazolium bromide) were purchased from Sigma-Aldrich (St. Louis, MO, USA), and gemcitabine was purchased from Selleck Chemicals (Houston, TX, USA). Resveratrol and gemcitabine were initially dissolved in Dimethyl Sulfoxide (DMSO) at stock concentrations of 50 mM and 10 mM, respectively. Working dilutions for resveratrol and gemcitabine were prepared in culture medium immediately before use, and DMSO was used as control in all experiments. The antibodies used in this study are listed in Supplementary Materials Table S1.

2.2. Cell Lines and Cell Culture

The human pancreatic cancer cell lines Panc-1 and BxPC-3 were purchased from the Type Culture Collection of the Chinese Academy of Sciences (Shanghai, China). Panc-1 and BxPC-3 were cultured in Dulbecco's Modified Eagle Medium (DMEM) or RPMI-1640, respectively, containing 10%

dialyzed heat-inactivated fetal bovine serum (FBS) (HyClone, Logan, UT, USA), 100 U/mL penicillin and 100 μg/mL streptomycin in a humidified atmosphere containing 5% CO_2 at 37 °C.

2.3. Cell Viability Assay

Cancer cell lines (Panc-1, BxPC-3) were plated into 96-well plates at a density of 5000 cells/well and treated with various concentrations (0, 25, 50, 100, and 200 μM) of resveratrol and various concentrations (0, 1, 2, 5, 10, and 20 μM) of gemcitabine for designated lengths of time (24, 48, and 72 h). After being transfected with siRNA for 48 h, cells were plated in 96-well plates at a density of 5000 cells/well and treated with 2 μM gemcitabine for 72 h. Cell viability was assessed by the MTT assay. Ten microliters of 5 mg/mL MTT was added into each well after media were removed and incubated at 37 °C for 4 h. Then, 100 μL DMSO was added to each well, and the optical density (OD) was measured at 490 nm on a multifunction microplate reader (POLARstar OPTIMA; BMG, Offenburg, Germany). The proliferation inhibition rate was calculated according to the following equation: Proliferation inhibition rate = (1 − OD sample/OD control) × 100%.

2.4. Apoptosis Assay

Cell apoptosis was assessed by flow cytometry with an Annexin V-FITC/7-AAD apoptosis detection kit from Becton, Dickinson and Company (BD) (Franklin Lakes, NJ, USA) according to the manufacturer's instructions. Briefly, cancer cells were seeded into 6-well plates at a density of 1×10^5 cells per well, after being starved overnight, and each treatment was applied for 48 h. Then, cells were trypsinized, washed with phosphate buffered saline (PBS) and stained with Annexin V and 7-AAD. The percentage of apoptotic cells was quantified by flow cytometry using a FACSCalibur (BD Biosciences, San Diego, CA, USA) instrument. The total apoptosis rate was calculated by summing the rate of populations stained with Annexin V-FITC+/7-AAD- (early apoptotic cells) and Annexin V-FITC+/7-AAD+ (late apoptotic cells).

2.5. Immunofluorescence Staining

Cells were fixed in 4% formaldehyde diluted in phosphate buffered saline (PBS) for 15 min, permeabilized with 0.3% Triton X-100, treated with blocking buffer (5% BSA in PBS), and then incubated overnight with the primary antibody at 4 °C. Cells were then incubated with the Red conjugated secondary antibody from Jackson Immunoresearch Laboratories (West Grove, PA, USA) for 1 h at room temperature. Slides were mounted and examined using a Zeiss Instruments confocal microscope.

2.6. Gene Silencing by Small Interfering RNA

Loss-of-function analysis was performed using siRNAs targeting AMPK and YAP, which were purchased from GenePharm (Shanghai, China). The siRNA sequences are provided in Supplementary Materials Table S2. Each siRNA (100 nM) was transfected into pancreatic cancer cells using Lipofectamine 2000 according to the manufacturer's instructions. The knockdown of each target gene was confirmed by Western blot analysis. The cells were used for subsequent experiments 48 h after transfection.

2.7. Western Blot Analysis

Total proteins were extracted by RIPA lysis buffer (Beyotime, Guangzhou, China), and the concentration of proteins was determined using the BCA protein assay kit (Pierce, Rockford, IL, USA) according to the manufacturer's instruction. The proteins were then subjected to SDS-PAGE using a 10% polyacrylamide gel with a 5% stacking gel. The proteins were subsequently transferred to polyvinylidene difluoride (PVDF) membranes. The membranes were blocked with 5% fat-free milk in Tris-buffered saline-Tween (TBS-T) for 2 h and then incubated with the primary antibodies (listed in Supplementary Materials Table S1) at 4 °C overnight. Then, the membranes were incubated with a secondary antibody (diluted 1:10,000) for 2 h at room temperature. Chemiluminescence detection of bound antibodies was performed using an enhanced chemiluminescence (ECL) PLUS system and a Molecular Imager ChemiDoc XRS System (Bio-Rad Laboratories, Hercules, CA, USA).

2.8. Real-Time PCR

Total RNA was extracted using the Fastgen1000 RNA isolation system (Fastgen, Shanghai, China) according to the manufacturer's protocol. Total RNA was reverse-transcribed into cDNA using the Prime Script RT reagent kit (TaKaRa, Dalian, China). Real-time PCR was used to quantitatively examine the expression of YAP, CTGF and CYR61 at the mRNA level. Real-time PCR was conducted according to a previous report [25]. The PCR primer sequences for YAP, CTGF, CYR61, and β-actin are shown in Supplementary Materials Table S3. The expression of each target gene was determined using β-actin as the normalization control. Relative gene expression was calculated using the $2^{-\Delta\Delta Ct}$ method [26].

2.9. Colony Formation Assay

One thousand cells were seeded into a 35-mm petri dish and allowed to adhere overnight. The next day, a different treatment was applied to the dishes for 24 h, after which the medium was replaced with drug-free medium. Cells were further cultured for two weeks to allow colonies to form. At the indicated time point, colonies were fixed with 4% paraformaldehyde and then stained with 0.1% crystal violet solution, rinsed, and then imaged. The number of colonies larger than 0.5 mm in diameter was counted using a microscope (Nikon Eclipse Ti-S, Tokyo, Japan) at a magnification of 400×.

2.10. Statistical Analysis

Each experiment was performed at least three times. Data are presented as means ± standard deviation. Differences were evaluated using Student's *t*-test, with $p < 0.05$ considered to be statistically significant.

3. Results

3.1. Resveratrol Inhibits the Proliferation of Pancreatic Cancer Cells

First, we examined the effects of resveratrol on the viability of cancer cells. Pancreatic cancer cells Panc-1 and BxPC-3 were treated with increasing doses of resveratrol (0, 25, 50, 100, and 200 μM). At the indicated time points (24, 48, and 72 h), the cell viability was assessed by the MTT assay. As shown in Figure 1, resveratrol decreased the growth of cancer cell lines in a dose- and time-dependent manner. The 50% inhibitory concentration (IC50) for both BxPC-3 and Panc-1 cells was approximately 50 μM resveratrol, which exhibited no cytotoxic effects on the BxPC-3 and Panc-1 cells. These results were in accord with our previous results. Therefore, cells were treated with 50 μM resveratrol in subsequent experiments.

3.2. Resveratrol Inhibits Clone Formation and Induces Apoptosis of Pancreatic Cancer Cells

To address the underlying mechanism governing the inhibitory effect of resveratrol (Res) on pancreatic cancer cell viability, we measured Res-induced apoptosis in BxPc-3 and Panc-1 cells by flow cytometry. The flow cytometric analyses were conducted after Panc-1 and BxPC-3 cells were treated with or without resveratrol (50 μM) for 48 h. As shown in Figure 2A,B, treatment of cancer cells with resveratrol caused an increase in the apoptotic population compared with that of the untreated control cells. Next, we detected the effect of resveratrol on the clone formation ability of cancer cells Panc-1 and BxPC-3. As shown in Figure 2C,D, treatment with 50 μM resveratrol markedly decreased the number of colonies compared with the untreated control cells. These results demonstrate that Res has a potent effect against clone formation and induces apoptosis of cancer cells.

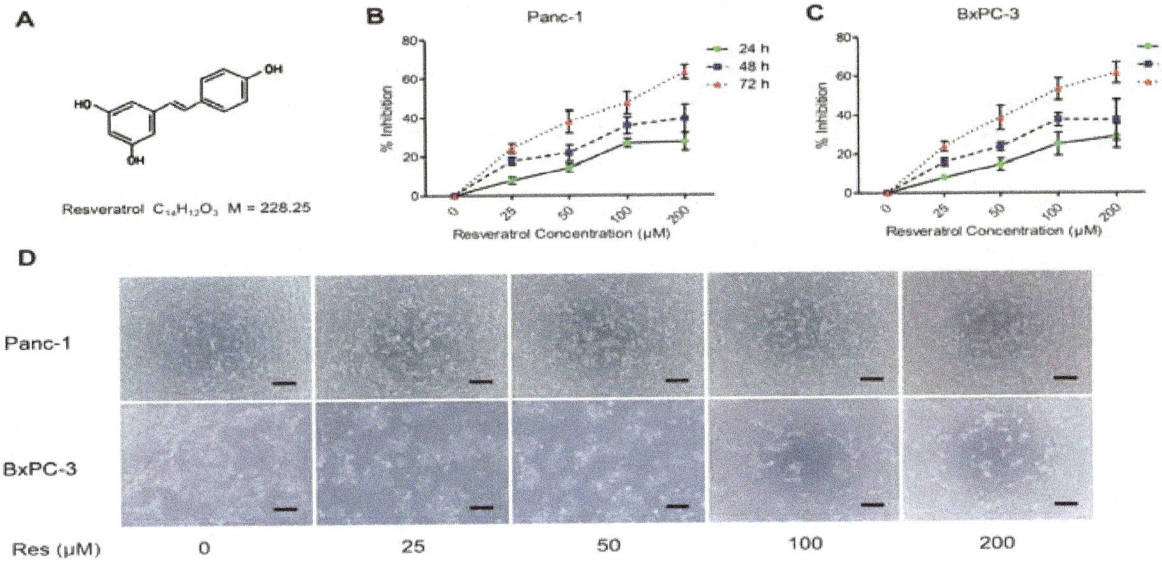

Figure 1. Resveratrol inhibits the proliferation of pancreatic cancer cells. (**A**) The structure of resveratrol (Res); (**B**,**C**) Panc-1 and BxPC-3 pancreatic cancer cells were treated with increasing concentrations of resveratrol (0, 25, 50, 100, and 200 μM) for 24 h, 48 h, or 72 h to analyze the inhibition ratio for cancer cell proliferation; (**D**) Micrographs of Panc-1 and BxPC-3 cells after being treated with the indicated concentrations of resveratrol for 48 h; representative images were captured (magnification, 100×; Scar bar: 100 μm).

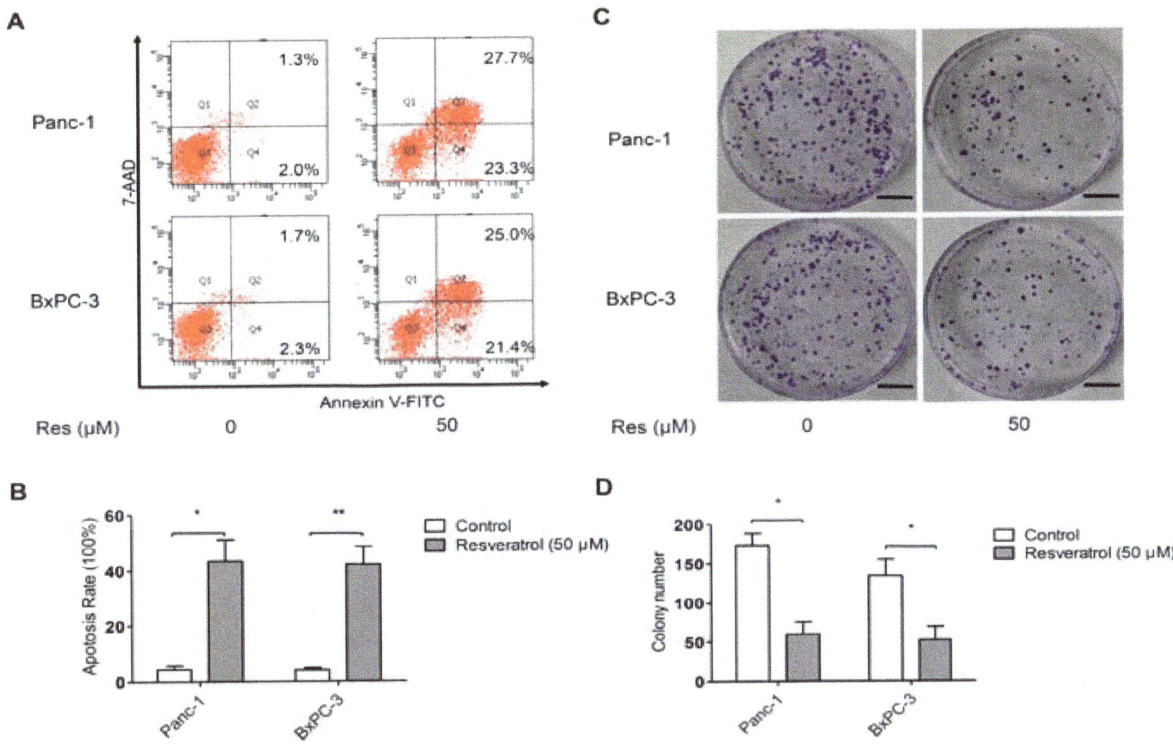

Figure 2. Resveratrol inhibits clone formation and induces apoptosis of pancreatic cancer cells. (**A**,**B**) The effects of resveratrol on Panc-1 and BxPC-3 cells apoptosis were detected by flow cytometry; (**C**,**D**) The effects of resveratrol on the colony-forming ability of Panc-1 and BxPC-3 cells. Images are representative of three independent experiments (Scale bar: 1 cm). Column: Mean, bar: SD, * $p < 0.05$, ** $p < 0.01$.

3.3. *Resveratrol Inhibits YAP Expression of Pancreatic Cancer Cells*

Increasing evidence has suggested that overexpression of YAP plays a key role in cancer cell survival and progression [27]. In particular, YAP can be phosphorylated at Ser127 and forms a more stable complex with the 14-3-3 proteins; therefore, it is retained in the cytoplasm and subject to degradation [28]. To determine whether resveratrol affects the YAP expression of cancer cells, Panc-1 and BxPC-3 cells were treated with resveratrol (0, 25, 50, and 100 μM) for 24 h. The protein expression of YAP and p-YAP (Ser127) in the pancreatic cancer cells exposed to resveratrol was evaluated by Western blot analysis. As shown in Figure 3A,B, resveratrol treatment up-regulated the level of p-YAP (Ser127), and the total level of YAP was significantly inhibited by resveratrol in a dose-dependent manner. Connective tissue growth factor (CTGF) and cysteine-rich angiogenic inducer 61 (CYR61) are two YAP-mediated downstream effectors that play an important role in tumor progression [29,30]. We therefore examined the expression of YAP, CTGF and CYR61 in response to treatment with resveratrol. The results showed that the mRNA levels of YAP, CTGF, and CYR61 were downregulated upon treatment with resveratrol (50 μM) (Figure 3C,D). Additionally, the nuclear translocation of YAP was decreased due to the effect of resveratrol, as demonstrated by immunofluorescence (Figure 3E). Together, these data indicate that resveratrol inhibits YAP expression of cancer cells via YAP phosphorylation at Ser127.

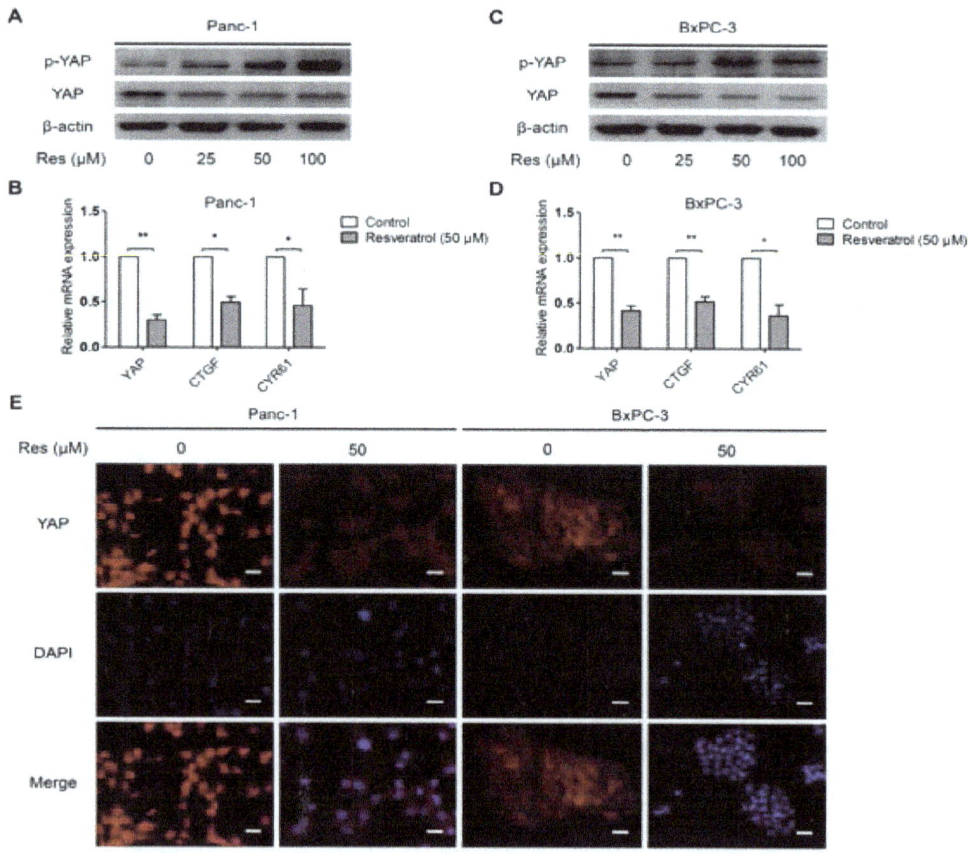

Figure 3. Resveratrol inhibits YAP expression of pancreatic cancer cells. (**A**,**B**) The effects of resveratrol on the protein expression of YAP and p-YAP (Ser127) were examined by Western blot analysis using β-actin as an internal loading control; (**C**,**D**) The effects of resveratrol on the mRNA expression of YAP, connective tissue growth factor (CTGF) and CYR61 were examined by real-time PCR with β-actin as the normalized reference gene. The data represent the results of three independent experiments; (**E**) Immunofluorescence staining of YAP in Panc-1 and BxPC-3 cells after treatment with resveratrol (50 μM) for 24 h. YAP staining is shown in red, and nuclear DNA staining by DAPI is shown in blue. (Magnification, 400×; Scale bar: 20 μm). Column: mean, bar: SD, * $p < 0.05$, ** $p < 0.01$.

3.4. Knockdown of AMPK Rescues Resveratrol Induced Suppression of YAP in Pancreatic Cancer Cells

Previous studies have established that resveratrol can activate the AMPK pathway [31]. The activation of AMPK leads to the suppression of YAP expression [32]. Based on the abovementioned promising findings, we speculated that the effect of resveratrol on cancer cell YAP inhibition may be mediated by AMPK signaling. To test this hypothesis, we further examined the effect of resveratrol on the activity of AMPK signaling. Immunoblotting results revealed that the phosphorylation level of AMPK (p-AMPK) in pancreatic cancer cells was significantly increased in response to resveratrol treatment in a dose-dependent manner (Figure 4A,B). To verify that resveratrol-inhibited YAP expression in cancer cells is mediated by AMPK signaling, siRNA technology was developed to knock down AMPK expression. We found that knocking down AMPK expression alone did not affect the expression of YAP or the phosphorylation level of p-YAP in Panc-1 and BxPC-3 cells (Figure 4C,D). However, resveratrol induced the activation of p-AMPK and p-YAP, and inhibition of YAP was restored by AMPK knockdown (Figure 4C,D). Additionally, the immunofluorescence results indicated that the nuclear translocation and total level of YAP was inhibited by resveratrol and that this inhibition effect was restored by AMPK knockdown (Figure 4E). Together, these data suggest that AMPK signaling is involved in resveratrol-suppressed YAP expression in pancreatic cancer cells.

3.5. Knockdown of YAP Increased Gemcitabine Sensitivity in Pancreatic Cancer Cells

First, we used the MTT assay to examine the effects of gemcitabine on the proliferation of the Panc-1 and BxPC-3 cell lines. As shown in Figure 5A,B, we found that BxPC-3 was sensitive whereas Panc-1 was resistant to gemcitabine, in accord with previous findings [33]. Therefore, we used Panc-1 in further experiments. To evaluate the effects of YAP on cell survival and resistance to chemotherapy, we treated Panc-1 cells, which express high levels of YAP natively and are resistant to gemcitabine, with 2 μM gemcitabine in the presence of either siControl or siYAP and confirmed the silencing of YAP in the cells using Western blot analysis (Figure 5H). MTT assay results showed that the proliferation capacity was lower in siYAP cells than in siControl cells after treating them with gemcitabine (Figure 5C). Furthermore, silencing of YAP increased the apoptotic response to treatment with gemcitabine (2 μM) in Panc-1 cells (Figure 5D,E). The clone ability was significantly decreased after silencing YAP, and siYAP enhanced the gemcitabine inhibition effect on clone ability (Figure 5F,G). Together, these data suggest that YAP silencing enhances the sensitivity of gemcitabine in gemcitabine-resistant pancreatic cancer cells.

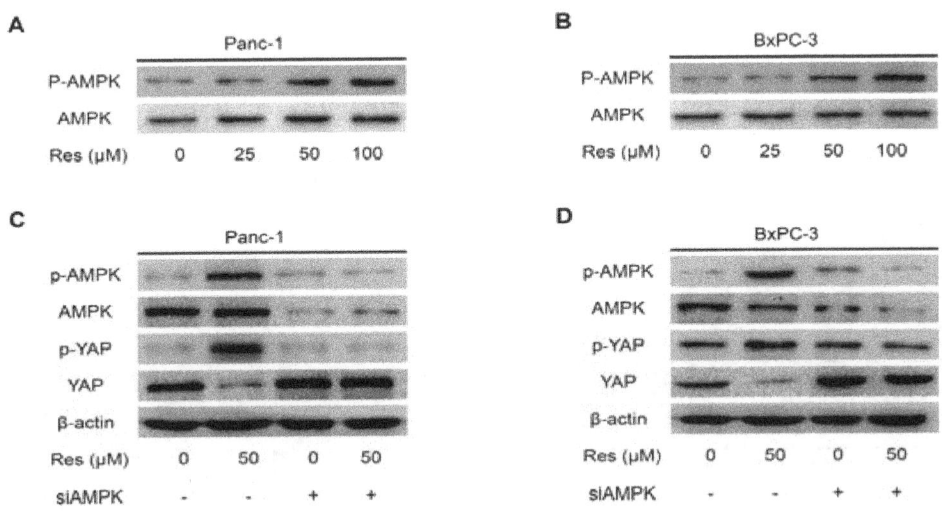

Figure 4. *Cont.*

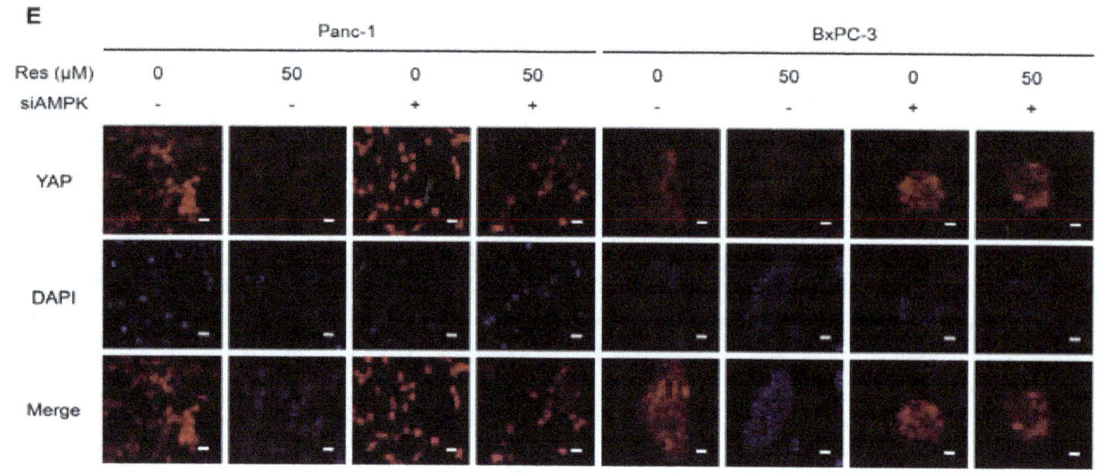

Figure 4. Knockdown of AMP-activated protein kinase (AMPK) rescues resveratrol-induced suppression of YES-associated protein (YAP) of pancreatic cancer cells. (**A**,**B**) The effects of resveratrol on the activation of AMPK (Thr172) in Panc-1 and BxPC-3 cells were measured by Western blot analysis; (**C**,**D**) After transfection with siAMPK or siControl for 48 h, Panc-1 and BxPC-3 cells were treated with resveratrol (50 μM) for 24 h. The protein expression levels of YAP, p-YAP (Ser127), AMPK and p-AMPK (Thr172) were examined by Western blot analysis using β-actin as an internal loading control; (**E**) YAP in Panc-1 and BxPC-3 cells was stained for immunofluorescence after transfection with siAMPK or siControl for 48 h and then treated with resveratrol (50 μM) for 24 h. YAP staining is shown in red, and nuclear DNA staining by DAPI is shown in blue (Magnification, 400×; Scale bar: 20 μm).

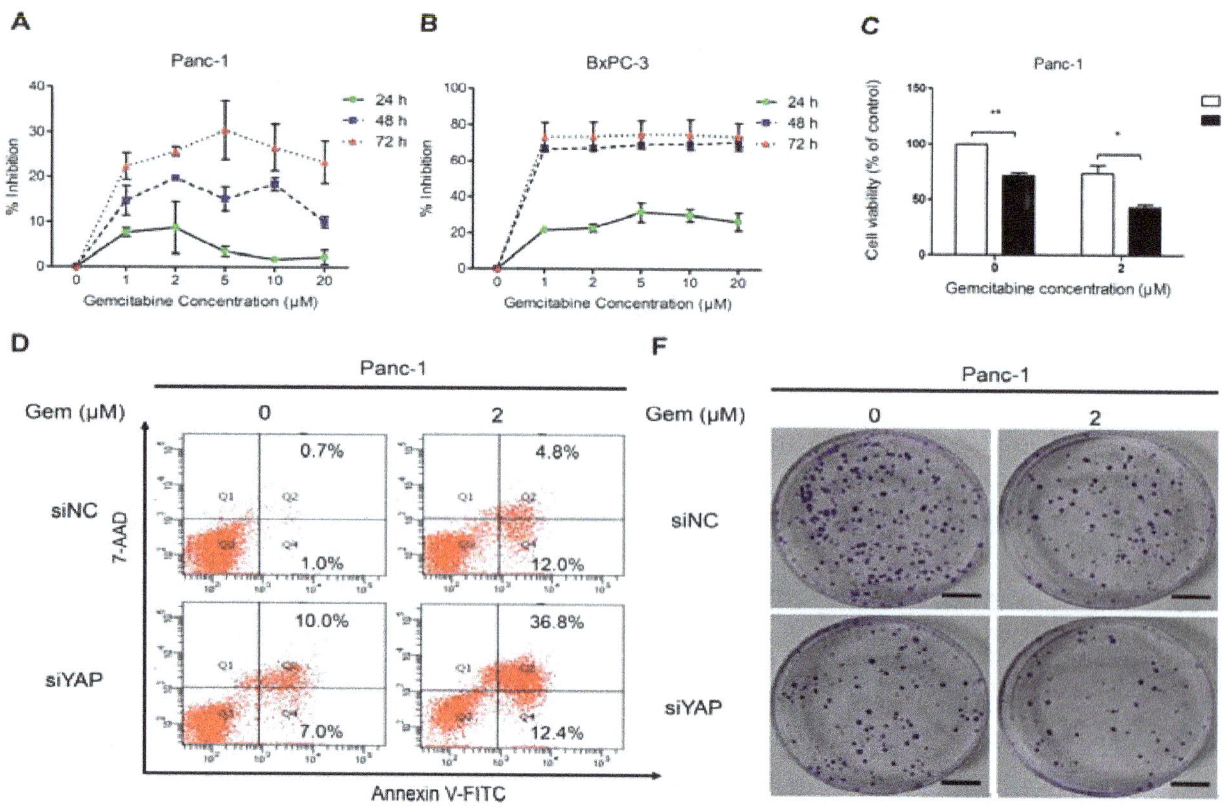

Figure 5. *Cont.*

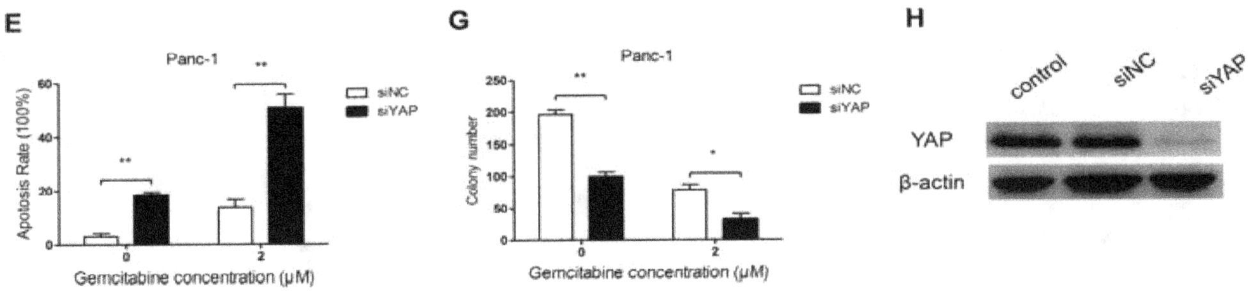

Figure 5. Knockdown of YAP increases gemcitabine sensitivity in pancreatic cancer cells. (**A**,**B**) Panc-1 and BxPC-3 cells were treated with increasing concentrations of gemcitabine (0, 1, 2, 5, 10, and 20 μM) for 24 h, 48 h, or 72 h to analyze the inhibition ratio for cancer cell proliferation; (**C**) After being transfected with siControl or siYAP for 48 h, cells were plated in 96-well plates and treated with 2 μM gemcitabine for 72 h. Cell viability was assessed by the MTT assay; (**D**,**E**) The effects of siControl or siYAP on Panc-1 cancer cells apoptosis after treatment with 2 μM gemcitabine for 48 h was detected by flow cytometry; (**F**,**G**) The effects of siControl or siYAP combined with gemcitabine on the colony-forming ability of Panc-1 cells. Images are representative of three independent experiments (Scale bar: 1 cm); (**H**) The efficiency of siRNAs targeting YAP in Panc-1cells was evaluated by Western blot analysis. Column: Mean, bar: SD, * $p < 0.05$, ** $p < 0.01$.

3.6. Inhibition of YAP Activity by Resveratrol Enhanced the Sensitivity of Pancreatic Cancer Cells to Gemcitabine

To determine whether resveratrol increases the susceptibility of Panc-1 cells to gemcitabine, we treated Panc-1 cells with 50 μM resveratrol and 2 μM gemcitabine. The MTT assay results showed that the proliferation capacity was significantly lower in the resveratrol and gemcitabine therapy group than in the resveratrol alone or gemcitabine alone group (Figure 6A). The protein expression of YAP and p-YAP (Ser127) in Panc-1 exposed to resveratrol and gemcitabine was evaluated by Western blot analysis. As shown in Figure 6B, resveratrol treatment up-regulated the level of p-YAP (Ser127), and the total level of YAP was significantly inhibited by resveratrol. However, gemcitabine had no effect on YAP expression. Next, we measured the apoptosis rate in Panc-1 cells by flow cytometry. Flow cytometric analyses were conducted after Panc-1 cells were treated with or without resveratrol (50 μM) and gemcitabine (2 μM) for 48 h. As shown in Figure 6C,D, treatment of cancer cells with resveratrol caused an increase in apoptotic population compared with the untreated control cells, but almost all cells underwent apoptosis in the resveratrol and gemcitabine combined therapy group. Next, we detected the clone formation ability of Panc-1 cancer cells after treatment with resveratrol and gemcitabine. As shown in Figure 6E,F, treatment with resveratrol and gemcitabine markedly decreased the number of colonies compared with the number measured for the gemcitabine or resveratrol alone cells. Taken together, these results demonstrate that resveratrol has a potent effect in enhancing the sensitivity of pancreatic cancer cells to gemcitabine by inhibiting YAP expression.

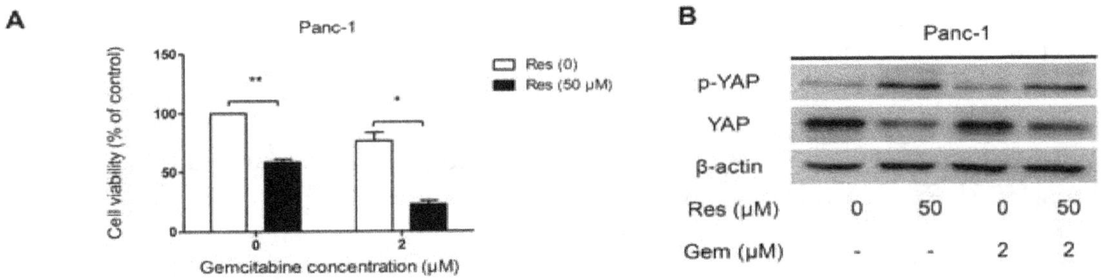

Figure 6. *Cont.*

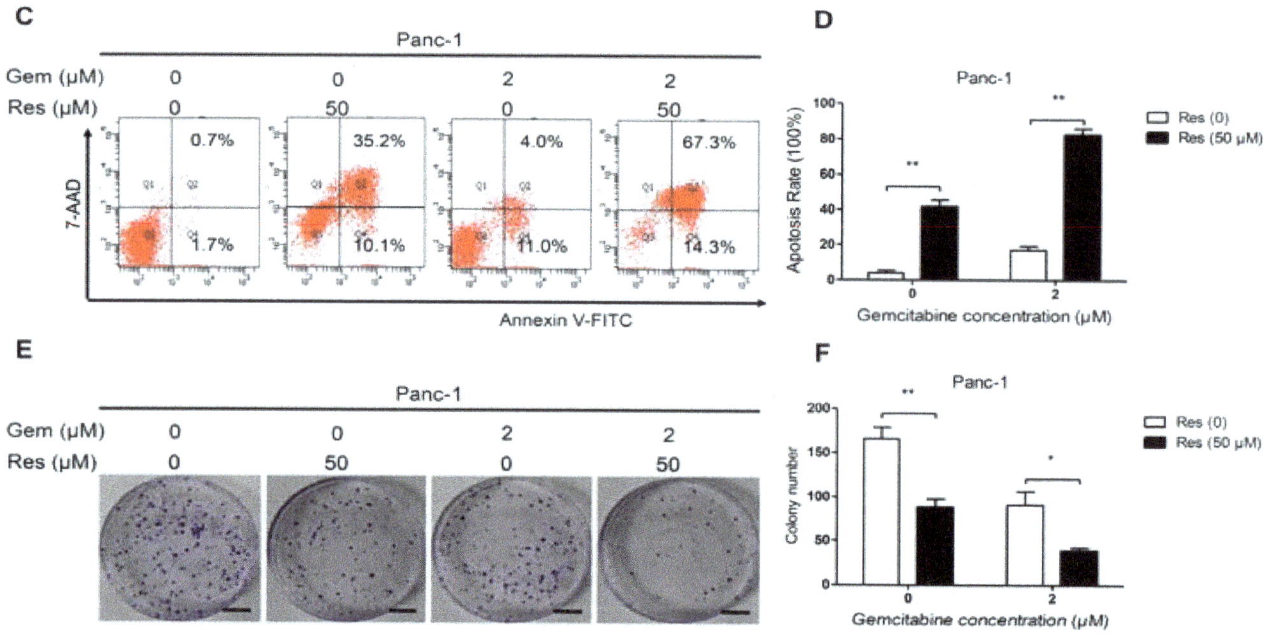

Figure 6. Inhibition of YAP activity by resveratrol enhances the sensitivity of pancreatic cancer cells to gemcitabine. (**A**) Panc-1 cells were treated with gemcitabine (2 μM) and resveratrol (50 μM) for 72 h. Cell viability was assessed by the MTT assay; (**B**) Panc-1 cells were treated with gemcitabine (2 μM) and resveratrol (50 μM) for 24 h. The protein expression levels of YAP and p-YAP (Ser127) were examined by Western blot analysis using β-actin as an internal loading control; (**C**,**D**) Panc-1 cells were treated with gemcitabine (Gem) (2 μM) and resveratrol (50 μM) for 48 h. Apoptosis was detected by flow cytometry; (**E**,**F**) The combined effects of Res and Gem on Panc-1 cell clones' colony-forming ability was detected. Images are representative of three independent experiments (Scale bar: 1 cm). Column: Mean, bar: SD, * $p < 0.05$, ** $p < 0.01$.

4. Discussion

In this study, we observed that resveratrol inhibited pancreatic cancer cell proliferation and clone formation and induced cell apoptosis, which was accompanied by the activation of p-AMPK and p-YAP and a decreased level of YAP in BxPc-3 and Panc-1 cells. Moreover, the results suggest that AMPK signaling is essential in resveratrol-suppressed YAP expression in pancreatic cancer cells. Furthermore, we found that YAP silencing enhances the sensitivity of gemcitabine in gemcitabine-resistant Panc-1 cancer cells. Resveratrol has a synergistic effect with gemcitabine in Panc-1 cells by inhibiting YAP expression. Our findings suggest that resveratrol is a potential drug for adjuvant therapy or a complementary alternative medicine for the management of pancreatic cancers via activation of AMPK and inhibition of YAP.

Despite great advances in modern medicine over the past several years, pancreatic cancer is still associated with an extremely high mortality rate [1]. Currently, gemcitabine [3] and FOLFIRINOX [4] are considered first-line drugs for treating pancreatic cancer, but their efficacy is still low because of a seriously adverse reaction and because acquired drug resistance limits their cytotoxic efficacy. Therefore, we must find a novel target for enhancing current chemotherapy to improve the outcomes of patients with pancreatic cancer.

Resveratrol is a natural polyphenolic phytoalexin that is widely found in plants and in traditional Chinese medicines [16,17]. Resveratrol has been shown to directly inhibit the proliferation and viability of human pancreatic cancer cells in vitro in a dose- and time-dependent manner [22]. Accordingly, our results demonstrated that resveratrol inhibited cell proliferation and clone formation and induced cell apoptosis. Interestingly, we found that Panc-1 and BxPC-3 cells respond differently to gemcitabine (BxPC-3 being more sensitive). But their biochemical and functional response to resveratrol appears to be the same. As we know, BxPC-3 and Panc-1 cells have many differences such as K-*ras* mutation types (BxPC-3 is a K-*ras* wild cell while Panc-1 is a K-*ras* mutant cell) [34] and epithelial-mesenchymal transition (EMT) regulated genes (E-cadherin and Zeb-1) [35] which could affect gemcitabine sensitivity in pancreatic cancer cells. Our previous reports have shown that resveratrol could inhibit the EMT of pancreatic cancer cells via suppression of the PI3K/Akt/NF-kappaB pathway in Panc-1 and BxPC-3 cells [22]. Furthermore, resveratrol could also inhibit pancreatic cancer stem cell characteristics in human and Kras (G12D) transgenic mice by inhibiting pluripotency maintaining factors and epithelial-mesenchymal transition [36]. However, the specific mechanism needs to be further explored.

The AMPK system is traditionally considered a sensor of cellular energy status and a regulator of metabolism [37]. Recent studies have provided novel evidence that AMPK may function as a suppressor of cell proliferation. Indeed, activation of AMPK has been shown to benefit a variety of malignant tumors by inhibiting the proliferation of tumor cells [38,39]. In this respect, our results demonstrated that resveratrol could activate AMPK (Thr172) and suppress the proliferation of pancreatic cancer cells, indicating the anti-proliferative action of AMPK in pancreatic cancer cells. The effect of AMPK on cell proliferation appears to be mediated through multiple mechanisms, mainly the regulation of cell cycle progression, inhibition of protein synthesis, and de novo fatty acid biosynthesis [40,41]. Previous reports have suggested that AMPK activation stabilizes and increases AMOTL1 steady-state protein levels, contributing to YAP inhibition [42]. Accordingly, our results demonstrated that resveratrol induces YAP cytoplasmic retention and S127 phosphorylation and inhibits YAP transcriptional activity and YAP-dependent transformation via activation of AMPK. Knockdown of AMPK rescues resveratrol-induced suppression of YAP in pancreatic cancer cells. Some reports have suggested that glucose starvation and energy stress could result in phosphorylation of YAP and contribute to its inactivation [43]. Harris et al. [44] demonstrated that resveratrol could inhibit glycogen synthesis, which may serve as the underlying mechanism in the inhibition of YAP. However, Jung-Soon Mo [32] and his colleagues also found that AMPK inhibits YAP activity through phosphorylation of serine 94. Whether resveratrol could induce YAP phosphorylation at serine 94 need further investigation.

As an oncogene, YAP is abundantly expressed in many types of cancers [15,27], and tremendous progress has been made toward our understanding of the roles of YAP in tumorigenesis, size control, and stem cell renewal and differentiation [45,46]. However, YAP's function in chemotherapeutic drug response is largely unknown in pancreatic cancer cells. Ciamporcero et al. [47] demonstrated that YAP overexpression protected, whereas YAP knockdown sensitized, urothelial cell carcinoma (UCC) cells to chemotherapy and radiation effects by increasing the accumulation of DNA damage and apoptosis. Verteporfin, a pharmacological YAP inhibitor, could inhibit tumor cell proliferation and restore sensitivity to cisplatin. In our study, we found that the chemotherapeutic sensitivity of pancreatic cancer to gemcitabine can be increased by YAP inhibition in vitro. YAP may participate in regulating the chemosensitivity of pancreatic cancer to chemotherapy. As a dietary and synthetic agent that is a pharmacological YAP inhibitor, resveratrol may exhibit greater efficacy and lower toxicity for the prevention and treatment of pancreatic cancer. However, its more specific mechanisms and safety require further investigation.

5. Conclusions

In conclusion, the present study demonstrated that resveratrol suppressed the proliferation and cloning ability and induced the apoptosis of pancreatic cancer cells. These multiple biological effects might result from the activation of AMPK (Thr172), thus, inducing YAP cytoplasmic retention and S127 phosphorylation, and inhibiting YAP transcriptional activity by resveratrol. YAP silencing by siRNA or resveratrol could enhance the sensitivity of gemcitabine in pancreatic cancer cells. These results suggest that resveratrol is a potential anticancer agent for the treatment of pancreatic cancer. However, whether other mechanisms are involved in the anti-tumor effects of resveratrol and its safety in humans warrant further study.

Acknowledgments: This study was supported by grants from the National Natural Science Foundation of China (No. 81402971) and the Clinical Innovation Funds of the 1st Affiliated Hospital of XJTU (No. 14ZD05, No. 14ZD06, No. 15ZD02, No. 15ZD03, No. 15ZD07 and No. 15ZD15).

Author Contributions: Z.J. designed and performed the experiments, analyzed and interpreted the data, and wrote the manuscript. X.C. and K.C. participated in the design of the study and performed the statistical analysis. C.Z., M.L., L.S., L.G., W.D., and Z.W. contributed to the conception of the study and the revision of the article. J.M. and Q.M. contributed to the conception and design of the study, the revision of the manuscript, and the final approval of the version to be published. All authors read and approved the final manuscript.

References

1. Siegel, R.L.; Miller, K.D.; Jemal, A. Cancer statistics, 2016. *CA Cancer J. Clin.* **2016**, *66*, 7–30. [CrossRef] [PubMed]
2. Bosetti, C.; Bertuccio, P.; Negri, E.; La Vecchia, C.; Zeegers, M.P.; Boffetta, P. Pancreatic cancer: Overview of descriptive epidemiology. *Mol. Carcinog.* **2012**, *51*, 3–13. [CrossRef] [PubMed]
3. Tamburrino, A.; Piro, G.; Carbone, C.; Tortora, G.; Melisi, D. Mechanisms of resistance to chemotherapeutic and anti-angiogenic drugs as novel targets for pancreatic cancer therapy. *Front. Pharmacol.* **2013**, *4*, 56. [CrossRef] [PubMed]
4. Conroy, T.; Desseigne, F.; Ychou, M.; Bouche, O.; Guimbaud, R.; Becouarn, Y.; Adenis, A.; Raoul, J.L.; Gourgou-Bourgade, S.; de la Fouchardiere, C.; et al. FOLFIRINOX versus gemcitabine for metastatic pancreatic cancer. *N. Engl. J. Med.* **2011**, *364*, 1817–1825. [CrossRef] [PubMed]
5. Edgar, B.A. From cell structure to transcription: Hippo forges a new path. *Cell* **2006**, *124*, 267–273. [CrossRef] [PubMed]
6. Huang, J.; Wu, S.; Barrera, J.; Matthews, K.; Pan, D. The Hippo signaling pathway coordinately regulates cell proliferation and apoptosis by inactivating Yorkie, the Drosophila Homolog of YAP. *Cell* **2005**, *122*, 421–434. [CrossRef] [PubMed]
7. Yimlamai, D.; Christodoulou, C.; Galli, G.G.; Yanger, K.; Pepe-Mooney, B.; Gurung, B.; Shrestha, K.; Cahan, P.; Stanger, B.Z.; Camargo, F.D. Hippo pathway activity influences liver cell fate. *Cell* **2014**, *157*, 1324–1338. [CrossRef] [PubMed]
8. Yu, F.X.; Zhao, B.; Guan, K.L. Hippo Pathway in Organ Size Control, Tissue Homeostasis, and Cancer. *Cell* **2015**, *163*, 811–828. [CrossRef] [PubMed]
9. Von, E.B.; Jaenicke, L.A.; Kortlever, R.M.; Royla, N.; Wiese, K.E.; Letschert, S.; McDuffus, L.A.; Sauer, M.; Rosenwald, A.; Evan, G.I.; et al. A MYC-Driven Change in Mitochondrial Dynamics Limits YAP/TAZ Function in Mammary Epithelial Cells and Breast Cancer. *Cancer Cell* **2015**, *28*, 743–757.
10. Dubois, F.; Keller, M.; Calvayrac, O.; Soncin, F.; Hoa, L.; Hergovich, A.; Parrini, M.C.; Mazieres, J.; Vaisse-Lesteven, M.; Camonis, J.; et al. RASSF1A Suppresses the Invasion and Metastatic Potential of Human Non-Small Cell Lung Cancer Cells by Inhibiting YAP Activation through the GEF-H1/RhoB Pathway. *Cancer Res.* **2016**, *76*, 1627–1640. [CrossRef] [PubMed]
11. Yagi, H.; Asanoma, K.; Ohgami, T.; Ichinoe, A.; Sonoda, K.; Kato, K. GEP oncogene promotes cell proliferation through YAP activation in ovarian cancer. *Oncogene* **2016**, *35*, 4471–4480. [CrossRef] [PubMed]
12. Wang, J.; Ma, L.; Weng, W.; Qiao, Y.; Zhang, Y.; He, J.; Wang, H.; Xiao, W.; Li, L.; Chu, Q.; et al. Mutual interaction between YAP and CREB promotes tumorigenesis in liver cancer. *Hepatology* **2013**, *58*, 1011–1020. [CrossRef] [PubMed]
13. Yuan, Y.; Li, D.; Li, H.; Wang, L.; Tian, G.; Dong, Y. YAP overexpression promotes the epithelial-mesenchymal transition and chemoresistance in pancreatic cancer cells. *Mol. Med. Rep.* **2016**, *13*, 237–242. [CrossRef] [PubMed]
14. Morvaridi, S.; Dhall, D.; Greene, M.I.; Pandol, S.J.; Wang, Q. Role of YAP and TAZ in pancreatic ductal adenocarcinoma and in stellate cells associated with cancer and chronic pancreatitis. *Sci. Rep.* **2015**, *5*, 16759. [CrossRef] [PubMed]
15. Zhao, Y.; Khanal, P.; Savage, P.; She, Y.M.; Cyr, T.D.; Yang, X. YAP-induced resistance of cancer cells to antitubulin drugs is modulated by a Hippo-independent pathway. *Cancer Res.* **2014**, *74*, 4493–4503. [CrossRef] [PubMed]

16. Borriello, A.; Bencivenga, D.; Caldarelli, I.; Tramontano, A.; Borgia, A.; Pirozzi, A.V.; Oliva, A.; Della, R.F. Resveratrol and cancer treatment: Is hormesis a yet unsolved matter. *Curr. Pharm. Des.* **2013**, *19*, 5384–5393. [CrossRef] [PubMed]
17. Xu, Q.; Zong, L.; Chen, X.; Jiang, Z.; Nan, L.; Li, J.; Duan, W.; Lei, J.; Zhang, L.; Ma, J.; et al. Resveratrol in the treatment of pancreatic cancer. *Ann. N. Y. Acad. Sci.* **2015**, *1348*, 10–19. [CrossRef] [PubMed]
18. Zhang, H.; Morgan, B.; Potter, B.J.; Ma, L.; Dellsperger, K.C.; Ungvari, Z.; Zhang, C. Resveratrol improves left ventricular diastolic relaxation in type 2 diabetes by inhibiting oxidative/nitrative stress: in vivo demonstration with magnetic resonance imaging. *Am. J. Physiol. Heart Circ. Physiol.* **2010**, *299*, H985–H994. [CrossRef] [PubMed]
19. Hu, F.W.; Tsai, L.L.; Yu, C.H.; Chen, P.N.; Chou, M.Y.; Yu, C.C. Impairment of tumor-initiating stem-like property and reversal of epithelial-mesenchymal transdifferentiation in head and neck cancer by resveratrol treatment. *Mol. Nutr. Food Res.* **2012**, *56*, 1247–1258. [CrossRef] [PubMed]
20. Buhrmann, C.; Shayan, P.; Popper, B.; Goel, A.; Shakibaei, M. Sirt1 Is Required for Resveratrol-Mediated Chemopreventive Effects in Colorectal Cancer Cells. *Nutrients* **2016**, *8*, 145. [CrossRef] [PubMed]
21. Roy, S.K.; Chen, Q.; Fu, J.; Shankar, S.; Srivastava, R.K. Resveratrol inhibits growth of orthotopic pancreatic tumors through activation of FOXO transcription factors. *PLoS ONE* **2011**, *6*, e25166. [CrossRef] [PubMed]
22. Li, W.; Ma, J.; Ma, Q.; Li, B.; Han, L.; Liu, J.; Xu, Q.; Duan, W.; Yu, S.; Wang, F.; et al. Resveratrol inhibits the epithelial-mesenchymal transition of pancreatic cancer cells via suppression of the PI-3K/Akt/NF-kappaB pathway. *Curr. Med. Chem.* **2013**, *20*, 4185–4194. [CrossRef] [PubMed]
23. Li, W.; Cao, L.; Chen, X.; Lei, J.; Ma, Q. Resveratrol inhibits hypoxia-driven ROS-induced invasive and migratory ability of pancreatic cancer cells via suppression of the Hedgehog signaling pathway. *Oncol. Rep.* **2016**, *35*, 1718–1726. [CrossRef] [PubMed]
24. Qin, Y.; Ma, Z.; Dang, X.; Li, W.; Ma, Q. Effect of resveratrol on proliferation and apoptosis of human pancreatic cancer MIA PaCa-2 cells may involve inhibition of the Hedgehog signaling pathway. *Mol. Med. Rep.* **2014**, *10*, 2563–2567. [PubMed]
25. Ma, Q.; Zhang, M.; Wang, Z.; Ma, Z.; Sha, H. The beneficial effect of resveratrol on severe acute pancreatitis. *Ann. N. Y. Acad. Sci.* **2011**, *1215*, 96–102. [CrossRef] [PubMed]
26. Schmittgen, T.D.; Livak, K.J. Analyzing real-time PCR data by the comparative C(T) method. *Nat. Protoc.* **2008**, *3*, 1101–1108. [CrossRef] [PubMed]
27. Hall, C.A.; Wang, R.; Miao, J.; Oliva, E.; Shen, X.; Wheeler, T.; Hilsenbeck, S.G.; Orsulic, S.; Goode, S. Hippo pathway effector Yap is an ovarian cancer oncogene. *Cancer Res.* **2010**, *70*, 8517–8525. [CrossRef] [PubMed]
28. Basu, S.; Totty, N.F.; Irwin, M.S.; Sudol, M.; Downward, J. Akt phosphorylates the Yes-associated protein, YAP, to induce interaction with 14–3-3 and attenuation of p73-mediated apoptosis. *Mol. Cell* **2003**, *11*, 11–23. [CrossRef]
29. Dong, J.; Feldmann, G.; Huang, J.; Wu, S.; Zhang, N.; Comerford, S.A.; Gayyed, M.F.; Anders, R.A.; Maitra, A.; Pan, D. Elucidation of a universal size-control mechanism in Drosophila and mammals. *Cell* **2007**, *130*, 1120–1133. [CrossRef] [PubMed]
30. Lu, L.; Li, Y.; Kim, S.M.; Bossuyt, W.; Liu, P.; Qiu, Q.; Wang, Y.; Halder, G.; Finegold, M.J.; Lee, J.S.; et al. Hippo signaling is a potent in vivo growth and tumor suppressor pathway in the mammalian liver. *Proc. Natl. Acad. Sci. USA* **2010**, *107*, 1437–1442. [CrossRef] [PubMed]
31. Yi, C.O.; Jeon, B.T.; Shin, H.J.; Jeong, E.A.; Chang, K.C.; Lee, J.E.; Lee, D.H.; Kim, H.J.; Kang, S.S.; Cho, G.J.; et al. Resveratrol activates AMPK and suppresses LPS-induced NF-kappaB-dependent COX-2 activation in RAW 264.7 macrophage cells. *Anat. Cell Biol.* **2011**, *44*, 194–203. [CrossRef] [PubMed]
32. Mo, J.S.; Meng, Z.; Kim, Y.C.; Park, H.W.; Hansen, C.G.; Kim, S.; Lim, D.S.; Guan, K.L. Cellular energy stress induces AMPK-mediated regulation of YAP and the Hippo pathway. *Nat. Cell Biol.* **2015**, *17*, 500–510. [CrossRef] [PubMed]
33. Cao, J.; Yang, J.; Ramachandran, V.; Arumugam, T.; Deng, D.; Li, Z.; Xu, L.; Logsdon, C.D. TM4SF1 Promotes Gemcitabine Resistance of Pancreatic Cancer in vitro and in vivo. *PLoS ONE* **2015**, *10*, e0144969. [CrossRef] [PubMed]
34. Shao, T.; Zheng, Y.; Zhao, B.; Li, T.; Cheng, K.; Cai, W. Recombinant expression of different mutant K-ras gene in pancreatic cancer Bxpc-3 cells and its effects on chemotherapy sensitivity. *Sci. China Life Sci.* **2014**, *57*, 1011–1017. [CrossRef] [PubMed]

35. Arumugam, T.; Ramachandran, V.; Fournier, K.F.; Wang, H.; Marquis, L.; Abbruzzese, J.L.; Gallick, G.E.; Logsdon, C.D.; McConkey, D.J.; Choi, W. Epithelial to mesenchymal transition contributes to drug resistance in pancreatic cancer. *Cancer Res.* **2009**, *69*, 5820–5828. [CrossRef] [PubMed]
36. Shankar, S.; Nall, D.; Tang, S.N.; Meeker, D.; Passarini, J.; Sharma, J.; Srivastava, R.K. Resveratrol inhibits pancreatic cancer stem cell characteristics in human and KrasG12D transgenic mice by inhibiting pluripotency maintaining factors and epithelial-mesenchymal transition. *PLoS ONE* **2011**, *6*, e16530. [CrossRef] [PubMed]
37. Foretz, M.; Taleux, N.; Guigas, B.; Horman, S.; Beauloye, C.; Andreelli, F.; Bertrand, L.; Viollet, B. Regulation of energy metabolism by AMPK: A novel therapeutic approach for the treatment of metabolic and cardiovascular diseases. *Med. Sci.* **2006**, *22*, 381–388.
38. Ming, M.; Sinnett-Smith, J.; Wang, J.; Soares, H.P.; Young, S.H.; Eibl, G.; Rozengurt, E. Dose-Dependent AMPK-Dependent and Independent Mechanisms of Berberine and Metformin Inhibition of mTORC1, ERK, DNA Synthesis and Proliferation in Pancreatic Cancer Cells. *PLoS ONE* **2014**, *9*, e114573. [CrossRef] [PubMed]
39. Hadad, S.M.; Hardie, D.G.; Appleyard, V.; Thompson, A.M. Effects of metformin on breast cancer cell proliferation, the AMPK pathway and the cell cycle. *Clin. Transl. Oncol.* **2014**, *16*, 746–752. [CrossRef] [PubMed]
40. Ma, J.; Duan, W.; Han, S.; Lei, J.; Xu, Q.; Chen, X.; Jiang, Z.; Nan, L.; Li, J.; Chen, K.; et al. Ginkgolic acid suppresses the development of pancreatic cancer by inhibiting pathways driving lipogenesis. *Oncotarget* **2015**, *6*, 20993–21003. [CrossRef] [PubMed]
41. Lin, V.C.; Tsai, Y.C.; Lin, J.N.; Fan, L.L.; Pan, M.H.; Ho, C.T.; Wu, J.Y.; Way, T.D. Activation of AMPK by pterostilbene suppresses lipogenesis and cell-cycle progression in p53 positive and negative human prostate cancer cells. *J. Agric. Food Chem.* **2012**, *60*, 6399–6407. [CrossRef] [PubMed]
42. De Ran, M.; Yang, J.; Shen, C.H.; Peters, E.C.; Fitamant, J.; Chan, P.; Hsieh, M.; Zhu, S.; Asara, J.M.; Zheng, B.; et al. Energy stress regulates hippo-YAP signaling involving AMPK-mediated regulation of angiomotin-like 1 protein. *Cell Rep.* **2014**, *9*, 495–503. [CrossRef] [PubMed]
43. Wang, W.; Xiao, Z.D.; Li, X.; Aziz, K.E.; Gan, B.; Johnson, R.L.; Chen, J. AMPK modulates Hippo pathway activity to regulate energy homeostasis. *Nat. Cell Biol.* **2015**, *17*, 490–499. [CrossRef] [PubMed]
44. Harris, D.M.; Li, L.; Chen, M.; Lagunero, F.T.; Go, V.L.; Boros, L.G. Diverse mechanisms of growth inhibition by luteolin, resveratrol, and quercetin in MIA PaCa-2 cells: A comparative glucose tracer study with the fatty acid synthase inhibitor C75. *Metabolomics* **2012**, *8*, 201–210. [CrossRef] [PubMed]
45. Hong, W.; Guan, K.L. The YAP and TAZ transcription co-activators: Key downstream effectors of the mammalian Hippo pathway. *Semin. Cell Dev. Biol.* **2012**, *23*, 785–793. [CrossRef] [PubMed]
46. Yu, F.X.; Guan, K.L. The Hippo pathway: Regulators and regulations. *Genes Dev.* **2013**, *27*, 355–371. [CrossRef] [PubMed]
47. Ciamporcero, E.; Shen, H.; Ramakrishnan, S.; Yu, K.S.; Chintala, S.; Shen, L.; Adelaiye, R.; Miles, K.M.; Ullio, C.; Pizzimenti, S.; et al. YAP activation protects urothelial cell carcinoma from treatment-induced DNA damage. *Oncogene* **2016**, *35*, 1541–1553. [CrossRef] [PubMed]

Permissions

All chapters in this book were first published by MDPI; hereby published with permission under the Creative Commons Attribution License or equivalent. Every chapter published in this book has been scrutinized by our experts. Their significance has been extensively debated. The topics covered herein carry significant findings which will fuel the growth of the discipline. They may even be implemented as practical applications or may be referred to as a beginning point for another development.

The contributors of this book come from diverse backgrounds, making this book a truly international effort. This book will bring forth new frontiers with its revolutionizing research information and detailed analysis of the nascent developments around the world.

We would like to thank all the contributing authors for lending their expertise to make the book truly unique. They have played a crucial role in the development of this book. Without their invaluable contributions this book wouldn't have been possible. They have made vital efforts to compile up to date information on the varied aspects of this subject to make this book a valuable addition to the collection of many professionals and students.

This book was conceptualized with the vision of imparting up-to-date information and advanced data in this field. To ensure the same, a matchless editorial board was set up. Every individual on the board went through rigorous rounds of assessment to prove their worth. After which they invested a large part of their time researching and compiling the most relevant data for our readers.

The editorial board has been involved in producing this book since its inception. They have spent rigorous hours researching and exploring the diverse topics which have resulted in the successful publishing of this book. They have passed on their knowledge of decades through this book. To expedite this challenging task, the publisher supported the team at every step. A small team of assistant editors was also appointed to further simplify the editing procedure and attain best results for the readers.

Apart from the editorial board, the designing team has also invested a significant amount of their time in understanding the subject and creating the most relevant covers. They scrutinized every image to scout for the most suitable representation of the subject and create an appropriate cover for the book.

The publishing team has been an ardent support to the editorial, designing and production team. Their endless efforts to recruit the best for this project, has resulted in the accomplishment of this book. They are a veteran in the field of academics and their pool of knowledge is as vast as their experience in printing. Their expertise and guidance has proved useful at every step. Their uncompromising quality standards have made this book an exceptional effort. Their encouragement from time to time has been an inspiration for everyone.

The publisher and the editorial board hope that this book will prove to be a valuable piece of knowledge for researchers, students, practitioners and scholars across the globe.

List of Contributors

Amaya Azqueta
Department of Pharmacology and Toxicology, Faculty of Pharmacy, University of Navarra, C/Irunlarrea 1, 31009 Pamplona, Spain
IdiSNA, Navarra Institute for Health Research Spain

Andrew Collins
Department of Nutrition, Institute of Basic Medical Sciences, University of Oslo, Blindern, 0316 Oslo, Norway

Fazlullah Khan, Kamal Niaz, Faheem Maqbool, Fatima Ismail Hassan and Mohammad Abdollahi
Pharmaceutical Sciences Research Center, International Campus, Tehran University of Medical Sciences, Tehran 1417614411, Iran
Department of Toxicology and Pharmacology, Faculty of Pharmacy, Tehran University of Medical Sciences, Tehran 1417614411, Iran

Kalyan C. Nagulapalli Venkata and Anupam Bishayee
Department of Pharmaceutical Sciences, College of Pharmacy, Larkin Health Sciences Institute, Miami, FL 33169, USA

Seyed Mohammad Nabavi
Applied Biotechnology Research Center, Baqiyatallah University of Medical Sciences, Tehran 1435916471, Iran

Ahmed Abdal Dayem, Hye Yeon Choi, Gwang-Mo Yang, Kyeongseok Kim, Subbroto Kumar Saha and Ssang-Goo Cho
Department of Stem Cell & Regenerative Biotechnology, Incurable Disease Animal Model and Stem Cell Institute (IDASI), Konkuk University, Gwangjin-gu, Seoul 05029, Korea

Anna Boss and Gareth Marlow
Discipline of Nutrition, FM & HS, University of Auckland Medical School, Auckland 1142, New Zealand

Matthew P. G. Barnett
Food Nutrition & Health Team, Food & Bio-based Products Group, AgResearch Limited, Grasslands Research Centre, Tennent Drive, Palmerston North 4442, New Zealand

Aleksandra Niedzwiecki, Mohd Waheed Roomi, Tatiana Kalinovsky and Matthias Rath
Dr. Rath Research Institute, 1260 Memorex Drive, Santa Clara, CA 95050, USA

Fuchsia Gold-Smith and Karen Bishop
Auckland Cancer Society Research Center, Faculty of Medical and Health Sciences, University of Auckland, Private Bag 92019, Auckland 1142, New Zealand

Alyssa Fernandez
Faculty of Medical and Health Sciences, University of Auckland, Private Bag 92019, Auckland 1142, New Zealand

Van-Long Truong, Se-Yeon Ko and Woo-Sik Jeong
Department of Smart Food and Drug, College of Biomedical Science & Engineering, Inje University, Gimhae 50834, Korea

Mira Jun
Department of Food and Science & Nutrition, Dong-A University, Busan 49315, Korea

Giuseppina Mandalari
Dipartimento di Scienze Chimiche, Biologiche, Farmaceutiche ed Ambientali, University of Messina, Sal. Sperone 31, 98166 Messina, Italy
The Model Gut, Institute of Food Research, Norwich Research Park, Colney Lane, Norwich NR4 7UA, UK

Carlo Bisignano, Maria Martorana, Antonella Smeriglio and Domenico Trombetta
Dipartimento di Scienze Chimiche, Biologiche, Farmaceutiche ed Ambientali, University of Messina, Sal. Sperone 31, 98166 Messina, Italy

Maria Vardakou and Richard Faulks
The Model Gut, Institute of Food Research, Norwich Research Park, Colney Lane, Norwich NR4 7UA, UK

Meixia Chen, Qingli Luo, Shuming Mo, Yubao Lyu, Ying Wei and Jingcheng Dong
Department of Integrative Medicine, Huashan Hospital, Fudan University, Shanghai 200040, China

Jinfeng Wu
Department of Dermatology, Huashan Hospital, Fudan University, Shanghai 200040, China

Yue Zhou, Jie Zheng, Ya Li, Dong-Ping Xu and Yu-Ming Chen
Guangdong Provincial Key Laboratory of Food, Nutrition and Health, School of Public Health, Sun Yat-sen University, Guangzhou 510080, China

Sha Li
School of Chinese Medicine, The University of Hong Kong, Hong Kong, China

Hua-Bin Li
Guangdong Provincial Key Laboratory of Food, Nutrition and Health, School of Public Health, Sun Yat-sen University, Guangzhou 510080, China
South China Sea Bioresource Exploitation and Utilization Collaborative Innovation Center, Sun Yat-sen University, Guangzhou 510006, China

Zhengdong Jiang, Xin Chen, Ke Chen, Liankang Sun, Luping Gao, Cancan Zhou, Meng Lei, Wanxing Duan, Zheng Wang and Qingyong Ma
Department of Hepatobiliary Surgery, First Affiliated Hospital of Xi'an Jiaotong University, Xi'an 710061, China

Jiguang Ma
Department of Anesthesiology, First Affiliated Hospital of Xi'an Jiaotong University, Xi'an 710061, China

Index

www.ingramcontent.com/pod-product-compliance
Lightning Source LLC
LaVergne TN
LVHW080930210926
848485LV00004B/770